Tropomyosin

ADVANCES IN EXPERIMENTAL MEDICINE AND BIOLOGY

Recent Volumes in this Series

Volume 636
MOLECULAR MECHANISMS IN SPERMATOGENESIS
Edited by C. Yan Cheng

Volume 637
MOLECULAR MECHANISMS IN XERODERMA PIGMENTOSUM
Edited by Shamin Ahmad and Fumio Hanaoka

Volume 638
SOMITOGENESIS
Edited by Miguel Maroto and Neil Whittock

Volume 639
BREAST FEEDING: EARLY INFLUENCES ON LATER HEALTH
Edited by Gail Goldberg

Volume 640
MULTICHAIN IMMUNE RECOGNITION RECEPTOR SIGNALING
Edited by Alexander Sigalov

Volume 641
CELLULAR OSCILLATORY MECHANISMS
Edited by Miguel Maroto and Nicholas A.M. Monk

Volume 642
THE SARCOMERE AND SKELETAL MUSCLE DISEASE
Edited by Nigel G. Laing

Volume 643
TAURINE 7
Edited by Junichi Azuma

Volume 644
TROPOMYOSIN
Edited by Peter Gunning

Tropomyosin

Edited by

Peter Gunning, PhD

Oncology Research Unit, Department of Pharmacology
School of Medical Sciences, University of New South Wales
Sydney, New South Wales, Australia

Springer Science+Business Media, LLC
Landes Bioscience

Springer Science+Business Media, LLC
Landes Bioscience

Printed in the USA

Springer Science+Business Media, LLC, 233 Spring Street, New York, New York 10013, USA
http://www.springer.com

Please address all inquiries to the publishers:
Landes Bioscience, 1002 West Avenue, Austin, Texas 78701, USA
Phone: 512/ 637 5060; FAX: 512/ 637 6079
http://www.landesbioscience.com

Tropomyosin, edited by Peter Gunning, Landes Bioscience / Springer Science+Business Media, LLC
dual imprint / Springer series: Advances in Experimental Medicine and Biology

ISBN: 978-0-387-85765-7

Library of Congress Cataloging-in-Publication Data

Tropomyosin / edited by Peter Gunning.
    p. ; cm. -- (Advances in experimental medicine and biology ; v. 644)
  Includes bibliographical references and index.
  ISBN 978-0-387-85765-7
1. Tropomyosins. I. Gunning, Peter, 1950- II. Series.
  [DNLM: 1. Tropomyosin. W1 AD559 v.644 2008 / WE 500 T856 2008]
  QP552.M93T76 2008
  572'.633--dc22
                          2008032000

PREFACE

A recent review of one of my grant applications commented on the 'rediscovery of tropomyosin'. I was tempted to write back in my rebuttal to the reviewer that I didn't realise it had been lost. Uncharacteristic maturity prevailed and I resisted the temptation, but I was struck by the underlying observation that research on the structure and function of tropomyosin has been somewhat invisible, particularly in terms of the cytoskeleton isoforms. So, how can it be that one of the two major components of the actin filament has been so thoroughly overlooked? I suspect that the answer is disappointingly pedestrian. Whereas the biochemistry of the 1980s revealed the potential of tropomyosin isoforms to diversify the function of actin filaments, the subsequent disenchantment with isoform biology in general in the 1990s inhibited growth of this field. With the development of more sophisticated experimental approaches we are now seeing a growing realisation of the importance of tropomyosin in regulating actin filaments beyond its pivotal role in muscle contraction.

The opportunity to edit this book came at a time when we had written several reviews on different aspects of tropomyosin function and I had just finished the background reading for a comprehensive review of tropomyosin biology. I realised that the field was simply beyond the capacity of any one person to do the field justice. Therefore it was a comparatively easy task to look at all the major aspects of tropomyosin biology and identify the leaders in each area. Unfortunately, it was not possible for all the major contributors to the field to write chapters; however, every chapter is written by an expert in the area. It says something of those who work in the field that everyone who was approached enthusiastically agreed to contribute a chapter. Everyone recognised the importance of pulling the field together through this book and ensuring that each chapter would review the current status of their area and provide an insight into future research directions.

I am particularly grateful to Sarah Hitchcock-DeGregori, David Wieczorek, Mario Gimona and David Helfman who worked through the concept of the book with me. They were very generous with their time and suggestions, and this is much appreciated.

I am struck by how much I have learned reading these chapters, and the same view has been expressed to me by essentially all authors. All the authors have made the different areas very accessible and provide a current view of the field. It is my expectation that this will serve as the core source on this topic into the foreseeable future. It has captured the first 60 years of work in this field and shone a light into the immediate future. I hope that it is as useful to you as it has been to all of the authors.

Finally, I want to thank Ron Landes for the opportunity to edit this book and the team at Landes Bioscience, particularly Cynthia Conomos, Celeste Carlton, Megan Klein and Erin O'Brien, for their help and patience. It has been a great pleasure to work on this with you.

Peter Gunning, PhD

ABOUT THE EDITOR...

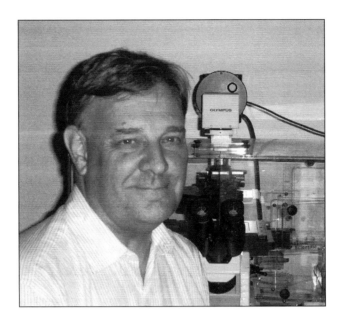

PETER GUNNING, PhD, is Head of the Oncology Research Unit, Department of Pharmacology, School of Medical Sciences, at the University of New South Wales located in Sydney, Australia. The primary focus of his research is the regulation of cell and tissue architecture and its modification in cancer. He is a member of numerous professional organisations and has served on the Boards of the NSW Cancer Council and Bio-Link Partners and as Chairman of the NSW Cancer Council and NSW Cancer Institute Research Committees. Peter received his academic degrees from Monash University, Melbourne, Australia.

PARTICIPANTS

Manisha Bajpai
Department of Medicine
Division of Gastroenterology
    and Hepatology
Crohn's and Colitis Center
    of New Jersey
UMDNJ-Robert Wood Johnson
    Medical School
New Brunswick, New Jersey
USA

James R. Bamburg
Department of Biochemistry
    and Molecular Biology
Colorado State University
Fort Collins, Colorado
USA

Roger Craig
Department of Cell Biology
University of Massachusetts
    Medical School
Worcester, Massachusetts
USA

Kiron M. Das
Division of Gastroenterology
    and Hepatology
Department of Medicine
Crohn's and Colitis Center
    of New Jersey
UMDNJ-Robert Wood Johnson
    Medical School
New Brunswick, New Jersey
USA

M. El-Mezgueldi
Department of Biochemistry
University of Leicester
Leicester
UK

Robbin D. Eppinga
Department of Biology
University of Iowa
Iowa City, Iowa
USA

Patrick Flynn
Graduate Program in Cell
    and Developmental Biology
Leonard M. Miller School
    of Medicine
University of Miami
Miami, Florida
USA

Mario Gimona
Unit of Actin Cytoskeleton Regulation
Consorzio Mario Negri Sud
Department of Cell Biology
    and Oncology
Santa Maria Imbaro
Italy

Robert D. Goldman
Department of Cell and Molecular
    Biology
Feinberg School of Medicine
Northwestern University
Chicago, Illinois
USA

Clare Gooding
Department of Biochemistry
University of Cambridge
Cambridge
UK

Staffan Grenklo
Department of Microbiology,
   Tumor Biology, and Cell Biology
Karolinska Institutet
Stockholm
Sweden

Peter Gunning
Oncology Research Unit
Department of Pharmacology
School of Medical Sciences
University of New South Wales
Sydney, New South Wales
Australia

Edna C. Hardeman
Department of Anatomy
School of Medical Sciences
University of New South Wales
Sydney, New South Wales
Australia

David M. Helfman
Department of Cell Biology
   and Anatomy
Sheila and David Fuente Graduate
   Program in Cancer Biology
Sylvester Comprehensive Cancer
   Center
Leonard M. Miller School
   of Medicine
University of Miami
Miami, Florida
USA

Louise Hillberg
Department of Microbiology,
   Tumor Biology, and Cell Biology
Karolinska Institutet
Stockholm
Sweden

Sarah E. Hitchcock-DeGregori
Department of Neuroscience
   and Cell Biology
Robert Wood Johnson Medical School
Piscataway, New Jersey
USA

Ganapathy Jagatheesan
Department of Molecular Genetics,
   Biochemistry, and Microbiology
University of Cincinnati Medical
   Center
Cincinnati, Ohio
USA

Anthony J. Kee
Muscle Development Unit
Children's Medical Research Institute
and
Faculty of Medicine
University of Sydney
Sydney
Australia

Protiti Khan
Graduate Program in Cell
   and Developmental Biology
Leonard M. Miller School
   of Medicine
University of Miami
Miami, Florida
USA

Alla S. Kostyukova
Department of Neuroscience
   and Cell Biology
Robert Wood Johnson Medical School
Piscataway, New Jersey
USA

Thomas B. Kuhn
Department of Chemistry
University of Alaska Fairbanks
Fairbanks, Alaska
USA

William Lehman
Department of Physiology
   and Biophysics
Boston University School of Medicine
Boston, Massachusetts
USA

Jim Jung-Ching Lin
Department of Biology
University of Iowa
Iowa City, Iowa
USA

Uno Lindberg
Department of Microbiology,
   Tumor Biology, and Cell Biology
Karolinska Institutet
Stockholm
Sweden

Steve Marston
National Heart and Lung Institute
Imperial College London
London
UK

Claire Martin
Oncology Research Unit
The Children's Hospital at Westmead
Westmead, New South Wales
Australia

Keith R. McCrae
Department of Medicine
Division of Hematology
   and Oncology
School of Medicine
Case Western Reserve University
Cleveland, Ohio
USA

Maria Nyåkern-Meazza
Department of Microbiology,
   Tumor Biology, and Cell Biology
Karolinska Institutet
Stockholm
Sweden

Geraldine O'Neill
Oncology Research Unit
The Children's Hospital
   at Westmead
Westmead, New South Wales
and
Discipline of Pediatrics
   and Child Health
University of Sydney
Sydney, New South Wales
Australia

E. Michael Ostap
Department of Physiology
University of Pennsylvania School
   of Medicine
Philadelphia, Pennslyvania
USA

David Pruyne
Department of Molecular Biology
and Genetics
Cornell University
Ithaca, New York
USA

Sudarsan Rajan
Department of Molecular Genetics,
   Biochemistry, and Microbiology
University of Cincinnati Medical
   Center
Cincinnati, Ohio
USA

Li-Sophie Zhao Rathje
Department of Microbiology,
   Tumor Biology, and Cell Biology
Karolinska Institutet
Stockholm
Sweden

Ali Saeed
Sheila and David Fuente Graduate
   Program in Cancer Biology
Leonard M. Miller School of Medicine
University of Miami
Miami, Florida
USA

Galina Schevzov
Oncology Research Unit
The Children's Hospital
   at Westmead
Westmead, New South Wales
and
Discipline of Pediatrics
   and Child Health
University of Sydney
Sydney, New South Wales
Australia

Clarence E. Schutt
Department of Chemistry
Princeton University
Princeton, New Jersey
USA

Christopher W.J. Smith
Department of Biochemistry
University of Cambridge
Cambridge
UK

Nadine Thézé
Université Victor Segalen Bordeaux
Bordeaux
France

Pierre Thiébaud
Université Victor Segalen Bordeaux
Bordeaux
France

Larry S. Tobacman
Departments of Medicine, Physiology
   and Biophysics
University of Illinois at Chicago
Chicago, Illinois
USA

Bernadette Vrhovski
Oncology Research Unit
The Children's Hospital
   at Westmead
Westmead, New South Wales
Australia

C.-L. Albert Wang
Boston Biomedical Research Institute
Watertown, Massachusetts
USA

Kerri S. Warren
Department of Biology
University of Iowa
Iowa City, Iowa
USA

David F. Wieczorek
Department of Molecular Genetics,
   Biochemistry, and Microbiology
University of Cincinnati Medical
   Center
Cincinnati, Ohio
USA

CONTENTS

Section I. Genes and Their Expression

4. TROPOMYOSIN GENE EXPRESSION IN VIVO AND IN VITRO ... 43

Galina Schevzov and Geraldine O'Neill

Section II. Protein Structure

5. TROPOMYOSIN: FUNCTION FOLLOWS STRUCTURE ... 60

Sarah E. Hitchcock-DeGregori

6. DIMERIZATION OF TROPOMYOSINS ... 73

Mario Gimona

Section III. Role in Muscle Function

Section IV. Tropomyosin in Human Disease

Section V. Tropomyosin Directed Regulation of the Cytoskeleton

14. TROPOMYOSIN FUNCTION IN YEAST 168

David Pruyne

15. ISOFORM SORTING OF TROPOMYOSINS 187

Claire Martin and Peter Gunning

16. HUMAN TROPOMYOSIN ISOFORMS IN THE REGULATION OF CYTOSKELETON FUNCTIONS 201

Jim Jung-Ching Lin, Robbin D. Eppinga, Kerri S. Warren and Keith R. McCrae

Section VI. Mechanisms of Tropomyosin Function

20. TROPOMYOSINS AS DISCRIMINATORS OF MYOSIN FUNCTION 273

E. Michael Ostap

21. TROPOMODULIN/TROPOMYOSIN INTERACTIONS REGULATE ACTIN POINTED END DYNAMICS 283

Alla S. Kostyukova

Section VII. Conclusion

22. EMERGING ISSUES FOR TROPOMYOSIN STRUCTURE, REGULATION, FUNCTION AND PATHOLOGY 293

Peter Gunning

CHAPTER 1

Introduction and Historical Perspective

Peter Gunning*

Abstract

Tropomyosin is a coiled coil dimer which forms a polymer along the major groove of the majority of actin filaments. It is therefore one of the two primary components of the actin filament. Our understanding of the biological function of tropomyosin has been driven almost entirely by its role in striated muscle. This reflects both its original discovery as part of the thin filament in skeletal muscle and its pivotal role in regulating muscle contraction. In contrast, its role in the function of the cytoskeleton of all cells has been poorly understood due, at least in part, to the technical challenge of deciphering the function of a large number of isoforms. This book has brought together many of the leading researchers who have defined the function of tropomyosin in both normal and pathological conditions. Each author brings their own perspective in a series of stand alone reviews of the areas of tropomyosin research they have played a major role in defining.

Introduction

The opportunity to edit a book on tropomyosin arose at a time when I had just completed my reading in preparation for writing the recent review, 'Tropomyosin-based regulation of the actin cytoskeleton in time and space'[1] for Physiological Reviews. It was clear to me that the scope and significance of tropomyosin research would greatly benefit from bringing together leaders in the field to comprehensively cover all the different aspects of this research. Indeed, it is not possible for a single author to cover in sufficient depth both the current state of knowledge and the future directions of research in a field of this breadth. The overall layout of the book draws heavily on that of recent reviews[1-6] and on very helpful discussions with Sarah Hitchcock-DeGregori, David Wieczorek, Mario Gimona and David Helfman. Because of space considerations not all major contributors to the field could be included as authors but conversely, all research topics have been authored by leaders in that field.

Discovery and Context of Tropomyosin Research

Tropomyosin was originally discovered as a structural component of the skeletal muscle contractile apparatus.[7,8] Because of its physical properties it was originally believed to be a precursor of myosin and hence was named 'tropomyosin'.[7] The first thirty years of tropomyosin research focussed on its role in striated muscle function. Tropomyosin is a coiled coil dimer which forms a head to tail polymer along the length of the major grooves in the actin filament. The recognition that tropomyosin regulates the interaction of the head of the myosin motor with the actin filament has formed not only the basis for our understanding of the regulation of muscle contraction[9,10] but has also set the context for our understanding of the function of tropomyosin.[5] This has led to

*Peter Gunning—Oncology Research Unit, Department of Pharmacology, School of Medical Sciences, University of New South Wales Sydney, NSW 2052, Australia.
Email: p.gunning@unsw.edu.au

Tropomyosin, edited by Peter Gunning. ©2008 Landes Bioscience and Springer Science+Business Media.

a remarkable wealth of knowledge concerning the molecular function of tropomyosin in muscle contraction but has hampered the growth of our understanding of tropomyosin function in the context of the cytoskeleton. Even our naming of tropomyosin's, muscle and nonmuscle, fails to recognise the nature of the cytoskeleton itself.

In 2008, it is hard to understand the extent to which the discovery of 'nonmuscle contractile proteins' in the 1970s was considered highly controversial. This, in large part, reflects the way in which the concept of contraction driven by contractile proteins did not easily translate into the functional context of nonmuscle cells at that time. Fibroblasts, for example, do not contain structures resembling the repeating arrays of contractile proteins found in striated muscle. In parallel, there was no appreciation of the functional diversity to which evolution has recruited the actin filament system. This was over 20 years before the human genome project would reveal that evolutionary diversity is driven primarily by the formation of protein variants rather than the formation of entirely new types of proteins.[11-13]

Initial studies of cytoskeletal tropomyosin focussed on its incorporation into the fibroblast stress fibre.[14] The discovery of the plethora of tropomyosin isoforms raised the potential importance of these isoforms in diversifying actin filament function.[15-17] Protein chemistry studies of tropomyosin isoforms from a number of laboratories supported this view of tropomyosins as isoform specific regulators of actin filament function.[18-21] In retrospect, it is interesting to note that whereas protein chemistry provided a compelling case for isoform specific function, the difficulty in demonstrating isoform specific function of structural proteins by gene transfection slowed the development of the field throughout the 1990s.

In 2008, it is increasingly clear that the actin cytoskeleton is centrally involved in a variety of functions in all eukaryotic cells. Many of these functions require diversity of function of the actin filaments themselves. For example, the leading edge of a migrating cell requires multiple populations of actin filaments with different turnover kinetics and affinities for different actin binding proteins.[22] In contrast, the filaments within an actin stress fibre require greater stability than those in the leading edge, a resistance to actin severing proteins and an ability to generate tension through interaction with conventional myosin motors.[23] This diversity of actin filament function is most easily reconciled with the existence of multiple types of actin filament populations which are characterised by different isoform (actin and tropomyosin) composition and/or different interactions with actin binding proteins.[1,2] Tropomyosin is becoming increasingly recognised as a pivotal contributor to this diversity of filament function.[1]

With the advantage of hindsight, this book has been designed to present a systematic analysis of tropomyosin structure and function. Each author has been asked to review a specific area of research where they have made a major contribution. While each chapter is self contained, cross referencing to other chapters identifies additional sources of more detailed information on particular issues.

Genes and Their Expression (Chapters 2-4)

The complexity of tropomyosin gene evolution and alternative splicing is a challenge for those both in and outside the field. Chapter 2 was designed to present the evolution of the genes and the generation of isoforms by alternative splicing in an easy to understand manner. It covers the major phyla and presents a number of surprising observations, particularly concerning abrupt changes in the use of the different genes between closely related species and the relationship between isoform number and functional complexity of the organism. The tropomyosin genes have served as a paradigm for understanding mechanisms which regulate alternative splicing and Chapter 3 covers the current view of this process in the two best studied models. The mutually exclusive splicing of exons 2a and 2b in the α-Tm gene and exons 6a and 6b in the β-Tm gene provide insights not only into the role of associated cis-sequences but also the role of different trans-acting factors. Finally, Chapter 4 reviews the expression of tropomyosin isoforms both between different cell types and during development of higher eukaryotes. Some general principles of isoform specific regulation are identified and the relationship between tropomyosin supply and actin polymer formation explored in striated muscle and the cytoskeleton.

Protein Structure (Chapters 5, 6)

Tropomyosin has historically served as the classic coiled coil protein and Chapter 5 covers recent advances in our understanding of the structure of the tropomyosin dimer. Of particular interest is the recent insight into the structure of the overlap between adjoining dimers in the filament. The chapter also addresses the relationship between structure and the functional differences between tropomyosin isoforms. Because tropomyosin is a dimer there is the potential to form a large number of different dimers. Chapter 6 reviews the principles which govern the preferential formation of specific tropomyosin dimers. These two chapters reveal the remarkable subtlety between what on the surface seems a very simple family of structurally similar molecules and the contrasting diversity of their biological functions.

Role in Muscle Function (Chapters 7-9)

One of the more surprising features of tropomyosin is that the affinity of the dimer for the actin filament is so low as to discount it as an actin binding protein. Rather, it more resembles a polymer 'floating' over the surface of the major grooves in the actin polymer. At the same time, the tropomyosin polymer coordinates the response of the actin filament along its length to ensure coordinated interactions of the thin actin filament with the thick myosin filament. This is a core conceptual problem which underpins the function of skeletal and cardiac muscle. The challenge of understanding the assembly of the tropomyosin polymer depends on its cooperative binding to actin which is explained in Chapter 7. This cooperative binding goes to the heart of the tropomyosin actin interaction. Chapter 8 reviews the state of our current understanding of the role of tropomyosin in the regulation of striated muscle contraction. While the current models provide an elegant view of the role of tropomyosin in this process, the chapter also draws attention to the weaknesses in our understanding of contraction. Unlike striated muscle, smooth muscle uses a much less regular structure to achieve contraction and Chapter 9 demonstrates how smooth muscle substitutes caldesmon for the troponin complex to control tropomyosin regulation of the actin-myosin interaction. This provides an excellent example of how evolution has recruited different members of multigene families to specialise the process of contraction in different tissues with different functional requirements.

Tropomyosin in Human Disease (Chapters 10-13)

The involvement of tropomyosin in a range of human diseases continues to grow and it is to be expected that there is more to be found. Indeed this arose during the preparation of Chapter 12 and hence the scope had to be expanded. The earliest recognition of an association between tropomyosin and human disease was the observation that changes in the profile of tropomyosin isoforms show a characteristic change in cancer cells. Chapter 10 reviews the evidence for a direct role of tropomyosin as a regulator of cancer and the emerging view that this involves changes in the oncogenic signalling properties of these cells. Mutations in striated muscle tropomyosins have now been identified as disease causing in a numbers of human conditions. Chapter 11 reviews the role of αfast-Tm mutations in hypertrophic and dilated cardiomyopathies and the use of animal models to understand the mechanisms underlying these conditions. Mouse models are also used to demonstrate the functional differences between muscle tropomyosins. Similarly, Chapter 12 reviews the role of mutations in αslow-Tm and β-Tm underlying nemaline myopathy and the recent discovery of additional myopathies caused by these genes. Analysis of an animal model has revealed the impact of a disease causing mutation on dimer preference with resulting alteration in thin filament composition. These reviews serve to emphasise the impact of the subtle differences in muscle tropomyosins on actin filament function. Finally, Chapter 13 covers the role of the cytoskeletal Tm5 isoform as an autoantigen in ulcerative colitis. Surprisingly, evidence is mounting that some Tm5 is present on the surface of intestinal epithelial cells which mediates the impact of these autoantibodies in the colon.

Tropomyosin Directed Regulation of the Cytoskeleton (Chapters 14-16)

Genetic analysis of the role of tropomyosin in the cytoskeleton was first achieved in yeast and Chapter 14 reviews how the power of yeast genetics has defined key principles of tropomyosin function. This chapter demonstrates the importance of tropomyosin not only in terms of regulating cell shape but also intracellular transport. In mammals functionally distinct populations of actin filaments can often be identified by different isoforms of tropomyosin and Chapter 15 reviews the extent to which this is found in different cell types. The relationship between localised cellular signalling and the localised accumulation of specific tropomyosins is considered as a mechanism for the spatial specialisation of actin filament function. The implications of this work for the specialised function of specific actin filament populations in human cells are considered in Chapter 16. A variety of experimental approaches have demonstrated that tropomyosin isoforms define functionally distinct populations of actin filaments and that tropomyosin plays a pivotal role in determining the functional properties of specific filaments.

Mechanisms of Tropomyosin Function (Chapters 17-21)

A substantial body of data now supports the view that tropomyosin isoforms can determine the functional role of specific actin filaments. In some respects it is ironical that the protein chemistry of the 1980s is more relevant now than when it was originally published. This is because the context has changed and the isoform specific role of tropomyosins is now well established. Chapter 17 reviews the role of tropomyosin isoforms in regulating the activity of the actin binding proteins gesolin and cofilin against different populations of actin filaments. This is discussed in terms of their relationship to different conformational states of the actin filament. This theme is extended in Chapter 18 where the relationship between the actin severing proteins ADF/Cofilin and specific tropomyosins are considered not only in terms of competition but also as potential collaborators in an isoform specific manner. Of particular interest is the impact of ADF/Cofilin and different tropomyosins on the kinetic properties of specific populations of actin filaments. Similarly, Chapter 19 reviews the isoform specific effects of cytoskeletal caldesmon on tropomyosin containing actin filaments to provide a calcium sensitive mechanism to differentially regulate different populations of actin filaments in the cytoskeleton. As might be expected from its role in skeletal muscle different tropomyosins also have the capacity to discriminate between different myosin motors and Chapter 20 explores the significance of this function of tropomyosins. This chapter looks at the potential relationship between myosin and tropomyosin diversity in specifying the functional role of specific actin filaments. Finally, Chapter 21 reviews the impact of the different tropomodulins on the stability of actin filaments containing different tropomyosins. It is now clear that different combinations of tropomyosins and tropomodulins can regulate the turnover of different actin filaments. In conclusion, it appears that the different tropomyosins have the capacity to regulate the impact of the different actin binding proteins on actin filament function which has resulted in a remarkable diversification of the actin cytoskeleton.

Acknowledgements

It is a pleasure to acknowledge and thank the authors of this book who have provided insightful reviews of the different aspects of this field. I wish to thank the NHMRC for their support of my research via project grant funding and I am a Principal Research Fellow of the NHMRC. I also wish to acknowledge and thank the Oncology Children's Foundation for their support. Finally, I would like to express my thanks to Ron Landes for the opportunity to edit this book and to Cynthia Conomos, Celeste Carlton and Megan Klein for all their help.

References

1. Gunning P, O'Neill G, Hardeman E. Tropomyosin-based regulation of the actin cytoskeleton in time and space. Physiol Rev 2008; 88:1-35.
2. Gunning PW, Schevzov G, Kee AJ et al. Tropomyosin isoforms: divining rods for actin cytoskeleton function. Trends Cell Biol 2005; 15(6):333-341.
3. Gordon AM, Homsher E, Regnier M. Regulation of contraction instriated muscle. Physiol Rev 2000; 80:853-924.
4. Geeves MA, Holmes KC. The molecular mechanism of muscle contraction. Adv Protein Chem 2005: 71:161-193.
5. Perry SV. Vertebrate tropomyosin: distribution, properties and function. J Muscle Res Cell Motil 2001; 22:5-49.
6. Pawlak G, Helfman DM. Cytoskeletal changes in cell transformation and tumorigenesis. Curr Opin Genet Dev 2001; 11(1):41-47.
7. Bailey K. Tropomyosin a new asymmetric protein of muscle. Nature 1946; 157:368
8. Bailey K. Tropomyosin: a new asymmetric protein of the muscle fibril. Biochem J 1948; 43:271-279.
9. Huxley HE. Structural changes in the actin- and myosin-containing filaments during contraction. Cold Spring Harb Symp Quant Biol 1972; 37:361-376.
10. Parry DA, Squire JM. Structural role of tropomyosin in muscle regulation: analysis of the x-ray diffraction patterns from relaxed and contracting muscles. J Mol Biol 1973; 75:33-55.
11. Lander ES, Linton LM, Birren B et al. Initial sequencing and analysis of the human genome. Nature 2001; 409:860-921.
12. Venter JC, Adams MD, Myers EW et al. The sequence of the human genome. Science 2001; 291:1304-1351.
13. Gunning PW. Protein isoforms and isozymes. Nature Encyclopedia Human Genome 2003; 835-839.
14. Lazarides E. Tropomyosin antibody: the specific localization of tropomyosin in nonmuscle cells. J Cell Biol 1975; 65:549-561.
15. Matsumura F, Lin J-J, Yamashiro-Matsumura S et al. Differential expression of tropomyosin forms in the microfilaments isolated from normal and transformed rat cultured cells. J Biol Chem 1983; 258:13954-13964.
16. Hendricks M, Weintraub H. Multiple tropomyosin polypeptides in chicken embryo fibroblasts: differential repression of transcription by rous sarcoma virus transformation. Mol Cell Biol 1984; 4:1823-1833.
17. Lin JJ, Helfman DM, Hughes SH et al. Tropomyosin isoforms in chicken embryo fibroblasts:purification, characterization, changes in Rous sarcoma virus-transformed cells. J Cell Biol 1985; 100: 692-703.
18. Bernstein BW, Bamburg JR. Tropomyosin binding to F-actin protects the F-actin from disassembly by brain actin-depolymerizing factor (ADF). Cell Motil 1982; 2:1-8.
19. Broschat KO, Burgess DR. Low Mr tropomyosin isoforms from chicken brain and intestinal epithelium have distinct actin-binding properties. J Biol Chem 1986; 261:13350-13359.
20. Ishikawa R, Yamashiro S, Matsumura F. Differential modulation of actin-severing activity of gelsolin by multiple isoforms of cultured rat cell tropomyosin. Potentiation of protective ability of tropomyosins by 83-kDa nonmuscle caldesmon. J Biol Chem 1989; 264:7490-7497.
21. Fanning AS, Wolenski JS, Mooseker MS et al. Differential regulation of skeletal muscle myosin-II and brush border myosin-I enzymology and mechanochemistry by bacterially produced tropomyosin isoforms. Cell Motil Cytoskeleton 1994; 29:29-45.
22. Cooper HL. Actin dynamics: tropomyosin provides stability. Curr Biol 2002; 12:R523-R525.
23. Bryce NS, Schevzov G, Ferguson V et al. Specification of actin filament function and molecular composition by tropomyosin isoforms. Mol Biol Cell 2003; 14:1002-1016.

CHAPTER 2

Structure and Evolution of Tropomyosin Genes

Bernadette Vrhovski, Nadine Thézé and Pierre Thiébaud*

Abstract

Tropomyosins constitute a family of highly related actin-binding proteins found in the animal kingdom from yeast to human. In vertebrates, they are encoded by a multigene family where each member can produce several isoforms through alternative splicing and for some of them with alternate promoters. Tropomyosin isoform diversity has considerably increased during evolution from invertebrates to vertebrates and stems from the duplication of ancestral genes. The advance of genomic sequence information on various animals has expanded our knowledge on the structure of tropomyosin genes in different phyla and subphyla. We present the organisation of tropomyosin genes in different major phyla and the phylogenetic comparison of their structure highlights the evolution of this multigene family.

Introduction

Tropomyosins (Tm) are ubiquitous, highly conserved proteins found in eukaryotic cells that play an indispensable role in a diversity of processes that include among others, cytokinesis, cell motility, cell transformation or more highly specialized function like myofibrillar contraction.[1,2] Tropomyosins have been found in all eukaryotic phyla except plants and show an increased complexity in terms of protein isoforms from lower eukaryotes to vertebrates which exhibit a multiplicity of isoforms. This isoform diversity is produced by a combination of multiple Tm encoding genes, alternative splicing of primary transcripts and for some of them alternative promoter usage.[3] The rationale for such protein diversity is still unknown but it has been shown that the production of Tm isoforms in some species is developmentally regulated and that Tm isoforms are functionally distinct.[1,2,4] It appears that the complexity of Tm isoform diversity is clearly related to the increased complexity of animals during evolution stemming from unicellular eukaryotic cells like yeast to highly organized multicellular organism such as vertebrates. The structure of several Tm genes has been elucidated, in a first approach, by analysis of a combination of cDNA and genomic clones and PCR on genomic DNA. Since the genome sequencing of numerous highly evolutionarily distant organisms is under completion, the presence of Tm genes in these genomes and their structural organization can be now evaluated. Moreover the availability of EST sequences for many species completes the picture we have on Tm gene expression and we can infer about gene numbers in those species. In this chapter, we review our knowledge about tropomyosin gene number and structure in various organisms. Because tropomyosins are present in different eukaryotes as divergent as fungi and human, we have decided not to report on every species where Tm genes have been characterized but rather focused on major species that are important in evolutionary analysis in order to understand the origin and evolution of the Tm gene family.

*Corresponding Author: Pierre Thiébaud—UMR 5164—CNRS, Université Victor Segalen Bordeaux 2, 146, rue Léo Saignat, 33076 Bordeaux Cedex, France. Email: pierre.thiebaud@u-bordeaux2.fr

Tropomyosin, edited by Peter Gunning. ©2008 Landes Bioscience and Springer Science+Business Media.

Structure of Tropomyosin Genes

The structural organization of tropomyosin genes has been inferred from genomic clones isolated from different species and from databank sequences. We describe what is known about *Tm* genes number and structure in relevant species along the phylogenic tree of the animal kingdom (Fig. 1). *Tm* genes have been found in eukaryotic unicellular organisms and also in several invertebrates model organisms but the best knowledge we have about this multigene family is deduced from vertebrates studies.

Eukaryotic Unicellular Organisms

Tropomyosin genes have been characterized in two fungi species, the budding yeast *Saccharomyces cerevisiae* and the fission yeast *Schizosaccharomyces pombe* (see Chapter 14). These constitute the earliest Tm isoforms identified in the evolution of the eukaryotic lineage. In *S. cerevisiae* there are two *Tm* genes, *TPM1* and *TPM2*, that encode 199 and 166 amino acid (aa) proteins respectively with 64.5% sequence identity.[5,6] The two proteins show distinct functions and are not interchangeable. The two genes appear probably through a yeast-specific gene duplication both encoding single isoforms. In *S. pombe*, Tm is the product of the *cdc8* gene and

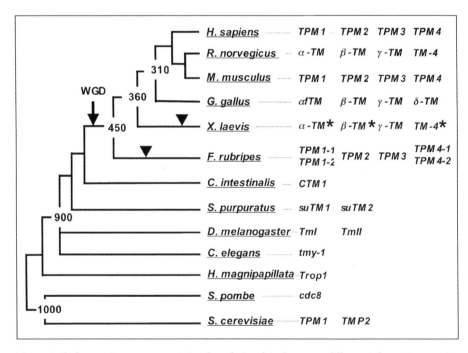

Figure 1. Phylogenetic tree summarizing the relationships between different informative species and the tropomyosin genes identified in those species. Divergence times in millions of years ago are shown.[8] The whole duplications of genomes that have been proposed to occur in the vertebrate lineage are indicated (WGD). The genome duplication that has occurred in fishes and amphibians lineages is indicated by black triangles. The duplicated *Xenopus laevis* genes inferred from cDNAs sequence analysis are indicated by an asterisk (*). The nomenclature of the tropomyosin genes is as follows : *H. sapiens,* HGNC database; *R. norvegicus;*[44,48,52] *M. musculatus,* MGI database; *G. gallus;*[36,40] *X. laevis;*[32,33,35] *F. rubripes;*[28] *C. intestinalis;*[25] *S. purpuratus,* SUGP at http://sugp.caltech.edu/; *D. melanogaster,* Flybase; *C. elegans;*[16] *H. magnipapillata;*[9] *S. cerevisiae;*[6] *S. pombe.*[7] Regarding nonfully sequenced species, one cannot rule out the possibility that some other members of *Tm* genes family are still to be found.

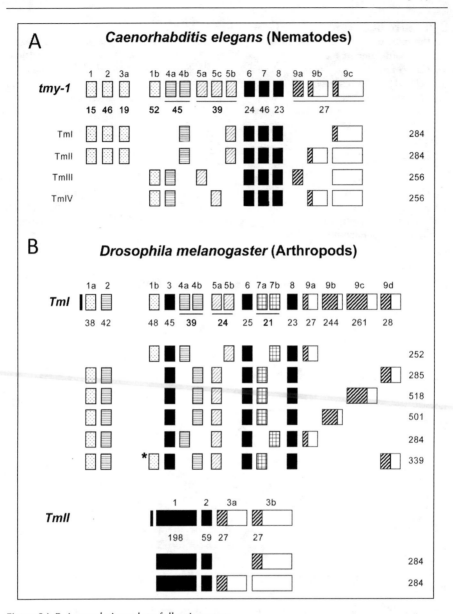

Figure 2A,B. Legend viewed on following page.

codes for a 161aa protein that shows only 42% identity with *S. cerevisiae* proteins.[7] This is not surprising given the great sequence divergence of the two yeast species that are separated by about 1 gya.[8] However, the yeast proteins display the typical characteristics of tropomyosin including the hydrophobic-hydrophilic pseudoheptapeptide repeats. In both species, *Tm* genes contain no introns like the vast majority of yeast genes.

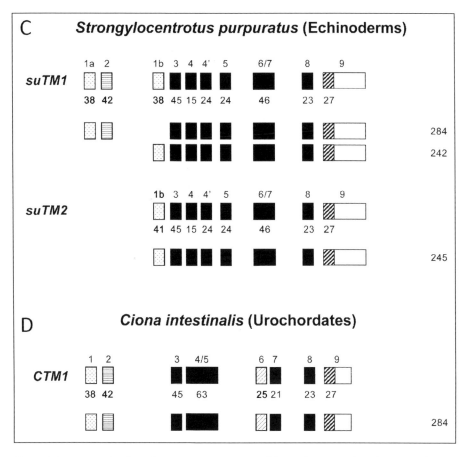

Figure 2. Exon organisation of tropomyosin genes and the isoforms produced in invertebrates. A) nematodes represented by *C.elegans* ; B) arthropods represented by *D. melanogaster* ; C) echinoderms represented by *S. purpuratus;* D) urochordates represented by *C. intestinalis*. Exons are represented by boxes. The 5′ untranslated leader exon in *D. melanogaster* genes is represented by a thick vertical bar. The 3′ untranslated regions are represented by a white box. The gene name is shown in italics and the number of the exon above and size in aa below the boxes. Exons subject to alternate usage are shaded the same. Isoforms known to be produced from each gene are shown and the size in aa is shown on the right. The nomenclature for the exons of the *C. elegans* gene is refered to previous report.[15,16] The nomenclature for the exons of the *D. melanogaster* genes has been adapted from previous reports.[17,22] in order to illustrate the internal alternative exons and the distinct carboxy terminal exons. The carboxy terminal exons 9a, 9b, 9c and 9d in the invertebrates genes are not related to those described in the vertebrates genes (see text and legend Fig. 3). *Exon 1b in the 339 aa isoform contains 54 aa instead of 48 aa because of the splicing of exon 2 to exon 1b that has occurred 18 nucleotides upstream of the initiation codon of exon 1b.

Invertebrates

Cnidarians

The cnidarians belong to the diploblats phylum and are animals that display only two main layers, the ectoderm and the endoderm, thus representing the most basic metazoan phylum. *Tm* cDNAs have been cloned from *Hydra magnipapillata* (class of hydrozoa) and from the marine medusa *Podocoryne carne*.[9,10] In *H. magnipapillata*, a cDNA clone encoding a 253 aa tropomyosin has been identified. From genomic southern blot and PCR analysis, it has been found that the corresponding gene (*Trop1*) is present in a single copy in the genome and lacks introns.[9] The protein shows the characteristic feature of repeating pseudoheptapeptide pattern of nonpolar and polar residues. Two cDNA clones, *Tpm1* and *Tpm2*, have been isolated in the marine medusa *P. carne* and they encode Tm isoforms of 242 and 251 aa respectively.[10] Both proteins share 19% identity suggesting they are produced by a duplication event that occurred early in metazoan evolution in the phylum Cnidaria. No alternative isoforms of the two cDNA clones have been identified. While the *Tpm1* gene is widely expressed, *Tpm2* gene expression is restricted to striated muscle of the medusa.

Nematodes

With the advance of genome sequencing, the traditional phylogeny based on morphology and embryology has been replaced by a molecular based phylogeny and a metazoan phylogenetic tree has been established. According to this phylogeny, nematodes and arthropods are placed in the same group of ecdysozoans that belongs to the phylum of protostomes.[11] Several cDNA clones encoding tropomyosin proteins have been characterized in a number of species of nematodes. Those proteins are highly related showing 85-90% identity between them and about 60% identity with human tropomyosins.[12-14] The complete gene structure and isoform diversity production have been established for the organism model *Caenorhabditis elegans*.[15,16] There is a single *Tm* gene (named *tmy-1* or lev-11) in the genome of the *C. elegans* (Fig. 2A). The gene spans more than 14 kb, contains two alternate promoters and has 15 exons with three groups of alternatively spliced exons. Four major different isoforms, named CeTmI-IV, that are produced by the gene have been described.[15,16] CeTmI and CeTmII, which are produced by the distal promoter, are 284 aa long and differ by the 27 aa encoding exon at their carboxyl terminus. They show 64 to 68% identity with the *Drosophila* muscle tropomyosin and about 50% with rabbit skeletal muscle isoforms. When comparing the carboxyl-terminus of CeTMI and CeTMII (exon 9) with the skeletal and cytoskeletal isoforms from *Drosophila* and mammals, it appears that CeTMI represents a skeletal isoform while CeTMII represents a cytoskeletal isoform. CeTmIII and CeTmIV are produced by the internal promoter and are 256 aa long and represent cytoskeletal isoforms. A unique feature of the *C. elegansTm* gene, compared to other *Tm* genes, is the alternative splicing of exon 4 and the choice of three alternatives for exon 5. Seven additional transcripts generated by the *tmy-1* gene are found in databanks (www.wormbase.org) and they encode proteins of 151 to 193 amino acids but their relevance is unknown. One cannot exclude that additional isoforms might be produced by the *tmy-1* gene.

Arthropods

Among arthropods, the fruitfly *Drosophila melanogaster* is one of the major animal models studied and tropomyosin gene structure and expression has been well documented. cDNA and genomic clone analysis have showed that there are two *Tm* genes in *D. melanogaster*, namely *TmI* (also known as gene 1) and *TmII* (also known as gene 2) that are closely linked on chromosome 3 and generate at least 8 proteins (Fig. 2B) that show about 47% identity with vertebrate Tm.[17-22] *TmI* gene is about 26 kb long and is the more complex of the two *Tm* genes. It contains 17 exons (including an untranslated leader exon) with two promoters, three internal alternative exons and four distinct carboxy terminal exons. Unlike vertebrate *Tm* genes, the *D. melanogasterTmII* gene does not contain alternatively spliced exons 2 and 6 but instead contains alternate exons 4, 5, 7 and 9. Contrary to what is found in the vertebrates, exon 9a encodes the carboxy terminus of a cytosketal isoform, while exons 9b, 9c and 9d encode the carboxy temini of striated mucle tropomyosins. At least six distinct mRNAs are produced by the *TmI* gene encoding polypeptides ranging from 252 to 518 aa.[22] The distal promoter is considered as a muscle promoter and is active in muscle cells of the embryo, larva and adult while the internal one is considered as an housekeeping-type promoter. Six additional transcripts and polypeptides potentially generated by the *TmI* are found in databanks (e.g., Flybase) but their significance is unknown.

The *TmII* gene is 5 kb long and comprises five exons (including an untranslated leader exon), of which the last is alternatively spliced to give rise to two 284 amino acid proteins showing distinct carboxyl-terminal regions of 27 aa.[19] The two *D. melanogaster Tm* genes have in common the presence of an untranslated leader exon that is not found in vertebrate genes.

Echinoderms

Echinoderms constitute a phylum of marine invertebrates that belong, like chordates and urochordates to Deuterostomes. Among echinoderms, the sea urchin has been widely used as a major organism model in developmental biology and the genome of the species *Strongylocentrotus purpuratus* has been recently sequenced and annotated.[23] Because sea urchin is a non chordate deuterostome, it will give insights about the gene families it does and does not share with chordate deuterostomes and animals of other superphyla. Two *Tm* genes, named *suTM1* and *suTM2*, can be identified in the recently sequenced genome of *S. purpuratus*.[23] (Fig. 2C). The *suTM1* gene is composed of 10 exons and comprises two promoters. The distal promoter is used to produce a 284 aa Tm isoform while the internal one produces a 242 aa isoform, both isoforms showing 37-38% identity with the vertebrate α and β striated isoforms. When compared with the vertebrate *Tm* gene, it appears that the 39 aa containing exon 4 of the vertebrate gene is split into two exons of 15 and 24 aa in the *suTM1* gene while exons 6 and 7 in vertebrate genes are fused in the sea urchin gene to give a unique 46 aa exon. The *suTM2* gene codes for a 245 aa protein and has the same pattern of splicing and same size of exons as the *suTM1* gene except for exon 1b which is 3 aa longer in the *suTM2* gene. The protein encoded by the *suTM2* gene has 33% identity with the low molecular weight Tm produced by the *suTM1* gene and only 24% with α and β vertebrate tropomyosins.

Urochordates

Urochordates (also known as tunicates) belong to the phylum of deuterostomes and constitute with vertebrates and cephalochordates one major subphylum of the chordates that includes animals possessing a notochord. Phylogenetic studies indicate that urochordates represent a sister group of vertebrates and therefore constitutes a good system for exploring the evolutionary origin of the chordates lineage from which all vertebrates sprouted.[24] Within the urochordates, the ascidian *Ciona intestinalis*, whose tadpole exhibit the general architecture of vertebrates embryos, has emerged as a model organism and its genome has been recently sequenced and assembled. A cDNA clone encoding a 284 aa tropomyosin has been isolated from the body wall muscle of *C. Intestinalis* and identified as the *CTM1* gene (Fig. 2D). The *C. intestinalis* Tm has 72% identity with either the α or β vertebrate skeletal muscle tropomyosin and 52% identity with the *Drosophila* muscle Tm.[25] Genomic data indicates that the *CTM1* gene is a single copy gene that is 4.4 kb long and comprises 8 exons but shows no evidence of alternatively spliced exons.

Vertebrates

Tm genes have been cloned or identified in databases in the major sub-phyla of vertebrates, namely fishes, amphibians, avians and mammalians. Four distinct genes are found in vertebrates and they can produce, through alternative promoters, mutually alternatively spliced exons and different carboxyl termini more that 40 isoforms.[1-3,26] There is not a unified nomenclature for the vertebrate *Tm* genes and each of the genes has been named, when first described, after the protein they encode. The α (also known as *TPM1*) and β (also known as *TPM2*) genes are named after striated muscle α and β-Tm isoforms respectively. The *TMnm* (also referred to *as* γ-*Tm* or *TPM3*) and the *TM-4* (also known as δ-*Tm* or *TPM4*) genes have been named after human fibroblast *TM30nm* and the rat fibroblast *TM-4* respectively. The *Tm* gene nomenclature in the human genome project is *TPM1-4*. As shown in Figure 3, we have kept the original name by which they have been first identified and described by different groups. One structural feature of all the vertebrate *Tm* genes is their highly conserved exon-intron structural organization with the number and order of exons being, except in a few cases, strictly conserved. Furthermore, for each exon the class of junction is the same. The different exons have been named 1a to 9d in order to facilitate simple comparison between genes.

Fishes

The Japanese pufferfish (*Fugu rubripes*) and the zebra fish (*Danio rerio*) and are two widely used model species whose genome sequencing has been undertaken. In both species, *Tm* genes have been identified through cDNA cloning, expressed sequence tags (ESTs) and genomic sequence database. The most comprehensive picture we have today about *Tm* genes structure and number in fish is that of *Fugu rubripes*. Six genes, namely *TPM1* to *TPM4*, have been found in the genome of *F. rubripes* (Fig. 3A) and four of them correspond to duplicated paralogs.[27,28] *TPM1-1*, with its paralog *TPM1-2* and *TPM4-1*, with its paralog *TPM4-2*, correspond to the mammalian α-*Tm* and δ-*Tm* respectively. *TPM2* and *TPM3* arc single copy genes and correspond to the mammalian β-*Tm* and γ-*Tm* respectively. *TPM1-1* is structurally equivalent to the amphibian, avian or mammalian α-*Tm* genes with two promoters and two mutually alternatively spliced exons (2a:2b, 6a:6b) but contains three different carboxyl termini instead of four in the avian and mammalian genes. The duplicated *TPM1-2* differs from its paralog *TPM1-1* by the absence of exons 2a and 6a. *TPM2* is equivalent to its counterpart vertebrate β-*TM* genes with the exception that it has no exon 6a. *TPM3*, in contrast to avian and mammalian γ-*Tm* genes has a single promoter and no mutually alternatively spliced exon 6a. *TPM4-1* and *TPM4-2* genes have an identical structure to the amphibian and avian δ-*Tm* genes with two promoters and two alternative carboxyl termini. One striking feature of the fishes *Tm* genes is the absence of exon 9c which in avians and mammalians encodes a brain specific exon.

Amphibians

Amphibians have long been considered as animal models in developmental biology and *Xenopus laevis* has emerged more recently as a preferred one. However, due to its tetraploid status it is the genome of the closely related diploid *Xenopus tropicalis* whose genome sequence has been undertaken.[29] Three *Tm* genes have been identified in *X. laevis* through cDNA and genomic clone analysis and the presence of a fourth gene has been deduced from the inspection of EST database (Fig. 3B). The *Xenopus laevis* α-*Tm* gene is 35 kb long and possesses 14 exons, two alternate promoters, two sets of alternatively spliced exons (2a:2b and 6a:6b) and three distinct carboxyl termini 9a:9b:9d.[30-32] The gene generates skeletal and smooth muscle isoforms together with cytoskeletal isoforms. The main structural difference with its avian and mammalian counterparts is the absence of the brain specific exon 9c. The amphibian β-*Tm* gene is structurally related to the mammalian ortholog with one promoter, an internal alternatively spliced set of exons and two different carboxyl termini 9a:9d.[33,34] Like the mammalian gene it produces striated and smooth muscle Tm isoforms. The *TM4* gene is structurally equivalent to its avian ortholog with two alternate promoters and two distinct carboxyl termini. It can produce a 284 aa muscle isoform and a 248 aa cytoskeletal isoform.[35] EST sequence analysis indicates that the *TM4* gene can also produce a mRNA from the distal promoter and that includes the carboxyl terminus 9d. As previously mentioned, *X. laevis* is a tetraploid species where most if not all the genes characterized in that species exist in two copies per haploid genome. A close inspection of EST databases indicates that there are two α-*Tm*, two β-*Tm* and two *TM-4* expressed genes in *X. laevis* and cDNA sequence comparison suggest that the duplicated genes have the same structure. From EST sequences in databases it appears that there is a fourth *Tm* gene, equivalent to *TPM3* (γ-*Tm*) also present (BC043980, Fig. 3B). The cDNA corresponding to that gene encodes a 250 aa low molecular weight isoform but there is no evidence for additional alternatively spliced isoforms produced by the gene.

Avians

Tm cDNAs and genomic sequences have been isolated and characterized from chicken (*Gallus gallus*) and quail (*Coturnix coturnix*). The structure of the α*fTM* and β-*TM* genes from *G. gallus* has been established from cDNAs and genomic clones and those of the δ-*TM* gene is deduced from cDNAs sequences.[36-41] The structure of the γ-*Tm* gene is deduced from isoforms found in EST databases (Fig. 3C). The avian α*fTM* gene has the same structure as its mammalian ortholog. It covers 20 kb and consists of 15 exons, including two sets of internally alternatively spliced exons (2a:2b; 6a:6b) and it possesses two alternate promoters. It can produce at least nine isoforms

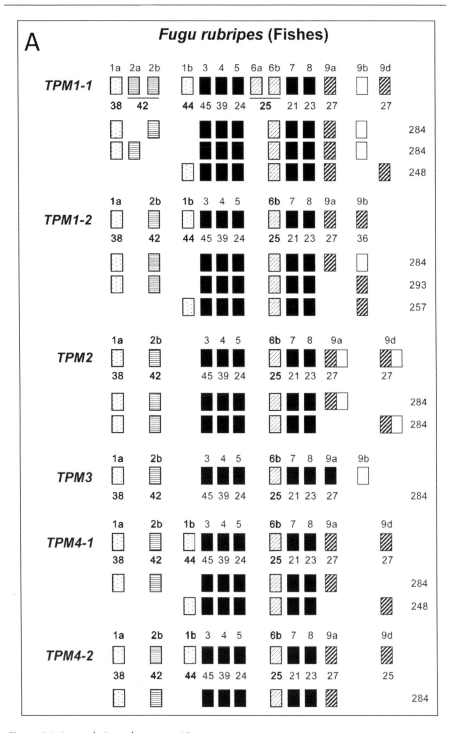

Figure 3A. Legend viewed on page 16.

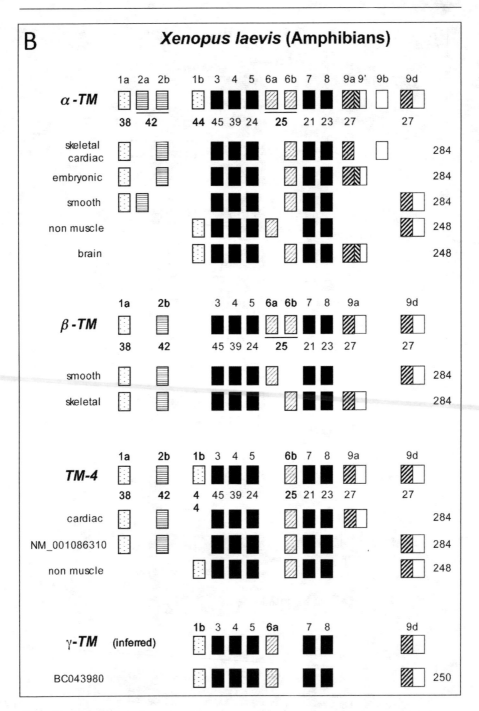

Figure 3B. Legend viewed on page 16.

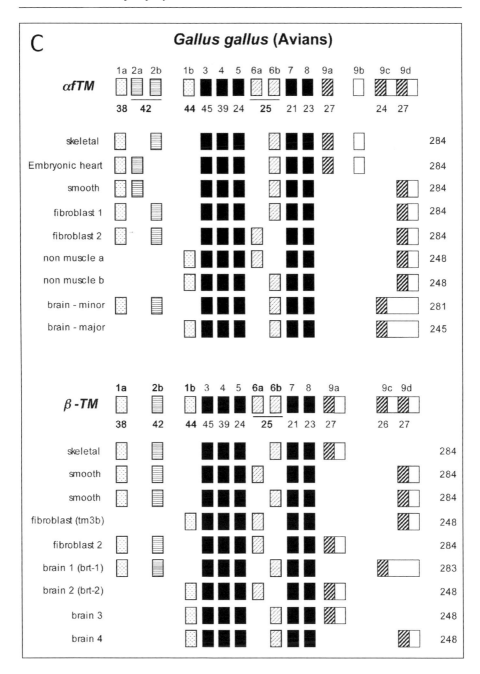

Figure 3C. Legend viewed on following page.

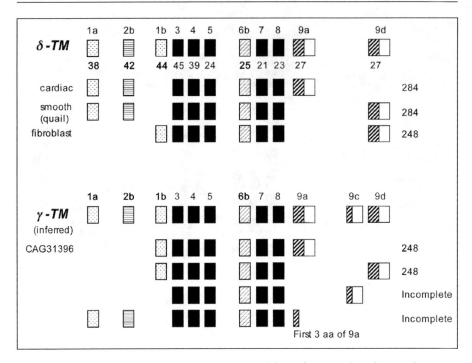

Figure 3. Exon organisation of tropomysosin genes and the isoforms produced in vertebrates. A) fishes represented by *F.rubripes*; B) amphibians represented by *X. laevis;* C) avians represented by *G. gallus*. Exons are represented by boxes. The 3'untranslated regions are represented by a white box. The gene name is shown in italics and the number of the exon above and size in aa below the boxes. Exons subject to alternate usage are shaded the same. Isoforms known to be produced from each gene are shown and the size in aa is shown on the right. Only one known isoform is produced by *TPM3* of *F. rubripes* and therefore is not shown below the gene. In the case of the γ-*Tm* gene for *X. laevis* and *G. gallus* the organisation of the exons is inferred from sequences in the EST database as no gene information is available. As our knowledge of this gene is incomplete there may be other exons present which have not yet been found. Exons have been numbered according to previous reports[3,45] in order to facilitate comparison between genes. Exons 9a 9b, 9c and 9d are equivalent when considering fishes, amphibians, avians or mammalians genes.

and the carboxyl terminus of the different isoforms is encoded by three distinct alternative exons 9a:9c:9d.[36,37] Among them, exon 9c is specifically expressed in brain cells as has been found for the mammalian gene. One striking feature of the chicken α*fTM* gene, compared to its vertebrates orthologs, is that exon 2a has been found in an mRNA (Embryonic heart in Fig. 3C) expressed solely in embryonic heart.[42] A similar mRNA has been described in *Fugu rubripes* but none expression data are available.[28]The chicken β-*TM* gene spans 13 kb and possesses 13 exons generating at least 9 isoforms.[38-40] One major difference between the avian gene and the mammalian β-*TM* gene is the presence of two alternate promoters, the internal one being used to produce a 248 aa cytoskeletal isoform.[40]There are also many more known isoforms from the avian β-*Tm* than have been found in mammalians. The γ-*TM* gene, according to EST sequences is composed of at least 12 exons with three alternative carboxyl termini but show no evidence of internal alternatively spliced exons. At least four isoforms appear to be produced and two of them are incomplete (Fig. 3C). The avian δ-*TM* gene is structurally equivalent to the amphibian *TM-4* gene with 11 exons, two alternate promoters and two distinct carboxyl termini. It produces a cardiac and a smooth muscle isoform of 284 aa and a cytoskeletal 248 aa Tm.[41]

Mammalians

Most of our knowledge concerning the mammalian *Tm* gene structure comes from cDNAs and genomic clones that have been isolated in rodents (rat and mouse) and human. The picture has been then completed with the help of genomic and EST sequence databases that record the genomic sequences and/or expression of *Tm* genes in several additional mammalian species. For simplicity we have used the mouse *Tm* genes as representative of mammals although there are differences between species as mentioned in the text (Fig. 4) (see also Chapter 16).

α-Tropomyosin Gene (TPM1)

The α-*tropomyosin* gene is the most complex mammalian *tropomyosin* gene and its structure has been first elucidated from rat genomic clones analysis.[43-45]The rat α-*Tm* gene spans about 28 kb and comprises 15 exons and includes two alternative promoters, two internally mutually exclusive exons (2a:2b and 6a:6b) and four alternatively spliced 3'exons (9a-9d) that encode four different carboxyl termini. The mouse and human α-*Tm* (*TPM1*) genes are about 27 kb and 29 kb respectively and show a similar structure (Fig. 4). In addition to the production of at least four cytoskeletal isoforms, the α-*Tm* gene can produce skeletal and smooth muscle specific isoforms where exon 2a is unique to smooth muscle.[46,47] Three distinct brain isoforms are also produced by the gene and two of them contain the unique carboxyl terminus encoded by the brain specific exon 9c.[45] For a comparison with the human gene, see Chapter 16.

β-Tropomyosin Gene (TPM2)

The mammalian β *tropomyosin* gene ranges from 8 kb in human (*TPM2*) to 9 kb in mouse (*TPM2*) and 10kb in rat (β-*TM*). The gene spans 11 exons and contains a single promoter, a unique mutually exclusive internal exon (6a:6b) and two distinct carboxyl termini (9a:9d) (Fig. 4). It produces two 284 aa tropomyosin proteins corresponding to the skeletal β-Tm isoform and the smooth muscle β-Tm isoform which is identical to the cytoskeletal TM1 isoform.[48,49] An additional product has been detected in humans (Chapter 16).

γ-Tropomyosin Gene (TPM3)

The structure of the γ-*tropomyosin* gene has been first described in human. The human gene (named *TM30nm*), spans about 42 kb and comprises 14 exons with two promoters, a single mutually exclusive internal exon (6a:6b) and four carboxyl-termini encoded by distinct alternatively spliced exons.[50] The mouse gene (*TPM3*) and the rat gene (γ-*TM*) cover 28 kb and 27 kb respectively. The γ-*TM* gene encodes a 284 aa residues tropomyosin present in slow twitch skeletal muscle and several low molecular weight cytoskeletal tropomyosins. For instance, the rat gene has been described to produce at least ten cytoskeletal isoforms that ranges from 177 to 248 aa residues and that are expressed in a complex pattern.[51] The mouse γ-*TM* gene can produce at least 11 cytoskeletal isoforms (Fig. 4).

δ-Tropomyosin Gene (TPM4)

The complete structure of the mammalian δ-*Tm* gene has been first described for the rat gene (also known as *TM-4* gene). The gene spans 16 kb and comprises 8 exons but shows no alternatively spliced exons. Instead, the presence of "vestigial" exons similar in sequence to exons 2b and 9a of the rat β-*Tm* genes have been found in the gene but mutations has rendered them non-functional.[52] The mouse δ-*Tm* gene (TPM4) is structurally equivalent to the rat gene and covers 18 kb (Fig. 4). Database analysis reveals different situations for the structural organization of δ-*Tm* genes in other mammalian species. For instance, the human gene spans about 35 kb and displays a distal promoter. Moreover it possesses an exon 2b and can generate a 284 aa protein containing a carboxyl end encoded by exon 9d and that is similar to the smooth muscle Tm isoform produced by the quail δ-*Tm* gene (also see Chapter 16). An intact exon 9a is also found in human but not yet been found to be used in any transcripts.

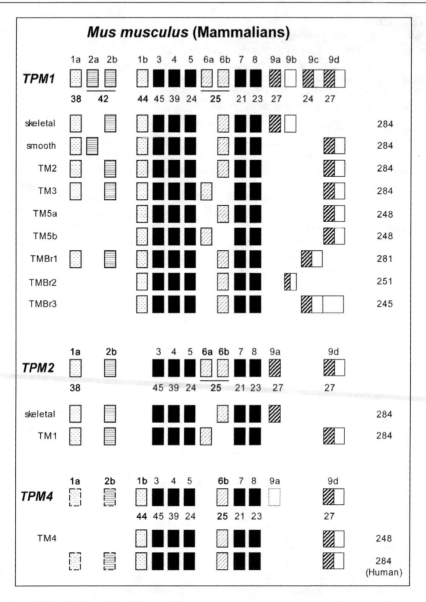

Figure 4. Legend viewed on following page.

Evolution of the Tropomyosin Genes

The number of tropomyosin isoforms found in different species of the animal kingdom is directly related to the number of encoding genes and whether or not those genes are subject to alternative splicing. In the early eukaryotic lineage such as in yeast, only one or two Tm isoform are found and they are encoded by single genes that show no alternatively spliced isoforms (see Chapter 14). This is the same for the diploblast phylum, illustrated by cnidarians, where the identified *Tm* genes possess no introns. In the tripoblast lineages that include the protostomes and

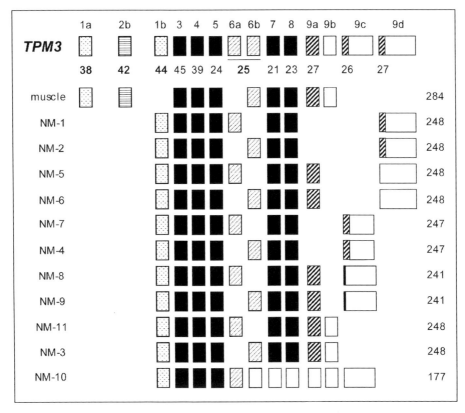

Figure 4. Exon organisation of tropomyosin genes and the isoforms produced in mammals, represented by mouse *M. musculus*.[2] Exons are represented by boxes. The 3′untranslated regions are represented by a white box. The gene name is shown in italics and the number of the exon above and size in aa below the boxes. Exons subject to alternate usage are shaded the same. Isoforms known to be produced from each gene are shown and the size in aa is shown on the right. The *TPM4* gene organisation varies in different species (see Chapter 16). Exons 1a and 2b are not present in mouse but are shown here as they exist in human to produce the isoform shown (Ensembl Peptide ID ENSP00000345230 in www.ensembl.org/homo_sapiens/). Exons have been numbered according to previous report[2] in order to facilitate comparison between genes. Exons 9a 9b, 9c and 9d are equivalent when considering mammalians, fishes, amphibians or avians genes.

deuterostomes phyla, tropomyosin isoform diversity has increased through the combination of gene duplication and alternative splicing.

Gene Duplication

During its 2 billion years of evolution, the eukaryotic genome has undergone several processes that has led to an increase in the phenotypic complexity of animals. One of these processes is the whole genome duplication that occurred at different steps during evolution.[53] On the basis of genome size, gene family analysis and the availability of sequenced genomes, it has been proposed that two rounds (2R) of whole genome duplication (WGD) has occurred in the lineage leading to vertebrates (Fig. 5)[54] This hypothesis is exemplified by several gene families that were found to have expanded from a single member in invertebrates to four members in vertebrates. For instance, many single-copy genes in *Drosophila* have four vertebrate orthologs, consistent with

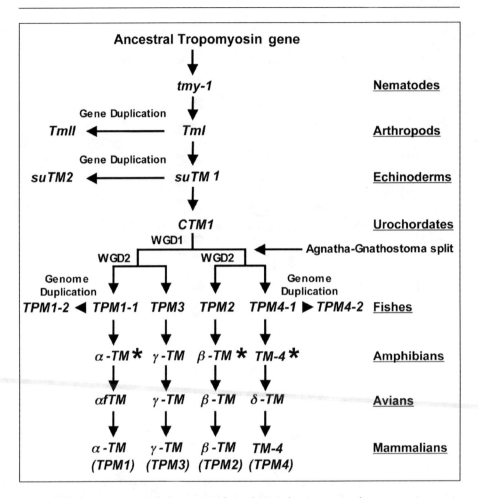

Figure 5. Tropomyosin gene phylogeny. We hypothesize that an ancestral tropomyosin gene is the common ancestor to all bilateria *Tm* genes and which gave rise to the present *tmy-1* gene in the nematode *C. elegans*, the *TmI* gene in the arthropod *D. melanogaster*, the *suTM1* gene in the echinoderm *S. purpuratus* and in the urochordate *C. intestinalis CTM1* genes. Additional *Tm* genes in arthropods *(TmII)* and echinoderms *(SuTM2)* resulted from gene duplications. Two whole genome duplications (WGD1 and WGD2) from the ancestral gene produced the four vertebrates *Tm* genes. Further genome duplications in fish gives rise to *TPM1-2* and *TPM4-2*. In amphibians, the duplication of the α-*TM*, β-*TM* and *TM-4* is indicated by an asterisk (*).

the notion of two rounds of genome duplication in vertebrates.[55] The two *Drosophila Tm* genes, *TmI* and *TmII*, have a different exon-intron organization and they probably arose through a gene duplication event of either an individual gene or a genomic segment followed by a massive loss of introns resulting in the 5 kb *TmI* gene that contains only three introns.[17] Because the *Drosophila TmI* gene has an exon-intron structure identical to its vertebrate orthologs (see Fig. 6A), we can postulate in agreement with the 2R hypothesis, that it represents the ancestor *Tm* gene from which the four vertebrates orthologs are derived. Considering the sea urchin *Tm* genes, the *suTM2* gene probably represents a duplication event that occurred in the echinoderm lineage. Because the unique *Tm* gene that is present in both the nematode *C. elegans* and the urochordate *C. intestinalis*

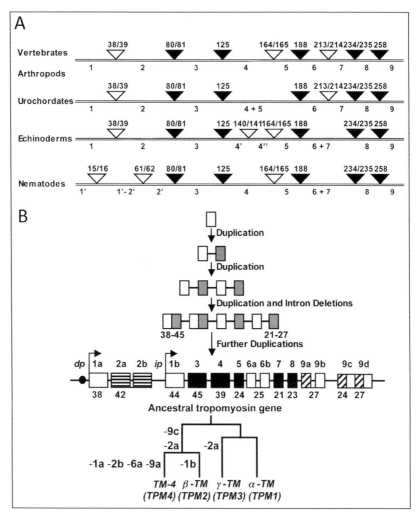

Figure 6. Evolution of the tropomyosin genes structure. A) Comparison of positions of introns in *Tm* genes of various organisms. The horizontal bar represents tropomyosin protein with the amino terminus at the left and the carboxy terminus at the right. The positions of conserved introns in all organisms are indicated by black triangles relative to the amino acid sequence of the protein. Variable introns positions are indicated by an open triangle. Numbers above the triangles indicate the position numbers of the amino acid residues at which introns interrupt the sequence. Exons are numbered below the horizontal bar with respect to the vertebrate striated α-Tm protein. Data on gene structures were taken from the following sources : vertebrates,[40,45,50] arthropods.[22] nematodes.[16] Data on urochordates and echinoderms are from genomic sequencing data. B) Proposed evolution origin of the vertebrate *Tm* genes (upper) and in the mouse and rat rodents (lower). A series of duplication of an ancestral exon, with an average size of 21 amino acid, combined with intron deletions led to a minimal ancestral tropomyosin gene [adapted from ref. 44]. The distal (*dp*) and the internal (*ip*) promoters are indicated together with the evolutionary conserved module of 30-bp identified in the vertebrates α-*Tm* genes [68](black circle). Duplication events of the ancestral gene give rise in vertebrates to the lines with α-*Tm* and γ-*Tm* genes on one side and the β-*Tm* and *TM-4* genes on the other. Selective loss of the exons 1a, 1b, 2a, 6a, 9a and 9c during the course of speciation have generated the rodent specific *Tm* genes.

genomes has a highly conserved structural organization with the vertebrate *Tm* orthologs, one can hypothesize that the four vertebrates genes are derived from a unique ancestral *tropomyosin* gene after two genome duplications.

A phylogenic tree analysis made with the 176 aa region corresponding to common exons 3:4:5:6b:7:8 of vertebrates tropomyosins indicates that the first genome duplication (WGD1) resulted in one line leading to the α-*Tm* and γ-*Tm* genes and another line leading to the β-*Tm* and δ-*Tm* genes (Fig. 5). The second genome duplication (WGD2) has led to the four contemporary vertebrates genes[28,52] (Fig. 5). Phylogenetic analysis has postulated that the two periods of gene duplication arose during urochordate-vertebrate transition, one before and one after the Agnata-Gnathostoma split as suggested by the analysis of several lamprey and hagfish genes.[56] This is consistent with the presence of a unique *Tm* gene in *Ciona intestinalis* that occupies a phylogenetic position prior to Agnata-Gnathostoma radiation. The additional *Tm* genes found in the *Fugu rubripes* and *Xenopus laevis* genomes are related to the tetrapolyploidisation events that occurred in the fish and amphibian lineages. Whole genomic sequence data analysis of the two related pufferfish genomes (*Fugu rubripes* and *Tetraodon nigroviridis*) indicate that a genome duplication occurred in the teleost fish lineage about 350 Mya, subsequent to its divergence from mammals.[57,58] Regarding *Xenopus laevis Tm* genes, cDNA clones analysis and available EST sequences strongly suggest that the α-*Tm*, β-*Tm* and *TM-4* genes are duplicated.[32,33,35] This has been observed for many *Xenopus laevis* genes and is consistent with the recent tetraploidization event that occurred ~40 million years ago in the amphibian lineage.[59] Numerous gene families found in vertebrates genomes do not follow the 2R rule suggesting that many genes were loosened from constraint after the genome duplications and experienced an accelerated rate of sequence change before returning to single copy.[60] This is not the case of *Tm* genes probably due to constraints imposed on their essential function as actin binding proteins.

Evolution of Exon-Intron Structure, Alternative Splicing and Alternate Promoters

The structure of the *Tm* genes is highly conserved between evolutionarily distant species like invertebrates and vertebrates. This is strikingly apparent when comparing the exon-intron organization of the arthropod *Drosophila melanogaster TmII* gene with its vertebrates orthologs (Fig. 6A). In all known vertebrate *Tm* genes, the position of the introns relative to the coding sequence is totally conserved with those of the *Drosophila TmII* gene and respects, at the nucleotide level, the same phase of interruption (Fig. 6A).[22,43] This conservation is also observed within the distantly related taxa of urochordates (*Ciona intestinalis*), echinoderms (*Strongylocentrotus purpuratus*) and nematodes (*Caenorhabditis elegans*) although with differences. For instance in the *Ciona intestinalis* CTM1 gene, the intron at position 164/165 is absent therefore generating a 63 aa exon encoded by the joining of exon 4 with exon 5. In the sea urchin *Strongylocentrotus purpuratus* gene *su*TM1, it is the intron at position 213/214 that is absent while there is an additional intron that splits the 39 aa exon 4 of vertebrate genes into two exons of 16 and 23 aa. In the nematode *Caenorhabditis elegans tmy-1* gene, the first 80 aa sequence is encoded by three exons while in other species it is encoded by only two exons. However, this conservation of intron position is still remarkably high when considering such distant species. The exon-intron structure of human and mouse ortholog genes is largely conserved but this is not the case for other taxonomic groups and it has been shown that there was an extensive loss of introns in some of the eukaryotic lineages with a recent intron gain in the vertebrates lineage.[61,62] As a comparison, the six highly conserved mammalian *actin* genes have only three out of seven identical exon-intron boundaries and none of them is conserved in *Drosophila melanogaster* or *Caenorhabditis elegans* genes.[63]

The tropomyosin molecule possesses an α-helical coiled coil structure and consists of a repeating heptapeptide extending throughout the entire length.[64] Muscle tropomyosins bind to seven actin monomers with a binding site spaced approximately every 40 aa while low-molecular weight proteins bind six actin monomers. On the basis of structural organization of the gene and the non random location of exon-intron boundaries, it has been suggested that the *Tm* originated by repeated duplications of an ancestral 21 aa long sequence.[43,44] (Fig. 6B). Tandem exon duplication has been postulated for the generation of many alternatively spliced exons and constitutes a major way of functional diversification of proteins.[65] In the case of *Tm* genes, the duplication of the 21 aa ancestral exon with the loss of intron between duplicated exons would explain the generation of exons with an average of 42 aa exons. Although there are some discrepancies between the size of the ancestral exon and those observed in different *Tm* genes, ranging from either 21 to 27 or 38-45, this could be explained by a junctional exon sliding process.[66] The duplication of an ancestral exon is the basis for the modular and repetitive structure of the Tm molecule that has been highly conserved throughout evolution and present in the ancestral gene before the radiation of protostomes and deuterostomes about 900 Mya.

Alternative splicing is a major process for isoform diversity production and has contributed to the evolution of modern genomes.[67] Most if not all the *Tm* genes from nematodes to mammals are differentially spliced and the degree of divergence between pairs of alternatively spliced exons within a gene is greater than that among isoform specific exons between evolutionary distant species. This suggests that the alternatively spliced exons in Tm is an ancient trait and present before radiation of nematodes. As shown in Figures 2, 3 and 4 the regions of alternatively spliced exons differ between invertebrates and vertebrates. The region encoded by alternative exon 6b and 9a in vertebrate genes are important for troponin T interaction in striated muscle cells, while alternative exon 1a and 9a are important for head to tail polymerisation between Tm molecules. Alternative regions of the *Tm* genes have therefore evolved in order to carry out specialized functions. Among the alternatively spliced exons, some are specific to vertebrate lineages such as exon 2a which is only found in the vertebrate smooth muscle isoform generated by the α-Tm gene. The exon 9c is a "brain" specific exon found in Tm isoforms expressed in the brain and generated by the α-*Tm* and γ-*Tm* genes. The exon 9c has not been found in amphibian or fish genomes suggesting it could correspond to a recent duplication event. The "subfunctionalization" paradigm proposed for the evolution of duplicates genes is applicable to the exon duplication proposed for the *Tm* genes. The *Tm* genes have therefore evolved between invertebrates and vertebrates to produce alternative regions supporting cell-type or developmental stage specific specialized functions. Because of their functional importance these alternative regions have been under evolutionary constraint and preserved during evolution of the different lineages. When considering the overall organization of *Tm* genes in different species it appears that a selective loss of exons for several *Tm* genes has occurred during speciation events and this is particularly evident in the mammalian lineage. A comparative analysis of the structural organization of mammalian *Tm* genes suggests that, in the rodent lineage, the β-*Tm*, γ-*Tm* and TM-4 genes are derived from the ancestral gene through a successive loss of alternative exons while the α-*Tm* has conserved all the alternative exons and has a similar structural organization to that of the ancestral gene (Fig. 6B). The rodent *TM-4* gene has lost exons 1a, 2a/2b, 6a, 9a/9c while the β-*TM* gene has lost exons 2a, 1b and 9c. The γ-*TM* gene that is in the same lineage as the α-*TM* gene has only lost exon 2a. The lost of exons 1a, 2a and 2b or exon 1b leads to the absence of distal and internal promoters respectively. This loss of exon is lineage specific because whole sequence genomic data indicates that the human *TPM4* gene has conserved exon 1a (Fig. 4).

Because of their functional importance, coding sequences show a higher evolutionary conservation than intronic or genomic sequences that flank exons. This is the case for both the internal and distal promoter of the vertebrate *Tm* genes except for a highly conserved 30-bp region that is unique to all known α-*TM* genes. This region has been shown to be essential for the muscle α-*TM* gene expression through the binding of the transcription factor TEF-1.[68]

Concluding Remarks

Tropomyosin isoform diversity has increasingly evolved during metazoan evolution through a combination of gene duplication and complex alternative splicing. Because of its essential function as an actin binding protein, the repetitive structure that shapes the protein has been crafted into a modular gene where each exon constitutes the repetitive unit. This ancestral gene was probably already present at the origin of the Bilateria phylum before the beginning of the Cambrian. The evolutionarily conserved structure of *Tm* genes reflects an absolute structural requirement imposed on the protein and which has been under selective pressure. During evolution of the animal kingdom the number of Tm isoforms produced in different species has reached its maximum in mammals where the four *Tm* genes are expressed in a complex pattern during development and in adult tissues (see Chapter 4). This complexity reflects the various specialized functions that has been acquired by the proteins in response to the increased complexity of organisms and that is exemplified by the appearance of a brain specific exon in higher vertebrates.

Acknowledgements

Work in the laboratory of Nadine Thézé and Pierre Thiébaud has been supported by the University V. Segalen Bordeaux 2 and the CNRS.

References

1. Pittenger MF, Kazzaz JA, Helfman DM. Functional properties of nonmuscle tropomyosin isoforms. Curr Opin Cell Biol 1994; 6(1):96-104.
2. Gunning PW, Schevzov G, Kee AJ et al. Tropomyosin isoforms: divining rods for actin cytoskeleton function. Trends Cell Biol 2005; 15(6):333-341.
3. Lees-Miller JP, Helfman DM. The molecular basis for tropomyosin isoform diversity. Bioessays 1991; 13(9):429-437.
4. Vrhovski B, Schevzov G, Dingle S et al. Tropomyosin isoforms from the gamma gene differing at the C-terminus are spatially and developmentally regulated in the brain. J Neurosci Res 2003; 72(3):373-383.
5. Liu HP, Bretscher A. Disruption of the single tropomyosin gene in yeast results in the disappearance of actin cables from the cytoskeleton. Cell 1989; 57(2):233-242.
6. Drees B, Brown C, Barrell BG et al. Tropomyosin is essential in yeast, yet the TPM1 and TPM2 products perform distinct functions. J Cell Biol 1995; 128(3):383-392.
7. Balasubramanian MK, Helfman DM, Hemmingsen SM. A new tropomyosin essential for cytokinesis in the fission yeast S. pombe. Nature 1992; 360(6399):84-87.
8. Hedges SB. The origin and evolution of model organisms. Nat Rev Genet 2002; 3(11):838-849.
9. Lopez de Haro MS, Salgado LM, David CN et al. Hydra tropomyosin TROP1 is expressed in head-specific epithelial cells and is a major component of the cytoskeletal structure that anchors nematocytes. J Cell Sci 1994; 107(Pt 6):1403-1411.
10. Groger H, Callaerts P, Gehring WJ et al. Gene duplication and recruitment of a specific tropomyosin into striated muscle cells in the jellyfish Podocoryne carnea. J Exp Zool 1999; 285(4):378-386.
11. Adoutte A, Balavoine G, Lartillot N et al. The new animal phylogeny: reliability and implications. Proc Natl Acad Sci USA 2000; 97(9):4453-4456.
12. Frenkel MJ, Savin KW, Bakker RE et al. Characterization of cDNA clones coding for muscle tropomyosin of the nematode Trichostrongylus colubriformis. Mol Biochem Parasitol 1989; 37(2):191-199.
13. Nakada T, Nagano I, Wu Z et al. Molecular cloning and expression of the full-length tropomyosin gene from Trichinella spiralis. J Helminthol 2003; 77(1):57-63.
14. Jenkins RE, Taylor MJ, Gilvary NJ et al. Tropomyosin implicated in host protective responses to microfilariae in onchocerciasis. Proc Natl Acad Sci USA 1998; 95(13):7550-7555.
15. Anyanful A, Sakube Y, Takuwa K et al. The third and fourth tropomyosin isoforms of Caenorhabditis elegans are expressed in the pharynx and intestines and are essential for development and morphology. J Mol Biol 2001; 313(3):525-537.
16. Kagawa H, Sugimoto K, Matsumoto H et al. Genome structure, mapping and expression of the tropomyosin gene tmy-1 of Caenorhabditis elegans. J Mol Biol 1995; 251(5):603-613.
17. Karlik CC, Fyrberg EA. Two Drosophila melanogaster tropomyosin genes: structural and functional aspects. Mol Cell Biol 1986; 6(6):1965-1973.
18. Basi GS, Boardman M, Storti RV. Alternative splicing of a Drosophila tropomyosin gene generates muscle tropomyosin isoforms with different carboxy-terminal ends. Mol Cell Biol 1984; 4(12):2828-2836.
19. Basi GS, Storti RV. Structure and DNA sequence of the tropomyosin I gene from Drosophila melanogaster. J Biol Chem 1986; 261(2):817-827.
20. Hanke PD, Lepinske HM, Storti RV. Characterization of a Drosophila cDNA clone that encodes a 252-amino acid nonmuscle tropomyosin isoform. J Biol Chem 1987; 262(36):17370-17373.
21. Hanke PD, Storti RV. Nucleotide sequence of a cDNA clone encoding a Drosophila muscle tropomyosin II isoform. Gene 1986; 45(2):211-214.

22. Hanke PD, Storti RV. The Drosophila melanogaster tropomyosin II gene produces multiple proteins by use of alternative tissue-specific promoters and alternative splicing. Mol Cell Biol 1988; 8(9):3591-3602.

23. Sodergren E, Weinstock GM, Davidson EH et al. The genome of the sea urchin Strongylocentrotus purpuratus. Science 10 2006; 314(5801):941-952.

24. Corbo JC, Di Gregorio A, Levine M. The ascidian as a model organism in developmental and evolutionary biology. Cell 2001; 106(5):535-538.

25. Meedel TH, Hastings KE. Striated muscle-type tropomyosin in a chordate smooth muscle, ascidian body-wall muscle. J Biol Chem 1993; 268(9):6755-6764.

26. Perry SV. Vertebrate tropomyosin: distribution, properties and function. J Muscle Res Cell Motil 2001; 22(1):5-49.

27. Ikeda D, Toramoto T, Ochiai Y et al. Identification of novel tropomyosin 1 genes of pufferfish (Fugu rubripes) on genomic sequences and tissue distribution of their transcripts. Mol Biol Rep 2003; 30(2):83-90.

28. Toramoto T, Ikeda D, Ochiai Y et al. Multiple gene organization of pufferfish Fugu rubripes tropomyosin isoforms and tissue distribution of their transcripts. Gene 2004; 331:41-51.

29. Graf JD, Kobel HR. Genetics of Xenopus laevis. Methods Cell Biol 1991; 36:19-34.

30. Gaillard C, Theze N, Lerivray H et al. A novel tropomyosin isoform encoded by the Xenopus laevis alpha-TM gene is expressed in the brain. Gene 1998; 207(2):235-239.

31. Gaillard C, Theze N, Hardy S et al. Alpha-tropomyosin gene expression in Xenopus laevis: differential promoter usage during development and controlled expression by myogenic factors. Dev Genes Evol 1998; 207(7):435-445.

32. Hardy S, Fiszman MY, Osborne HB et al. Characterization of muscle and non muscle Xenopus laevis tropomyosin mRNAs transcribed from the same gene. Developmental and tissue-specific expression. Eur J Biochem 1991; 202(2):431-440.

33. Hardy S, Thiebaud P. Isolation and characterization of cDNA clones encoding the skeletal and smooth muscle Xenopus laevis beta tropomyosin isoforms. Biochim Biophys Acta 1992; 1131(2):239-242.

34. Gaillard C, Lerivray H, Theze N et al. Differential expression of two skeletal muscle beta-tropomyosin mRNAs during Xenopus laevis development. Int J Dev Biol 1999; 43(2):175-178.

35. Hardy S, Theze N, Lepetit D et al. The Xenopus laevis TM-4 gene encodes nonmuscle and cardiac tropomyosin isoforms through alternative splicing. Gene 1995; 156(2):265-270.

36. Lemonnier M, Balvay L, Mouly V et al. The chicken gene encoding the alpha isoform of tropomyosin of fast-twitch muscle fibers: organization, expression and identification of the major proteins synthesized. Gene 1991; 107(2):229-240.

37. Lindquester GJ, Flach JE, Fleenor DE et al. Avian tropomyosin gene expression. Nucleic Acids Res 1989; 17(5):2099-2118.

38. Forry-Schaudies S, Maihle NJ, Hughes SH. Generation of skeletal, smooth and low molecular weight nonmuscle tropomyosin isoforms from the chicken tropomyosin 1 gene. J Mol Biol 1990; 211(2):321-330.

39. Libri D, Lemonnier M, Meinnel T et al. A single gene codes for the beta subunits of smooth and skeletal muscle tropomyosin in the chicken. J Biol Chem 1989; 264(5):2935-2944.

40. Libri D, Mouly V, Lemonnier M et al. A nonmuscle tropomyosin is encoded by the smooth/skeletal beta-tropomyosin gene and its RNA is transcribed from an internal promoter. J Biol Chem 1990; 265(6):3471-3473.

41. Fleenor DE, Hickman KH, Lindquester GJ et al. Avian cardiac tropomyosin gene produces tissue-specific isoforms through alternative RNA splicing. J Muscle Res Cell Motil 1992; 13(1):55-63.

42. Zajdel RW, Denz CR, Lee S et al. Identification, characterization and expression of a novel alpha-tropomyosin isoform in cardiac tissues in developing chicken. J Cell Biochem 2003; 89(3):427-439.

43. Ruiz-Opazo N, Nadal-Ginard B. Alpha-tropomyosin gene organization. Alternative splicing of duplicated isotype-specific exons accounts for the production of smooth and striated muscle isoforms. J Biol Chem 1987; 262(10):4755-4765.

44. Wieczorek DF, Smith CW, Nadal-Ginard B. The rat alpha-tropomyosin gene generates a minimum of six different mRNAs coding for striated, smooth and nonmuscle isoforms by alternative splicing. Mol Cell Biol 1988; 8(2):679-694.

45. Lees-Miller JP, Goodwin LO, Helfman DM. Three novel brain tropomyosin isoforms are expressed from the rat alpha-tropomyosin gene through the use of alternative promoters and alternative RNA processing. Mol Cell Biol 1990; 10(4):1729-1742.

46. Goodwin LO, Lees-Miller JP, Leonard MA et al. Four fibroblast tropomyosin isoforms are expressed from the rat alpha-tropomyosin gene via alternative RNA splicing and the use of two promoters. J Biol Chem 1991; 266(13):8408-8415.

47. Ruiz-Opazo N, Weinberger J, Nadal-Ginard B. Comparison of alpha-tropomyosin sequences from smooth and striated muscle. Nature 1985; 315(6014):67-70.
48. Helfman DM, Cheley S, Kuismanen E et al. Nonmuscle and muscle tropomyosin isoforms are expressed from a single gene by alternative RNA splicing and polyadenylation. Mol Cell Biol 1986; 6(11):3582-3595.
49. MacLeod AR, Houlker C, Reinach FC et al. A muscle-type tropomyosin in human fibroblasts: evidence for expression by an alternative RNA splicing mechanism. Proc Natl Acad Sci USA 1985; 82(23):7835-7839.
50. Clayton L, Reinach FC, Chumbley GM et al. Organization of the hTMnm gene. Implications for the evolution of muscle and nonmuscle tropomyosins. J Mol Biol 1988; 201(3):507-515.
51. Dufour C, Weinberger RP, Schevzov G et al. Splicing of two internal and four carboxyl-terminal alternative exons in nonmuscle tropomyosin 5 premRNA is independently regulated during development. J Biol Chem 1998; 273(29):18547-18555.
52. Lees-Miller JP, Yan A, Helfman DM. Structure and complete nucleotide sequence of the gene encoding rat fibroblast tropomyosin 4. J Mol Biol 1990; 213(3):399-405.
53. Holland PW. Gene duplication: past, present and future. Semin Cell Dev Biol 1999; 10(5):541-547.
54. Panopoulou G, Hennig S, Groth D et al. New evidence for genome-wide duplications at the origin of vertebrates using an amphioxus gene set and completed animal genomes. Genome Res 2003; 13(6A):1056-1066.
55. Spring J. Vertebrate evolution by interspecific hybridisation—are we polyploid? FEBS Lett 1997; 400(1):2-8.
56. Escriva H, Manzon L, Youson J et al. Analysis of lamprey and hagfish genes reveals a complex history of gene duplications during early vertebrate evolution. Mol Biol Evol 2002; 19(9):1440-1450.
57. Jaillon O, Aury JM, Brunet F et al. Genome duplication in the teleost fish Tetraodon nigroviridis reveals the early vertebrate proto-karyotype. Nature 2004; 431(7011):946-957.
58. Aparicio S, Chapman J, Stupka E et al. Whole-genome shotgun assembly and analysis of the genome of Fugu rubripes. Science 2002; 297(5585):1301-1310.
59. Hellsten U, Khokha MK, Grammer TC et al. Accelerated gene evolution and subfunctionalization in the pseudotetraploid frog Xenopus laevis. BMC Biol 2007; 5:31.
60. Dehal P, Boore JL. Two rounds of whole genome duplication in the ancestral vertebrate. PLoS Biol 2005; 3(10):e314.
61. Rogozin IB, Wolf YI, Sorokin AV et al. Remarkable interkingdom conservation of intron positions and massive, lineage-specific intron loss and gain in eukaryotic evolution. Curr Biol 2003; 13(17):1512-1517.
62. Malko DB, Makeev VJ, Mironov AA et al. Evolution of exon-intron structure and alternative splicing in fruit flies and malarial mosquito genomes. Genome Res 2006; 16(4):505-509.
63. Kusakabe T, Araki I, Satoh N et al. Evolution of chordate actin genes: evidence from genomic organization and amino acid sequences. J Mol Evol 1997; 44(3):289-298.
64. Smillie LB. Structure and functions of tropomyosins from muscle and nonmuscle sources. Trends Biochem Sci 1979; 4:151-155.
65. Kondrashov FA, Koonin EV. Origin of alternative splicing by tandem exon duplication. Hum Mol Genet 2001; 10(23):2661-2669.
66. Stoltzfus A, Logsdon JM Jr et al. Intron "sliding" and the diversity of intron positions. Proc Natl Acad Sci USA 1997; 94(20):10739-10744.
67. Xing Y, Lee C. Alternative splicing and RNA selection pressure—evolutionary consequences for eukaryotic genomes. Nat Rev Genet 2006; 7(7):499-509.
68. Pasquet S, Naye F, Faucheux C et al. Transcription enhancer factor-1-dependent expression of the alpha-tropomyosin gene in the three muscle cell types. J Biol Chem 2006; 281(45):34406-34420.

CHAPTER 3

Tropomyosin Exons as Models for Alternative Splicing

Clare Gooding and Christopher W.J. Smith*

Abstract

Three of the four mammalian tropomyosin (Tm) genes are alternatively spliced, most commonly by mutually exclusive selection from pairs of internal or 3' end exons. Alternative splicing events in the *TPM1, 2 and 3* genes have been analysed experimentally in various levels of detail. In particular, mutually exclusive exon pairs in the βTm (*TPM2*) and αTm (*TPM1*) genes are among the most intensively studied models for striated and smooth muscle specific alternative splicing, respectively. Analysis of these model systems has provided important insights into general mechanisms and strategies of splicing regulation.

Introduction

Along with the other major contractile proteins, tropomyosins were among the first mammalian proteins for which cDNA and genomic sequences became available. They thereby provided early examples of the phenomenon of tissue-specific alternative premRNA splicing. One gene no longer gave rise to a single lone mRNA and protein. Instead, multiple mRNAs encoding distinct protein isoforms, tailored to the requirements of different cell-types, could arise from individual genes. Early speculations suggested that alternative splicing might be peculiarly prevalent in contractile systems.[1] The current view, informed by global methods of transcriptome analysis, is that alternative splicing is the rule rather than the exception.[2-4] The majority of human genes are alternatively spliced and if anything alternative splicing is more common in the nervous system than in other tissues.[5] Nevertheless, due to their early discovery, alternatively spliced exons in tropomyosin genes have long been used as model systems in which to understand the regulation of alternative splicing. While the molecular mechanisms of individual tropomyosin alternative splicing events are still incompletely understood, work on these systems has provided important general insights into splicing mechanisms and their regulation.

Mammalian tropomyosin genes (*TPM1-4* in humans) undergo three main types of alternative splicing (Fig. 1):

    i. alternative 5' end exons used in conjunction with different promoters. These allow the *TPM1* and 3 genes to generate HMW (~284 aa) and LMW (~245 aa) Tm isoforms.

    ii. alternative 3' end exons with associated 3' end processing and polyA addition sites (*TPM1-3*), which encode differing C-terminal ends and 3' untranslated regions (3' UTRs).

    iii. mutually exclusive splicing of internal exons, encoding alternative peptide segments at the N-terminal end (*TPM1*) or in the centre of the protein (*TPM1, 2 and 3*).

*Corresponding Author: Christopher W.J. Smith—Department of Biochemistry, University of Cambridge, CB2 1GA, UK. Email: cwjs1@cam.ac.uk

Tropomyosin, edited by Peter Gunning. ©2008 Landes Bioscience and Springer Science+Business Media.

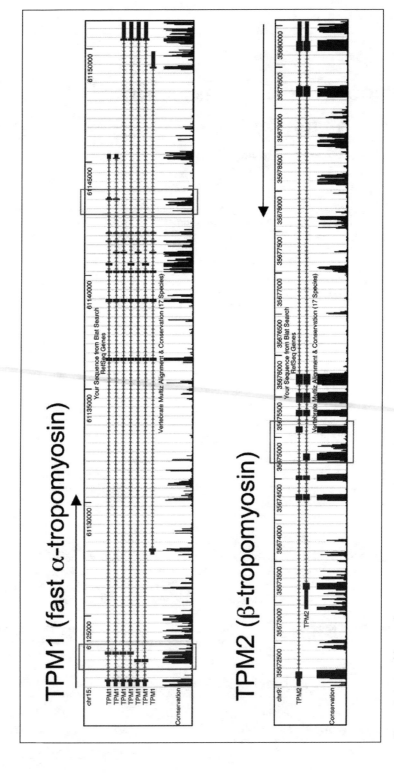

Figure 1. Legend located on next page.

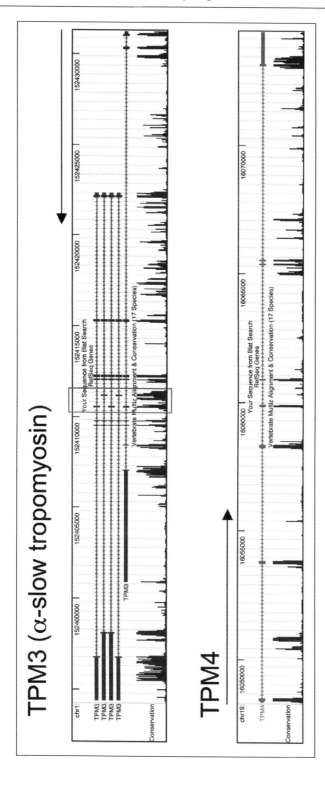

Figure 1. Organization of human tropomyosin genes, *TPM1-4*. For each gene a screen-shot from the UCSC Genome Browser,[81] shows the known Refseq isoforms (7 for *TPM1*, 2 for *TPM2*, 5 for *TPM3* and 1 for *TPM4*). The 17 vertebrate species conservation track is shown at the bottom. Conservation is mainly restricted to exons, but conserved intronic regions are sometimes indicative of regulatory elements that control splicing. The polarity of each gene (5' to 3') is indicated by the arrows above. Note that the *TPM2* gene occupies only 7.5 kb, while the *TPM1, 2 and 4* genes extend for ~30-35 kb. Boxes highlight alternative splicing events that have been investigated experimentally. Note that although Refseq shows only a single TPM4 isoform encoding a LMW Tm, a HMW isoform can also be produced using an upstream promoter and can be viewed using the Ensembl and UCSC gene prediction tracks of the Genome Browser.

The tissue specificity of these different alternative splicing events varies. Many of them are regulated with striated muscle specificity i.e., striated muscles undergo one splicing pattern, while all other cells undergo the alternative pattern. In contrast, mutually exclusive exons 2a and 2b of αTm (*TPM1*) are spliced with smooth muscle specificity.

Our aim in this chapter is to discuss what has been learned about how particular alternative splicing events in vertebrate tropomyosin genes are regulated and the general insights that have been provided about mechanisms of premRNA splicing and its regulation. We start with a brief overview of the process of premRNA splicing.

Splicing Mechanism

The process of premRNA splicing is orchestrated by the spliceosome—a multi-subunit ribonucleoprotein machine of similar size and complexity to the ribosome—which assembles on splice site elements at the boundaries between exons and introns.[6,7] The consensus splice site elements, present in all introns are (Fig. 2A):

- the 5' splice site (5'ss), a 9nt sequence that is complementary to U1 snRNA
- the 3' splice site (3'ss), recognized by splicing factor U2AF35
- the polypyrimidine tract (PPT) just upstream of the 3'ss, recognized by splicing factor U2AF65
- the branch point (BP) sequence usually just upstream of the PPT, recognized first by splicing factor SF1 and then by U2 snRNA.

These sequences are initially recognized by the factors mentioned above in early prespliceosomal complexes, after which the remaining spliceosome components bind to assemble the complete spliceosome. Following some conformational rearrangements, the two chemical steps of splicing occur (Fig. 2C). First, the 2'-OH of the branch point adenosine attacks the phosphate group at the 5'ss. As a result, the phosphodiester bond between the 5' exon and intron is broken and at the same time a new 5'-2' bond is formed between the 5' end of the intron and the branch point. In the second step, the 3'OH at the end of the 5' exon attacks the 3' splice site, leading to ligation of the two exons and release of the intron in the so-called "lariat" configuration.

A conceptual problem with the preceding brief summary is that splice sites vary considerably and some have sequences that are remote from the consensus. Only the GU and AG dinucleotides at the ends of introns are nearly invariant and in many cases the authentic sites match the consensus sequence less well than multiple "cryptic" sites in the introns. In short, the information content of the consensus splice sites is insufficient to distinguish authentic splice sites from the multiple cryptic splice sites.[6] The answer to this paradox is provided by the existence of a wide range of auxiliary regulatory elements located in both exons and introns and known as splicing enhancers and silencers (reviewed in 3,4,8). Enhancers provide binding sites for activator proteins, commonly members of the SR protein family, while silencers bind repressor proteins, which are often members of the hnRNP family.[3] Commonly, the splicing of individual exons is under the influence of multiple positive and negative influences. The dynamic balance between these inputs determines the extent to which an exon is spliced.

Analysis of Alternative Splicing Mechanisms

Analysis of alternative splicing, like other levels of gene expression, involves identification and characterization first of *cis*-regulatory elements in the RNA. These include the properties, relative locations and strengths of consensus splice site elements as well as enhancers, silencers and secondary structures. The second crucial component are the *trans*-acting factors, which are usually proteins but can be RNAs,[9] that affect the splicing pattern. Having assembled a "parts list" the remaining challenge is to characterize how the regulatory mechanisms promote or inhibit particular splicing events.

The commonest alternative splicing events are so-called cassette exons, which are individual exons that can be included or skipped from mRNA independently of other exons. The Tm genes more commonly exhibit mutually exclusive splicing of pairs of exons, which encode interchangeable peptide segments and have provided some of the best studied examples of this type of splicing. Analysis of mutually exclusive splicing usually aims to address the basis of the mutually exclusive behaviour and

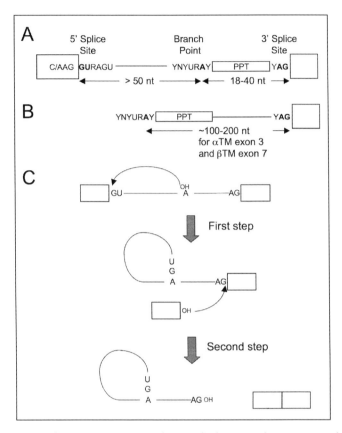

Figure 2. Consensus splice site sequences and steps of splicing A) The consensus elements for splicing are shown. Exons are shown as boxes and the intron as a line. Invariant bases (GU at the 5′ splice site, A at the branch point and AG at the 3′ splice site, are shown in bold). R = purine, Y = pyrimidine. PPT = polypyrimidine tract. At least 50 nt are required between the 5′ splice site and branch point and conventionally the branch point is 18-40 nt upstream of the 3′ splice site. B) As first illustrated by αTm exon 2b and βTm exon 6b, the branch point can be located far upstream of the 3′ splice site.[12,14-15-50] In these cases the polypyrimidine tract (PPT) is located adjacent to the BP and the region between the BP and the 3′ splice site is devoid of AG dinucleotides. Repressive regulatory elements lie between the PPT and 3′ splice site of both αTm exon 2b and βTm exon 6b. C) The two chemical steps of splicing. In the first step the 2′ OH of the branch point adenosine attacks the 5′ splice site, leading to breakage of the bond between the 5′ exon and intron and creation of a new 2′-5′ bond between the branch point and the 5′ end of the intron. Step 2 involves attack by the newly exposed 3′OH of the upstream exon upon the 3′ splice site. As a result the two products are the spliced mRNA and the excised intron in the typical "lariat" configuration.

of the selection of the individual exons in different cell types. If the gene is widely expressed in a variety of cell types, it may be apparent that selection of one exon represents a "default" splicing choice, while the the other exon represents a regulated choice that typically occurs in a restricted cell-type. Such "default" and "regulated" patterns may also be revealed by expression of minigene constructs in a variety of cell types in cell culture or in transgenic animals. In fact, default vs regulated splicing may be an oversimplified conceptual framework; the precise splicing pattern often appears to be the outcome of a dynamic interplay between multiple positive and negative influences.

In the following sections we describe some of the detailed analyses that have been carried out on Tm alternative splicing and conclude by emphasizing some common themes and general concepts that have arisen from these studies.

β-Tropomyosin—Tpm2

β-Tm has two alternative splicing events—an internal pair of mutually exclusive exons (6a and 6b) and a mutually exclusive pair of 3' end exons (9a and 9d) each with its own 3' end processing and polyadenylation site (Fig. 1). Both events are regulated with striated muscle specificity; exons 6b and 9a are selected in myotubes and muscle, while exons 6a and 9d are selected in myoblasts and other cell types. The internal pair of mutually exclusive exons have been studied extensively by Helfman's group for the rat gene (in the published literature they are usually referred to as exons 6 and 7) and by Joëlle Marie's and Mark Fiszman's groups for the chicken gene. This pair of exons provides one of the best models for striated muscle specific splicing (see Fig. 3 for summary). While many of the findings from the two species are in concordance, some features seem to be species specific. This is underlined by the fact that minigenes transfected into myogenic cells from a different class of organism (e.g., mammalian minigene in avian cells) are not spliced appropriately, primarily due to differences in the elements associated with exon 6a.[10,11] With this caveat in mind, important findings have nevertheless emerged from analysis of splicing of both rat and chicken RNAs in the standard HeLa nuclear extract system for in vitro analysis of splicing.

One of the first striking findings in this system was that βTm exon 6b has an unconventional arrangement of its 3' splice site elements. The branchpoint (BP), which is usually located within ~40 nt of the associated exon (Fig. 2A), in this case is much further upstream (Fig. 2B). In the rat gene, three BPs at -144 to -153 were mapped,[12,13] while the chicken BP was at -105.[14] In both cases and in αTm exon 2b with a BP at -175, an extended PPT was located adjacent to the BP rather than next to the 3' splice site. The downstream exon and 3' splice site were not required until the second step of splicing.[12,14,15] Unlike αTm exon 2b (see below), the βTm exon 6b BP is sufficiently distant from the upstream mutually exclusive exon 6a to the extent that its location does not enforce mutually exclusive behaviour. Indeed, under some experimental circumstances exons 6a and 6b are able to splice to each other, showing that there is not an absolute physical impediment to their splicing together.[14,16] The precise mechanism by which these exons are maintained as mutually exclusive remains elusive. The most plausible suggestion is that the regulation of the two exons is usually sufficiently tightly coordinated to prevent inappropriate splicing together (see below).

The basis of the nonmuscle splicing pattern has been the major focus of attention in this system. The muscle-specific exon 6b is actively repressed in nonmuscle cells and is not spliced even when exon 6a splice sites are inactivated.[17] The basis of this repression has been extensively investigated. In both the chicken and rat genes two key silencer elements were located within exon 6b itself and in the upstream intron.[12,14,17,18] In the chicken gene these repressor elements were initially proposed to act mainly via formation of repressive RNA secondary structure,[19,20] While a role for secondary structure was also suggested for the rat gene,[12] later evidence was more consistent with repression being mediated by binding of repressor proteins. A repressive "intron regulatory element" between exon 6b and the upstream polypyrimidine tract was identified by mutagenesis.[12,17] and was later shown to be a binding site for the hnRNP protein Polypyrimidine Tract Binding protein (PTB).[21] This was an important finding that went against prevailing opinion that PTB was a positively acting splicing factor,[22-25] indicating for the first time that it was in fact a repressor. PTB bound not only to the intronic silencer element, but also with higher affinity to the BP associated polypyrimidine tract further upstream. However, deletions at the latter location impaired splicing because the PPT is required for splicing, even though it may harbour overlapping repressor binding sites.[12,14] Unequivocal in vivo support for PTB's role as a regulator of βTm came very recently with RNAi experiments.[26-28] Knockdown of both PTB and its paralog nPTB (which itself is upregulated upon PTB knockdown) in HeLa cells led to a nearly complete switch to splicing of exon 6b and also exon 9a.[27] Using the chicken gene, Sauliere et al[26] showed that cooperative binding of PTB blocked splicing by competing with binding of the splicing factor U2AF$_{65}$ at the PPT.[26] Another pyrimidine-rich element, referred to as S4 (S4, Fig. 3),

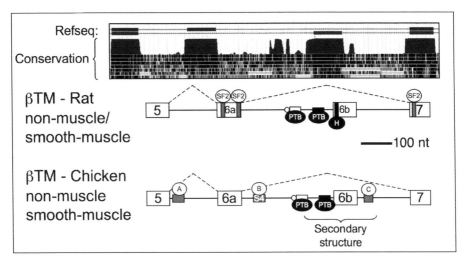

Figure 3. Alternative splicing of βTm exons 6a and 6b. The cartoons depict βTm exons 5-6a-6b-7 (referred to as 5-6-7-8 elsewhere) drawn to scale, with some of the characterized regulators. Black shapes represent repressor proteins that bind to silencer elements (also black). The branch point and PPT of exon 6b are indicated by the small white circle and rectangle respectively. Note that the PPT in this case is also a repressor binding site. White shapes represent activator proteins that bind to enhancers (coloured grey). The region implicated in secondary structure formation in chicken is indicated by the brackets. Both cartoons show the state in which exon 6b is repressed. Proteins binding at the three enhancer sequences are denoted A, B and C. A—proteins unknown; B—exon 6a activators binding at S4 element include SF2, hnRNP K, exon 6a repressors include SC35, exon 6b repressors include PTB; C—activators include SF2, SC35, repressors include hnRNPA1. The UCSC browser screen-shot above is based upon the human TPM2 gene and includes Refseq and vertebrate conservation tracks (below). A mirror-image of the original screen shot is shown so that the polarity is 5′ to 3′, left to right. Original text has therefore been removed. Note the conserved intronic regions flanking exon 6b.

is located 37 nt downstream of chicken exon 6a and has striking bifunctional activity. It acts both as a direct silencer of exon 6b and as an enhancer of exon 6a.[29,30] The S4 elements binds various proteins including PTB,[31] which could account for its repressive influence on exon 6b.

A second key element is a G-rich exon splicing silencer (ESS) at the 5′ end of exon 6b, which binds a second hnRNP protein, hnRNP H.[32] In vitro depletion and addback provided the first demonstration that hnRNP H can act as a splicing repressor. A number of other proteins were identified that bind to the region upstream of exon 6b, but none of these were demonstrated to have a role in the regulation of exon 6b selection.[33]

RNA secondary structure has also been proposed as a major contributor to repression of chicken βTm exon 6b.[14,18-20,34] Structure predictions and mapping demonstrated a structure extending from ~90 nt upstream to ~60 nt downstream of exon 6b. Various in vivo and in vitro experiments support the negative influence of at least parts of this structure.[18,19,34] In particular, splicing of exon 6b to 7 is inhibited by the structure.[19,34] However, the maximal form of the proposed structure also encompasses elements that in single stranded form have subsequently been shown to bind protein regulators. The pyrimidine-rich section of the upstream intron has repressive activity independent of the ability to form secondary structure,[30] consistent with a role in binding PTB.[26] Although a similar structure was proposed for the rat gene, subsequent experiments have not supported its involvement. Transfection of HeLa cells with increasing quantities of minigene reporter led to some splicing of exon 6b, which is consistent with repression by *trans*-acting factors but not secondary structure.[17] Moreover, the effects of mutations are also more consistent with repressive sequences acting by binding PTB and hnRNP H.[21,32] Secondary structure has been shown in various systems to influence alternative splicing, most commonly by hiding splice site elements, although it can also play activating roles in some circumstances (reviewed in 35). The simplest explanation for the inhibitory effects of the βTm secondary structure would be sequestration of splice site or enhancer sequences, which function in single-stranded form. However, in some circumstances U1 snRNP is able to bind to the 5' splice site of exon 6b, even though splicing remains repressed by repressive secondary structure, so its mode of action may be more complex.[34]

In addition to the preceding repressive influences, a repetitive A/UGGG downstream element acts as an enhancer of exon 6b splicing and binds to a 55 kDa protein.[36] Subsequent analysis showed that various antagonistic activating (SF2, SC35) and repressive (hnRNPA1) proteins could bind to this element and thereby influence exon 6b splicing.[37]

Various factors activate exon 6a in nonmuscle cells. In the rat gene, exon 6a has inherently suboptimal 3' and 5' splice sites, which can be readily strengthened by mutagenesis.[38] Exon splicing enhancers in exons 6a and 7, which bind the splicing activator SF2/ASF, are important to activate the 3' splice site of exon 6a.[38,39] The activity of the exon 7 enhancers accounts for the early observation that splicing of exon 6a or 6b to exon 5 only took place if the downstream splice to exon 7 had first occurred.[40] Two pyrimidine-rich sequences in each of the introns flanking chicken exon 6a also activate its inclusion and account for the species specificity of βTm splicing.[10,11] The first is 25 nt downstream of exon 5.[11] The second is the previously mentioned S4 element just downstream of exon 6a, which independently represses exon 6b and activates exon 6a.[29,30,41] The element promotes U1 snRNP binding to the 5' splice site of exon 6a, by binding either SF2/ASF[41] or hnRNP K.[31] Interestingly, a second "SR family" splicing regulator—SC35—antagonizes SF2 at this enhancer element, effectively acting as a repressor of exon 6a.[41] It is an interesting possibility that by both activating 6a and repressing 6b, the S4 element may play a key role in preventing the splicing together of the two mutually exclusive exons.[31]

While the basis of the selection of exon 6a in nonmuscle cells is reasonably well understood, the way in which exon 6b is selected in muscle cells has received less experimental attention, in part connected with the difficulty of obtaining active muscle nuclear extracts for biochemical analysis. Transfection of various chicken βTm minigenes in quail myotubes showed that exon 6b becomes de-repressed upon myogenic differentiation. Significantly, there is no concomitant repression of exon 6a, which is spliced efficiently in myotubes upon transfection of constructs from which exon 6b has been deleted.[42] Rather, exon 6b wins in competition with exon 6a for splicing to flanking constitutive exons. In principle, alterations in the activies of a number of the factors responsible for the nonmuscle splicing pattern could be involved in the switch to the muscle pattern. Consistent with the evidence for loss of repression,[42] reduction in the activity of the repressor PTB likely contributes to the switch to muscle specific splicing. Knockdown of PTB in HeLa cells leads to a partial switch from selection of exon 6a to exon 6b with both construct and endogenous βTm RNA.[26,27] However, knockdown of PTB is compensated in part by upregulation of the related repressor nPTB.[27,28] If both PTB and nPTB are knocked down, the switch in splicing to exon 6b is almost complete. Indeed skeletal β-Tm was identified by quantitative proteomic analysis of HeLa cells knocked down for both PTB and nPTB.[27] Levels of PTB expression are lower in striated muscle than in many other tissues and although nPTB mRNA is present at similar levels in myoblasts and myotubes, increasing levels of the micro-RNA miR-133 lead to complete translational repression of nPTB and possibly PTB.[43] Since PTB and nPTB are known to repress a number of muscle specific exons, micro-RNA mediated repression of their expression provides an attractive explanation for how exon selection could be switched. It is also possible that alterations in the levels of the other repressor—hnRNP H—might also be involved in the switch to muscle specific splicing. Another possibility is the involvement of CELF proteins, which are known to antagonize PTB in the troponin-T[44] and α-actinin genes.[45] Preliminary evidence indicates that CELF proteins promote exon 6b splicing while muscle-blind like (MBNL) proteins

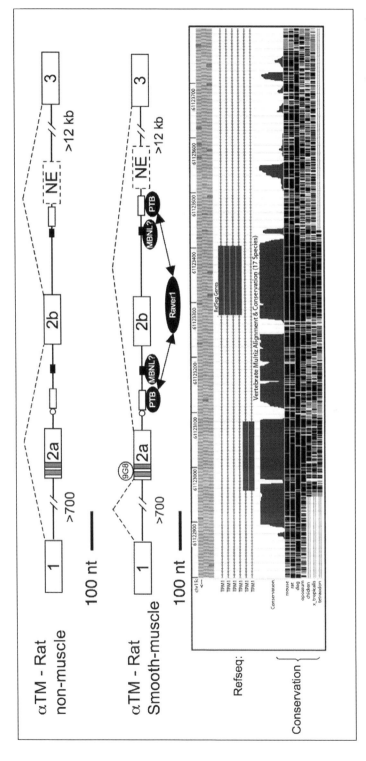

Figure 4. Alternative splicing of αTm exons 2a and 2b. The cartoons depict αTm exons 1-2a-2b-3 (usually referred to as exons 1-2-3-4) drawn to scale, with some of the characterized regulators. Cross-hatch lines indicate large sections of the flanking introns that are not indicated to scale. Black shapes represent repressor proteins that bind to silencer elements (also black) and the corepressor protein raver1. The branch point and PPT of exon 3 are indicated by the small white circle and rectangle respectively. Note that the PPT in this case is also a repressor binding site. White shapes represent activator proteins that bind to enhancers (coloured grey). The UCSC browser screen-shot above is based upon the human TPM1 gene and includes Refseq and vertebrate conservation tracks (below). Note that large sections of the intron between exons 2 and 3 are highly conserved including the branch point, PPT and binding sites for PTB and possibly MBNL proteins. The proposed "nonsense exon"[75] is indicated as the rectangle with dashed outline.

repress (J. Marie, unpublished observations). Antagonism between CELF and MBNL proteins has been observed in other systems[46](see αTm below).

Interestingly, a complete switch in selection from βTm exon 9d to exon 9a was also observed upon PTB + nPTB knockdown in HeLa cells.[27] Exon 9a has many of the familiar sequence characteristics of a PTB-repressed exon, with predicted distant BPs at -122 and -100 and multiple optimal PTB-binding motifs between the exon and the BPs. It therefore appears that repression of exon 9a by PTB is important to maintain the nonmuscle splicing pattern for this pair of exons too and can help to explain how splicing of the two pairs of mutually exclusive βTm exons is closely coordinated.

α-Tropomyosin Exons 2a and 2b

The αfast Tm gene (αTm or *TPM1*) undergoes several AS events leading to at least 8-12 mRNA and protein isoforms.[47,48] The event that has undergone most intense investigation is the mutually exclusive splicing of rat αTm exons 2a and 2b (usually referred to in published literature as exons 2 and 3), which shows smooth-muscle rather than striated-muscle specificity (Fig. 4). Exon 2a is used principally in smooth muscle, while exon 2b is used in many other cell types including striated muscle.[48,49] Based primarily upon overexpression of minigene constructs in cell lines, the view was established that exon 2b selection represented a "default" choice that occurred everywhere except smooth muscle, the latter representing a "regulated" splicing environment.[25] In fact, RT-qPCR analysis of αTm splicing across a range of mouse tissues showed high proportions of exon 2a use in tissues such as spleen and liver, which transcribe αTm at low levels. However, analysis of transgenic mouse lines with different levels of expression of an αTm minigene suggested that smooth muscle tissues and bladder in particular, were the only ones that could sustain skipping of exon 2b (which effectively equates to inclusion of exon 2a) even at high expression levels.[49] This suggests that the concept of a default (nonsmooth muscle) and a regulated smooth muscle splicing pattern does have a mechanistic basis and that smooth muscle has higher levels of the relevant splicing regulators than other cell types.

Mutually exclusive behaviour of αTm exons 2a and 2b has a simple explanation. The BP of exon 2b is so close to the 5' splice site of exon 2a that spliceosomes cannot assemble between these two sites due to steric interference.[50] This was not at first apparent because the intron between exons 2a and 2b is over 200 nt, which is well above the minimal ~70 nt size of a mammalian intron. However, the exon 2b branch point was unusual in being very distant (175 nt upstream) from its associated 3' splice site. At around the same time distant BPs were also mapped upstream of βTm exon 6b (see above), although in that case the BP was not sufficiently close to the upstream exon to explain mutually exclusive behaviour. Indeed this seemingly neat explanation for mutually exclusive splicing does not seem to apply in the majority of cases.[51] Rather, the unifying principle is that in all analyzed cases, repressive regulatory elements lie between the exon and the upstream BP.

Default selection of exon 2b arises from competition between exons 2a and 2b for the flanking splice sites. Exon 2b has stronger consensus splice sites. In particular the distant branch point of exon 2b has an adjacent 50 nt polypyrimidine tract which is functionally much stronger than the PPT of exon 2a[25] and binds U2AF65 with a 100-fold higher affinity.[52] If exon 2b is deleted from constructs, exon 2a can be spliced efficiently in nonSM cells.[25] Indeed exon 2a has stronger splicing enhancers than exon 2b.[53,54] The SR activator protein 9G8 is responsible for activation of exon 2a via these ESEs and it can be antagonized by hnRNPs H and F.[55]

Most ongoing attention on this system has focused upon the regulated switching of exon selection, which primarily involves repression of exon 2b, as indicated by deletion of exon 2a from minigene constructs. Exon 2b still shows increased levels of skipping in transfected smooth muscle cells.[56] It remains possible that there is also a contribution by cell-specific activation of exon 2a.[53,55] However, the behaviour of reporter minigenes in transgenic mice argues that repression of exon 2b is the dominant regulatory mechanism in vivo.[49] Mapping of essential negative regulatory elements indicates that binding sites for Polypyrimidine Tract Binding protein (PTB) as well as clusters of UGC or CUG repeats are required on each side of the exon.[56-59] The PTB binding sites consist of

UCUU or similar motifs within a pyrimidine tract[59] and lie both within the PPT adjacent to the exon 2b branch point, as well as in a second pyrimidine tract ~200 nt downstream of exon 2b. The UGC/CUG clusters on each side of exon 2b lie slightly closer to the exon than the PPTs. None of these negative regulatory elements mediate a strictly cell-specific effect. That is to say, if exon 2b skipping in nonSM cells is activated, for example by mutation of the branch point, the elevated level of exon skipping in nonSM cells remains dependent upon the defined negative regulatory elements. This implies that the factors that bind to these elements are present in other cell types, although they may be more abundant, or more active in smooth muscle. PTB is certainly not restricted to smooth muscle, but is widely expressed and represses many exons that are spliced in striated muscle and brain.[28,60] PTB repression of αTm exon 2b has been demonstrated by a variety of approaches including overexpression, RNAi knockdown, artifical tethering to RNA and in vitro depletion and addback of recombinant protein.[27,58,59,61-63] However, αTm exon 2b is unique among the PTB-repressed exons that have been investigated, in that the PTB-mediated repression occurs in a cell restricted manner. In most cases, PTB represses an exon in a wide variety of cell types, but in a specific cell type the repression is relieved, as for βTm exon 6b (see above). Part of the clue to the SM specific enhanced repression by PTB could lie in the nature of the factors that bind to the UGC/CUG elements. Two families of proteins known to interact with sequences like this are the CELF family[64] and the muscleblind like (MBNL) family[46] (see also βTm above). Disturbances in the levels of both protein families mediate the molecular pathology of Myotonic Dystrophy.[65] Overexpressed CELF proteins appear to have either no effect on exon 2b, or actually promote its inclusion, suggesting that they are not repressors of exon 2b.[57] The MBNL proteins have opposite effects to CELF proteins in some model systems[46] and preliminary evidence suggests that they repress αTm exon 2b and bind to the UGC/CUG clusters (CG & CWJS unpublished observations). Another factor implicated in repression of exon 2b is the PTB interacting protein raver1.[66] Cotransfection of raver1 expression constructs strongly promotes skipping of exon 2b and this repression activity involves the ability to interact with PTB.[67,68] Indeed, raver1 has between 2-4 peptide motifs that could interact with separate PTB molecules.[67] This suggests that one of the functions of raver1 might be to form a bridge between PTB molecules bound at the distantly separated PPTs flanking exon 2b. Raver1 is also not smooth muscle specific, although in cultured PAC1 smooth muscle cells it is in the nucleus. In contrast, in striated muscle cells it relocates to the cytoplasm upon differentiation, where it interacts with cytoskeletal proteins such as vinculin and actinin.[66,69] Splicing of exon 2b is also influenced by another RNA binding protein RBM4,[70] which tends to promote exon 2b inclusion by antagonizing PTB.

While a number of important regulators of αTm exon 2b have been characterized, the qualitative and quantitative differences in the factors between smooth muscle and other tissues responsible for the switch in splicing remain to be elucidated.

Other Tm Splicing Events

A number of other Tm alternative splicing events have been studied. Most are striated-muscle specific and share some common features with the well-studied examples above.

Alternative splicing of the central pair of mutually exclusive NM and SK exons in the human αslowTm gene (*TPM3*), equivalent to exons 6a and 6b of βTm, also occurs with striated muscle specificity.[71,72] Analysis has mainly been carried out in nonmuscle (COS) cells and has indicated that the skeletal muscle specific SK exon is repressed even when the NM exon is inactivated by mutation. Repression is mediated via sequences in the SK exon itself.[71] The RNA binding protein hnRNP G represses the SK exon and can be antagonized by the splicing activator Tra2β.[72] Like the βTm exons, in some circumstances the two mutually exclusive exons can be induced to splice together. This is consistent with the fact that while the SK exon branch point is located 79 nt upstream, it is not close enough to the NM exon to interfere with splicing (see αTm, above).

Alternative splicing of exon 9A9' of the *Xenopus TPM1* gene has been investigated in oocytes and embryos.[73,74] Exon 9A9' is skipped in nonmuscle cells, included as an internal exon in adult striated muscle and as a 3' end exon with its own polyA site in myotome. This exon also has a distant branch point 274 nt upstream and is repressed by PTB. The region between the exon and the branch point has a number of high affinity PTB binding sites. Repression of PTB expression by morpholino antisense oligos leads to inclusion of 9A9′ in nonmuscle cells, while overexpression of PTB in muscle leads to skipping of 9A9′. In this case, PTB appears to directly inhibit both splicing and polyadenylation at exon 9A9′.[74]

A final example is a non peptide-coding putative exon—denoted as "NE" (Nonsense Exon) in Figure 4—in the αTm gene.[75] This 107 nt exon lies 234 nt downstream of αTm exon 2b, just beyond the negative elements that are necessary for exon 2b skipping. The exon is flanked by splice sites but is never observed in cDNAs or ESTs and so would normally be designated a "pseudo-exon". However, this apparent pseudo-exon is conserved in mammals and is also readily activated by simple point mutations. If spliced into αTm mRNA it would introduce stop codons, thereby leading to degradation of the mRNA by Nonsense Mediated Decay (NMD), which might account for its lack of appearance in ESTs. Single point mutations that activated this exon would effectively lead to a null *TPM1* allele. It seems unlikely that such a potentially deleterious sequence would be maintained from rodents to humans unless it has a conserved function. The initial αTm minigene expressed in transgenic mice contained this "nonsense exon" and it was seen to be included with some tissue specificity, with highest inclusion levels in the heart.[49] One possibility is that its inclusion serves as a posttranscriptional mechanism to limit αTm expression in muscle. A surprisingly large number of mammalian alternative splicing events produce mRNAs that are degraded by NMD, suggesting that alternative splicing may play a widespread but largely hidden role in quantitative regulation of transcript levels.[76,77]

Concluding Remarks: Common Themes, General Insights and Future Directions

The preceding discussion makes clear that despite the elapse of 20 years since Tm alternative splicing events were first characterized, the underlying mechanisms by which these events are regulated remain incompletely understood. Despite this, much progress has been made and a number of themes of general importance have been uncovered by analysis of these model systems of alternative splicing. The steric interference mechanism to enforce mutually exclusive splicing, as characterized in αTm, clearly does not apply in all cases. However, with the availability of genome and EST databases it is possible to find other examples where it almost certainly operates. For example, the predicted branch point of *SCN5a* exon 7 is sufficiently close to the mutually exclusive exon 6 to prevent the two exons from splicing together. The bifunctional enhancer/silencer S4 element between βTm exons 6a and 6b represents another possible way to enforce mutually exclusive behaviour. A similar dual function element has been identified between a pair of mutually exclusive exons in the *FGFR2* premRNA,[78] suggesting that this too could be a common strategy.

The unconventional distant BP arrangement common to so many Tm alternative exons is also found elsewhere. Following the original characterization of distant BPs in Tm genes, a method for globally identifying such exons was developed, based upon the extended upstream regions devoid of AG dinucleotides.[79] This has allowed the identification of many such exons in a variety of genes. The Tm examples suggest that the purpose of such an arrangement may be primarily to accommodate the presence of repressive regulatory elements between the exon and BP. Likewise, the splicing regulators PTB and hnRNP H, first characterized by their repressor roles in Tm splicing, have subsequently been found to regulate many other splicing events (e.g., 27,28). In some other cases PTB has been found to repress by binding to silencer elements between the exon and a distant BP.[27]

The outstanding questions that remain to be answered principally focus upon the alterations in regulatory factors that are responsible for tissue-specific switching of splicing. In the case of βTm, how is the repression present in nonmuscle cells relieved or antagonized? RNAi experiments in HeLa cells and neurons suggest that reduction in PTB levels may be sufficient.[27,28,43] However, many other regulatory proteins have been implicated and alterations in their activities may also be important. In the case of αTm exon 2b, the converse question is posed: how is PTB-mediated repression specifically upregulated in smooth muscle cells? The answer to this question no doubt lies partly in the identification of the particular isoforms of MBNL, raver1 or other proteins that act as corepressors with PTB in smooth muscle cells. Another related question is why in this system alone PTB-mediated repression only occurs in a restricted cell type? This may be related to the large distance separating the regulatory elements on each side of the exon.

The answers to these outstanding questions may be provided in part by the same cell transfection and in vitro biochemical approaches that have been used to date. However, a new range of global methods for analysis of alternative splicing (e.g., alternative splicing sensitive microarrays) has the promise to allow important progress to be made (reviewed in 3,4). A particularly useful way forward will be the use of microarrays that can at the same time interrogate large numbers of alternative splicing events, as well as the expression levels (and splicing patterns) of all known splicing regulators (e.g., see ref. 80). In principle this should allow correlations to be drawn between coregulated sets of splicing events and particular complements of splicing regulators. In general, the newer global approaches, whether computational or wet-experimental, have the potential to reveal details of the regulatory circuitry—the combinations of arrangements of *cis* regulatory motifs and complements of trans factors that mediate particular programmes of splicing regulation. However, understanding the molecular mechanisms by which regulatory programmes operate will still require the same kind of detailed molecular analysis of individual model systems as has been carried out over the preceding 20 years.

Acknowledgements

Work in the authors' lab is funded by the Wellcome Trust (programme grant 077877) and by EURASNET, an EU FP6 Network of Excellence. We thank Joëlle Marie for helpful comments on the manuscript and for communicating unpublished results.

References

1. Nadal-Ginard B, Smith CW, Patton JG et al. Alternative splicing is an efficient mechanism for the generation of protein diversity: contractile protein genes as a model system. Adv Enzyme Regul 1991; 31:261-286.
2. Black DL. Protein diversity from alternative splicing: a challenge for bioinformatics and postgenome biology. Cell 2000; 103(3):367-370.
3. Matlin AJ, Clark F, Smith CW. Understanding alternative splicing: towards a cellular code. Nat Rev Mol Cell Biol 2005; 6(5):386-398.
4. Blencowe BJ. Alternative splicing: new insights from global analyses. Cell 2006; 126(1):37-47.
5. Black DL, Grabowski PJ. Alternative premRNA splicing and neuronal function. Prog Mol Subcell Biol 2003; 31:187-216.
6. Burge CB, Tuschl T, Sharp PA. Splicing of precursors to mRNA by the spliceosomes. In: Gestetland RF, Cech TR, Atkins JF, eds. The RNA World. 2nd ed. Cold Spring Harbor: Cold Spring Harbor Laboratory Press, 1999; 525-560.
7. Jurica MS, Moore MJ. Pre-mRNA splicing: awash in a sea of proteins. Mol Cell 2003; 12(1):5-14.
8. Cartegni L, Chew SL, Krainer AR. Listening to silence and understanding nonsense: exonic mutations that affect splicing. Nat Rev Genet 2002; 3(4):285-298.
9. Kishore S, Stamm S. The snoRNA HBII-52 regulates alternative splicing of the serotonin receptor 2C. Science 2006; 311(5758):230-232.
10. Balvay L, Pret AM, Libri D et al. Splicing of the alternative exons of the chicken, rat and Xenopus beta tropomyosin transcripts requires class-specific elements. J Biol Chem 1994; 269(31):19675-19678.
11. Pret AM, Fiszman MY. Sequence divergence associated with species-specific splicing of the nonmuscle beta-tropomyosin alternative exon. J Biol Chem 1996; 271(19):11511-11517.
12. Helfman DM, Roscigno RF, Mulligan GJ et al. Identification of two distinct intron elements involved in alternative splicing of beta-tropomyosin premRNA. Genes Dev 1990; 4(1):98-110.
13. Helfman DM, Ricci WM. Branch point selection in alternative splicing of tropomyosin premRNAs. Nucleic Acids Res 1989; 17(14):5633-5650.
14. Goux-Pelletan M, Libri D, d'Aubenton-Carafa Y et al. In vitro splicing of mutually exclusive exons from the chicken beta-tropomyosin gene: role of the branch point location and very long pyrimidine stretch. EMBO J 1990; 9(1):241-249.
15. Smith CW, Porro EB, Patton JG et al. Scanning from an independently specified branch point defines the 3' splice site of mammalian introns. Nature 1989; 342(6247):243-247.

16. Libri D, Marie J, Brody E et al. A subfragment of the beta tropomyosin gene is alternatively spliced when transfected into differentiating muscle cells. Nucleic Acids Res 1989; 17(16):6449-6462.

17. Guo W, Mulligan GJ, Wormsley S et al. Alternative splicing of beta-tropomyosin premRNA: cis-acting elements and cellular factors that block the use of a skeletal muscle exon in nonmuscle cells. Genes Dev 1991; 5(11):2096-2107.

18. Libri D, Goux-Pelletan M, Brody E et al. Exon as well as intron sequences are cis-regulating elements for the mutually exclusive alternative splicing of the beta tropomyosin gene. Mol Cell Biol 1990; 10(10):5036-5046.

19. Clouet d'Orval B, d'Aubenton Carafa Y, Sirand-Pugnet P et al. RNA secondary structure repression of a muscle-specific exon in HeLa cell nuclear extracts. Science 1991; 252(5014):1823-1828.

20. Libri D, Piseri A, Fiszman MY. Tissue-specific splicing in vivo of the beta-tropomyosin gene: dependence on an RNA secondary structure. Science 1991; 252(5014):1842-1845.

21. Mulligan GJ, Guo W, Wormsley S et al. Polypyrimidine tract binding protein interacts with sequences involved in alternative splicing of beta-tropomyosin premRNA. J Biol Chem 1992; 267(35):25480-25487.

22. Patton JG, Mayer SA, Tempst P et al. Characterization and molecular cloning of polypyrimidine tract-binding protein: a component of a complex necessary for premRNA splicing. Genes Dev 1991; 5(7):1237-1251.

23. Gil A, Sharp PA, Jamison SF et al. Characterization of cDNAs encoding the polypyrimidine tract-binding protein. Genes Dev 1991; 5(7):1224-1236.

24. Garcia-Blanco MA, Jamison SF, Sharp PA. Identification and purification of a 62,000-dalton protein that binds specifically to the polypyrimidine tract of introns. Genes Dev 1989; 3(12A):1874-1886.

25. Mullen MP, Smith CW, Patton JG et al. Alpha-tropomyosin mutually exclusive exon selection: competition between branchpoint/polypyrimidine tracts determines default exon choice. Genes Dev 1991; 5(4):642-655.

26. Sauliere J, Sureau A, Expert-Bezancon A et al. The polypyrimidine tract binding protein (PTB) represses splicing of exon 6B from the beta-tropomyosin premRNA by directly interfering with the binding of the U2AF65 subunit. Mol Cell Biol 2006; 26(23):8755-8769.

27. Spellman RH, Llorian M, Smith CWJ. Functional redundancy and cross-regulation between the splicing regulator PTB and its paralogs nPTB and ROD1. Mol Cell 2007; 27(3).

28. Boutz PL, Stoilov P, Li Q et al. A post-transcriptional regulatory switch in polypyrimidine tract-binding proteins reprograms alternative splicing in developing neurons. Genes 2007; 21(13):1636-1652.

29. Balvay L, Libri D, Gallego M et al. Intronic sequence with both negative and positive effects on the regulation of alternative transcripts of the chicken beta tropomyosin transcripts. Nucleic Acids Res 1992; 20(15):3987-3992.

30. Gallego ME, Balvay L, Brody E. cis-acting sequences involved in exon selection in the chicken beta-tropomyosin gene. Mol Cell Biol 1992; 12(12):5415-5425.

31. Expert-Bezancon A, Le Caer JP, Marie J. Heterogeneous nuclear ribonucleoprotein (hnRNP) K is a component of an intronic splicing enhancer complex that activates the splicing of the alternative exon 6A from chicken beta-tropomyosin premRNA. J Biol Chem 2002; 277(19):16614-16623.

32. Chen CD, Kobayashi R, Helfman DM. Binding of hnRNP H to an exonic splicing silencer is involved in the regulation of alternative splicing of the rat beta-tropomyosin gene. Genes Dev 1999; 13(5):593-606.

33. Grossman JS, Meyer MI, Wang YC et al. The use of antibodies to the polypyrimidine tract binding protein (PTB) to analyze the protein components that assemble on alternatively spliced premRNAs that use distant branch points. RNA 1998; 4(6):613-625.

34. Sirand-Pugnet P, Durosay P, Clouet d'Orval BC et al. Beta-Tropomyosin premRNA folding around a muscle-specific exon interferes with several steps of spliceosome assembly. J Mol Biol 1995; 251(5):591-602.

35. Buratti E, Baralle FE. Influence of RNA secondary structure on the premRNA splicing process. Mol Cell Biol 2004; 24(24):10505-10514.

36. Sirand-Pugnet P, Durosay P, Brody E et al. An intronic (A/U)GGG repeat enhances the splicing of an alternative intron of the chicken beta-tropomyosin premRNA. Nucleic Acids Res 1995; 23(17):3501-3507.

37. Expert-Bezancon A, Sureau A, Durosay P, et al. hnRNP A1 and the SR proteins ASF/SF2 and SC35 have antagonistic functions in splicing of beta-tropomyosin exon 6B. J Biol Chem 2004; 279(37):38249-38259.

38. Tsukahara T, Casciato C, Helfman DM. Alternative splicing of beta-tropomyosin premRNA: multiple cis-elements can contribute to the use of the 5'- and 3'-splice sites of the nonmuscle/smooth muscle exon 6. Nucleic Acids Res 1994; 22(12):2318-2325.

39. Selvakumar M, Helfman DM. Exonic splicing enhancers contribute to the use of both 3' and 5' splice site usage of rat beta-tropomyosin premRNA. RNA 1999; 5(3):378-394.

40. Helfman DM, Ricci WM, Finn LA. Alternative splicing of tropomyosin premRNAs in vitro and in vivo. Genes Dev 1988; 2(12A):1627-1638.

41. Gallego ME, Gattoni R, Stevenin J et al. The SR splicing factors ASF/SF2 and SC35 have antagonistic effects on intronic enhancer-dependent splicing of the beta-tropomyosin alternative exon 6A. EMBO J 1997; 16(7):1772-1784.

42. Libri D, Balvay L, Fiszman MY. In vivo splicing of the beta tropomyosin premRNA: a role for branch point and donor site competition. Mol Cell Biol 1992; 12(7):3204-3215.
43. Boutz P, Chawla G, Stoilov P et al. MicroRNAs involved in muscle development regulate the expression of the alternative splicing factor nPTB. Genes Dev 2007.
44. Charlet BN, Logan P, Singh G et al. Dynamic antagonism between ETR-3 and PTB regulates cell type-specific alternative splicing. Mol Cell 2002; 9(3):649-658.
45. Gromak N, Matlin AJ, Cooper TA et al. Antagonistic regulation of alpha-actinin alternative splicing by CELF proteins and polypyrimidine tract binding protein. RNA 2003; 9(4):443-456.
46. Ho TH, Charlet BN, Poulos MG et al. Muscleblind proteins regulate alternative splicing. EMBO J 2004; 23(15):3103-3112.
47. Lees-Miller JP, Goodwin LO, Helfman DM. Three novel brain tropomyosin isoforms are expressed from the rat alpha-tropomyosin gene through the use of alternative promoters and alternative RNA processing. Mol Cell Biol 1990; 10(4):1729-1742.
48. Wieczorek DF, Smith CW, Nadal-Ginard B. The rat alpha-tropomyosin gene generates a minimum of six different mRNAs coding for striated, smooth and nonmuscle isoforms by alternative splicing. Mol Cell Biol 1988; 8(2):679-694.
49. Ellis PD, Smith CW, Kemp P. Regulated tissue-specific alternative splicing of enhanced green fluorescent protein transgenes conferred by alpha-tropomyosin regulatory elements in transgenic mice. J Biol Chem 2004; 279(35):36660-36669.
50. Smith CW, Nadal-Ginard B. Mutually exclusive splicing of alpha-tropomyosin exons enforced by an unusual lariat branch point location: implications for constitutive splicing. Cell 1989; 56(5):749-758.
51. Smith CW. Alternative splicing—when two's a crowd. Cell 2005; 123(1):1-3.
52. Zamore PD, Patton JG, Green MR. Cloning and domain structure of the mammalian splicing factor U2AF. Nature 1992; 355(6361):609-614.
53. Dye BT, Buvoli M, Mayer SA et al. Enhancer elements activate the weak 3' splice site of alpha-tropomyosin exon 2. RNA 1998; 4(12):1523-1536.
54. Roberts GC, Gooding C, Smith CW. Smooth muscle alternative splicing induced in fibroblasts by heterologous expression of a regulatory gene. EMBO J 1996; 15(22):6301-6310.
55. Crawford JB, Patton JG. Activation of alpha-tropomyosin exon 2 is regulated by the SR protein 9G8 and heterogeneous nuclear ribonucleoproteins H and F. Mol Cell Biol 2006; 26(23):8791 8802.
56. Gooding C, Roberts GC, Moreau G et al. Smooth muscle-specific switching of alpha-tropomyosin mutually exclusive exon selection by specific inhibition of the strong default exon. EMBO J 1994; 13(16):3861-3872.
57. Gromak N, Smith CW. A splicing silencer that regulates smooth muscle specific alternative splicing is active in multiple cell types. Nucleic Acids Res 2002; 30(16):3548-3557.
58. Gooding C, Roberts GC, Smith CW. Role of an inhibitory pyrimidine element and polypyrimidine tract binding protein in repression of a regulated alpha-tropomyosin exon. RNA 1998; 4(1):85-100.
59. Perez I, Lin CH, McAfee JG, Patton JG. Mutation of PTB binding sites causes misregulation of alternative 3' splice site selection in vivo. RNA 1997; 3(7):764-778.
60. Spellman R, Rideau A, Matlin A et al. Regulation of alternative splicing by PTB and associated factors. Biochem Soc Trans 2005; 33(Pt 3):457-460.
61. Lin CH, Patton JG. Regulation of alternative 3' splice site selection by constitutive splicing factors. RNA 1995; 1(3):234-245.
62. Robinson F, Smith CW. A splicing repressor domain in polypyrimidine tract-binding protein. J Biol Chem 2006; 281(2):800-806.
63. Wollerton MC, Gooding C, Robinson F et al. Differential alternative splicing activity of isoforms of polypyrimidine tract binding protein (PTB). RNA 2001; 7(6):819-832.
64. Ladd AN, Charlet N, Cooper TA. The CELF family of RNA binding proteins is implicated in cell-specific and developmentally regulated alternative splicing. Mol Cell Biol 2001; 21(4):1285-1296.
65. Faustino NA, Cooper TA. Pre-mRNA splicing and human disease. Genes Dev 2003; 17(4):419-437.
66. Huttelmaier S, Illenberger S, Grosheva I et al. Raver1, a dual compartment protein, is a ligand for PTB/hnRNPI and microfilament attachment proteins. J Cell Biol 2001; 155(5):775-786.
67. Rideau AP, Gooding C, Simpson PJ et al. A peptide motif in Raver1 mediates splicing repression by interaction with the PTB RRM2 domain. Nat Struct Mol Biol 2006; 13(9):839-848.
68. Gromak N, Rideau A, Southby J et al. The PTB interacting protein raver1 regulates alpha-tropomyosin alternative splicing. EMBO J 2003; 22(23):6356-6364.
69. Zieseniss A, Schroeder U, Buchmeier S et al. Raver1 is an integral component of muscle contractile elements. Cell Tissue Res 2007; 327(3):583-594.
70. Lin JC, Tarn WY. Exon selection in alpha-tropomyosin mRNA is regulated by the antagonistic action of RBM4 and PTB. Mol Cell Biol 2005; 25(22):10111-10121.

71. Graham IR, Hamshere M, Eperon IC. Alternative splicing of a human alpha-tropomyosin muscle-specific exon: identification of determining sequences. Mol Cell Biol 1992; 12(9):3872-3882.
72. Nasim MT, Chernova TK, Chowdhury HM et al. HnRNP G and Tra2beta: opposite effects on splicing matched by antagonism in RNA binding. Hum Mol Genet 2003; 12(11):1337-1348.
73. Hamon S, Le Sommer C, Mereau A et al. Polypyrimidine tract-binding protein is involved in vivo in repression of a composite internal/3′ -terminal exon of the Xenopus alpha-tropomyosin Pre-mRNA. J Biol Chem 2004; 279(21):22166-22175.
74. Le Sommer C, Lesimple M, Mereau A et al. PTB regulates the processing of a 3′-terminal exon by repressing both splicing and polyadenylation. Mol Cell Biol 2005; 25(21):9595-9607.
75. Grellscheid SN, Smith CW. An apparent pseudo-exon acts both as an alternative exon that leads to nonsense-mediated decay and as a zero-length exon. Mol Cell Biol 2006; 26(6):2237-2246.
76. Hillman RT, Green RE, Brenner SE. An unappreciated role for RNA surveillance. Genome Biol 2004; 5(2):R8.
77. Lareau LF, Green RE, Bhatnagar RS et al. The evolving roles of alternative splicing. Curr Opin Struct Biol 2004; 14(3):273-282.
78. Carstens RP, McKeehan WL, Garcia-Blanco MA. An intronic sequence element mediates both activation and repression of rat fibroblast growth factor receptor 2 premRNA splicing. Mol Cell Biol 1998; 18(4):2205-2217.
79. Gooding C, Clark F, Wollerton MC et al. A class of human exons with predicted distant branch points revealed by analysis of AG dinucleotide exclusion zones. Genome Biol 2006; 7(1):R1.
80. Relogio A, Ben-Dov C, Baum M et al. Alternative splicing microarrays reveal functional expression of neuron-specific regulators in Hodgkin lymphoma cells. J Biol Chem 2004.
81. Kent W, Sugnet C, Furey T et al. The Human Genome Browser at UCSC. Genome Res 2002; 12:996-1006.

CHAPTER 4

Tropomyosin Gene Expression in Vivo and in Vitro

Galina Schevzov* and Geraldine O'Neill

Abstract

The evolution from unicellular to multicellular organisms of increasing complexity is paralleled by increased numbers of tropomyosin (Tm) genes and increasing numbers of isoforms encoded by each gene. The regulation of Tm isoform expression is intimately associated with the morphological changes that take place during development and cell differentiation. The tissue- and cell- specific Tm expression patterns are regulated at multiple levels, allowing precise spatial and temporal regulation of Tm expression. In this chapter, we review the Tm isoform expression pattern during differentiation of different tissue types and from this data infer some general principles regarding Tm expression patterns during differentiation. Finally, we review the mechanisms that account for the highly regulated repertoire of Tm isoform expression.

Introduction

Following the discovery in 1948 of Tm in rabbit skeletal muscle,[1] Tm has now been found in a wide range of organisms spanning yeast to humans. Tm belongs to a multigene family of related actin binding proteins and isoform diversity is generated via the use of alternative promoters and splicing of the primary RNA transcripts from multiple genes (see Chapter 3 for more details). The number of genes appears to increase with the complexity of the organism and so to does the number of isoforms encoded by these genes (Table 1)(see Chapter 2 for more details). In all, the four mammalian Tm genes encode greater than 40 Tm variants classified into two major groups according to their molecular weights, high molecular weight (HMW) and low molecular weight (LMW). The HMW Tms are approximately 284 amino acids in length and have an apparent molecular weight on SDS gels of between 33 and 40 kDa and the LMW isoforms are approximately 247 amino acids in length with an apparent molecular weight of 28 to 34 kDa. HMW Tms are further classified according to their tissue specificity. Thus HMW isoforms are divided into striated muscle specific (α and βTm), smooth muscle (αTm, also referred to as Tm 6[2]) brain-specific (TmBr1 and TmBr3) and Tms associated with early development/proliferation (Tm1, Tm2 and Tm3). Examples of LMW isoforms are the nonmuscle Tm5NM1—11 encoded by the γTm gene, Tm5a and Tm5b encoded by the αTm gene and Tm4 from the δTm gene.[3,4] The presence of multiple genes and alternative exon splicing is the principle mechanism determining the qualitative regulation of Tm isoform expression (see Chapter 3 for more detail). A variety of other modes of regulation control the quantitative expression of Tm isoforms and are discussed in later sections of this article.

*Corresponding Author: Galina Schevzov—Oncology Research Unit, The Children's Hospital at Westmead, Locked Bag 4001, Westmead, NSW 2145, Discipline of Paediatrics and Child Health, University of Sydney, Sydney, NSW 2006, Australia. Email: galinas@chw.edu.au

Tropomyosin, edited by Peter Gunning. ©2008 Landes Bioscience and Springer Science+Business Media.

Table 1. Tm genes found in different organisms and isoforms

Organism	Tm Gene Name	Proposed Number of Tm Isoforms
Fungi *(Schizosaccharomyces pombe*[59]	cdc8TM	1
Saccharomyces cerevisiae)[57]	TPM1	1
	TPM2	1
Invertebrates		
Nematode *(Caenorhabditis elegans)*[123,124]	tmy-1/lev-11	4
Insect *(Drosophila melanogaster)*[125,126]	TmI	2
	TmII	6
Tunicate *(Ciona intestinalis)*[127]	CTm1	1
Vertebrates		
Amphibian *(Xenopus laevis)*[128-132]	α-Tm	5
	β-Tm	2
	Tm-4	3
Avian (Chicken, quail)[133-137]	α	8
	β (Tm-1)	9
	cardiac[a]	3
	Tm_{nm}	1
Mammal (rat, mouse, rabbit, human[b])[30,138-143]	αTm	29
	βTm	2
	γTm	10
	δTm	1

[a]The chicken cardiac gene is homologous to rat Tm4, human TPM4. [b]In the human the α, β, γ and δ genes are referred to as TPM1, TPM2, TPM3 and TPM4 respectively.

Temporal Alterations in Tm Isoform Expression during Development

Morphological alterations during cellular differentiation are closely associated with the remodeling of the actin cytoskeleton and this is accompanied by prominent changes in the expression of specific Tm isoforms. It is clear that Tm gene products are required for embryonic development as genetic deletion of the αTm gene results in embryonic lethality between days 9.5 and 13.5[5] and even more strikingly, it proved impossible to isolate any homozygous γTm knockout embryos, suggesting that the products of this gene are absolutely required for early embryogenesis.[6] The detection of individual Tm isoforms has been confounded by the high sequence homology between isoforms making it difficult to generate isoform-specific antibodies. However, the derivation and use of panels of Tm isoform antibodies (Table 2) to screen tissue expression has facilitated the identification of discrete Tm isoform expression patterns. Below, we review tissue and cell differentiation events in which the Tm isoform expression profile has been characterized.

Early Embryogenesis

During early development there are numerous shape and motility changes that occur and thus it is not surprising to find that there are a wide variety of Tm isoforms expressed during embryogenesis. Constitutively expressed isoforms in both developing mouse embryos and in vitro differentiated embryonic stem cells include Tm4, Tm5, the striated muscle βTm and smooth muscle αTm.[7] In contrast, striated αTm is not present until day 5 in the differentiated embryonic stem cells and day 7.5 of the developing embryo. During later stages of development, myocardial cells spontaneously contract and the primitive cardiac tube forms accompanied by expression of both striated muscle HMW Tms α and βTm. Similarly, the Tm profile changes in murine preimplantation conceptuses as they develop from fertilized eggs to the 8 cell stage.[8]

Table 2. List of Tm antibodies

Antibody Name	Exon Specificity	Tm Gene	Tm Isoform Recognition
TM311[144]	Exon 1a	α, β, γTm	Tm6, 1, 2, 3 α, β, γ muscle Tm
α/2a[23]	Exon 2a	αTm	Smooth muscle Tm
anti-rTM9c[26]	Exon 9c	αTm	TmBr1, TmBr3
α-9c[27]	Exon 9c	αTm	TmBr1, TmBr3
WSα/9c[28]	Exon 9c	αTm	TmBr1, TmBr3
α/9c (Mab)[31]	Exon 9c	αTm	TmBr3
α/9d[145]	Exon 9d	αTm	Tm6, 1, 2, 3, 5a, 5b
Pep3-43[146]	Exon 1b	αTm	Tm5a, 5b, Br2, Br3
Anti-TM1[147]	Exon 6a	βTm	Tm1
CG3[148]	Exon 1b	γTm	All Tm5NM products
LC1[60]	Exon 1b	γTm (human)	Human Tm5NM1, NM2
γ/9a[31]	Exon 9a	γTm	Tm5NM3, 5, 6, 8, 9, 11 α, β, γ muscle Tm
TC22-4mAb[149]	Exon 9c	γTm	Tm5NM4, 7
γ/9c[31]	Exon 9c	γTm	Tm5NM4, 7
γ/9d[56]	Exon 9d	γTm	Tm5NM1, 2
δ-9d[26]	Exon 9d	δTm	Tm1, Tm4
WD4/9d[150]	Exon 9d	δTm	Tm4
Sarcomeric Tm (CH1)[151]	Exon 9a	α, β, γ Tm	α, β, γ muscle Tm, does not recognize 9a-containing Tm5NMs

Striated Muscle Development

Within mammalian striated muscle the two predominant α and β striated muscle Tms are present in different molar ratios depending on the muscle type.[9-12] αTm predominates in fast-twitch adult skeletal muscle, whereas slow-twitch skeletal muscle displays increased βTm and γTm (also referred to as αTm slow).[13,14] The hearts of rodents and chickens primarily contain a single α isoform.[9,15] Both mRNA and protein profiling have demonstrated that HMW nonmuscle Tm isoforms are repressed during muscle differentiation and the muscle adopts muscle specific HMW Tm expression.[16] However, in both in vitro and in vivo systems the expression of LMW nonmuscle isoforms are retained (Tm4 and Tm5NM1) albeit at significantly lower levels than that seen for the muscle counterparts.[16,17]

Smooth Muscle Cell Differentiation

Unlike skeletal and cardiac muscle cells that differentiate irreversibly, smooth muscle cells (SMC) retain a high degree of plasticity. SMC cultured in vitro can transition between a differentiated or "contractile" phenotype to a less differentiated and highly proliferative "synthetic" phenotype, accompanied by cell shape and cytoskeletal changes. In contractile SMC two HMW Tm isoforms are expressed, the unique smooth muscle αTm (also referred to as Tm6) and Tm1.[10,13] The addition of serum to SMC in culture promotes the transition to the less differentiated synthetic state. Under these conditions both isoforms are downregulated in SMC from a variety of animal species[18-20] and expression of the early development/proliferation HMW isoforms Tm2 and Tm3 is elevated.[18] SMC in the synthetic state also display elevated expression of LMW Tm4.[21,22] Surprisingly, the unique smooth muscle αTm isoform, Tm6, is not constitutively expressed in smooth muscle cells and appears to be a later marker of smooth muscle maturation.[23]

Brain Development

A highly ordered repertoire of Tm isoforms is expressed in the developing mammalian brain. These include TmBr1, TmBr2, TmBr3, Tm5a and Tm5b from the αTm gene; multiple products from the γTm gene; and Tm4 from the δTm gene is present in all neuronal cells. TmBr3 is specific to mature neurons, TmBr2 to glial cells (astrocytes and oligodendrocytes) and TmBr1 to astrocytes. Primary cultures of rat astrocytes initially show transcripts encoding Tm1, Tm2, Tm5a, Tm4, TmBr1 and TmBr2. As the cells differentiate and mature, the levels of Tm1, Tm4 and Tm5a decrease, Tm2 and TmBr1 remain unchanged and TmBr2 increases.[24] Examination during postnatal development of the rat cerebellum demonstrates that the expression of Tm isoforms present in neurons is closely regulated during development. Tm4 transcript levels are high in the young versus old rat cerebellum and correspondingly protein levels are increased early in the development of the rat cerebellum in areas where neurites are growing. Later in the adult, Tm4 localizes at postsynaptic sites in the cerebellar cortex. In contrast TmBr3 expression occurs later[25] and that of TmBr1 later still.[26-28] TmBr3 was also found in presynaptic terminals in the adult rat brain.[26] In mouse brain, HMW Tm (Tm1, 2, 3) expression is restricted to the germinal ventricular zone, a region rich in neuroblasts. As the neuroblasts mature and move through to the inner ventricular zone, there is a decrease in expression of these early development/proliferation HMW Tms.[29] The loss of these HMW Tms is concomitant with increased neurite outgrowth.

Comprehensive analysis of the rat brain identified a total of 10 mRNAs encoded by the γTm gene.[30] Evaluation of these mRNA splice variants clearly showed that these transcripts were temporally regulated during brain development. Exon 9d containing transcripts were significantly decreased, exon 9a transcripts were increased and exon 9c transcripts remained constant during development.[30] It was later confirmed that the pattern of protein expression parallels that seen at the mRNA level.[31] Thus, overall output from the γTm gene is constant but the choice of the C-terminus is developmentally regulated.

Granulosa Cell Differentiation

Granulosa cells surround the mammalian ovary follicle and when isolated from immature rats and induced to differentiate, undergo dramatic changes in their actin cytoskeleton and cell-cell interactions. The changes in the actin cytoskeleton correlate with a pronounced decrease in several nonmuscle Tm isoform mRNAs, with the greatest reduction occurring in the early development/proliferation HMW (Tm1, 2, 3) isoforms. This pattern of decreased Tm isoform expression is also seen in the developing ovary.[32] Furthermore, a temporal change in the expression of Tm4 coincides with differentiation of a rat ovarian granulosa cell line with follicle stimulating hormone and rat ovarian follicular development.[33]

Lens Cell Differentiation

A primary chick lens cell culture system was used to study Tm expression during differentiation and morphogenesis. During lens cell differentiation F-actin reorganizes from an epithelial-type cytoskeleton with actin stress fibers in polygonal arrays that intersect with an adherens belt of F-actin, to a cortical F-actin network. During early lens differentiation the predominant Tm isoforms are HMW (36~34 kDa). As cells proceed to a more differentiated state these HMW Tms are lost and the predominant isoform is a LMW Tm (~28 kDa). Supporting these data, LMW Tms predominate in lens fibre cells in vivo. The shift in Tm isoform content suggests that the LMW tropomyosin may preferentially organize actin filaments in the cortical cytoskeleton.[34]

Maturation of Chicken Digestive Organs

Development of different chicken digestive organs including esophagus, gizzard and intestine is also accompanied by changes in the relative amounts of Tm isoforms. Two-dimensional gel electrophoresis demonstrated the existence of 4 HMW Tms (E1-E4), HMW muscle isoforms α and βTm and 5 LMW (E5-E9) as early as 7 days. As organ maturation proceeds, expression of both HMW (E1-E4) and LMW Tms gradually decreases and after hatching the predominant Tm isoforms are the muscle specific HMW α and βTms.[35-37]

Other Differentiated Cell Types

A common pattern of Tm expression has also emerged from the study of terminally differentiated cell types. Mouse macrophages lack HMW Tm1, 2 and 3 but express LMW Tm4 and 5.[38,39] Human erythrocytes and leukocytes express the LMW Tm5NM1 isoform encoded by the γTm gene and Tm5b encoded by the αTm gene and most likely lack the early development/proliferation HMW Tms.[40-42] Lastly, osteoclasts derived from murine bone marrow or from the macrophage cell line RAW264.7 also express low levels of HMW Tms (Tm1, 2, 3) but relatively high levels of LMW Tms such as Tm4, Tm5NM1 and Tm5a.[43]

Tm Isoform Expression in Cancer

As described above, Tm expression has been shown to be tissue specific and temporally regulated in a qualitative and quantitative manner. This observed strict regulation strongly suggests that de-regulation in Tm isoform expression might be predicted to cause altered cell function. Indeed, cancer cells acquire a unique Tm expression profile characterized by the down regulation of the HMW Tm isoforms (Tm1, 2, 3)[44,45] (see Chapter 10 for more details). The distinguishable features of cancer cells are an altered actin cytoskeleton and anchorage independent growth. Re-expression of HMW Tms in various transformed cell types in vitro can lead to the restoration of actin stress fibers and anchorage dependant growth (see Table 1 of ref. 45).

A Common Pattern of Tm Expression during Cell Differentiation

The preceding sections describing the survey of Tm expression during differentiation and development illustrate the tissue- and differentiation state- specific regulation of Tm isoform diversity. Moreover, some general principles of Tm expression emerge from this data. First we note a general trend for significant down-regulation of the early development/proliferation HMW Tms (Tm1, 2, 3) accompanying terminal differentiation of cell types that initially express these Tms (Table 3, Fig. 1). Importantly, studies of smooth muscle cells induced to de-differentiate show restored expression

Table 3. Alterations in Tm isoform expression following differentiation

Cell/Tissue Type	Expression of HMW Tms	Expression of LMW Tms
Embryogenesis[7]	+ αTm, βTm	+ Tm4, Tm5NM1
Granulosa cells[32,33]	↓ HMW Tms	+ LMW Tms
		↑ Tm4
Lens cells[34]	↓ HMW Tms	+ LMW Tms
Chicken digestive organs[35-37]	↓ HMW E1-E4	↓ LMW E5-E9
	↑ αTm, βTm	
Neurogenesis[25-31]	↓ Tm1, Tm2, Tm3	+ Tm4, Tm5NM1-10
	↑ TmBr-1	TmBr3
Skeletal muscle[9,10,13,14-16]	↓ Tm1, Tm2, Tm3	↓ Tm4, Tm5NM1
	↑ αTm, βTm, γTm	
Smooth muscle cell (synthetic to contractile phenotype)[13,18,19,21,22]	↓ Tm1, Tm2, Tm3	+ Tm4
	↑ αTm, βTm, γTm	
Erythrocyte[40,41]	− Tm1, Tm2, Tm3	+ Tm5NM1, Tm5b
Leukocytes[42]	− Tm1, Tm2, Tm3	+ Tm5NM1, Tm5b
Macrophages[38,39]	− Tm1, Tm2, Tm3	+ Tm4, Tm5

The studies presented in this table summarises the Tm isoform expression both at the transcript and protein level following the developmental differentiation of the mentioned cell or tissue types. The symbols denote: (−) absence, (+) presence, (↓) decrease in Tm expression, (↑) increase in Tm expression.

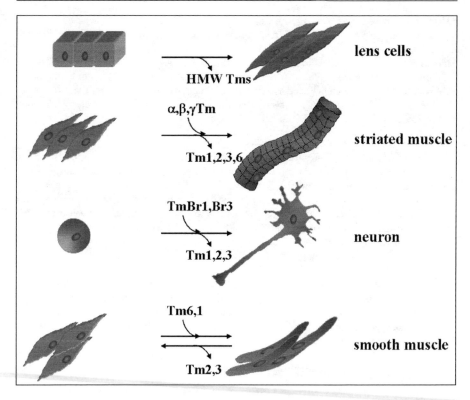

Figure 1. Alterations in the expression of the early development/proliferation HMW Tms (Tm1, 2 and 3) during morphogenesis. The observed morphological changes occuring during cellular differentiation are characterized by the loss of expression of the HMW Tms (Tm1, 2, 3).

of HMW Tms, thus providing further evidence that loss of HMW Tms is likely to be a critical event in cellular differentiation. Terminally differentiated cells exit the cell-cycle and there is evidence supporting a role for Tms in different aspects of cell-cycle regulation (reviewed by ref. 45). Thus it is tempting to speculate that the reduced expression of HMW Tms 1, 2 and 3 during differentiation may be linked to exit from the cell-cycle.

A second general principle to emerge from the survey of Tm expression during differentiation and development is that two LMW Tms are ubiquitously expressed: Tm4 encoded by the δTm gene and Tm5NM1 encoded by the γTm gene are detected in a wide range of tissues from brain to stomach,[2] including skeletal muscle where these isoforms localize to a specific subcellular compartment within the sarcomere.[16,17,46]

Functional Significance of Regulated Isoform Expression

Finally, specific Tms are up-regulated in differentiated tissues and it is likely that this represents specialized tissue functions of the Tm isoforms. In muscle, Tm is associated with the troponin complex that regulates the calcium sensitive interaction of actin and myosin, ultimately leading to contraction[13,47-49] (see also Chapters 8, 9 and 10 for more details). However, the lack of a troponin complex within both smooth and nonmuscle cells makes the role of Tm in these cell types less immediately obvious (Chapter 10). Within these cell types the two calcium-sensitive mechanisms controlling the interaction of actin and myosin are caldesmon and myosin light chain kinase, respectively.[50,51] The different mechanisms regulating contractility thus might require the expression of distinct Tm isoforms.[52,53] Moreover, nonmuscle Tm isoforms are implicated in a wide range of biological functions including intracellular granule movements,[54] Golgi function,[55,56] polarized cell growth and secretion,[57,58] cytokinesis,[59,60] cell morphogenesis[53] and endocytosis[61] (see Chapters 15-21 for more details). For this reason, we have proposed that specific Tm isoforms can impart distinct functional properties to the actin microfilaments leading to specialized biological roles.[3,4] To summarize, many differentiating cells down-regulate HMW Tms, maintain expression of Tm4 and Tm5NM1 and up-regulate expression of Tms that are likely to perform tissue-specific functions. In future, it will be most instructive to determine the function of each of these isoforms in the differentiation process.

Mechanisms Regulating Tm Expression

Tm isoform diversity is generated by 3 distinct mechanisms: (1) there are 4 mammalian genes encoding Tms; (2) 3 of the 4 genes are under the control of 2 alternative promoters and; (3) the transcripts from 3 of the 4 genes are subject to extensive alternative splicing (see Chapter 2 for more detail). Although transcript and protein data is available describing the Tm isoform profile in different tissues and cell types in a range of organisms as shown above, the molecular mechanisms that ultimately regulate this expression are poorly understood. Potential regulatory mechanisms that confer both tissue specific and cell specific Tm isoform regulation are discussed below.

Evidence for Transcriptional Regulation

During myogenesis the Drosophila *TmI* and *TmII* genes are under the control of at least 2 muscle enhancer regions, located within the first intron of these genes. These enhancer regions contain multiple muscle type specific positive and negative *cis*-acting elements which together determine the final extent of gene expression.[62,63] These muscle enhancers contain a consensus myocyte-specific enhancer factor 2 (MEF2) binding site (AT-rich sequence). However, even though MEF2 is necessary for the regulation of the Drosophila *TmI* gene in the somatic body-wall muscles of embryos, larvae and adults, this factor does not appear to be required for the expression of the *Tm1* gene in visceral muscle and heart.[64,65] Thus MEF2 dependent gene transcription of Tm is tissue specific. Analyses of the 5' flanking region of the chicken βTm gene have identified several *cis*-acting sequences, including E box, a CArG box and a C box responsible for transcriptional regulation in quail myoblasts cultured in vitro.[66] Similarly, using an in vitro C2C12 myoblast culture system, a 99bp enhancer sequence was identified in the rat αTm gene that could confer tissue and developmental specific expression.[67] In another model system, the Xenopus αTm gene carries a 284-bp promoter region that confers maximal activity in 3 muscle types (skeletal, cardiac and smooth). Among several cis-elements found within this region, an intact MCAT sequence was crucial for the correct temporal and spatial expression of the αTm gene. Since this site can bind transcription enhancer factor-1 present in muscle cells both in vitro and in vivo, this data strongly indicates that the specific muscle transcriptional regulation of the vertebrate αTm gene depends on this factor.[68]

Evidence for Translational Regulation

Quantitative comparison of the transcripts and protein levels of muscle Tm isoforms, αTm, βTm and γTm (αTm_{slow}), from both fast and slow-twitch muscles has revealed that translational mechanisms regulate production of muscle Tm protein. In both muscle types the translation of the βTm message is less efficient when compared with αTm and αTm_{slow} transcripts.[14] Gene knockout experiments have provided evidence that sarcomeric Tm is also regulated at the level of translation. While homozygous ablation of the αTm gene in mouse heart leads to embryonic lethality, the heterozygous animals display a 50% reduction in αTm mRNA but the total levels of the αTm protein are unaffected. The heterozygous mice display no phenotypic changes relative to the controls.[5,69] Similarly, transgenic over-expression of skeletal muscle βTm in the heart is compensated by a reduction in the levels of endogenous αTm. Thus a homeostasis of the total level of muscle Tm is maintained.[70] Similarly, transgenic over-expression of αTm_{slow} carrying an amino acid substitution (Met9Arg) in skeletal muscle coincides with the down regulation of the corresponding endogenous isoform.[71] Moreover, down-regulation of endogenous αTm protein also follows transgenic over-expression of αTm encoding mutations associated with familial hypertrophic cardiomyopathy.[72,73] Based on these studies, it is postulated that translational compensation ensures that the expression level of the total sarcomeric protein pool remains unaltered, hence maintaining the strict protein stoichiometry of the sarcomere.[74] In contrast, Drosophila melanogaster displays haplo-insufficiency of muscle Tm.[75]

Unlike the compensatory mechanism described above that regulates the expression of sarcomeric Tms, cytoskeletal Tms expression is not fixed. Extensive protein analysis of cytoskeletal Tm expression in tissues from both transgenic mice overexpressing cytoskeletal Tms or knock-out mice, demonstrate a lack of translational compensation among the cytoskeletal Tms.[76] As depicted in the model (Fig. 2), a feed-back regulatory mechanism controls the protein pool of sarcomeric

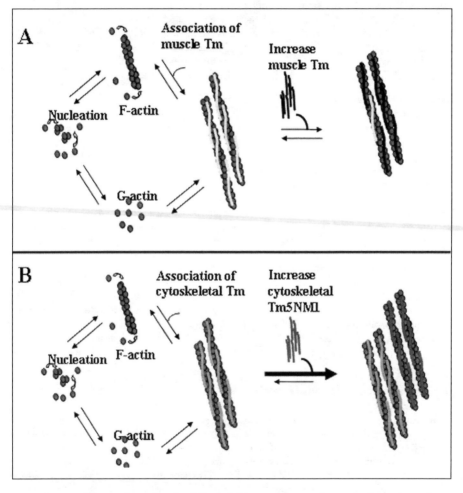

Figure 2. A model to account for the differential incorporation of ectopically expressed sarcomeric and cytoskeletal Tms into actin filaments. A) Within the actin filaments of striated muscle a feed-back mechanism regulates sarcomeric Tm expression. Ectopically expressed sarcomeric Tm is substituted for the endogenous sarcomeric Tm and thus a constant pool of Tm and actin is maintained. B) In contrast, no feed-back regulatory mechanism controls the expression of cytoskeletal Tm. Additional Tm5NM1 steers the equilibrium of G to F-actin in the direction of increased filament formation.

Tms. Such a mechanism ensures that a precise protein stoichiometry is maintained amongst the structural proteins in the sarcomere. Hence, following an increase in the expression of sarcomeric Tm, the expression of the endogenous sarcomeric Tm is downregulated and thus a constant pool of Tm and actin is maintained. In the case of the cytoskeletal Tms, additional Tm5NM1 drives the equilibrium of G to F-actin in the direction of increased filament formation. Thus the population of actin filaments containing cytoskeletal Tms is not fixed and can accommodate altered levels of Tm protein thus promoting more flexible cytoskeletal dynamics. This divergent regulation of Tm isoform expression in the muscle sarcomere versus the actin cytoskeleton in nonmuscle cells provides a mechanism to regulate actin filament structures with distinct functional requirements.

The Composition or Structure of Actin Filaments Can Impact on Tm Expression

Early studies have demonstrated that changes in actin isoform composition can influence the expression of Tm isoforms. Transfection of a mutant form of βactin correlated with an altered actin cytoskeleton and a corresponding decrease in the synthesis of HMW Tms (Tm1, 2, 3).[77,78] Similarly, changes in actin isoform composition via increased γactin and the down regulation of βactin led to a significant decrease in both the transcript and protein levels of Tm2.[79] Disruption of actin filaments following exposure of primary cultured astrocytes to cytochalasin D also promoted increased levels of Tm mRNA (Tm1 and Tm4), without altering either Tm2 or TmBr2.[80] In the case of normal rat kidney cells (NRK) HMW Tm protein turn over occurred at a higher rate than the LMW Tms when cells were exposed to cytochalasin B.[81] Thus, the stable accumulation of Tm isoforms can be influenced by the composition and/or the structural organization of the actin filaments and failure of Tm to incorporate into actin filaments leads to Tm degradation.

Mitogenic and Nonmitogenic Agents Can Impact on Tm Expression

As a general rule, repression of specific Tm isoforms is associated with mitogen deprivation, whereas exposure to mitogens restores expression. Serum deprivation of cultured rat astrocytes led to a halving in the transcript levels of Tm1, Tm 2, Tm4, TmBr1 and TmBr2.[80] Serum stimulation of previously serum-deprived in vitro cultures of rat aortic smooth muscle cells caused the levels of the early development/proliferation HMW Tms (Tm2, Tm3) to increase two fold while levels of smooth muscle αTm (Tm6) remained unaltered.[82] Importantly, the observed increase in the HMW Tms correlated with the stimulation of cell proliferation. In chicken gizzard SMC the specific transcriptional expression of the βTm gene was found to be mediated via serum response factor interaction with the CArG box sequence together with its coactivator Barx1b.[83] Moreover, addition of serum to quiescent cultures of fibroblasts induced the expression of the αTm gene that encodes HMW Tms 1, 2 and 3 in this cell type.[84] Nerve growth factor induced morphological differentiation of PC12 cells and the induction of the neuron-specific HMW Tm transcripts, TmBr1 and TmBr3.[85] Finally, the induction of morphological changes of three-week-old rat astrocytes from astroblasts to star-shaped process-bearing cells leads to repression of HMW Tms.[86]

Transforming growth factor-β (TGF-β) is a potent multifunctional regulator of cell growth and differentiation has been previously shown to restore the actin cytoskeleton, inhibit anchorage-independent growth and regulate invasion of certain transformed cells. Transformation suppression by TGF-β in sensitive cells is thought to occur via the induction of HMW Tms, shown in normal rat kidney, human lung carcinoma and metastatic breast cancer cells.[87-89] In contrast, TGF-α is often upregulated in carcinomas and has been proposed to be a mediator of transformation through autocrine stimulation. Exposure to TGF-α suppresses the synthesis of the HMW Tms (Tm1, 2, 3) without altering that of the LMW Tm4 and Tm5 isoforms in normal rat kidney and fibroblast cell lines.[81,90]

Nonmitogenic factors have also been shown to alter Tm expression. Increased intracellular levels of cAMP correlate with decreased HMW Tms and no significant changes in the levels of the LMW Tms. This has been observed in thyroid epithelial cells,[91] cultured rat vascular smooth muscle cells[92] and cultured rat astrocytes.[80,86] In most cases the decrease in HMW Tm expression was associated with morphological differentiation and the inability of the cells to proliferate.

Interestingly, α-tocopherol (vitamin E) treatment of serum stimulated vascular smooth muscle cells was also shown to induce the expression of HMW Tms.[93]

Signaling Pathways Known to Be Involve in Tm Regulation

The study of the possible mechanisms that trigger cellular transformation has shed some light on the signaling pathways by which Tm expression might be regulated, although whether the signaling pathways below operate in normal cells remains to be explored. Malignant transformation by oncogenes and tumor viruses results in characteristic alterations of the actin cytoskeleton together with the down-regulation of the HMW Tms (Tm1, 2, 3) (see Chapter 10 for more detail). The LMW Tms remain either unchanged or in some studies have been shown to increase in expression.[94-96] Mitogen-activated protein kinase (MAPK) pathways feature prominantly in the transduction of externally-derived signals. Mutations in components of MAPK signaling such as mutations in Ras and Raf oncogenes are known to lead to transformation and are commonly associated with altered Tm expression. The activation of Ras is mediated by interaction with multiple down stream effectors. Raf is a Ras effector which phosphorylates and activates MEK1/2, in turn activating the extracellular signal-regulated kinase (ERK) culminating in the activation of the Jun N-terminal and p38 kinases. A role for MEK in Tm regulation has been inferred from studies in c-jun-transformed FR3T3 cells where down regulation of HMW Tms is mediated through an autocrine pathway disrupted by inhibition of MEK.[97] Similarly, inhibition of MEK leads to re-expression of Tms (Tm1, 2, 3) in Ras-transformed NRK (normal rat kidney) and RIE (rat intestinal epithelial) cells.[98,99] Moreover, inhibition of the Ras-ERK pathway restores TGF-β induction of HMW Tms in metastatic breast cancer cells.[89] Surprisingly, other studies conclude that the down regulation of HMW Tms occurs via MEK-independent pathways such as in Ras and Raf-transformed NIH 3T3 cells[100,101] and transformed MDA-MB-231 breast cancer cells.[102] These conflicting reports demonstrate that although MEK and its down stream effectors may play a role in Tm regulation the contribution of MEK is likely to be complex.

Silencing of Tm Expression via DNA Methylation

A common mechanism known to silence gene expression is DNA methylation of gene promoters. Due to the common repression of HMW Tms isoforms reported in different cancer cells, cytosine methylation of both the αTm (encodes Tm2 and 3) and βTm (encodes Tm1) gene promoters has been explored. Azadeoxycytidine treatment to de-methylate promoters in Ras transformed cell lines restored protein expression of Tm1, 2 and 3.[99] In breast cancer cell lines elevated levels of Tm1 protein were seen following the combined treatment of azadeoxycytidine and trichostatin A.[103] This indicates that hypermethylation and chromatin remodeling are likely mechanisms mediating the repression of the βTm gene in the transformed breast cancer cell lines that were studied. Importantly, the authors also report that such drug treatment had no impact on the expression of LMW Tms encoded by the γTm and δTm genes. This work has been extended to show that induction of the αTm gene products by TGF-β requires prior treatment of the human breast cancer cell lines with azadeoxycytidine to remove methyl groups from the DNA.[104] In this study minimal impact on transcripts of the βTm gene was observed, further demonstrating the differential regulation of the Tm genes.

Posttranslational Modifications

Acetylation of the N-terminal methionine of mammalian Tm is required in order to associate with actin by modulating the structure of the N-terminus that facilitates head-to-tail interactions of Tm dimers.[105,106] However, unacetylated forms of βTm[107] and αTm smooth[108] were found to bind well to actin. Furthermore, an AlaSer dipeptide fused to the N-terminus of Tm is sufficient to replace the function of the N-terminal acetyl group in head-to-tail polymerization and the ability to inhibit myosin ATPase.[105,109]

On the other hand phosphorylation of Tm has been demonstrated to regulate actin filament function and ultimately remodelling of the actin cytoskeleton. Evidence for the presence of phosphorylated forms of Tm has been found both in skeletal and cardiac muscle from a variety of different sources including frog, rabbit and chicken.[15,110-115] The penultimate residue at the carboxyl terminal end, serine 283, on both α and βTm was found to be the phosphorylated residue. Interestingly, the degree of phosphorylation coincides with the maturation of the muscle such that a higher level is observed in embryonic developing muscle but not observed in regenerating or denervated muscle.[15,113-116] The phosphorylation of αTm in rabbit muscle enhances the ability of Tm to polymerize head-to-tail and promotes activation of myosin Mg^{2+}-ATPase by facilitating actomyosin interaction.[117,118] Similarly, acetylcholine induces protein kinase C—mediated and calcium-dependent phosphorylation of Tm in colonic smooth muscle cells. In the case of smooth muscle Tm phosphorylation is believed to sustain contraction.[119] Sarcomeric Tm phosphorylation is also observed in Drosophila indirect flight muscle. In this model phosphorylation is apparent in mature flies but not in recently emerged flies that are incapable of flight.[120] A more recent study shows that dephosphorylation of αTm in murine heart leads to depressed contractility, this is mediated via activation of p38-MAPK.[121] Thus it is proposed that the functional consequence of phosphorylation of sarcomeric Tm is to alter the structural and functional properties of the muscle contractile apparatus.

Non-sarcomeric Tms have also been shown to be phosphorylated. Tm1 phosphorylation leads to bundling of stress fibers, increase in cellular contractility and ultimately membrane blebbing.[122] Tm2 phosphorylation by phosphoinositide 3-kinase on residue Ser 61 regulates β-adrenergic receptor endocytosis.[61]

Conclusions

The tissue and cell specific expression of Tm isoforms strongly suggests that either each individual or group of isoforms is required to perform a specific biological function. The distinct morphological changes observed following cellular differentiation are intimately associated with changes in the organisation of the actin cytoskeleton and specific changes in the complement of Tm isoforms expressed. Analysis of the Tm isoform expression during the development of different cell lineages has demonstrated characteristic loss of a group of HMW Tms associated with terminal differentiation and this is accompanied by enhanced expression of other Tm isoforms associated with tissue specific functions. The challenge that faces us now is to integrate the functional roles of the Tm isoforms with the regulatory pathways that produce the required qualitative and quantitative changes in Tm isoform expression during differentiation and development.

Acknowledgements

The authors wish to acknowledge the support of the National Health and Medical Research Council of Australia and the Oncology Children's Foundation. Geraldine O'Neill is supported by a NSW Cancer Council Career Development Award.

References

1. Bailey K. Tropomyosin: a new asymmetric protein component of the muscle fibril. Biochem J 1948; 43(2):271-279.
2. Schevzov G, Vrhovski B, Bryce NS et al. Tissue-specific tropomyosin isoform composition. J Histochem Cytochem 2005; 53(5):557-570.
3. Gunning PW, Schevzov G, Kee AJ et al. Tropomyosin isoforms: divining rods for actin cytoskeleton function. Trends Cell Biol 2005; 15(6):333-341.
4. Gunning PW, O'Neill GM, Hardeman EC. Tropomyosin-based regulation of the actin cytoskeleton in time and space. Physiol Rev 2008; 88(1):1-35.
5. Blanchard EM, Iizuka K, Christe M et al. Targeted ablation of the murine alpha-tropomyosin gene. Circ Res 1997; 81(6):1005-1010.
6. Hook J, Lemckert F, Qin H et al. Gamma tropomyosin gene products are required for embryonic development. Mol Cell Biol 2004; 24(6):2318-2323.
7. Muthuchamy M, Pajak L, Howles P et al. Developmental analysis of tropomyosin gene expression in embryonic stem cells and mouse embryos. Mol Cell Biol 1993; 13(6):3311-3323.
8. Clayton L, Johnson MH. Tropomyosin in preimplantation mouse development: identification, expression and organization during cell division and polarization. Exp Cell Res 1998; 238(2):450-464.

9. Cummins P, Perry SV. The subunits and biological activity of polymorphic forms of tropomyosin. Biochem J 1973; 133(4):765-777.
10. Cummins P, Perry SV. Chemical and immunochemical characteristics of tropomyosins from striated and smooth muscle. Biochem J 1974; 141(1):43-49.
11. Salviati G, Betto R, Danieli BD. Polymorphism of myofibrillar proteins of rabbit skeletal-muscle fibres. An electrophoretic study of single fibres. Biochem J 1982; 207(2):261-272.
12. Bronson DD, Schachat FH. Heterogeneity of contractile proteins. Differences in tropomyosin in fast, mixed and slow skeletal muscles of the rabbit. J Biol Chem 1982; 257(7):3937-3944.
13. Lees-Miller JP, Helfman DM. The molecular basis for tropomyosin isoform diversity. Bioessays 1991; 13(9):429-437.
14. Pieples K, Wieczorek DF. Tropomyosin 3 increases striated muscle isoform diversity. Biochemistry 2000; 39(28):8291-8297.
15. Montarras D, Fiszman MY, Gros F. Characterization of the tropomyosin present in various chick embryo muscle types and in muscle cells differentiated in vitro. J Biol Chem 1981; 256(8):4081-4086.
16. Gunning P, Gordon M, Wade R et al. Differential control of tropomyosin mRNA levels during myogenesis suggests the existence of an isoform competition-autoregulatory compensation control mechanism. Dev Biol 1990; 138(2):443-453.
17. Kee AJ, Schevzov G, Nair-Shalliker V et al. Sorting of a nonmuscle tropomyosin to a novel cytoskeletal compartment in skeletal muscle results in muscular dystrophy. J Cell Biol 2004; 166(5):685-696.
18. Kashiwada K, Nishida W, Hayashi K et al. Coordinate expression of alpha-tropomyosin and caldesmon isoforms in association with phenotypic modulation of smooth muscle cells. J Biol Chem 1997; 272(24):15396-15404.
19. Girjes AA, Keriakous D, Cockerill GW et al. Cloning of a differentially expressed tropomyosin isoform from cultured rabbit aortic smooth muscle cells. Int J Biochem Cell Biol 2002; 34(5):505-515.
20. Halayko AJ, Salari H, MA X et al. Markers of airway smooth muscle cell phenotype. Am J Physiol 1996; 270(6 Pt 1):L1040-L1051.
21. Yamawaki-Kataoka Y, Helfman DM. Isolation and characterization of cDNA clones encoding a low molecular weight nonmuscle tropomyosin isoform. J Biol Chem 1987; 262(22):10791-10800.
22. Abouhamed M, Reichenberg S, Robenek H et al. Tropomyosin 4 expression is enhanced in dedifferentiating smooth muscle cells in vitro and during atherogenesis. Eur J Cell Biol 2003; 82(9):473-482.
23. Vrhovski B, McKay K, Schevzov G et al. Smooth muscle-specific alpha tropomyosin is a marker of fully differentiated smooth muscle in lung. J Histochem Cytochem 2005; 53(7):875-883.
24. Had L, Faivre-Sarrailh C, Legrand C et al. The expression of tropomyosin genes in pure cultures of rat neurons, astrocytes and oligodendrocytes is highly cell-type specific and strongly regulated during development. Brain Res Mol Brain Res 1993; 18(1-2):77-86.
25. Faivre-Sarrailh C, Had L, Ferraz C et al. Expression of tropomyosin genes during the development of the rat cerebellum. J Neurochem 1990; 55(3):899-906.
26. Had L, Faivre-Sarrailh C, Legrand C et al. Tropomyosin isoforms in rat neurons: the different developmental profiles and distributions of TM-4 and TMBr-3 are consistent with different functions. J Cell Sci 1994; 107(Pt 10):2961-2973.
27. Stamm S, Casper D, Lees-Miller JP et al. Brain-specific tropomyosins TMBr-1 and TMBr-3 have distinct patterns of expression during development and in adult brain. Proc Natl Acad Sci USA 1993; 90(21):9857-9861.
28. Weinberger R, Schevzov G, Jeffrey P et al. The molecular composition of neuronal microfilaments is spatially and temporally regulated. J Neurosci 1996; 16(1):238-252.
29. Hughes JA, Cooke-Yarborough CM, Chadwick NC et al. High-molecular-weight tropomyosins localize to the contractile rings of dividing CNS cells but are absent from malignant pediatric and adult CNS tumors. Glia 2003; 42(1):25-35.
30. Dufour C, Weinberger RP, Schevzov G et al. Splicing of two internal and four carboxyl-terminal alternative exons in nonmuscle tropomyosin 5 premRNA is independently regulated during development. J Biol Chem 1998; 273(29):18547-18555.
31. Vrhovski B, Schevzov G, Dingle S et al. Tropomyosin isoforms from the gamma gene differing at the C-terminus are spatially and developmentally regulated in the brain. J Neurosci Res 2003; 72(3):373-383.
32. Ben Ze'ev A, Baum G, Amsterdam A. Regulation of tropomyosin expression in the maturing ovary and in primary granulosa cell cultures. Dev Biol 1989; 135(1):191-201.
33. Grieshaber NA, Ko C, Grieshaber SS et al. Follicle-stimulating hormone-responsive cytoskeletal genes in rat granulosa cells: class I beta-tubulin, tropomyosin-4 and kinesin heavy chain. Endocrinology 2003; 144(1):29-39.
34. Fischer RS, Lee A, Fowler VM. Tropomodulin and tropomyosin mediate lens cell actin cytoskeleton reorganization in vitro. Invest Ophthalmol Vis Sci 2000; 41(1):166-174.

35. Hosoya M, Miyazaki J, Hirabayashi T. Tropomyosin isoforms in developing chicken gizzard smooth muscle. J Biochem (Tokyo) 1989; 105(5):712-717.
36. Xie L, Miyazaki J, Hirabayashi T. Identification and distribution of tropomyosin isoforms in chicken digestive canal. J Biochem (Tokyo) 1991; 109(6):872-878.
37. Xie L, Hirabayashi T, Miyazaki J. Histological distribution and developmental changes of tropomyosin isoforms in three chicken digestive organs. Cell Tissue Res 1992; 269(3):391-401.
38. Nakamura Y, Sakiyama S, Takenaga K. Suppression of syntheses of high molecular weight nonmuscle tropomyosins in macrophages. Cell Motil Cytoskeleton 1995; 31(4):273-282.
39. Fattoum A, Hartwig JH, Stossel TP. Isolation and some structural and functional properties of macrophage tropomyosin. Biochemistry 1983; 22(5):1187-1193.
40. Sung LA, Lin JJ. Erythrocyte tropomodulin binds to the N-terminus of hTM5, a tropomyosin isoform encoded by the gamma-tropomyosin gene. Biochem Biophys Res Commun 1994; 201(2):627-634.
41. Sung LA, Gao KM, Yee LJ et al. Tropomyosin isoform 5b is expressed in human erythrocytes: implications of tropomodulin-TM5 or tropomodulin-TM5b complexes in the protofilament and hexagonal organization of membrane skeletons. Blood 2000; 95(4):1473-1480.
42. Dunn SA, Mohteshamzadeh M, Daly AK et al. Altered tropomyosin expression in essential hypertension. Hypertension 2003; 41(2):347-354.
43. McMichael BK, Kotadiya P, Singh T et al. Tropomyosin isoforms localize to distinct microfilament populations in osteoclasts. Bone 2006.
44. Stehn JR, Schevzov G, O'Neill GM et al. Specialisation of the tropomyosin composition of actin filaments provides new potential targets for chemotherapy. Curr Cancer Drug Targets 2006; 6(3):245-256.
45. O'Neill GM, Stehn J, Gunning PW. Tropomyosins as interpreters of the signalling environment to regulate the local cytoskeleton. Seminars in Cancer Biology 2008; 18:35-44.
46. Vlahovich N, Schevzov G, Nair-Shaliker V et al. Tropomyosin 4 defines novel filaments in skeletal muscle associated with muscle remodelling/regeneration in normal and diseased muscle. Cell Motil Cyotskeleton 2008:65:73-85.
47. Smillie LB. Structure and functions of tropomyosins from muscle and nonmuscle sources. Trends in Biochemical Sciences 1979; 4(7):151-155.
48. Payne MR, Rudnick SE. Tropomyosin. Structural and functional diversity. Cell Muscle Motil 1985; 6:141-184.
49. Pittenger MF, Kazzaz JA, Helfman DM. Functional properties of nonmuscle tropomyosin isoforms. Curr Opin Cell Biol 1994; 6(1):96-104.
50. Adelstein RS, Pato MD, Conti MA. The role of phosphorylation in regulating contractile proteins. Adv Cyclic Nucleotide Res 1981; 14:361-373.
51. Wang CL. Caldesmon and smooth-muscle regulation. Cell Biochem Biophys 2001; 35(3):275-288.
52. Fanning AS, Wolenski JS, Mooseker MS et al. Differential regulation of skeletal muscle myosin-II and brush border myosin-I enzymology and mechanochemistry by bacterially produced tropomyosin isoforms. Cell Motil Cytoskeleton 1994; 29(1):29-45.
53. Bryce NS, Schevzov G, Ferguson V et al. Specification of actin filament function and molecular composition by tropomyosin isoforms. Mol Biol Cell 2003; 14(3):1002-1016.
54. Pelham RJ Jr, Lin JJ, Wang YL. A high molecular mass nonmuscle tropomyosin isoform stimulates retrograde organelle transport. J Cell Sci 1996; 109(Pt 5):981-989.
55. Heimann K, Percival JM, Weinberger R et al. Specific isoforms of actin-binding proteins on distinct populations of Golgi-derived vesicles. J Biol Chem 1999; 274(16):10743-10750.
56. Percival JM, Hughes JA, Brown DL et al. Targeting of a tropomyosin isoform to short microfilaments associated with the Golgi complex. Mol Biol Cell 2004; 15(1):268-280.
57. Drees B, Brown C, Barrell BG et al. Tropomyosin is essential in yeast, yet the TPM1 and TPM2 products perform distinct functions. J Cell Biol 1995; 128(3):383-392.
58. Pruyne DW, Schott DH, Bretscher A. Tropomyosin-containing actin cables direct the Myo2p-dependent polarized delivery of secretory vesicles in budding yeast. J Cell Biol 1998; 143(7):1931-1945.
59. Balasubramanian MK, Helfman DM, Hemmingsen SM. A new tropomyosin essential for cytokinesis in the fission yeast S. pombe Nature 1992; 360(6399):84-87.
60. Warren KS, Lin JL, McDermott JP et al. Forced expression of chimeric human fibroblast tropomyosin mutants affects cytokinesis. J Cell Biol 1995; 129(3):697-708.
61. Naga Prasad SV, Jayatilleke A, Madamanchi A et al. Protein kinase activity of phosphoinositide 3-kinase regulates beta-adrenergic receptor endocytosis. Nat Cell Biol 2005; 7(8):785-796.
62. Gremke L, Lord PC, Sabacan L et al. Coordinate regulation of Drosophila tropomyosin gene expression is controlled by multiple muscle-type-specific positive and negative enhancer elements. Dev Biol 1993; 159(2):513-527.

63. Meredith J, Storti RV. Developmental regulation of the Drosophila tropomyosin II gene in different muscles is controlled by muscle-type-specific intron enhancer elements and distal and proximal promoter control elements. Dev Biol 1993; 159(2):500-512.

64. Lin MH, Nguyen HT, Dybala C et al. Myocyte-specific enhancer factor 2 acts cooperatively with a muscle activator region to regulate Drosophila tropomyosin gene muscle expression. Proc Natl Acad Sci USA 1996; 93(10):4623-4628.

65. Lin SC, Storti RV. Developmental regulation of the Drosophila Tropomyosin I (TmI) gene is controlled by a muscle activator enhancer region that contains multiple cis-elements and binding sites for multiple proteins. Dev Genet 1997; 20(4):297-306.

66. Toutant M, Gauthier-Rouviere C, Fiszman MY et al. Promoter elements and transcriptional control of the chicken tropomyosin gene [corrected]. Nucleic Acids Res 1994; 22(10):1838-1845.

67. Herrera VL, Ruiz-Opazo N. Regulation of alpha-tropomyosin and N5 genes by a shared enhancer. Modular structure and hierarchical organization. J Biol Chem 1990; 265(16):9555-9562.

68. Pasquet S, Naye F, Faucheux C et al. TEF-1 dependent expression of the alpha-tropomyosin gene in the three muscle cell types. J Biol Chem 2006; 281(45):34406-34420.

69. Rethinasamy P, Muthuchamy M, Hewett T et al. Molecular and physiological effects of alpha-tropomyosin ablation in the mouse. Circ Res 1998; 82(1):116-123.

70. Muthuchamy M, Grupp IL, Grupp G et al. Molecular and physiological effects of overexpressing striated muscle beta-tropomyosin in the adult murine heart. J Biol Chem 1995; 270(51):30593-30603.

71. Corbett MA, Akkari PA, Domazetovska A et al. An alphaTropomyosin mutation alters dimer preference in nemaline myopathy. Ann Neurol 2005; 57(1):42-49.

72. Muthuchamy M, Pieples K, Rethinasamy P et al. Mouse model of a familial hypertrophic cardiomyopathy mutation in alpha-tropomyosin manifests cardiac dysfunction. Circ Res 1999; 85(1):47-56.

73. Prabhakar R, Boivin GP, Grupp IL et al. A familial hypertrophic cardiomyopathy alpha-tropomyosin mutation causes severe cardiac hypertrophy and death in mice. J Mol Cell Cardiol 2001; 33(10):1815-1828.

74. Palermo J, Gulick J, Colbert M et al. Transgenic remodeling of the contractile apparatus in the mammalian heart. Circ Res 1996; 78(3):504-509.

75. Molloy J, Kreuz A, Miller R et al. Effects of tropomyosin deficiency in flight muscle of Drosophila melanogaster. Adv Exp Med Biol 1993; 332:165-171.

76. Schevzov G, Fath T, Vrhovski B et al. Divergent regulation of the sarcomere and the cytoskeleton. J Biol Chem 2008;283(1):275-283.

77. Leavitt J, Ng SY, Varma M et al. Expression of transfected mutant beta-actin genes: transitions toward the stable tumorigenic state. Mol Cell Biol 1987; 7(7):2467-2476.

78. Ng SY, Erba H, Latter G et al. Modulation of microfilament protein composition by transfected cytoskeletal actin genes. Mol Cell Biol 1988; 8(4):1790-1794.

79. Schevzov G, Lloyd C, Hailstones D et al. Differential regulation of tropomyosin isoform organization and gene expression in response to altered actin gene expression. J Cell Biol 1993; 121(4):811-821.

80. Ferrier R, Had L, Rabie A et al. Coordinated expression of five tropomyosin isoforms and beta-actin in astrocytes treated with dibutyryl cAMP and cytochalasin D. Cell Motil Cytoskeleton 1994; 28(4):303-316.

81. Warren RH. TGF-alpha-induced breakdown of stress fibers and degradation of tropomyosin in NRK cells is blocked by a proteasome inhibitor. Exp Cell Res 1997; 236(1):294-303.

82. Hirano K, Hirano M, Eto W et al. Mitogen-induced up-regulation of nonsmooth muscle isoform of alpha-tropomyosin in rat aortic smooth muscle cells. Eur J Pharmacol 2000; 406(2):209-218.

83. Nakamura M, Nishida W, Mori S et al. Transcriptional activation of beta-tropomyosin mediated by serum response factor and a novel Barx homologue, Barx1b, in smooth muscle cells. J Biol Chem 2001; 276(21):18313-18320.

84. Ryseck RP, MacDonald-Bravo H, Zerial M et al. Coordinate induction of fibronectin, fibronectin receptor, tropomyosin and actin genes in serum-stimulated fibroblasts. Exp Cell Res 1989; 180(2):537-545.

85. Weinberger RP, Henke RC, Tolhurst O et al. Induction of neuron-specific tropomyosin mRNAs by nerve growth factor is dependent on morphological differentiation. J Cell Biol 1993; 120(1):205-215.

86. Canonne-Hergaux F, Zwiller J, Aunis D. cAMP and bFGF negatively regulate tropomyosin expression in rat cultured astroblasts. Neurochem Int 1994; 25(6):545-553.

87. Masuda A, Takenaga K, Kondoh F et al. Role of a signal transduction pathway which controls disassembly of microfilament bundles and suppression of high-molecular-weight tropomyosin expression in oncogenic transformation of NRK cells. Oncogene 1996; 12(10):2081-2088.

88. Tada A, Kato H, Takenaga K et al. Transforming growth factor beta1 increases the expressions of high molecular weight tropomyosin isoforms and vinculin and suppresses the transformed phenotypes in human lung carcinoma cells. Cancer Lett 1997; 121(1):31-37.

89. Bakin AV, Safina A, Rinehart C et al. A critical role of tropomyosins in TGF-beta regulation of the actin cytoskeleton and cell motility in epithelial cells. Mol Biol Cell 2004; 15(10):4682-4694.
90. Cooper HL, Bhattacharya B, Bassin RH et al. Suppression of synthesis and utilization of tropomyosin in mouse and rat fibroblasts by transforming growth factor alpha: a pathway in oncogene action. Cancer Res 1987; 47(16):4493-4500.
91. Roger PP, Rickaert F, Lamy F et al. Actin stress fiber disruption and tropomyosin isoform switching in normal thyroid epithelial cells stimulated by thyrotropin and phorbol esters. Exp Cell Res 1989; 182(1):1-13.
92. Ohara O, Nakano T, Teraoka H et al. cAMP negatively regulates mRNA levels of actin and tropomyosin in rat cultured vascular smooth muscle cells. J Biochem (Tokyo) 1991; 109(6):834-839.
93. Aratri E, Spycher SE, Breyer I et al. Modulation of alpha-tropomyosin expression by alpha-tocopherol in rat vascular smooth muscle cells. FEBS Lett 1999; 447(1):91-94.
94. Hendricks M, Weintraub H. Tropomyosin is decreased in transformed cells. Proc Natl Acad Sci USA 1981; 78(9):5633-5637.
95. Matsumura F, Lin JJ, Yamashiro-Matsumura S et al. Differential expression of tropomyosin forms in the microfilaments isolated from normal and transformed rat cultured cells. J Biol Chem 1983; 258(22):13954-13964.
96. Cooper HL, Feuerstein N, Noda M et al. Suppression of tropomyosin synthesis, a common biochemical feature of oncogenesis by structurally diverse retroviral oncogenes. Mol Cell Biol 1985; 5(5):972-983.
97. Ljungdahl S, Linder S, Franzen B et al. Down-regulation of tropomyosin-2 expression in c-Jun-transformed rat fibroblasts involves induction of a MEK1-dependent autocrine loop. Cell Growth Differ 1998; 9(7):565-573.
98. Pawlak G, Helfman DM. Posttranscriptional down-regulation of ROCKI/Rho-kinase through an MEK-dependent pathway leads to cytoskeleton disruption in Ras-transformed fibroblasts. Mol Biol Cell 2002; 13(1):336-347.
99. Shields JM, Mehta H, Pruitt K et al. Opposing roles of the extracellular signal-regulated kinase and p38 mitogen-activated protein kinase cascades in Ras-mediated downregulation of tropomyosin. Mol Cell Biol 2002; 22(7):2304-2317.
100. Janssen RA, Veenstra KG, Jonasch P et al. Ras- and Raf-induced down-modulation of nonmuscle tropomyosin are MEK-independent. J Biol Chem 1998; 273(48):32182-32186.
101. Janssen RA, Kim PN, Mier JW et al. Overexpression of kinase suppressor of Ras upregulates the high-molecular-weight tropomyosin isoforms in ras-transformed NIH 3T3 fibroblasts. Mol Cell Biol 2003; 23(5):1786-1797.
102. Seddighzadeh M, Linder S, Shoshan MC et al. Inhibition of extracellular signal-regulated kinase 1/2 activity of the breast cancer cell line MDA-MB-231 leads to major alterations in the pattern of protein expression. Electrophoresis 2000; 21(13):2737-2743.
103. Bharadwaj S, Prasad GL. Tropomyosin-1, a novel suppressor of cellular transformation is downregulated by promoter methylation in cancer cells. Cancer Lett 2002; 183(2):205-213.
104. Varga AE, Stourman NV, Zheng Q et al. Silencing of the Tropomyosin-1 gene by DNA methylation alters tumor suppressor function of TGF-beta. Oncogene 2005; 24(32):5043-5052.
105. Monteiro PB, Lataro RC, Ferro JA et al. Functional alpha-tropomyosin produced in Escherichia coli. A dipeptide extension can substitute the amino-terminal acetyl group. J Biol Chem 1994; 269(14):10461-10466.
106. Urbancikova M, Hitchcock-DeGregori SE. Requirement of amino-terminal modification for striated muscle alpha-tropomyosin function. J Biol Chem 1994; 269(39):24310-24315.
107. Pittenger MF, Kistler A, Helfman DM. Alternatively spliced exons of the beta tropomyosin gene exhibit different affinities for F-actin and effects with nonmuscle caldesmon. J Cell Sci 1995; 108 (Pt 10):3253-3265.
108. Cho Young-Joo. The carboxyl terminal amino acid residues glutamine276-threonine277 are important for actin affinity of the unacetylated smooth a-tropomyosin. Journal of biochemistry and molecular biology 2000; 33(6):531-536.
109. Maytum R, Geeves MA, Konrad M. Actomyosin regulatory properties of yeast tropomyosin are dependent upon N-terminal modification. Biochemistry 2000; 39(39):11913-11920.
110. Ribolow H, Barany M. Phosphorylation of tropomyosin in live frog muscle. Arch Biochem Biophys 1977; 179(2):718-720.
111. Mak A, Smillie LB, Barany M. Specific phosphorylation at serine-283 of alpha tropomyosin from frog skeletal and rabbit skeletal and cardiac muscle. Proc Natl Acad Sci USA 1978; 75(8):3588-3592.
112. O'Connor CM, Balzer DR Jr, Lazarides E. Phosphorylation of subunit proteins of intermediate filaments from chicken muscle and nonmuscle cells. Proc Natl Acad Sci USA 1979; 76(2):819-823.
113. Heeley DA, Moir AJ, Perry SV. Phosphorylation of tropomyosin during development in mammalian striated muscle. FEBS Lett 1982; 146(1):115-118.

114. Heeley DH, Dhoot GK, Perry SV. Factors determining the subunit composition of tropomyosin in mammalian skeletal muscle. Biochem J 1985; 226(2):461-468.
115. Dabrowska R, Nowak E, Drabikowski W. Some functional properties of nonpolymerizable and polymerizable tropomyosin. J Muscle Res Cell Motil 1983; 4(2):143-161.
116. Montarras D, Fiszman MY, Gros F. Changes in tropomyosin during development of chick embryonic skeletal muscles in vivo and during differentiation of chick muscle cells in vitro. J Biol Chem 1982; 257(1):545-548.
117. Heeley DH, Watson MH, Mak AS et al. Effect of phosphorylation on the interaction and functional properties of rabbit striated muscle alpha alpha-tropomyosin. J Biol Chem 1989; 264(5):2424-2430.
118. Heeley DH. Investigation of the effects of phosphorylation of rabbit striated muscle alpha alpha-tropomyosin and rabbit skeletal muscle troponin-T. Eur J Biochem 1994; 221(1):129-137.
119. Somara S, Pang H, Bitar KN. Agonist-induced association of tropomyosin with protein kinase Calpha in colonic smooth muscle. Am J Physiol Gastrointest Liver Physiol 2005; 288(2):G268-G276.
120. Mateos J, Herranz R, Domingo A et al. The structural role of high molecular weight tropomyosins in dipteran indirect flight muscle and the effect of phosphorylation. J Muscle Res Cell Motil 2006; 27(3-4):189-201.
121. Vahebi S, Ota A, Li M et al. p38-MAPK induced dephosphorylation of alpha-tropomyosin is associated with depression of myocardial sarcomeric tension and ATPase activity. Circ Res 2007; 100(3):408-415.
122. Houle F, Rousseau S, Morrice N et al. Extracellular signal-regulated kinase mediates phosphorylation of tropomyosin-1 to promote cytoskeleton remodeling in response to oxidative stress: impact on membrane blebbing. Mol Biol Cell 2003; 14(4):1418-1432.
123. Kagawa H, Sugimoto K, Matsumoto H et al. Genome structure, mapping and expression of the tropomyosin gene tmy-1 of Caenorhabditis elegans. J Mol Biol 1995; 251(5):603-613.
124. Anyanful A, Sakube Y, Takuwa K et al. The third and fourth tropomyosin isoforms of Caenorhabditis elegans are expressed in the pharynx and intestines and are essential for development and morphology. J Mol Biol 2001; 313(3):525-537.
125. Karlik CC, Fyrberg EA. Two Drosophila melanogaster tropomyosin genes: structural and functional aspects. Mol Cell Biol 1986; 6(6):1965-1973.
126. Hanke PD, Storti RV. The Drosophila melanogaster tropomyosin II gene produces multiple proteins by use of alternative tissue-specific promoters and alternative splicing. Mol Cell Biol 1988; 8(9):3591-3602.
127. Meedel TH, Hastings KE. Striated muscle-type tropomyosin in a chordate smooth muscle, ascidian body-wall muscle. J Biol Chem 1993; 268(9):6755-6764.
128. Hardy S, Fiszman MY, Osborne HB et al. Characterization of muscle and non muscle Xenopus laevis tropomyosin mRNAs transcribed from the same gene. Developmental and tissue-specific expression. Eur J Biochem 1991; 202(2):431-440.
129. Hardy S, Theze N, Lepetit D et al. The Xenopus laevis TM-4 gene encodes nonmuscle and cardiac tropomyosin isoforms through alternative splicing. Gene 1995; 156(2):265-270.
130. Hardy S, Thiebaud P. Isolation and characterization of cDNA clones encoding the skeletal and smooth muscle Xenopus laevis beta tropomyosin isoforms. Biochim Biophys Acta 1992; 1131(2):239-242.
131. Gaillard C, Theze N, Lerivray H et al. A novel tropomyosin isoform encoded by the Xenopus laevis alpha-TM gene is expressed in the brain. Gene 1998; 207(2):235-239.
132. Gaillard C, Theze N, Hardy S et al. Alpha-tropomyosin gene expression in Xenopus laevis: differential promoter usage during development and controlled expression by myogenic factors. Dev Genes Evol 1998; 207(7):435-445.
133. MacLeod AR. Distinct alpha-tropomyosin mRNA sequences in chicken skeletal muscle. Eur J Biochem 1982; 126(2):293-297.
134. Libri D, Lemonnier M, Meinnel T et al. A single gene codes for the beta subunits of smooth and skeletal muscle tropomyosin in the chicken. J Biol Chem 1989; 264(5):2935-2944.
135. Libri D, Mouly V, Lemonnier M et al. A nonmuscle tropomyosin is encoded by the smooth/skeletal beta-tropomyosin gene and its RNA is transcribed from an internal promoter. J Biol Chem 1990; 265(6):3471-3473.
136. Toutant M, Fiszman MY, Lemonnier M. The muscle specific promoter of chick beta tropomyosin gene requires helix-loop-helix myogenic regulatory factors and ubiquitous transcription factors. C R Acad Sci III 1993; 316(8):711-715.
137. Forry-Schaudies S, Hughes SH. The chicken tropomyosin 1 gene generates nine mRNAs by alternative splicing. J Biol Chem 1991; 266(21):13821-13827.
138. Mak AS, Smillie LB, Stewart GR. A comparison of the amino acid sequences of rabbit skeletal muscle alpha- and beta-tropomyosins. J Biol Chem 1980; 255(8):3647-3655.

139. Denz CR, Narshi A, Zajdel RW et al. Expression of a novel cardiac-specific tropomyosin isoform in humans. Biochem Biophys Res Commun 2004; 320(4):1291-1297.
140. MacLeod AR, Houlker C, Reinach FC et al. A muscle-type tropomyosin in human fibroblasts: evidence for expression by an alternative RNA splicing mechanism. Proc Natl Acad Sci USA 1985; 82(23):7835-7839.
141. Cooley BC, Bergtrom G. Multiple combinations of alternatively spliced exons in rat tropomyosin-alpha gene mRNA: evidence for 20 new isoforms in adult tissues and cultured cells. Arch Biochem Biophys 2001; 390(1):71-77.
142. Beisel KW, Kennedy JE. Identification of novel alternatively spliced isoforms of the tropomyosin-encoding gene, TMnm, in the rat cochlea. Gene 1994; 143(2):251-256.
143. Lees-Miller JP, Yan A, Helfman DM. Structure and complete nucleotide sequence of the gene encoding rat fibroblast tropomyosin 4. J Mol Biol 1990; 213(3):399-405.
144. Nicholson-Flynn K, Hitchcock-DeGregori SE, Levitt P. Restricted expression of the actin-regulatory protein, tropomyosin, defines distinct boundaries, evaginating neuroepithelium and choroid plexus forerunners during early CNS development. J Neurosci 1996; 16(21):6853-6863.
145. Schevzov G, Gunning P, Jeffrey PL et al. Tropomyosin localization reveals distinct populations of microfilaments in neurites and growth cones. Mol Cell Neurosci 1997; 8(6):439-454.
146. Temm-Grove CJ, Jockusch BM, Weinberger RP et al. Distinct localizations of tropomyosin isoforms in LLC-PK1 epithelial cells suggests specialized function at cell-cell adhesions. Cell Motil Cytoskeleton 1998; 40(4):393-407.
147. Prasad GL, Meissner S, Sheer DG et al. A cDNA encoding a muscle-type tropomyosin cloned from a human epithelial cell line: identity with human fibroblast tropomyosin TM1. Biochem Biophys Res Commun 1991; 177(3):1068-1075.
148. Novy RE, Sellers JR, Liu LF et al. In vitro functional characterization of bacterially expressed human fibroblast tropomyosin isoforms and their chimeric mutants. Cell Motil Cytoskeleton 1993; 26(3):248-261.
149. Lin JL, Geng X, Bhattacharya SD et al. Isolation and sequencing of a novel tropomyosin isoform preferentially associated with colon cancer. Gastroenterology 2002; 123(1):152-162.
150. Hannan AJ, Gunning P, Jeffrey PL et al. Structural compartments within neurons: developmentally regulated organization of microfilament isoform mRNA and protein. Molecular & Cellular Neuroscience 1998; 11(5-6):289-304.
151. Lin JJ, Chou CS, Lin JL. Monoclonal antibodies against chicken tropomyosin isoforms: production, characterization and application. Hybridoma 1985; 4(3):223-242.

CHAPTER 5

Tropomyosin:
Function Follows Structure

Sarah E. Hitchcock-DeGregori*

Abstract

Tropomyosin is known as the archetypal coiled coil, being the first to be sequenced and modeled. Studies of the structure and dynamics of tropomyosin, accompanied by biochemical and biophysical analyses of tropomyosin, mutants and model peptides, have revealed the complexity and subtleties required for tropomyosin function. Interruptions in the canonical coiled coil allow for bends and regions of local instability that are required for tropomyosin to bind to the helical actin filament. This chapter highlights insights gained from recent structural studies as they relate to variations in tropomyosin's coiled-coil structure that are essential for binding to actin and the relationship of periodic repeats to actin molecules in the filament.

Introduction

The adage, "form follows function" as applied to architecture and product design, can be turned around as we consider tropomyosin. The naming of tropomyosin and its proposed α-helical coiled-coil structure came long before knowledge of its localization and function, beyond its muscle source and presumed myofibrillar origin. There are three excellent reviews on the discovery of tropomyosin and its coiled-coil structure.[1-3] The present review, not intended to be comprehensive, will emphasize how recent structural studies of tropomyosin and its fragments give insight into how subtle features built into the α-helical coiled coil allow tropomyosin to associate end-to-end along the actin filament and cooperatively regulate its function. This chapter includes an overview of tropomyosin's coiled-coil structure, illustrations of the roles atypical residues play in allowing axial flexibility and formation of the intermolecular "head-to-tail" complex and a discussion of insights the structural studies give into tropomyosin's fundamental functions, cooperative actin binding and regulation. While there are many tropomyosin isoforms (see Chapters 2,4 and 16), the discussion here will be restricted to vertebrate striated muscle α-tropomyosin, the form used for most structural studies.

The Tropomyosin Coiled Coil

Tropomyosin was first isolated and described as an asymmetric protein by Bailey in 1946[4] and recognized to belong to the α-helical *k-m-e-f* class of proteins by Astbury in an early X-ray study.[5] Based on these and other studies, Crick proposed a model for the α-helical coiled coil in which two α-helices with a seven-fold sequence periodicity associate to form a supercoil (Fig. 1). The hydrophobic residues at the first and fourth positions in the repeat (*a* and *d*, where the seven residues are *a, b, c, d, e, f, g*) pack in a "knobs" into "holes" fashion to hold the two chains together.[6] Elucidation of the first tropomyosin amino acid sequence,[7,8] completed in 1975 and fully published

*Sarah E. Hitchcock-DeGregori—Department of Neuroscience and Cell Biology, Robert Wood Johnson Medical School, 675 Hoes Lane, Piscataway, New Jersey 08854, USA.
Email: hitchcoc@umdnj.edu

Tropomyosin, edited by Peter Gunning. ©2008 Landes Bioscience
and Springer Science+Business Media.

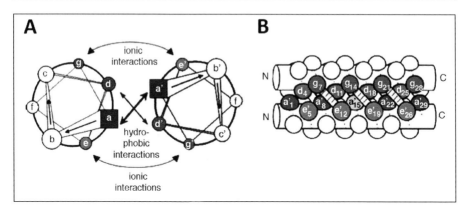

Figure 1. Model of a two-chained, parallel coiled coil such as that in tropomyosin (modified from Mason and Arndt[64]). A) Helical wheel representation viewing the helix axis from (www.molbiotech.uni-freiburg.de/ka/images/coiled-coil%20overview.jpg) the N terminus to the C terminus. B) Side view in which the helical backbones are represented by cylinders. The positions in the heptad are labeled *a* to *g* and *a′* to *g′* on the two helices. The interacting residues that stabilize the coiled coil are colored or shaded: *a* and *d* form the hydrophobic interface; and *e* and *g* pack against the hydrophobic core and can form interhelical salt bridges if oppositely charged; the *g* residue can form a salt bridge between the oppositely charged *e′* residue in the next heptad of the other helix.

in 1978,[9] confirmed Crick's anticipated heptapeptide repeat of hydrophobic residues and showed that the tropomyosin sequence is consistent with formation of an uninterrupted coiled coil along its entire length.[10,11] The pattern of charged residues in the *e* and *g* positions favors interhelical salt bridge formation when the chains are in register[11,12] (Fig. 1), an arrangement that was verified by chemical methods. Thus, tropomyosin became the archetypal coiled coil, but as we will see, it is not a paragon. The predicted "knobs" into "holes" packing of the coiled coil's hydrophobic interface and *e-g* saltbridges were initially proven in the GCN4 leucine zipper structure[13] and more recently in the first high resolution structure of a tropomyosin fragment.[14] The early studies are remarkable in their foresight and impact as we now recognize the wide distribution of the coiled-coil fold and its role in protein folding, oligomerization and assembly of proteins into higher order structures (reviewed in ref. 3).

Sarcomeric and HMW (high molecular weight) nonmuscle tropomyosins are 284 amino acids long and the two chains associate in parallel and in register to make a rod-shaped molecule approximately 20 Å in diameter and 400 Å long, the length of seven actin subunits in the filament (Fig. 4A). The parameters of tropomyosin's supercoil helix (in the crystals) differ from those of the actin filament helix; interaction requires plasticity. Tropomyosin is unusual in that there are no discontinuities in the diagnostic "coiled-coil" heptapeptide repeat by "skips" or "stutters" found in most other coiled coils of similar length (reviewed in ref. 3). However, detailed sequence analyses show that tropomyosin is by no means canonical along its length. Recent structural and functional studies have shown that tropomyosin's noncanonical regions contribute to the "flexibility" of the coiled coil and are critical for tropomyosin's most fundamental function, binding along the grooves of the helical actin filament.

The Tropomyosin Interface: Unstable Regions Interrupt Canonical Coiled Coil

Different types of "flexibility" contribute to the dynamics of the tropomyosin molecule; backbone, side-chain and inter-chain staggers can all increase the degrees of freedom of space sampling by the side-chains to optimize binding to the target, without having a major change in structure of the α-helical backbone. These points will be illustrated below with examples from high resolution tropomyosin structures. In addition, the least stable regions may be locally unfolded (or "molten globule") at physiological temperatures. Together, these forms of local flexibility can have global effects on the ability of a tropomyosin molecule to bind to its targets: another tropomyosin molecule, the actin filament, troponin and tropomodulin.

Despite the continuous coiled-coil conformation, it is well-established that stability is non-uniform along the length of the molecule. There are structurally distinct domains in the crystal structure that differ in stability and conformational flexibility, as well as variations in the inter-chain distance and the length of the coiled-coil pitch.[15,16] Intrinsic flexibility and the presence of multiple unfolding domains of differing stability and susceptibility to proteolysis are also documented in numerous biochemical and biophysical studies (see refs. 17-23). Regions of lower stability are known to be relevant to actin binding and regulatory function.[24-26]

The highest resolution in crystals of full-length tropomyosin is only 7 Å because of their high solvent content.[16,27,28] These structures established the overall undulating coiled-coil structure and illustrate the flexibility and bends in the crystal lattice along with the local variations in the pitch and molecular radius that reflect variation in the interface residues. The intermolecular junction is unresolved (to be discussed below). Atomic resolution NMR and crystal structures of tropomyosin fragments now span all but eight internal residues of the HMW striated muscle α-tropomyosin.[14,29-34] These structures give new insights into the complexity of the tropomyosin coiled coil as well as the source and significance of the dynamics.

One remarkable outcome of the structural studies is the variable and dynamic nature of the coiled-coil interface and its significance for binding along the helical actin filament. We can now appreciate how local destabilization caused by a poorly-packed interface with small hydrophobic or polar residues (such as Ser or Ala), or large, nonhydrophobic residues (such as Tyr or Glu) can have global effects on the structure. An unusual feature of tropomyosin among coiled coils is the high incidence of Ala at interface *d* positions,[35] as well as other "noncanonical" amino acids. A weak periodicity in residues with small versus large uncharged side chains was first noted by McLachlan and Stewart.[36] The "Ala clusters", featured by Brown et al,[14] are illustrated in Figure 2A. Alternating stabilizing and conserved destabilizing interface residues have been suggested to be important for in register folding of the two chains, overall stability and interhelical distance.[37] It is significant that some disease-causing mutations in tropomyosin alter the stability of the coiled-coil interface (see Chapters 11 and 12).

A major step forward in understanding the significance of conserved destabilizing "Ala clusters" came with the atomic resolution structure of residues 1-80, the first to contain an Ala cluster[14] (RCSB Protein Data Bank, accession code 1IC2). Brown and colleagues noticed that the coiled-coil radius was lower at the Ala cluster than in regions of canonical coiled coil, a feature that has been observed at the sites of all five Ala clusters in the other tropomyosin structures (RCSB Protein Data Bank, accession codes 2B9C; 2D9E).[29,34] Figure 2B illustrates the backbones in the region of the Ala cluster (Fig. 2B, left) that are axially staggered and closer together by ~2 Å than backbones of region with the interface leucines (Fig. 2B, right), compared in the central overlay. The effect of the interface residues on core packing is featured in the models in Figure 2C. The core of the Ala cluster region (Figs. 2B, left and 2C, left) is less well packed and the backbones are closer together as reflected in the smaller interhelical distance, compared to the model with a canonical coiled-coil interface of Leu and Val (Fig. 2C, center). The diameter and the packing reflect the character of the core side-chains; an interface with the larger destabilizing residues Asn and Gln is poorly packed (Fig. 2C, right), but the interhelical distance is similar to that of the larger hydrophobic side-chains.[38] In two of the five Ala cluster structures the axial stagger is followed by a specific axial bend.[14,29] Bends are not observed in all molecules or at all locations with Ala-rich interfaces, suggesting that the bends reflect molecular flexibility that can be influenced by crystal packing, rather than being fixed structures. The distribution of destabilizing Ala clusters along the length of the molecule led Brown and colleagues to suggest that they are de facto "skips" or "stutters," and that the bends provide flexibility required for tropomyosin to wind around the

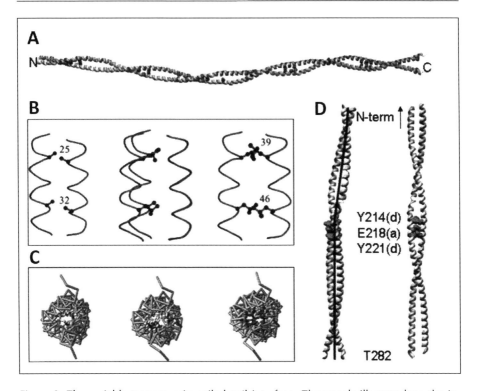

Figure 2. The variable tropomyosin coiled-coil interface. The panels illustrate how the interface residues of the coiled-coil influence packing and the interhelical distance. A) The side-chains of the interface Ala clusters on a ribbon model of the 7 Å structure[28] illustrate their quasi-periodic distribution. The model is oriented to highlight the bends in the crystal structure of the full-length tropomyosin molecule. B) Models of segments of the crystal structure of the first 80 residues of tropomyosin show the influence of the interface residues on packing, axial stagger and interhelical distance. The chains with an Ala cluster (left) are staggered, the interhelical distance is closer by ~2 Å and the interface is poorly packed compared to the canonical coiled coil interface (right); superimposed in the middle. Modified from Brown et al.[14] C) Models of a region of tropomyosin to show the effect of interface residues on core packing and interhelical distance as viewed through the core axis. The side-chains of three interface residues of each polypeptide are illustrated. Left: Ala, Ala, Ala; Middle: Leu, Val, Leu; Right: Asn, Gln, Asn. The side-chains are dark grey and aqua with hydrogens in white, oxygens in red and nitrogens in magenta. Modified from Singh and Hitchcock-DeGregori.[38] D) Model of the structure of the C-terminal third of tropomyosin, stabilized at the N terminus with a leucine zipper. The side-chains of the destabilizing interface residues, Tyr214-Glu218-Tyr221 are illustrated. The location of this interface at the site of a bend in the coiled-coil axis is illustrated at the left; the increased interhelical distance is illustrated at the right in a model rotated by 90 degrees. Based on a figure in Nitanai et al.[34]

helical actin filament and to carry out its dynamic role in thin filament regulation[14] (see Chapters by Tobacman, Lehman and Craig, Martson and El-Mezgueldi). The importance of an unstable interface, versus Ala residues or an axial stagger per se, is supported by mutagenesis studies in which destabilizing residues at the sites of Ala clusters were shown to be an essential requirement for cooperative actin binding by tropomyosin.[26,38]

The flexibility is illustrated in the 7 Å structure of full-length tropomyosin that contains two global bends (RCSB Protein Data Bank, accession code 1C1G)[28,34] (Fig. 2A). One of these is at a site with noncanonical, destabilizing residues (Y214, E218 and Y221 at *d, a, d* interface positions) shown in a high resolution structure of a tropomyosin fragment[34] where there is a poorly-packed interface and a high interhelical distance, higher than with a canonical Leu-Val interface (Fig. 2D). Nitanai and colleagues point out that the second bend in the full-length molecule is at D137, another poorly packed region with an Ala and an Asp at the interface and a peak interhelical distance.[29] The region between the bends at D137 and Y214 is important for actin binding,[25,26] for cooperative activation of the actin filament by myosin[39,40] and is the region where the troponin "core" that contains troponin C, troponin I and the C-terminal domain of troponin T binds, (reviewed in refs. 1, 2). One may imagine how segmental mobility of this region, regulated by the binding of Ca^{2+} to troponin C, or the binding of myosin heads to the actin filament, could be a critical feature of thin filament activation.

The most dramatic effect of a noncanonical coiled-coil interface on the structure is at the C terminus that forms the "overlap" complex with the N terminus responsible for end-to-end association of tropomyosin along the length of the actin filament. In two crystal structures, the C-terminal 22 residues splay apart and two molecules associate to form a nonnative antiparallel four helix bundle (RCSB Protein Data Bank, accession code entries 1QKL, 2D9E).[33,34] This flexibility is allowed by atypical interface residues, Q263 (*d*) and Y267 (*a*) that are not packed in a "knobs" into "holes" fashion and allow the C terminal chains to spread apart and form the intermolecular complex (Fig. 3B). In solution, the C-terminal structure is entirely different (PDB Entry 1MV4).[41] The C terminus is monomeric (two chains) and instead of splaying apart, after residue 269 the chains form an unusual linear, parallel arrangement with atypical hydrophobic interactions (Fig. 3B,D). As in the crystal structure, Q263 and Y267 are poorly packed and exhibit conformational flexibility. The flexibility is required for function since mutation of Q263 to Leu, a canonical interface residue, increases the stability and inhibits the ability of the C-terminal peptide to form a ternary complex with the N terminus of tropomyosin and troponin T.[31]

The Intermolecular Complex

Tropomyosin molecules associate end-to-end to form a continuous cable along both sides of the actin filament (Fig. 4A). The molecular length of tropomyosin calculated in crystals and paracrystals was shorter than expected for a full helical molecule of 284 residues, leading to the suggestion of an overlap of approximately 9 residues.[10,42] The requirement of the extreme ends for complex formation and normal actin affinity was originally established by carboxypeptidase digestion of the C terminus[43] and deletion mutagenesis of the N terminus.[44] Although the site of the molecular ends was identified in crystals of full-length tropomyosin, the structure was unresolved,[16,27,28] leaving open the question of how sequential tropomyosins and their proposed actin binding sites (see below) relate to each other and to the actin monomers in the filament. Atomic resolution structures and dynamics of the N terminus and C terminus have been obtained using model peptides[30,33,41] and the structure of an overlap complex formed using model peptides has been determined using NMR.[32]

As mentioned above, the helices in the C terminus are parallel in solution[41] or splayed apart to form an antiparallel complex with another C-terminal molecule in the crystal structure,[33-34] exemplifying the flexible hinge next to the beginning of the overlap region. In contrast, the N terminus is canonical coiled coil beginning with the N-acetylated N-terminal Met.[30] N-acetylation is required for coiled coil formation and for overlap complex formation.[45,46] The recombinant peptide used for the crystal structure of the first 80 amino acids is unacetylated and the first four residues are not in a helical coiled-coil conformation.[14]

The solution NMR structure of the overlap complex formed using model peptides is an almost symmetric, interleaved four-chained structure in which the C-terminal chains spread apart to form a cleft allowing insertion of 11 residues of the N-terminal coiled-coil[32] (RCSB Protein Data Bank, accession code 2G9J) (Fig. 3A,C). In the complex the planes of the two ends are rotated 90 degrees relative to each other (best visualized in Fig. 3C), a feature that has significant consequences for actin binding (see below). Most of the side-chain interactions at the interface of the overlap region

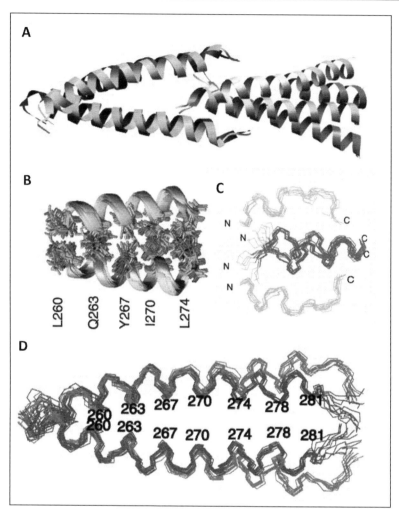

Figure 3. Solution NMR structure and dynamics of the tropomyosin overlap complex. A) Overlay of two ribbon models of the N-terminal/C-terminal complex illustrating the maximal variation between the calculated structures due to the flexibility of the interface of the complex. B) Structural changes in residues 260-270 of the C terminus upon complex formation. The backbone is depicted by a ribbon; the side-chains of interface residues L260, Q263, Y267, I270 and L274 are illustrated. Dark grey or brown: free C terminus; light grey or cyan, C-terminus in the complex. C) Ten structures of the N-terminal/C-terminal overlap complex of tropomyosin. C terminus, light grey or cyan; N terminus, dark grey or brown. The orientation illustrates the 90 degree rotation of the planes of the coiled coil relative to each other. D) Structural changes in the C-terminal domain upon complex formation: unbound, brown or dark grey; bound, cyan or light grey. Modified from Greenfield et al.[32]

involve intermolecular hydrophobic interactions of the canonical *a* and *d* interface positions, as well as between hydrophobic groups in noncanonical coiled coil positions. The structure differs from previously-proposed, asymmetric models of the tropomyosin junction.[10,47] The detailed structure of the complex also differs from that of a typical four-helix bundle in that the last five residues of the C terminus are not helical and have unusual packing interactions. The structure of the C

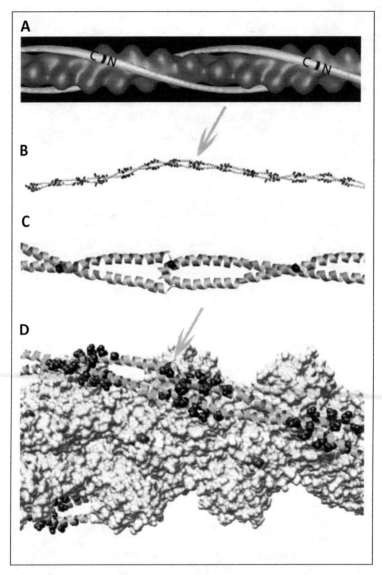

Figure 4. Binding of tropomyosin to the actin filament. A) Surface view of the thin filament showing actin and muscle tropomyosin. The image is based on a helical image reconstruction of electron micrographs of F-actin-tropomyosin-troponin, +Ca^{2+}.[65] Tropomyosin forms a continuous strand along both sides of the helical actin filament such that one tropomyosin molecule spans the length of seven actin subunits. The tropomyosin molecules are associated N terminus-to-C terminus, as indicated on the figure. The thin filament is oriented so that the N terminus of tropomyosin and "minus" or "pointed" end of the actin filament are at the left. Modified from a model prepared by Dr. William Lehman, Boston University School of Medicine, Boston, Massachusetts; modified from Hitchcock-DeGregori et al.[66] B) Model of two full-length molecules of the 7 Å tropomyosin structure joined together with the overlap complex illustrated in Figure 3. The arrow indicated the position of the overlap. The side-chains "consensus" residues are in black and have the similar orientations in the two molecules. Figure legend continued on next page.

Figure 4, continued. C) Detail of three "consensus" sites in the sequential molecules (periods 7, 1 and 2) to show that they have the similar orientations relative to the axis of the coiled coil. The C^α molecule of the first consensus residue in the three sites is marked. D) Model of the joined tropomyosins on a model of the regulated actin filament with EGTA. The side-chains of consensus the residues are shown in black and have similar relationships to the actin monomers in the filament. Residue K238 of actin in dark grey or red serves as a position marker on the actin filament. The axial position of the tropomyosin molecule on the actin filament is arbitrary and we make no inference as to the interaction between specific residues of tropomyosin and actin. Modified from and more completely described in Greenfield et al.[32]

terminus in the complex is similar to that seen in the crystal structures. Figure 3D compares the solution structure of the free C terminus to that in the complex.

A striking feature of the overlap complex structure is the conformational flexibility of the interface in the overlap region as well as in the region preceding the junction. The two models included in Figure 3A illustrate the maximal variation between ten calculated structures due to the flexibility of the interface of the overlap complex. The plasticity of the previously-mentioned residues Q263 and Y267 in the studies of the C terminus, as well as I270 (*d*), allows the chains to splay apart and bind the N terminus. Figure 3B shows the dynamic nature of the side-chains of interface residues L260, Q263, Y267, I270 and L274 in the region preceding the overlap complex upon complex formation (free, dark grey or brown; complex, light grey or cyan). Note for example that the side-chains of Q263 move away from the interface whereas those of Y267 move closer to the side-chains of I270 as the chains splay apart to bind the chains of the N-terminal coiled coil. The residues within the junctional interface are also dynamic and provide the plasticity that may be important for tropomyosin to bind to actin. Just as flexibility in internal regions of the molecule at sites of Ala clusters or other destabilizing residues is required to bind actin, the ability to bend at the junction between molecules is presumably essential for tropomyosin to form a cable that follows the long-pitch helix along the length of the filament.

Actin Binding Sites on Tropomyosin

Tropomyosin's paramount function is to bind to the actin filament; its regulatory functions follow. High molecular weight tropomyosins span the length of seven actin monomers in the filament (Fig. 4A). When seven-fold and fourteen-fold repeats that originate from gene duplication were first identified in the amino acid sequence, they were proposed to relate to actin binding sites along the length of one actin molecule.[11,12,36] These repeats are in addition to the heptapeptide repeat of hydrophobic residues and the weak periodicity of destabilizing interface residues in the amino acid sequence required for coiled coil formation and molecular flexibility. A fourteen-fold quasi-periodic repeat includes charged and nonpolar, non-interface residues poised to be involved in actin binding, versus coiled-coil formation. McLachlan and Stewart[36] proposed the periodicity to be seven pairs of alternating α- and β-zones that correspond to the two positions of tropomyosin on the actin filament in the then recently-introduced steric blocking model. They suggested that tropomyosin would roll in response to Ca^{2+} binding to troponin C allowing the two sets of sites, azimuthally located 90 degrees apart on the coiled coil, to occupy the blocked versus the open state on the thin filament.

In a later analysis Phillips[48] took into account the azimuthal position of the side-chains in the heptapeptide repeat of the helical coiled coil, whereas the earlier analyses were based on a linear amino acid sequence. He identified a seven-fold repeat of seven charged and nonpolar residues in *b*, *c* and *f* positions, that we refer to as "consensus" residues, that roughly correspond to McLachlan and Stewart's α-zones and are more regular than the β-zones. Because of the underlying heptapeptide repeat, the Phillips repeats are multiples of seven residues, either 35 or 42 residues long, with an average 39.3 residue length, as in the linear sequence analysis (Fig. 4B,D).

It has been inferred, based on the logic of simple symmetry, that since one tropomyosin spans the length of seven actin monomers in the actin filament there should be 3.5 turns of the supercoil, such that there is one actin periodic repeat per half turn.[2,36,42] It has long been appreciated that the pitch of the supercoil is variable along the length of the molecule and that the average pitch is ~140 Å, or about three turns of the supercoil per molecular length. Using the program TWISTER[49] that allows more accurate calculation of pitch, we found the 7 Å structure[28] has an average pitch of 149 Å for residues 2-274,[32] close to the 146 Å average pitch calculated for the structure of the mid-region of tropomyosin.[29] The standard deviation is large, reflecting the highly variable pitch. The molecular length of the tropomyosin molecule in the 7 Å structure, accounting for the 11 residues in the overlap complex, is 400 Å, close to the distance needed to span seven actin monomers at a radius of 40-42 Å in the filament.[50,51] With these considerations, the number of supercoil repeats per tropomyosin molecule is less than three, about 2.7, or ~5.5 half-turns of the supercoil. Sequential molecules joined together in the overlap complex are rotated 90 degrees with respect to each other, an arrangement that "corrects" for the non-integral number of half turns.[32] Another consequence is that the relationship of the repeats to actin is equivalent from one tropomyosin to the next along the actin filament.

Given that the number of periodic repeats (seven) differs from the number of half-turns of the supercoil (5.5), are the "consensus" residues in equivalent positions with respect to actin? Do the "consensus residues" form an actin binding site? Does the tropomyosin roll or slide on the filament to carry out its regulatory functions? None of these questions will be answered until there is a high resolution structure of actin in complex with tropomyosin; at this time it is neither available nor on the horizon. What we can say is that the solution NMR structure of the overlap complex was easily modeled into the unresolved intermolecular junction present in the 7 Å structure (Fig. 4B), but not into a tropomyosin model in which the ends are parallel.[52] The residues in the proposed actin binding sites in sequential molecules have equivalent azimuthal relationships on the coiled coil and to the actin monomers in a filament model[32] (Fig. 4B-D). These relationships would not be true with an even number of half turns of the supercoil, or if the planes of the coiled coils in the overlap complex were parallel. Because the repeats are 35 or 42 residues long, the axial spacing is variable. The bends and regions of local instability in the tropomyosin molecule as well as the variable pitch of the supercoil should allow the tropomyosin to accommodate local variations in the axial and azimuthal spacing of the periodic sites upon binding along the length of the actin filament. Indeed such accommodations are essential for the two molecules to associate, as illustrated by the inability to "dock" atomic models of the 7 Å tropomyosin structure onto the model of the actin filament over a distance of more than a few actin molecules. Flexibility of the actin filament may also be involved.

While there has been a lot of discussion of periodic actin binding sites, it should be emphasized that the fidelity is low and they are not easily recognizable as are, for example, a divalent cation binding sites in troponin C and other EF-hands. Mutagenesis of tropomyosin has, however, given support for the veracity of the Phillips periodic repeat of seven "consensus" residues. In period 5 (residues 165-188), the "consensus" residues coupled with an unstable coiled-coiled interface are essential for cooperative actin binding.[26] While the regions of tropomyosin do have specific functions and do not contribute equally to the overall affinity, discussed in,[25] they are quasi-equivalent with respect to actin affinity, with an emphasis on quasi. The period 1 or period 2 consensus regions can substitute for period 5 with respect to actin binding, as long as the interface is unstable.[53]

What Is the Structural Basis of Isoform Specificity?

The alternatively-expressed exons together with formation of heterodimers results in a large number of different tropomyosins; the specific localizations and functions of specific isoforms are discussed in other chapters (see Chapters 4, 6, 14, 16-22) and reviewed in Gunning et al.[54] The amino acid sequences are overall conserved and the coiled-coil structure is retained, yet the subtle structural differences can have profound effects on functional specificity. From in vitro and in vivo studies on the effects of single-site mutations and alternatively-expressed exons we know that seemingly small changes can influence protein folding, actin affinity, regulatory function and the cell's cytoskeleton, structure and motility in ways we cannot yet understand at the structural level. For example, the specific binding of troponin T to striated muscle tropomyosin[55] depends on the exon 9a-encoded sequence,[56,57] but an understanding of the specificity will require an atomic-resolution structure of the tropomyosin overlap complex with troponin T. In a more recent illustration, the basis of isoform-specific binding of LMW tropomyosins to tropomodulin has been primarily ascribed to a single residue that has little apparent effect on the tropomyosin structure, but a big affect on tropomodulin affinity,[58] discussed in the chapter by Kostyukova. Models based on existing structures and knowledge from model peptide studies[37,59] may give limited insight into how isoform-specific sequences may influence structure and stability.

We do understand the effect of isoform-specific sequence on structure of the alternate N-terminal sequences of LMW and HMW α-tropomyosins. As discussed above, the conserved HMW-tropomyosin N-terminus forms a coiled coil in solution[30] and the structure is retained in complex with the C terminus[32] (Fig. 4). The N terminus of LMW tropomyosins shares homology with the HMW sequence, but contains a variable N-terminal extension, five residues in α-tropomyosin that are nonhelical and flexible in solution.[60] Recombinant tropomyosins that contain LMW tropomyosin bind to actin with higher affinity than their HMW counterparts.[61,62] An overlap complex containing the LMW amino terminus and the nonmuscle/smooth muscle C terminus is more stable and more dynamic than the striated muscle overlap complex discussed earlier. The data indicate that the binding domain includes residues 1-17 of the N-terminus (compared to 11 residues in the striated muscle complex); the first five residues of the N terminus become helical and interact with the C terminus.[63] The longer and more flexible overlap complex may account for the observed higher actin affinity of tropomyosins containing these terminal sequences.

Summary and Perspective

In a sense we have known the structure of tropomyosin since 1953; determination of the amino acid sequence in the 1970s established it as the archetypal coiled coil. However, it has taken another generation to understand that this simple protein fold is far from plain. The availability of high resolution crystal and solution structures within the last decade has allowed major progress and the realization that tropomyosin's regions of noncanonical sequence have variable noncanonical structures and that tropomyosin's non-ideality is what allows it to function as a universal regulator of the actin filament. The irregularities in the coiled-coil structure, coupled with structural and folding studies of model coiled-coil peptides have led to a good understanding of how sequence contributes to the basic coiled-coil structure. Solution of the overlap complex structure answers the long unresolved question of the relationship between sequential tropomyosin molecules when they self-associate on the actin filament. Studies of designed mutations, as well as disease-causing mutations in humans, have given us an idea of the fundamental requirements for actin binding. The major step now is to learn the structures and dynamics of tropomyosin bound to its targets: actin, troponin and tropomodulin and possibly other proteins. Only then will we gain insight into how the different regions of tropomyosin are involved in the complex process of cooperative actin filament regulation.

Acknowledgements

I thank Dr. Norma J. Greenfield and Dr. Abhishek Singh for discussions, Dr. Singh for assistance in preparing Figure 2 and Ms. Lucy Kotylanskaya for comments on the manuscript. I am grateful to the NIH (GM36326) for long term support of our studies of tropomyosin structure and function.

References

1. Perry SV. Vertebrate tropomyosin: distribution, properties and function. J Muscle Res Cell Motil 2001; 22(1):5-49.
2. Brown JH, Cohen C. Regulation of muscle contraction by tropomyosin and troponin: how structure illuminates function. Adv Protein Chem 2005; 71:121-159.
3. Lupas AN, Gruber M. The structure of alpha-helical coiled coils. Adv Protein Chem 2005; 70:37-78.
4. Bailey K. Tropomyosin: a new asymmetric protein component of muscle. Nature 1946; 157:368-369.
5. Astbury WT, Reed R, Spark, LC. An X-ray and electron microscope study of tropomyosin. Biochem. J 1948; 43:282-287.

6. Crick FHC. The packing of alpha-helices. Simple coiled-coils. Acta Crystallographica. 1953; 6:689-697.
7. Hodges RS, Sodek J, Smillie LB et al. Tropomyosin: Amino acid sequence and coiled-coil structure. Cold Spring Harbor Symp. Quant Biol 1972; 37:299-310.
8. Sodek J, Hodges RS, Smillie LB et al. Amino-acid sequence of rabbit skeletal tropomyosin and its coiled-coil structure. Proc Natl Acad Sci USA 1972; 69(12):3800-3804.
9. Stone D, Smillie LB. The amino acid sequence of rabbit skeletal alpha-tropomyosin. The NH2-terminal half and complete sequence. J Biol Chem 1978; 253(4):1137-1148.
10. McLachlan AD, Stewart M. Tropomyosin coiled-coil interactions: evidence for an unstaggered structure. J Mol Biol 1975; 98(2):293-304.
11. Parry DA. Analysis of the primary sequence of alpha-tropomyosin from rabbit skeletal muscle. J Mol Biol 1975; 98(3):519-535.
12. McLachlan AD, Stewart M, Smillie LB. Sequence repeats in alpha-tropomyosin. J Mol Biol 1975; 98(2):281-291.
13. O'Shea EK, Klemm JD, Kim PS et al. X-ray structure of the GCN4 leucine zipper, a two-stranded, parallel coiled coil. Science 1991; 254(5031):539-544.
14. Brown JH, Kim KH, Jun G et al. Deciphering the design of the tropomyosin molecule. Proc Natl Acad Sci USA 2001; 98(15):8496-8501.
15. Phillips GN Jr, Fillers JP, Cohen C. Motions of tropomyosin. Crystal as metaphor. Biophys J 1980; 32(1):485-502.
16. Phillips GN Jr, Fillers JP, Cohen C. Tropomyosin crystal structure and muscle regulation. J Mol Biol 1986; 192(1):111-131.
17. Graceffa P, Lehrer SS. The excimer fluorescence of pyrene-labeled tropomyosin. A probe of conformational dynamics. J Biol Chem 1980; 255(23):11296-11300.
18. Potekhin SA, Privalov PL. Co-operative blocks in tropomyosin. J Mol Biol 1982; 159(3):519-535.
19. Betteridge DR, Lehrer SS. Two conformational states of didansylcystine-labeled rabbit cardiac tropomyosin. J Mol Biol 1983; 167(2):481-496.
20. Ueno H. Local structural changes in tropomyosin detected by a trypsin-probe method. Biochemistry 1984; 23(20):4791-4798.
21. Swenson CA, Stellwagen NC. Flexibility of smooth and skeletal tropomyosins. Biopolymers 1989; 28(5):955-963.
22. Ishii Y, Hitchcock-DeGregori S, Mabuchi K et al. Unfolding domains of recombinant fusion alpha alpha-tropomyosin. Protein Sci 1992; 1(10):1319-1325.
23. Phillips GN Jr, Chacko S. Mechanical properties of tropomyosin and implications for muscle regulation. Biopolymers 1996; 38(1):89-95.
24. Ishii Y, Lehrer SS. Fluorescence studies of the conformation of pyrene-labeled tropomyosin: effects of F-actin and myosin subfragment 1. Biochemistry 1985; 24(23):6631-6638.
25. Hitchcock-DeGregori SE, Song Y, Greenfield NJ. Functions of tropomyosin's periodic repeats. Biochemistry 2002; 41(50):15036-15044.
26. Singh A, Hitchcock-DeGregori SE. Dual requirement for flexibility and specificity for binding of the coiled-coil tropomyosin to its target, actin. Structure 2006; 14(1):43-50.
27. Whitby FG, Kent H, Stewart F et al. Structure of tropomyosin at 9 angstroms resolution. J Mol Biol 1992; 227(2):441-452.
28. Whitby FG, Phillips GN Jr. Crystal structure of tropomyosin at 7 Angstroms resolution. Proteins 2000; 38(1):49-59.
29. Brown JH, Zhou Z, Reshetnikova L et al. Structure of the mid-region of tropomyosin: bending and binding sites for actin. Proc Natl Acad Sci USA 2005; 102(52):18878-18883.
30. Greenfield NJ, Montelione GT, Farid RS et al. The structure of the N-terminus of striated muscle alpha-tropomyosin in a chimeric peptide: nuclear magnetic resonance structure and circular dichroism studies. Biochemistry 1998; 37(21):7834-7843.
31. Greenfield NJ, Palm T, Hitchcock-DeGregori SE. Structure and interactions of the carboxyl terminus of striated muscle alpha-tropomyosin: it is important to be flexible. Biophys J 2002; 83(5):2754-2766.
32. Greenfield NJ, Huang YJ, Swapna GV et al. Solution NMR Structure of the Junction between Tropomyosin Molecules: Implications for Actin Binding and Regulation. J Mol Biol 2006, 364:80-96.
33. Li Y, Mui S, Brown JH et al. The crystal structure of the C-terminal fragment of striated-muscle alpha-tropomyosin reveals a key troponin T recognition site. Proc Natl Acad Sci USA 2002; 99(11):7378-7383.
34. Nitanai Y, Minakata S, Maeda K et al. Crystal structures of tropomyosin: flexible coiled-coil. Adv Exp Med Biol 2007; 592:137-151.
35. Conway JF, Parry DA. Structural features in the heptad substructure and longer range repeats of two-stranded alpha-fibrous proteins. Int J Biol Macromol 1990; 12(5):328-334.

36. McLachlan AD, Stewart M. The 14-fold periodicity in alpha-tropomyosin and the interaction with actin. J Mol Biol 1976; 103(2):271-298.
37. Kwok SC, Hodges RS. Stabilizing and destabilizing clusters in the hydrophobic core of long two-stranded alpha-helical coiled-coils. J Biol Chem 2004; 279(20):21576-21588.
38. Singh A, Hitchcock-DeGregori SE. Local destabilization of the tropomyosin coiled coil gives the molecular flexibility required for actin binding. Biochemistry 2003; 42(48):14114-14121.
39. Landis C, Back N, Homsher E et al. Effects of tropomyosin internal deletions on thin filament function. J Biol Chem 1999; 274(44):31279-31285.
40. Hitchcock-DeGregori SE, Song Y, Moraczewska J. Importance of internal regions and the overall length of tropomyosin for actin binding and regulatory function. Biochemistry 2001; 40(7):2104-2112.
41. Greenfield NJ, Swapna GV, Huang Y et al. The structure of the carboxyl terminus of striated alpha-tropomyosin in solution reveals an unusual parallel arrangement of interacting alpha-helices. Biochemistry 2003; 42(3):614-619.
42. Phillips GN Jr, Lattman EE, Cummins P et al. Crystal structure and molecular interactions of tropomyosin. Nature 1979; 278(5703):413-417.
43. Johnson P, Smillie LB. Polymerizability of rabbit skeletal tropomyosin: effects of enzymic and chemical modifications. Biochemistry 1977; 16(10):2264-2269.
44. Cho YJ, Liu J, Hitchcock-DeGregori SE. The amino terminus of muscle tropomyosin is a major determinant for function. J Biol Chem 1990; 265(1):538-545.
45. Hitchcock-DeGregori SE, Heald RW. Altered actin and troponin binding of amino-terminal variants of chicken striated muscle alpha-tropomyosin expressed in Escherichia coli. J Biol Chem 1987; 262(20):9730-9735.
46. Greenfield NJ, Stafford WF, Hitchcock-DeGregori SE. The effect of N-terminal acetylation on the structure of an N-terminal tropomyosin peptide and alpha alpha-tropomyosin. Protein Sci 1994; 3(3):402-410.
47. Gaffin RD, Gokulan K, Sacchettini JC et al. Changes in end-to-end interactions of tropomyosin affect mouse cardiac muscle dynamics. Am J Physiol Heart Circ Physiol 2006; 291(2):H552-563.
48. Phillips GN Jr. Construction of an atomic model for tropomyosin and implications for interactions with actin. J Mol Biol 1986; 192(1):128-131.
49. Strelkov SV, Burkhard P. Analysis of alpha-helical coiled coils with the program TWISTER reveals a structural mechanism for stutter compensation. J Struct Biol 2002; 137(1-2):54-64.
50. Pirani A, Xu C, Hatch V et al, Lehman W. Single particle analysis of relaxed and activated muscle thin filaments. J Mol Biol 2005; 346(3):761-772.
51. Poole KJ, Lorenz M, Evans G et al. A comparison of muscle thin filament models obtained from electron microscopy reconstructions and low-angle X-ray fibre diagrams from non-overlap muscle. J Struct Biol 2006; 155(2):273-284.
52. Lorenz M, Poole KJ, Popp D et al. An atomic model of the unregulated thin filament obtained by X-ray fiber diffraction on oriented actin-tropomyosin gels. J Mol Biol 1995; 246(1):108-119.
53. Singh A, Hitchcock-DeGregori SE. Tropomyosin's periods are quasi-equivalent for actin binding but have specific regulatory functions. Biochemistry 2007; 46(51):14917-14927.
54. Gunning PW, Schevzov G, Kee AJ et al. Tropomyosin isoforms: divining rods for actin cytoskeleton function. Trends Cell Biol 2005; 15(6):333-341.
55. Pearlstone JR, Smillie LB. Binding of troponin-T fragments to several types of tropomyosin. Sensitivity to Ca^{2+} in the presence of troponin-C. J Biol Chem 1982; 257(18):10587-10592.
56. Cho YJ, Hitchcock-DeGregori SE. Relationship between alternatively spliced exons and functional domains in tropomyosin. Proc Natl Acad Sci USA 1991; 88(22):10153-10157.
57. Hammell RL, Hitchcock-DeGregori SE. The sequence of the alternatively spliced sixth exon of alpha- tropomyosin is critical for cooperative actin binding but not for interaction with troponin. J Biol Chem 1997; 272(36):22409-22416.
58. Kostyukova AS, Hitchcock-Degregori SE, Greenfield NJ. Molecular Basis of Tropomyosin Binding to Tropomodulin, an Actin-capping Protein. J Mol Biol 2007; 372(3):608-618.
59. Kwok SC, Hodges RS. Clustering of large hydrophobes in the hydrophobic core of two-stranded alpha-helical coiled-coils controls protein folding and stability. J Biol Chem 2003; 278(37):35248-35254.
60. Greenfield NJ, Huang YJ, Palm T et al. Solution NMR structure and folding dynamics of the N terminus of a rat nonmuscle alpha-tropomyosin in an engineered chimeric protein. J Mol Biol 2001; 312(4):833-847.
61. Pittenger MF, Helfman DM. In vitro and in vivo characterization of four fibroblast tropomyosins produced in bacteria: TM-2, TM-3, TM-5a and TM-5b are colocalized in interphase fibroblasts. J Cell Biol 1992; 118(4):841-858.

62. Moraczewska J, Nicholson-Flynn K, Hitchcock-DeGregori SE. The ends of tropomyosin are major determinants of actin affinity and myosin subfragment 1-induced binding to F-actin in the open state. Biochemistry 1999; 38(48):15885-15892.
63. Kostyukova AS, Hitchcock-DeGregori SE, Greenfield NJ. Molecular basis of tropomyosin binding to tropomodulin, an actin-capping protien. J Mol Biol. 2007. 372 (3);608-611.
64. Mason JM, Arndt KM. Coiled coil domains: stability, specificity and biological implications. Chembiochem 2004; 5(2):170-176.
65. Xu C, Craig R, Tobacman L, Horowitz R et al. Tropomyosin positions in regulated thin filaments revealed by cryoelectron microscopy. Biophys J 1999; 77(2):985-992.
66. Hitchcock-DeGregori SE, Greenfield NJ, Singh A. Tropomyosin: regulator of actin filaments. Adv Exp Med Biol 2007; 592:87-97.

CHAPTER 6

Dimerization of Tropomyosins

Mario Gimona*

Abstract

Tropomyosins consist of nearly 100% α-helix and assemble into parallel dimeric coiled-coils. Nonmuscle as well as muscle tropomyosins can form homodimers, however, expression of both muscle α and β tropomyosin subunits results in the preferential formation of stable α/β heterodimers in native muscle. The assembly preference of the muscle tropomyosin heterodimer can be understood in terms of its thermodynamically favorable energy distribution that provides increased stability over the homodimer. The simultaneous expression of multiple tropomyosin isoforms in nonmuscle cells (at least up to seven individual chains), however, points towards a more complex principle for determining dimer preference. The information for homo- and heterodimerization is contained within the tropomyosin molecule itself and the parameters for dimer selectivity are conferred in part by the alternatively spliced exons. However, it remains to be established if low molecular weight tropomyosin isoforms in nonmuscle cells engage in both homdimer and heterodimer formation in vivo. A thorough understanding of the selective dimer formation of the more than 40 tropomyosin isoforms is required to explain how subtle alterations in the sequence of one tropomyosin chain can result in the progression of diverse disease phenotypes.

Introduction

Tropomyosins (Tms) constitute a large and highly conserved family of dimeric, coiled-coil actin filament-binding proteins that are among the major components of the thin filaments of striated and smooth muscle and of the microfilaments of nonmuscle cells.[1,2] In vertebrate cells a combination of four genes, multiple promoters and alternative splicing mechanisms generate around 40 individual Tm forms[2-5] and the expression of different Tm isoforms is characteristic of specific cell types. In recent years our understanding of the relationship of Tm isoform expression and specific cell function has improved considerably, owing largely to the development of isoform-specific antibodies and through the use of GFP-tagged Tm isoforms.[6-9] Nevertheless, the precise functions of Tm isoforms in different cell types and various cellular processes remain to be determined in detail.

Tm functions exclusively as a dimer and monomers have not been observed to be stable in solution. The two Tm chains assemble into parallel and mostly in-register coiled-coil dimers.[10,11] Certain nonmuscle cell types express multiple different Tm chains simultaneously and in light of their high similarity both by sequence and structure a large variety of homo and heterodimers can be formed theoretically. From studies in muscle it is clear that homodimers and heterodimers carry diverging functions[12,13] and that imbalances in the formation of either dimer can lead to disease phenotypes such as nemaline myopathy[14,15] (see Chapter 12 by Hardeman). Key questions in the understanding of Tm function thus revolve around the issues of what mechanisms are responsible

*Mario Gimona—Unit of Actin Cytoskeleton Regulation, Consorzio Mario Negri Sud, Department of Cell Biology and Oncology, Via Nazionale 8a, 66030 Santa Maria Imbaro, Italy. Email: gimona@negrisud.it

Tropomyosin, edited by Peter Gunning. ©2008 Landes Bioscience and Springer Science+Business Media.

for the regulation of the assembly of homo- and heterodimers and whether cell type-specific factors are involved in this process.[16-18]

Rat embryo fibroblasts express up to seven nonmuscle Tm isoforms simultaneously,[4,19] three high molecular weight (HMW) Tms (β smooth muscle/Tm1, Tm2 and Tm3) and four low molecular weight (LMW) Tms (Tm4, Tm5NM1, Tm5a and Tm5b) of 284 and 248 amino acid residues in length, respectively (see Chapter 2). Skeletal and smooth muscle α and β Tm subunits assemble preferentially into the thermodynamically more stable α/β heterodimers.[20,21] Cardiac muscle expresses almost exclusively one α chain[4] and thus in the heart muscle α/α homodimers prevail. Tms from fibroblasts except Tm3 were shown to exist as homodimers[22] and thus additional parameters that determine the formation and stabilization of functional Tm dimers should exist in nonmuscle cells.

A series of studies in the mid 1990s identified that the specificity of dimer formation (homo- versus heterodimer) is partially determined by the thermodynamic stability of all possible protein-protein interactions, involving both intramolecular and intermolecular interactions. Investigation of the dimerization behavior of epitope tagged Tms in cultured cells led to the initial demonstration that the information for homo- and heterodimers is indeed contained within the Tm molecule itself and that the information for the selectivity is conferred in part by the alternatively spliced exons.[4,5,16,17] In this chapter I will summarize the current knowledge on the parameters that can influence dimer formation of Tms.

Homodimers and Heterodimers

Amino- and carboxyl-terminal regions, as well as internal regions contribute to the coiled-coil interactions of the Tm subunits.[12,13,22] The dimeric Tm molecule unfolds and dissociates in response to increasing temperature, indicating regions of varying stability or several states of partially unfolded molecules. The two major helix-coil transitions likely reflect the unfolding of independent domains.[23] However, the conformation of locally unfolded regions and the mechanism leading to the local unfolding of Tm remain to be resolved in detail. Expression of amino-terminally epitope-tagged muscle isoforms in nonmuscle cells leads to the formation of heterodimers between HMW muscle and nonmuscle Tms.[16] Muscle-specific factors cannot be involved in the process of formation and stabilization of heterodimers since this process takes place in a cultured nonmuscle cell. Nonmuscle-specific factors are also not sufficient for maintaining the homodimeric state of the endogenous nonmuscle Tms in the presence of the muscle isoforms. Notably, transgenic mice that express nonmuscle Tm3 specifically target this isoform to the Z-line-associated cytoskeleton as a homodimer,[24] without detectable heterodimerization with the muscle Tms.

A relationship between alternatively spliced exons and functional domains in Tms can be seen when the influence of exons 2a/b and 9a/d (see Chapter 2) of the smooth and striated α-Tms is analyzed.[25] Although the presence of exon 9a is correlated with Ca^{2+}-insensitive binding to troponin and that of exon 2a with changes in actin affinity, the individual exons were not recognizable as individual structural domains.[25]

Coordination between the N- and C-terminal regions of the Tm dimer is required for normal Tm function and this harmonization of several folded domains is critical for the formation of functionally relevant Tm dimers. Exons 3, 4, 5, 7 and 8 are common to all Tms, but are insufficient to warrant stable dimerization per se and heterodimers between LMW and HMW Tms are unstable. Whether or not changes in the sequences of these conserved domains could lead to perturbation of the dimeric interactions of Tm subunits is currently unknown.

The 284 residue long nonmuscle isoforms Tm1, Tm2 and Tm3 form exclusively homodimers, while the shorter Tm4, Tm5NM1, Tm5a and Tm5b form both homo and heterodimers.[16,17,19] Exons 1a and 1b in the α gene are highly similar and exon 1b, which is used in the LMW subunits of Tm4, Tm5NM1, Tm5a and Tm5b partially influences the dimerization properties of these isoforms. However, in a cellular context Tm5a and Tm5b do not form stable heterodimers with each other, but heterodimerize with Tm5NM1 and Tm4.[17] Tm5a and Tm5b share identical N-and C-terminal regions, as do Tm2 and Tm3 and differ only in the alternative use of exon 6a and 6b from the α gene, as do Tm2 and Tm3. This demonstrates that the combinatorial use of exons and not the sole presence or absence of individual exons dictates the stability of either dimer form. However, the basis underlying the exclusion of Tm5a/Tm5b heterodimers is far from being understood. At least for the HMW and LMW products of the α gene there is a clear contribution from the alternatively spliced exons to dimer preference, since the first 45 amino acids are required for assembly of the Tm4/Tm5NM1 heterodimer.[18]

The functional significance of expressing a multitude of Tm isoforms in nonmuscle cells and maintaining them as homo- or heterodimers remains to be fully understood. The higher actin-binding ability of strongly head-to-tail overlapping heterodimers of smooth muscle α and β Tm subunits reflects the necessity to maintain stable association with the muscle thin filament throughout the entire length of the actin filament. The α/β heterodimer exhibits a greater ability to bind cooperatively to F-actin, due to its stronger head-to-tail overlaps compared with α/α homodimers (see Chapter 7 by Tobacman for details). Tm heterodimers appear also to display a higher degree of flexibility than their homodimeric counterparts[26] and higher end-to-end association of Tm heterodimers in smooth muscle cells leads to the formation of elongated Tm polymers. By contrast, the low head-to-tail association of Tm homodimers can be seen as a necessary determinant for the more dynamic regulation of the actin cytoskeleton in nonmuscle cells. With the exception of cardiac muscle that expresses only a single α Tm isoform, muscle tissue usually contains α/β heterodimers,[27] which are thermodynamically favorable over the less stable β/β dimer, and also the α/α homodimers that show higher thermal stability.[28]

High and low MW Tms are unable to form a stable coiled coil together. Tm4 can form homodimers and heterodimers with Tm5NM1, Tm5a and Tm5b, but not with the HMW isoforms Tm1, Tm2 and Tm3 and any of the muscle Tms that readily form heterodimers with the otherwise preferentially homodimeric HMW nonmuscle isoforms Tm1, Tm2 and Tm3.[16,17] Although in general coiled coils between chains of non-identical length are possible the reason for the inability for Tms to do so becomes evident from a detailed comparison of the amino acid sequences (Fig. 1), the position of the alanine clusters and actin binding sites and the N-terminal acetylation patterns (see below for details on these parameters). LMW Tms from the α, γ and δ genes require an unusual alignment for proper comparison. The position of the polybasic ring at positions 5-7 in the HMW isoforms determines the position in the helical wheel arrangement (at positions e, f and g). If these residues are aligned according to a two dimensional linear heptad repeat alignment,[29] then the first 6 residues of the (mammalian) LMW Tms are out of phase as the wheel begins at the b position and the polybasic ring is at position 12-14. Such an alignment is, however, required to position the alanine clusters and actin binding regions in a similar manner to the HMW isoforms. With this alignment in place it becomes evident that the second alanine cluster and adjacent actin binding region are absent from the LMW isoforms, while the first and all C-terminal alanine clusters and actin binding regions overlap exactly with the HMW Tms, as does the trigger sequence in the C-terminus. It is thus plausible that even in the case of an initial attempt of coiled-coil assembly between an HMW and an LMW Tm, the N-terminal third of the molecule will be out-of-register, irrespective of a C-to-N terminal zipper mechanism, or if a best-fit model of individual subdomains drives the assembly.

It remains to be established if the heterodimers indeed exist in nonmuscle cells. In vivo, the (cooperative?) folding of α/β heterodimers from separate α and β chains is thermodynamically favored over the formation of homodimers. It was thus concluded that the formation of the dimers is guided exclusively by the Tm chains themselves, without contribution of additional biological factors,[30] albeit N-terminal acetylation is a requirement for physiological actin binding levels and may thus be indispensable for stabilization of the correct dimer assembly of each Tm isoform.

Coiled Coils and Trigger Sequences

Coiled-coils are highly versatile and ubiquitous assembly motifs that can be found in a wide range of structural and regulatory proteins. A most prominent characteristic of coiled coils is the heptad repeat, a 7-residue repeated sequence in which the first and fourth positions (termed a and d) are

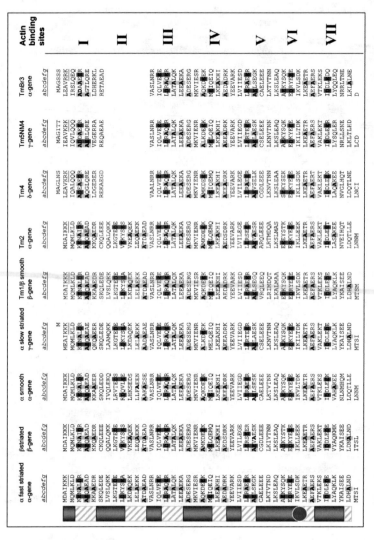

Figure 1. Linear heptad repeat alignment of HMW and LMW Tms. Note the 6-residue extensions in LMW Tms (Tm4, Tm5NM1 and TmBr3) and the absence of the consensus pattern corresponding to actin binding site II and to the second alanine cluster. a,b,c,d,e,f: positions in the heptad repeat. Amino acids forming the polybasic ring in the N-terminus are underlined. Grey boxes highlight alanine residues in the destabilizing alanine clusters. The hatched areas on the molecular ruler on the left indicate the positions of the alanine clusters in the helical Tm molecule. Red boxes highlight residues contributing to actin binding. The positions of the actin binding sites are indicated on the right (I-VII).

occupied by hydrophobic residues. The design rules for folding and assembly of coiled-coils are well understood and de-novo design of such proteins reproduces with considerable fidelity and preservation of function parallel and anti-parallel homo- and hetero-dimers, as well as trimers and tetramers.[31] In eukaryotic genomes almost 5% of all proteins contain coiled coil-forming sequences, a finding that suggests that coiled coil proteins engage in a wide variety of cellular processes[32-34] Coiled coils are autonomously folding units of amino acid sequence, typically consisting of two identical or largely similar sequences with high α helical propensity. The two α helical chains wrap around each other with a moderate super-helical twist.

The contour length of muscle Tms is about 400 Angstroms (or 40 nm). Together with the available crystal structures, solution NMR studies detected a flexible nature of the coiled coil (Fig. 2) and demonstrated that the coil is not homogenous but displays several undulating regions.[35] Parameters that drive this structural fluctuation are likely to drive coiled-coil interactions and stability and hence dimer specificity in Tms. Both internal and external parameters influence the stability of coiled-coils.[36] Intramolecular parameters include interchain and intrachain electrostatic effects, helical propensity and hydrophobicity outside the core positions (a and d) in the heptad repeat.[37] Positions a and d in the heptad repeat sequences of coiled coils are commonly occupied by nonpolar residues, whereas the e and g positions display presence of charged (acidic and basic) amino acid residues. Modification or removal of the N or C termini of Tms (by enzymatic digestion or mutagenesis) prevents head-to-tail interactions between Tm dimers and interactions with the actin filaments.[38] The most probable candidates that directly influence dimer specificity are the alanine-rich destabilizing clusters[39] (see below).

One common feature of coiled coil proteins is the presence of a short, autonomous helical folding unit, the "trigger sequence" that is indispensable for correct folding to occur at physiological temperatures (Fig. 3). Crucial determinants of both monomer helix and coiled coil structures are electrostatic interactions between the charged residues in the side chains.[40] In Tms the trigger sequence is located in the C-terminal portion of the molecule. In HMW Tms this region spans residues 226-238, which correspond to residues 190-202 in LMW isoforms and overlaps with the seventh alanine cluster.[18]

In LMW Tms the trigger sequence plays a significant role and is critical for the ability of Tm 4 to form homodimers—yet this region seems dispensable for the heterodimer formation with Tm5NM1.[18] Trigger sequences may thus not be an absolute requirement for all coiled coils, but they clearly increase the local stability of certain α helical sequences in coiled coil assemblies and increased molecular stability by trigger sequences may regulate the postribosomal folding time.[37] Such regions of increased stability may compensate for adjacent regions of lower stability and thus favor the overall stability of the coiled coil.

N-Terminal Acetylation

Both skeletal and smooth muscle Tms, require N-terminal acetylation for strong (physiological) actin binding affinity.[41-44] Although in the muscle α/β heterodimer the α chain contributes more to the actin binding than the β chain,[27] acetylation of the N-terminal methionine residue (N-Met) must be present on both chains in the Tm dimer. The absence of N-Met-acetylation results in an eight-fold reduction in actin affinity for β Tm and a 40-fold reduction for α Tm.[27] The C-terminus of the Tm dimer is splayed open (see Fig. 2) and can accommodate the tightly coiled N-terminus of an adjacent Tm dimer, provided that the Met in position one is acetylated (in vivo), or contains a compensating extension (see Chapter 5). Lack of acetylation in bacterially-expressed recombinant Tms can be compensated by fusion of an N-terminal Ala-Ser dipeptide (AS) to the Tm sequence, whereas muscle Tms with unmodified N-termini are unstable and mediate the destabilization of the entire coiled coil dimer.[41] However, N-terminal acetylation is not a requirement for either homo or heterodimer fomation. While the N-terminal Met of mammalian muscle Tms is acetylated in vivo and partially regulates actin binding, it was suggested that cytoplasmic Tms from fibroblast do not require such an N-terminal modification owing to the N-terminal extension in the sequences.[19] For clarity, however, it must be pointed out that these extensions are only present in some LMW

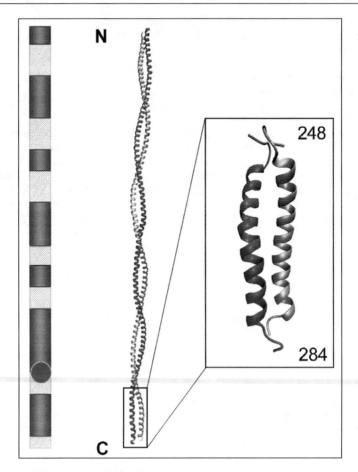

Figure 2. Molecular ribbon diagram of a HMW Tm dimer (PDB structure accession number 1c1g). The position on alanine-rich clusters (hatched areas) and the trigger sequence (solid circle) are indicated on the molecular ruler on the left. The C-terminal region encompassing residues 248-284 of exon 9a (PDB structure accession number 1 mv4) does not form a tight coiled coil structure.

isoforms, while cytoplasmic Tm1, Tm2 and Tm3 have identical N-terminal sequences to the muscle isoforms (Fig. 4) and conform to the consensus sequence for NatB-dependent acetylation.[45]

Although it is the N-terminal Met that is acetylated and in consequence stabilizes the coiled coil all the way to the N-terminal end, substrate specificity of the yeast Nα-terminal acetyl transferase includes the residue at position 2 and possibly also at position 3. In *Schizosaccharomyzes pombe* the only Tm, Cdc8, is acetylated in vivo and requires N-terminal acetylation for full functionality. In contrast to mammalian muscle Tms and to *Saccharomyces cerevisiae* TMP1 and TMP2, where an amino terminal AS extension rescues the absence of the N-Met acetylation, this fusion is, however, not sufficient to rescue actin binding in Cdc8.[44,46]

Studies in budding yeast have demonstrated that the mitochondrial distribution and morphology gene (Mdm20), together with the Nat3p subunit of the NatB N-terminal acetyl transferase complex cooperatively regulate Tm acetylation.[47,48] The human homolog of the yeast NatB complex is NATH, but the true nature and functionality of the mammalian Tm acetyl transferases is largely

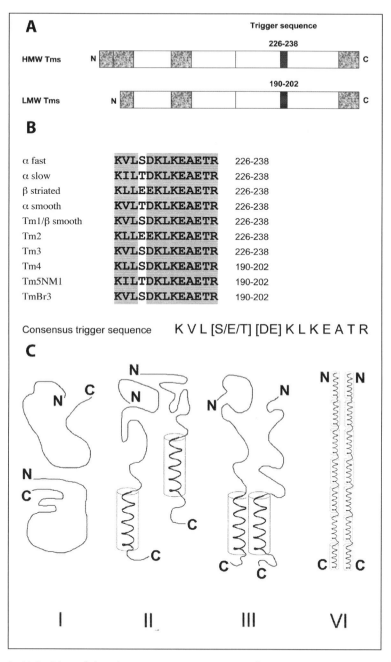

Figure 3. A) Position of the trigger sequence in HMW and LMW Tms. Grey areas indicate regions of alternatively spliced exons. B) Sequence comparison of the Tm isoforms shown in Figure 1. Numbers on the right indicate the position in the Tm sequence. C) Trigger sequences initiate and facilitate the formation of coiled coil Tm dimers. The autonomously folding trigger sequences that are located on the unfolded nascent polypeptide chain (I) form short helical regions in partially unfolded amino acid chains (II) and align the two chains (III) for in-register coiled coil dimer formation (IV) redrawn from reference 3I.

α *fast* striated   1 **MD**AIKKKMQMLKLDKENALD   :: 284
α *slow* striated   1 **MM**EAIKKKMQMLKLDKENALD   :: 284
β striated   1 **MD**AIKKKMQMLKLDKENAID   :: 284
α smooth   1 **MD**AIKKKMQMLKLDKENALD   :: 284

Tm1/β smooth   1 **MD**AIKKKMQMLKLDKENALD   :: 284
Tm2   1 **MD**AIKKKMQMLKLDKENAID   :: 284   HMW cytoplasmic Tms containing the NatB consenus sequence
Tm3   1 **MD**AIKKKMQMLKLDKENALD   :: 284

Tm4   1 MAGLNSLEAVKRKIQALQQQ   :: 248
Tm5NM4   1 MAGITTIEAVKRKIQVLQQQ   :: 248   LMW Tms lacking the NatB consensus sequence
TmBr3   1 MAGSSSLEAVRRKIRSLQEQ   :: 248

S. *cerevisiae* TPM1   1 **MD**KIREKLSNLKLE   :: 199
S. *cerevisiae* TPM2   1 **ME**KIKEKLNSLKLE   :: 161
Ss. *pombe* Cdc8   1 **MD**KLREKINAARAE   :: 161

■

Acetylation consensus sequences for NatB-complex-dependent N-terminal Met-acetylation.

Figure 4. Comparison of the N-terminal sequences of the Tm isoforms shown in Figure 1. Grey boxes highlight the consensus sequences for N-terminal Met acetylation. The NatB complex does not recognize the Met-Ala N-terminal sequence in LMW Tms, whereas the Met-Asp dipeptide in the cyto-plasmic HMW Tms Tm1, Tm2 and Tm3 follow the consensus for NatB recognition motifs.

obscure. Importantly, in either system any potential deacetylases that could play essential roles in regulating Tm dimer stability and turnover, remain to be identified.

Alanine Clusters and Protein Interaction Sites

In certain areas of the 400 Angstrom long Tm dimer the two chains of the coiled coil are axially out of register by about one Angstrom.[29] An axial shift breaks the twofold symmetry such that identical sequences along the Tm chain are in different environments in the dimer. Those places where the axially-shifted and in-register regions join one another, the dimer exposes sharp bends. Bending of a coiled coil by alternating clusters of alanine and leucine residues is considered a general principle of coiled coil dimer design. The core segments of the coiled coil are predominantly composed of alanine residues and contrast with the remaining canonical segments of Tms. The asymmetric design in a dimer of identical (or highly similar) sequences allows Tm molecules to adopt multiple bent conformations. The alanine clusters in the core of the dimer can promote this semi-flexible behavior of the Tm molecule, which appears to be a crucial prerequisite for the regulation of actomyosin interactions and muscle contraction.[29] HMW Tms contain seven clusters of d-position alanines, whereas LMW Tms contain only six (see Fig. 1). Remarkably, proper alignment of the d position clusters in LMW Tms requires a shift of the sequences by one position along the helical wheel and this shift implies that the N-terminal six residues in LMW Tms may not participate in the formation of a correct coiled coil.

Replacement of alternatively spliced exons alters the stability of the entire Tm molecule.[49] Exchange of exons 1a and 2a in smooth muscle Tm by exon 1b in Tm5a and 5b has no influence on the overall helical content of the protein chain, but has profound consequences on the head-to-tail interaction of the dimers and alters the calorimetric enthalpy of the thermal unfolding of the dimer, leading to increased stability of the resulting, shorter LMW Tm. Yet there is no simple correlation between specific exons or domains of Tm and the overall stability of the molecule. Rather, changes in the Tm sequence impact on long-range cooperative effects in the structure.[49]

Actin binding and regulation of actomyosin contractility in muscle and nonmuscle cells requires a balanced equilibrium between stability and flexibility. Enhanced dimer stability impacts negatively on actin affinity and also poorly folded or unstable Tms have lower actin affinities. Replacement of coiled coils with random coils locally destabilizes the coiled coil and reduces the affinity for actin. Deletions of individual and multiple central segments leads to loss of the force producing state of the actin filament, despite preserved actin binding. Thus the mid region of the Tm dimer is critical for the myosin-induced shift of the actin filament from the closed to the open state.[50]

The seven fold periodic repeat in the sequence of Tms is poorly conserved[50] and individual sequence repeats are not functionally equivalent: yet the detected periodicities overlap with the predicted number of actin binding sites in the various Tm isoforms (Fig. 1). Deletion of the fifth period devastates actin affinity, deletion of periods four and five, however, retain the ability to bind to actin, even in a cooperative manner. Deletion of periods three, four and five, or four, five and six also retain actin-binding activity. This suggests that the determinants of actin binding/affinity result from the preservation of the Tm dimer flexibility, as a consequence of local parameters of sequence, structure and stability of the dimeric fold.[50] Some of these parameters may in addition be influenced in vivo by a spatially and temporally regulated association with Tm-binding proteins. Reports indicating that under physiological temperature conditions significant proportions of the Tm dimer are not fully coiled coils[21,50] and may only poorly or incompletely dimerize lend additional support to such a scenario. The local unfolding sites that are seen at physiological temperature may coincide with the location and movement of destabilizing alanine clusters in the dimer core. Such unfolded regions may themselves provide binding or docking sites for Tm-binding proteins and can thus allow variable molecular flexibility of the dimer (also in the actin filament-bound form). In addition to the seven binding site-containing HMW Tms and the six site-containing LMW Tm isoforms, the even shorter yeast Tms are predicted to span the length of five (*S. cer.* TPM1), or four (*S. cer.* TPM2 and *S. pombe* Cdc8) actin monomers in the filament[50] (Chapter 14). In the sequences of these yeast Tms, however, there is no clear arrangement of alanine clusters and the regulation of dimer formation in this system awaits detailed analysis.

The major differences in sequence between striated muscle and smooth/nonmuscle Tms are largely confined to the C-terminus. The C-terminal seven residues of striated α Tm (270-279) are helical but do not participate in coiled-coil formation.[51] The interface residues of the last two heptad repeats have a high propensity of forming three stranded coiled coils[52] and NMR studies using the C-terminus of striated muscle α Tm revealed that residues 278-284 are nonhelical and flexible. This open conformation appears to be a requirement for successful cooperative head-to-tail overlap between the N-and C-terminal 9-11 residues of adjacent Tm dimers, at least for Tms containing exon 9a.[51,52]

The C-Terminus in Tm, Formin and Tropomodulin Interactions

Binding of Tm to formins, a family of actin nucleators, modulates actin barbed end filament capping. The flexible hinge near the C-terminus of the Tm dimer mediates interaction with the helical regions of the FH2 domain in mDia1 and mDia2. Instead of the helical N-terminus of an adjacent Tm dimer, the C-terminus appears to form a triple helical structure with formin. Tms and formin cooperate in the formation of stabilized, unbranched filaments in vivo[53] and this proposed helical insertion mechanism might represent the necessary process to guarantee the coordinated action of these two molecules along the actin filament. Strikingly, the relief of formin inhibition is isoform specific for both Tm and formin variants. Maximal inhibition has been detected between mDia2 and Tm2 and mDia1 and Tm5a, respectively.[53]

The "molecular ruler" that limits the length of erythrocyte membrane actin cytoskeleton filaments to an almost uniform length of 37 nm (spanning 12-13 actin monomers) contains LMW Tm and the filament end-capping molecule tropomodulin (Tmod; 54). This interaction is mediated specifically by Tm5(NM1?) and its potential heterodimeric partner Tm5b. The polybasic ring (KKK or KRK; see Fig. 1) at positions 7-14 in LMW Tms and 5-7 in HMW Tms) participates in the regulation of electrostatic forces with hydrophobic interactions and two KRK rings, one provided by each Tm monomer chain, form a ring around the N-terminus of the coiled coil dimer.[55,56] Molecular dynamics simulation studies have further revealed that the Tmod helix at residues 116-122 (containing the sequence LEE at residues 116-118) interacts with the KRK ring region and forms a stable triple helical complex (56 and Chapter 21).

Conclusions and Perspectives

The potential to form dimers of variable chain composition broadens the spectrum of potential cellular functions for Tms. Thus in a cell, the formation of dimers cannot be following random association principles and the formation of correct, functional dimers must be tightly regulated in addition by intracellular factors. Only correct dimers function properly in the context of a given cell type (as demonstrated for nemaline myopathy, where a shift from the α/β to a predominantly α/α homodimer occurs with considerable consequences for skeletal muscle regulation—see Chapter 12). A shift in the dimer species away from the preferred dimer likely perturbs the regulation of actin filaments and actomyosin interactions during force generation in muscle contraction and potentially impacts also on the distribution and regulation of nonmuscle cell contractility. A comprehensive molecular dynamics simulation of all theoretically possible Tm dimers may help to shed light on the complexity of Tm chain interactions.

Acknowledgements

I thank Dr. Alexander Spaar (CMNS, Santa Maria Imbaro, Italy) for valuable assistance with Figures 2 and 3C. The support from the European Union (Marie Curie Excellence grant 002573) is gratefully acknowledged.

References

1. Leavis PC, Gergely J. Thin filament proteins and thin filament-linked regulation of vertebrate muscle contraction. CRC Crit Rev Biochem 1984; 16:235-305.
2. Gunning PW, Shevzov G, Kee AJ et al. Tropomyosin isoforms: divining rods for actin cytoskeleton function. Trends Cell Biol 2005; 15:333-41.
3. Goodwin LO, Lees-Miller JP, Cheley S et al. Four fibroblast tropomyosin isoforms are expressed from the rat alpha-tropomyosin gene via alternative RNA splicing and the use of two promoters. J Biol Chem 1991; 266:8408-15.
4. Lees-Miller JP, Helfman DM. The molecular basis for tropomyosin isoform diversity. Bioessays 1991; 13:429-37.
5. Pittenger MF, Kazzaz JA, Helfman DM. Functional properties of nonmuscle tropomyosin isoforms. Curr Opin Cell Biol 1994; 6:96-104.
6. Nyakern-Meazza M, Narayan K, Schutt CE et al. Tropomyosin and gelsolin cooperate in controlling the microfilament system. J Biol Chem 2002; 277:28774-9.
7. Bryce NC, Shevzov G, Ferguson V et al. Specification of actin filament function and molecular composition by tropomyosin isoforms. Mol Biol Cell 2003; 14:1002-16.
8. Schevzov G, Bryce NS, Almonte-Baldonado R et al. Specific features of neuronal size and shape are regulated by tropomyosin isoforms. Mol Biol Cell 2005; 16:3425-37.
9. Hillberg L, Zhao Rathje LS, Nyakern-Meazza M et al. Tropomyosins are present in lamellipodia of motile cells. Eur J Cell Biol 2006; 85:399-409.
10. Graceffa P. In-register homodimers of smooth muscle tropomyosin. Biochemistry 1989; 28:1282-7.
11. Whitby FG, Kent H, Stewart F et al. Structure of tropomyosin at 9 angstroms resolution. J Mol Biol 1992; 227:441-52.
12. Sanders C, Burtnick LD, Smillie LB. Native chicken gizzard tropomyosin is predominantly a beta gamma-heterodimer. J Biol Chem 1986; 261:12774-8.
13. Lehrer SS, Qian Y, Hvidt S. Assembly of the native heterodimer of Rana esculenta tropomyosin by chain exchange. Science 1989; 246:926-8.
14. Laing NG, Wilton SD, Akkari PA et al. A mutation in the alpha tropomyosin gene TPM3 associated with autosomal dominant nemaline myopathy NEM1. Nat Genet 1995; 10:249.
15. Corbett MA, Akkari PA, Domazetovska A et al. An α-Tropomyosin mutation alters dimer preference in nemaline myopathy. Ann Neurol 2005; 57:42-9.
16. Gimona M, Watakabe A, Helfman DM. Specificity of dimer formation in tropomyosins: influence of alternatively spliced exons on homodimer and heterodimer assembly. Proc Natl Acad Sci USA 1995; 92:9776-80.
17. Temm-Grove CJ, Guo W, Helfman DM. Low molecular weight rat fibroblast tropomyosin 5 (TM-5): cDNA cloning, actin-binding, localization and coiledcoil interactions. Cell Motil Cytoskeleton 1996; 33:223-40.
18. Araya E, Berthier C, Kim E et al. Regulation of coiled-coil assembly in tropomyosins. J Struct Biol 2002; 137:176-83.
19. Pittenger MF, Helfman DM. In vitro and in vivo characterization of four fibroblast tropomyosins produced in bacteria: TM-2, TM-3, TM-5a and TM-5b are colocalized in interphase fibroblasts. J Cell Biol 1992; 118:841-58.
20. Brown HR, Schachat FH. Renaturation of skeletal muscle tropomyosin: implications for in vivo assembly. Proc Natl Acad Sci USA 1985; 82:2359-63.
21. Lehrer SS, Qian Y. Unfolding/refolding studies of smooth muscle tropomyosin. Evidence for a chain exchange mechanism in the preferential assembly of the native heterodimer. J Biol Chem 1990; 265:1134-8.
22. Matsumura F, Yamashiro-Matsumura S. Purification and characterization of multiple isoforms of tropomyosin from rat cultured cells. J Biol Chem 1985; 260:13851-9.
23. Hvidt S, Lehrer SS. Thermally induced chain exchange of frog alpha beta-tropomyosin. Biophys Chem 1992; 45:51-9.
24. Kee AJ, Schevzov, G, Nair-Shalliker V et al. Sorting of a nonmuscle tropomyosin to a novel cytoskeletal compartment in skeletal muscle results in muscular dystrophy. J Cell Biol 2004; 166:685-96.
25. Cho YJ, Hitchcock-DeGregori SE. Relationship between alternatively spliced exons and functional domains in tropomyosin. Proc Natl Acad Sci USA 1991; 88:10153-57.
26. Censullo R, Cheung HC Tropomyosin length and two-stranded F-actin flexibility in the thin filament. J Mol Biol 1994; 243:520-9.
27. Coulton A, Lehrer SS, Geeves MA. Functional homodimers and heterodimers of recombinant smooth muscle tropomyosin. Biochemistry 2006; 45:12853-8.
28. Lehrer SS, Stafford WF 3rd. Preferential assembly of the tropomyosin heterodimer: equilibrium studies. Biochemistry 1991; 30:5682-8.

29. Brown JH, Kim K-H, Jun G et al. Deciphering the design of the tropomyosin molecule. Proc Natl Acad Sci USA 2001; 98:8496-501.
30. Lehrer SS, Quian Y. Unfolding/refolding studies of smooth muscle tropomyosin. J Biol Chem 1990; 265:1134-8.
31. Kammerer RA, Schulthess T, Landwehr R et al. An autonomous folding unit mediates the assembly of two stranded coiled coils. Proc Natl Acad Sci USA 1998; 95:13419-24.
32. Lupas A, van Dyke M, Stock J. Predicting coiled coils from protein sequences. Science 1991; 252:1162-64.
33. Wolf E, Kim PS, Berger B. MultiCoil: a program for predicting two- and three-stranded coiled coils. Protein Sci 1997; 6:1179-89.
34. Liu J, Rost B. Comparing function and structure between entire proteomes. Protein Sci 2001; 10:1970-9.
35. Ishii Y, Hitchcock-DeGregori SE, Mabuchi K et al. Unfolding domains of recombinant fusion alpha alpha-tropomyosin. Protein Sci 1992; 1:1319-25.
36. Jancsò A, Graceffa P. Smooth muscle tropomyosin coiled-coil dimers. Subunit composition, assembly and end-to-end interaction. J Biol Chem 1991; 266:5891-7.
37. Lee DL, Lavigne P, Hodges RS. Are trigger sequences essential in the folding of two-stranded α-helical coiled-coils? J Mol Biol 2001; 306:539-53.
38. Morais AC, Ferreira ST. Folding and stability of a coiled-coil investigated using chemical and physical denaturing agents: Comparative analysis of polymerized and nonpolymerized forms of α-tropomyosin. Int J Biochem Cell Biol 2005; 37:1386-1395.
39. Nitanai Y, Minakata S, Maeda K et al. Crystal structure of tropomyosin: flexible coiled-coil. Adv Exp Med Biol 2007; 592:137-51.
40. Steinmetz MO, Jelesarov I, Matousek WM et al. Molecular basis of coiled-coil formation. Proc Natl Acad Sci USA 2007; 104:7062-67.
41. Monteiro PB, Lataro RC, Ferro JA et al. Functional alpha-tropomyosin produced in Escherichia coli. A dipeptide extension can substitute the amino-terminal acetyl group. J Biol Chem 1994; 269:10461-6.
42. Urbancikova M, Hitchcock-DeGregori SE. Requirement of amino-terminal modification for striated muscle alpha-tropomyosin function. J Biol Chem 1994; 269:24310-5.
43. Greenfield NJ, Stafford WF, Hitchcock-DeGregori SE. The effect of N-terminal acetylation on the structure of an N-terminal tropomyosin peptide and alpha alpha-tropomyosin. Protein Sci 1994; 3:402-10.
44. Skoumpla K, Coulton AT, Lehman W et al. Acetylation regulates tropomyosin function in the fission yeast Schizosaccharomyces pombe. J Cell Sci 2007; 120:1635-45.
45. Polevoda B, Sherman F. Composition and function of the eukaryotic N-terminal acetyltransferase subunits. Biochem Biophys Res Commun 2003; 308:1-11.
46. Polevoda B, Cardillo TS, Doyle TC et al. Nat3p and Mdm20p are required for function of yeast NatB Nα-terminal acetyltransferase and of actin and tropomyosin. J Biol Chem 2003; 278:30686-97.
47. Singer JM, Shaw JM. Mdm20 protein functions with Nat3 protein to acetylate Tpm1 protein and regulate tropomyosin-actin interactions in budding yeast. Proc Natl Acad Sci USA 2003; 100:7644-9.
48. Caesar R, Warringer J, Blomberg A. Physiological importance and identification of novel targets for the N-terminal acetyltransferase NatB. Eucaryotic Cell 2006; 5:268-78.
49. Kremneva E, Nikolaeva O, Maytum R et al. Thermal unfolding of smooth muscle and nonmuscle tropomyosin α-homodimers with alternatively spliced exons. FEBS J 2006; 273:588-600.
50. Hitchcock-DeGregori SE, Song Y, Greenfield NJ. Functions of tropomyosin's periodic repeats. Biochemistry 2002; 41:15036-44.
51. Greenfield NJ, Swapna GVT, Huang Y et al. The structure of the carboxyl terminus of striated α-tropomyosin in solution reveals an unusual parallel arrangement of interacting α-helices. Biochemistry 2003; 42:614-9.
52. Greenfield NJ, Palm T, Hitchcock-DeGregori SE. Structure and interactions of the carboxyl terminus of striated α-tropomyosin: it is important to be flexible. Biophys J 2002; 83:2754-66.
53. Wawro B, Greenfield NJ, Wear MA et al. Tropomyosin regulates elongation by formin at the fast-growing end of the actin filament. Biochemistry 2007; 46:8146-55.
54. McElhinny AS, Kolmerer B, Fowler VM et al. The N-terminal end of nebulin interacts with tropomodulin at the pointed ends of the thin filaments. J Biol Chem 2001; 276:583-92.
55. Vera C, Sood A, Gao KM et al. Tropomodulin-binding site mapped to residues 7-14 at the N-terminal heptad repeats of tropomyosin isoform 5. Arch Biochem Biophys 2000; 378:16-24.
56. Vera C, Lao J, Hamelberg D et al. Mapping the tropomyosin isoform 5 binding site on human erythrocyte tropomodulin: Further insights into E-Tmod/TM5 interaction. Arch Biochem Biophys 2005; 444:130-8.

CHAPTER 7

Cooperative Binding of Tropomyosin to Actin

Larry S. Tobacman*

Abstract

Tropomyosin molecules attach to the thin filament conjointly rather than separately, in a pattern indicating very high cooperativity. The equilibrium process drawing tropomyosins together on the actin filament can be measured by application of a linear lattice model to binding isotherm data and hypotheses on the mechanism of cooperativity can be tested. Each end of tropomyosin overlaps and attaches to the end of a neighboring tropomyosin, facilitating the formation of continuous tropomyosin strands, without gaps between neighboring molecules along the thin filament. Interestingly, the overlap complexes vary greatly in size and composition among tropomyosin isoforms, despite consistently cooperative binding to actin. Also, the tendency of tropomyosin to bind actin cooperatively rather than randomly does not correlate with the strength of end-to-end binding. By implication, tropomyosin's actin-binding cooperativity likely involves effects on the actin filament, as well as direct interactions between adjacent tropomyosins.

Introduction—Conjunction Junctions Have Anti-Gap Functions

The cooperativity of tropomyosin-actin binding derives primarily from a striking, qualitative aspect of tropomyosin structure: it is a very elongated protein. Muscle tropomyosins, the prototypical forms, are coiled-coils no less than 40 nm in span, stretching along the surface of seven actin monomers and even the shortest known tropomyosins extend four actins in length.[1-4] One might imagine that this feature, the contact of each molecule with multiple actins, would facilitate the full and homogeneous assembly of thin filaments, i.e., each actin monomer bound to tropomyosin. Paradoxically, the opposite is the case; the fact that each elongated tropomyosin occupies multiple actins is a feature that can in principle limit the saturation of the entire actin filament with tropomyosin. The issue is statistical.[5] If tropomyosin molecules bound to actin independently, no matter how tightly, the molecules would attach to and distribute on any thin filament randomly with respect to each other. Adjacent, neighboring tropomyosins might occasionally attach immediately end-to-end. But, more commonly gaps would form between them, gaps too short for another molecule to fit. For actin filaments to be saturated with tropomyosin, it is virtually essential that tropomyosin bind to actin cooperatively rather than randomly. Cooperative binding also has a secondary effect: it strengthens tropomyosin's overall affinity for actin (quite weak when single tropomyosin's bind to actin in a solitary manner). But, it is cooperative binding, rather than tight binding, that is essential for saturation of actin with tropomyosin.

If in principle there is a docking problem, a statistical obstacle to the continuous parking of tropomyosin along the actin filament, in practice tropomyosin molecules bind to actin conjointly,

---

*Larry S. Tobacman—Departments of Medicine and of Physiology & Biophysics, University of Illinois at Chicago, Chicago, IL, USA. Email: lst@uic.edu

Tropomyosin, edited by Peter Gunning. ©2008 Landes Bioscience and Springer Science+Business Media.

cooperatively, greatly facilitating the effectiveness of tropomyosin attachment to the thin filament. How is this accomplished? That is the subject of this review.

The Mechanism of Cooperative Tropomyosin-Actin Binding

The starting point for understanding the cooperative binding mechanism is end-to-end, tropomyosin-tropomyosin binding. Tropomyosins bind adjacently, without gaps, primarily because the N-terminus of one tropomyosin can directly adhere to the C-terminus of the next molecule along the actin filament. Three compelling lines of evidence support this. The first can be expressed as the consequence of calculation. That is, there is a compelling quantitative argument that tropomyosin could not bind cooperatively to actin, would instead bind with true negative cooperativity, were it not for permissive end-to-end interactions. This inference is based on the fact that tropomyosins are slightly longer than needed to span integer numbers of actin monomers. Muscle tropomyosins, for example, are 284 amino acids long, whereas approximately 274 residues are sufficient for an extended alpha helix molecule to span 7 actins. The 'extra' overlapping residues from the ends of adjacent tropomyosins must accommodate each other, or an anti-cooperative effect would ensue. The second argument that tropomyosins interact end-to-end is that the protein's solution behavior so indicates. Purified tropomyosin polymerizes under low ionic strength conditions, becoming highly viscous,[6] presumably involving molecule-to-molecule, N-terminus to C-terminus contacts that are similar to what occurs when tropomyosin is bound to actin. Finally, protein structure data establish the reality of tropomyosin-tropomyosin binding. Most compellingly in this regard, the atomic structure of such an end-to-end complex was elucidated by Greenfield, et al, using NMR.[7] Tropomyosin's COOH-terminus splays, allowing insertion of 11 residues of the NH$_2$-terminal coiled-coil in the resulting cleft. Described in detail elsewhere in this volume (see Chapter 5), the structure's notable features include rotation of the NH2-terminus relative to the COOH-terminus by ~90° and considerable structural flexibility. It seems only reasonable to conclude that end-to-end binding of this type is an important component of tropomyosin's actin-binding cooperativity.

In fact, end-to-end binding is such an intuitive and well supported explanation for cooperative binding of tropomyosin to actin, that even specialists in tropomyosin may be surprised to learn the strength of the evidence that other factors are equally important. This evidence suggests that, although end-to-end binding is required for cooperative attachment of tropomyosin to actin, the cause of the cooperativity is more complex and likely involves the actin lattice as well as end-to-end binding. The evidence on the nature of tropomyosin-tropomyosin end-to-end binding and on its role in cooperative attachment to actin, again is of three types: tropomyosin solution data, tropomyosin sequence data and tropomyosin-actin binding data.

End-to-End Binding of Tropomyosin in Solution

Consider the relevant solution behavior of tropomyosin, which supports the phenomenon of tropomyosin-tropomyosin interactions, but which also indicates these interactions are weak relative to most other examples of protein-protein binding. Precise data are sparse, reflecting the difficulty in measurement of this process. Nevertheless, important quantitative findings have been published. How can one measure the affinity of two tropomyosins for each other? Mere detection of end-to-end binding can be accomplished in a variety of ways, but reliable measurement is challenging. Biophysical detection of polymerization can be misleading as a measure of end-to-end binding, because dimers, trimers and short polymers are poorly detected. The most satisfactory experimental solution yet presented is Sousa and Farah's spectroscopic technique,[8] based on the fluorescence of an engineered tropomyosin mutant with Trp near the C-terminus, expressed in Trp auxotrophs upon induction in the presence of 5-hydroxytryptophan (5HW). Experiments combining polymerizeable and nonpolymerizeable tropomyosins, 5HW labeled and unlabeled either way, established that the 5HW fluorescence was sensitive to end-to-end binding. Protein concentration-dependent effects on fluorescence reported the varying fraction of tropomyosin C-termini that were bound to N-termini. From this, the end-to-end affinity was determined, with the analysis requiring the reasonable approximation that this affinity is similar for binding between two isolated molecules and binding between a molecule and a chain of molecules (polymerized tropomyosin of any length.). Notably, the measured affinity of the tropomyosin N-terminus for the tropomyosin C-terminus fell two orders of magnitude when the ionic strength increased modestly, from I = 0.045 to I = 0.095. Extrapolating to physiological conditions (I ≈ 0.18 M), the tropomyosin C-terminus to tropomyosin N-terminus affinity is approximately 3×10^3 M^{-1}.

The above results indicate that, for the only form of tropomyosin where there are extensive quantitative data, end-to-end affinity is relatively weak under physiological conditions, when assessed in the absence of actin. For tropomyosin molecules attached to actin however, tropomyosin-tropomyosin binding is not a bi-molecular process, but rather a uni-molecular process. (Thin filaments are the molecules, with tropomyosins attached to actin and either binding to each other or not.) For this reason alone there is no simple correspondence of one type of equilibrium constant for another. Furthermore, on the thin filament, tropomyosin ends might interact favorably or unfavorably with actin (this is unknown), as well as favorably with each other when immediately adjacent and can affect the underlying actin filament in ways that are hard to assess. The differences between end-to-end binding in solution and on the filament are more than a formalism; each involves a different set of processes.

From these data and these considerations one infers that tropomyosins bind end to end, facilitating cooperative attachment to actin, but that the quantitative consequence, the contribution to the tendency of tropomyosins to bind adjacently rather than randomly, is uncertain. Is this effect sufficient to explain the measured cooperativity in binding? On the one hand, the interactions are weak and one cannot dismiss this as isoform specific, because the isoform studied by Farah and coworkers, striated muscle alpha tropomyosin, binds to actin cooperatively. On the other hand, weak interactions might be all that is required. The conundrum is the difficulty in establishing whether such interactions are sufficient to explain the observed cooperativity in tropomyosin attachment to actin. Perhaps the primary functional role of end-to-end binding is to affect thin filament behavior once tropomyosin is bound, rather than to cause cooperative binding. To approach these issues, other types of data are needed.

The Highly Variable End-to-End Overlap Regions of Tropomyosin Isoforms

Tropomyosin binds relatively loosely to actin, with few if any close stereospecific contacts between the two proteins.[9,10] Correspondingly, except for preservation of the coiled-coil forming motif, tropomyosin is not known as a highly conserved protein. Furthermore, alternative splicing generates a multiplicity of isoforms from each tropomyosin gene and the alternative exons encoding residues near the N-terminus or at the C-terminus are a particular source of such variation.[11] Thus, the end-to-end overlap elements are among the least conserved regions of a relatively nonconserved protein. Obviously, this heterogeneity has potential significance for cooperative attachment of tropomyosin to actin.

To investigate this issue more thoroughly, in the service of this review, the N- and C-terminal residues comprising the overlap complexes of multiple forms of tropomyosin were identified (Fig. 1). For simplicity, only homo-dimers and homo-polymers were considered. This was accomplished in a three step process. First, a diverse set of tropomyosin sequences were analyzed and aligned relative to each other. Secondly, gaps of particular lengths (lengths required to span integer numbers of actin monomers) were inserted into some of the sequences as needed, i.e., into the sequences of tropomyosins that span fewer than seven actins. Finally, the overlap residues for each tropomyosin were identified by alignment with the C- and N-termini of 284 residue tropomyosins, particularly striated muscle tropomyosin.

Seven mammalian, one amphibian, five insect and three yeast tropomyosin protein sequences were selected for analysis, with the set chosen to include a wide variety of tropomyosin lengths (range 161-287) and termini, rather than to comprise a complete survey. Insect forms with very extended or unusual termini were excluded. ClustalW was used as an aid, with the analysis biased to identify the best corresponding continuous region of tropomyosin that comparably aligns along the actin filament axis, rather than assigning alignment primacy to evolutionary relationships. As expected for this well studied protein, with well characterized genomic and exon structure described elsewhere in this volume and which contains both heptad repeats and longer quasi-repeating motifs,[12] an unambiguous alignment resulted for the selected set of tropomyosins. Residues 81 to 251 from the various molecules (numbering as per 284-residue tropomyosins), aligned readily, excepting the yeast isoforms. This 170 residue region is not sufficiently interesting or novel to merit illustration here. However, because it comprises the bulk of the molecule, it must dictate corresponding axial positions of tropomyosin on actin, i.e., structural alignment within the thin filament. From this inference, the proximate C-termini of the isoforms were aligned relative to each other (Fig. 1) by simple extension of the 170 residue consensus alignment region. Alignments of the tropomyosins' N-termini relative to each other required an additional step: insertion of actin-spanning gaps of proper size: 39 residues for tropomyosins spanning 6 actins and still larger gaps for still shorter tropomyosins. (Note that 39 does not maximize sequence alignment per se, which would have required a gap that could maintain the phase of the coiled-coil heptad repeat motif, i.e., a gap that was an integer multiple of seven residues.)

For the more divergent *S. cerevisiae* and *S. pombe* isoforms, there is ambiguity in alignment to the vertebrate tropomyosin sequences. Unlike the other sequences, yeast tropomyosins have either one or two interruptions of the otherwise continuous heptad motif pattern, beginning about 70 residues from the N-terminus.[4] The three yeast sequences were aligned to each other as a separate group using ClustalW and then the group's 91 residues C-terminal to all of the heptad repeat interruptions were aligned to the C-terminal portion of the other tropomyosins. To align the yeast tropomyosin N-termini with the other molecules, gaps of either 78 or 116 residues were inserted, which properly accounts for their overall spans of either 4 or 5 actins, depending on the isoform.

In Figure 1 (top), the N-and C-termini of smooth muscle tropomyosin are shown schematically as 11 overlapping residues, corresponding to what is known to comprise[7] the overlap complex of tropomyosins sharing this overall sequence length (284 residues). Below in the same figure, the overlaps from 7 other tropomyosins are shown, exemplifying the different overlap 'lengths' (i.e., number of overlapping residues) identified by the alignment of all tropomyosins analyzed, but

Overlap Residues	Overlap Region	Tropomyosin Isoform	Total Residues
11	- - - M L D Q T L L E L N N M COOH NH2 M D A I K K K M Q M L K - - -	α-smooth muscle	284
8	- - - E L K L A L N E D COOH NH2 M D A I K K K M Q - - -	α-Tm-Br1	281
14	- - - R M S H L S E L C I C L L S S COOH NH2 M D A I K K K M Q M L K L D K - - -	α-a (AF372217)	287
14	- - - M H Q M L D Q T L L E L N N M COOH NH2 M A G S S S L E A V R R K I R - - -	α-Tm-5a&5b	248
17	- - - P S S R M S H L S E L C I C L L S S COOH NH2 M A G S S S L E A V R R K I R S L Q - - -	α-TmBr-2	251
11	- - - L T N E L K L A L N E D COOH NH2 M A G S S S L E A V R R - - -	α-TmBr-3	245
18	- - - G N K L L Q E E M E A T L H D I Q N M COOH NH2 M T T S I P Q G T L L D V L K K K M R - - - - - -	D. melanogaster Tm1-A	252
4	- - - S L E N L COOH NH2 M D K I R - - -	S. cerevisiae 1	199

Figure 1. Alignments of tropomyosin end-to-end overlap regions of representative isoforms. Alternative splicing of exons 1a/1b and of exons 9b/9c/9d produces α-tropomyosin isoforms with overlap regions that differ from each other as shown and that also differ from the representative yeast and insect isoforms shown. Schematically shown overlap regions vary considerably in composition and mass. Note that these overlaps' unknown three dimensional stuctures may not be fully helical and must include four polypetides, not two, since tropomyosin is dimeric. See text and also Chapter 2 for details.

here emphasizing isoforms derived from alternative splicing of α-tropomyosin gene transcripts (See Chapter 2). To accomplish this, all the N-termini in the figure are positioned (left to right) in the figure according to their alignments relative to the N-terminus of 284 residue smooth muscle tropomyosin. Similarly, the various C-termini are positioned relative to the smooth muscle tropomyosin C-terminus, which overlaps the smooth muscle N-terminus as shown. Thus, the figure presents both the approximate size of the overlaps, i.e., the number of residues involved and a schematic axial representation of these overlaps on actin relative to the position of the smooth muscle overlap complex on actin. In this last regard, the barbed end of the actin filament would be toward the right of an imaginary, horizontal thin filament axis.

The results indicate that tropomyosin end-to-end overlap complexes vary greatly in size, from approximately 4 to approximately 18 residues. In some cases, Gly and Pro residues suggest the chains are not helical to their termini. Nevertheless, it is clear that the overlapping helical regions differ considerably among isoforms. The functional consequences of this structural variation are two-fold. First, a very long overlap has implications for myosin binding to actin. For myosin to bind tightly to actin, tropomyosin must shift its azimuthal position on the thin filament.[13-15] A relatively long overlap complex will tend to enforce, much more than a 4-residue overlap, behavior of actin-attached tropomyosin as a continuous polymerized structure, thereby influencing cooperative attachment of myosin cross-bridges. Second, the considerable overlap variation from isoform to isoform, often present within the same cell, will affect the extent to which segregation vs copolymerization of tropomyosin isoforms onto actin filaments occurs. In some manner, the overlap variation must affect isoform distributions of actin-bound molecules, with the details within the realm of future, practicable experimentation.

On the other hand, the figure suggests that the differing overlap complexes share rather closely one overall characteristic: their similar axial positions on actin. Slight deviations to the left or right suggest, correspondingly, axial positions varying slightly toward the directions of the pointed and barbed ends of the actin filament, respectively. The figure indicates that, in general, these deviations are small relative to the spacing of successive actin monomers (~39 tropomyosin residues). Interestingly, in a 3-D axial alignment of (284 residue) muscle tropomyosin on actin proposed in 2006,[16] the overlap complex lies relatively far from the actin surface, because it overlies a region of low filament radius, near the junction between adjacent actin monomers. Thus, a variety of different overlap complexes, as implied by Figure 1, might be accommodated in this axial location.

Perhaps most interestingly from Figure 1, are the short overlaps of the yeast tropomyosins: they barely comprise a single, 3.6 residue turn of an alpha helix, which would seem to provide a modest mechanism for facilitation of cooperative tropomyosin binding to actin. Furthermore, the yeast tropomyosin overlap complex must be small, regardless of any imprecision in the Figure 1 estimation of the axial position of this complex along the actin filament relative to that of other, more closely inter-related tropomyosins. Coiled-coils of 161 or 199 residues, the lengths of the yeast tropomyosin isoforms,[3] span 4 or 5 actins, respectively, with few tropomyosin residues to spare for end-to-end overlaps between neighboring molecules. One might expect this to diminish cooperative attachment to actin, but sufficient cooperativity must exist for function in the cell. Experimentally, there are few measures of how cooperatively these yeast tropomyosins, in native form, bind to actin. However, there are experimental data demonstrating cooperativity for a recombinant version of the 161 residue *S. cerevisiae* isoform. (This version contains 163 residues, as it includes a dipeptide added to stabilize the helical end of the bacterially expressed, N-unacetylated protein.) This yeast tropomyosin binds to actin with considerable cooperativity, indistinguishable from the cooperativity observed with muscle tropomyosin.[17,4] Since tropomyosin binds to actin with cooperativity even when the overlap complex is small, since it binds cooperatively even when end-to-end contacts are weak (vide supra), judicious scrutiny is needed for any simple contention that the entirety of the cooperative mechanism is ascribable to tropomyosin-tropomyosin contacts. Other factors may also be contributing to the cooperativity.

The Linear Lattice Conception of Cooperative Tropomyosin Binding to Actin

Tropomyosin-actin binding is one of a class of biological phenomena in which relatively long ligands attach to their targets so as to span more than one equivalent binding site. McGhee and Von Hippel developed[5] a formalism for quantitative analysis of such linear lattice processes, processes which include not only the attachment of tropomyosin to actin, but also the action of certain general DNA binding proteins. In their linear lattice approach, reasonable biochemical assumptions can be combined with experimental data, i.e., binding curves, to measure two parameters: K_o, the affinity of the ligand for an isolated site on the lattice, (e.g., tropomyosin binding to an otherwise bare actin filament) and y, the cooperative fold-increase in affinity when binding is enhanced by favorable interactions (particularly but not exclusively, end-to-end contacts) with an immediately adjacent ligand that is already attached to the lattice. Equivalently, as shown in Figure 2, y is an equilibrium constant describing the repositioning of a bound tropomyosin from an isolated site on the thin filament to a site allowing contact with an adjacent tropomyosin (end-to-end binding). The cooperative free energy between tropomyosins equals $-RT \ln (y)$. With proper assumptions, described below, an exact binding equation can be written, taking into account all the statistical complications of gaps that potentially arise along the lattice, including gaps too short for a ligand to fit.

Unlike more standard binding processes, for linear lattice processes the extent of binding is not an explicit function of the free ligand concentration; there is no such mathematical expression. Instead, a closed form equation has been found in which binding is an implicit function of the free ligand concentration.[5,18] This is sufficient for numerical solutions; for any free concentration (L) of the ligand tropomyosin, of an isoform spanning an integral number (n) of actins, a numerical search can be used to identify the fractional saturation of the thin filament with tropomyosin (θ) so that the following equality is satisfied:

$$L = \frac{4\theta(1-\theta)^2[2(y-1)(1-\theta)]^{n-1}}{nK_0(1-(n+1)\theta/n+R)^2[(2y-1)(1-\theta)+\theta/n-R]^{n-1}(1-\theta)} \tag{1}$$

where,

$$R \equiv [(1-(n+1)\theta/n)^2 + 4y\theta(1-\theta)/n]^{1/2}$$

When this expression is used to fit experimental data for a tropomyosin of known span (in the case of muscle tropomyosin, for example, n = 7), unique values of K_o and y are readily found. Qualitatively, tropomyosin's apparent affinity is determined by the product yK_o, (50% saturation occurs when $L \approx 1/yK_o$) and the shape of a tropomyosin binding curve is determined by the cooperativity parameter, y. Examples are shown in Figure 3. The S-shaped direct plot and highly convex scatchard plot are equivalent graphical demonstrations of a cooperative process (filled squares in top and bottom panels). The McGhee-Von Hippel approach permits one to go beyond the qualitative determination of the presence of cooperativity, which is evident from either panel and instead achieve a more useful quantitative insight: based on curvefitting of the experiment shown, cardiac tropomyosin bound to actin 84-fold more tightly when attaching next to another tropomyosin than when binding to a bare site on the filament. Also shown, are several binding curves that do not match the data, but that would result if there were the same overall affinity, but a lower cooperativity. Because of the 'parking problem', binding would appear to be negatively cooperative if there were in fact no cooperativity, as shown by the convex scatchard plot for y = 1. A 4-fold cooperative effect produces a nearly linear scatchard plot, a pattern which ordinarily, for simpler phenomena than tropomyosin-actin attachment, indicates noncooperative hyperbolic binding.

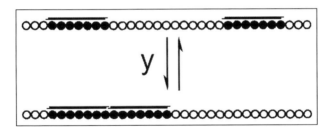

Figure 2. Schematic representation of tropomyosin's tendency to bind actin cooperatively. In the illustrated transition involving a section of an actin filament, one of two tropomyosin molecules is repositioned. When tropomyosins are directly adjacent, end-to-end contacts occur between neighboring molecules Filled circles indicate actins that are in direct contact with tropomyosin. Note y >> 1, producing cooperativity and also strengthening overall binding affinity.

A few assumptions of this analysis are worth noting. There are no data at present to establish that these assumptions are problematic for tropomyosin, but the assumptions are potentially important because they underlie any quantitative application of Eq. 1 to tropomyosin-actin binding data. First, actin is a two stranded lattice with respect to tropomyosin attachment, not a one stranded lattice, so use of the linear lattice model assumes that effects of one strand on the other strand are negligible with respect to tropomyosin-actin binding. Second, the linear lattice equation is derived with the assumption that only ligands immediately adjacent to each other have any effect on each other; a gap of one actin between tropomyosins for example, would result in binding identical to that occurring along an infinitely long bare stretch. This is valid if end-to-end binding is the only source of cooperativity. But, this assumption may be inexact if cooperativity is mediated to a significant extent by alterations in the actin lattice. Third, this is an equilibrium model. Its application assumes that tropomyosin's on- and off- rate constants are fast enough that equilibrium is approached under experimental conditions. This may be inexact, but is supported by the fact that binding data are not affected measurably by time of incubation. Finally, the model assumes that the finite length of actin filaments has no measurable effect. Complications due to the ends of filaments, where each tropomyosin has one rather than two adjacent, cooperative partners, or perhaps even hangs off the end of the actin filament, are (reasonably) assumed to be small, given the length of actin filaments.

Application of the Linear Lattice Formalism—
Insights and Mechanistic Implications from Measurements
of the Cooperativity of Tropomyosin-Actin Binding

The linear lattice analysis, using Eq. 1, makes it possible to perform quantitative structure-function studies of cooperative actin-tropomyosin binding. One can measure the equilibrium constant/cooperativity factor y and one can measure K_0, the component of overall binding affinity that does not involve cooperative contributions, under conditions of stronger or weaker end-to-end tropomyosin-tropomyosin binding. The results of such measurements can be summarized as follows: tropomyosin-actin binding generally depends upon end-to-end tropomyosin-tropomyosin interactions, but the strength of these end-to-end interactions correlates poorly with the cooperativity of binding. Under changing experimental conditions, K_0 varies by orders of magnitude, but y varies at most a few-fold, often in the opposite direction from expectation. This pattern plays out in three very different examples. (1) Tropomyosin retains but minimal ability to bind to actin if either the N- or C-terminus of tropomyosin is altered to abolish polymerizability.[19,20] Somewhat remarkably it is K_0 that is decreased by these structural changes. The effect on the value of y is hard to assess, except in the presence of troponin, in which case y is either unchanged or but slightly decreased by these alterations of the tropomyosin N and/or C-termini that are profoundly

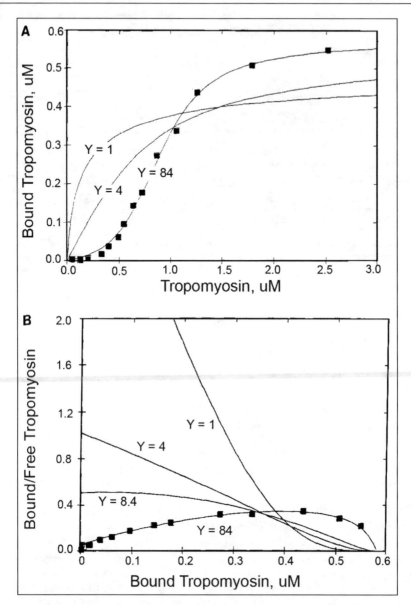

Figure 3. Cooperative binding of tropomyosin to actin. Direct (top) and Scatchard (bottom) plots of cardiac tropomyosin binding to actin. Best fit curves are with y = 84. The other curves, not matching the data, show the pattern that would be found with lower levels of cooperativity and with an unchanged value for the product yK_o, which is the apparent binding constant when cooperativity is high.

polymerization-disrupting.[21,22] (2) Similarly, troponin promotes the polymerization of (normal) tropomyosin[23,24] and in what might seem to be a corresponding effect, troponin strengthens tropomyosin-actin binding. However, linear lattice analysis suggests this effect is due to an increase in K_o.[17] Despite the tendency of troponin to polymerize tropomyosin, the cooperativity parameter y does not increase when troponin is added. (3) Finally, the value of y does not decrease when the ionic strength is increased, despite the sharply anti-polymerizing effect of salt. Rather, K_0 is decreased and y is unchanged or, opposite to expectation, moderately increased.[17,21,22]

The straightforward implication of such data would be that the cooperativity of tropomyosin-actin binding is not simply attributable to end-to-end tropomyosin-tropomyosin interactions. It would follow that alterations in actin are involved as a prominent component of the mechanism of cooperativity. This is shown schematically in Figure 2, in which the phenomena underlying the equilibrium constant y include not only end-to-end tropomyosin polymerization, but also a decrease in the number of boundaries between actins contacting (filled circles) and not contacting (open circles) tropomyosin. When tropomyosin is repositioned from an isolated site to site that is directly adjacent to another tropomyosin, so that end-to-end binding occurs, this also changes the number of boundaries: as shown schematically the number decreases from four to two (seen in the Figure by inspection; the number of sites where open circles are adjacent to filled circles.) Does this matter energetically; are such boundaries unfavorable, with a free energy cost and therefore contribute to the measured cooperativity? At present there is no direct experimental evidence whether this is the case. Rather, it seems the most reasonable inference from the data described in this review.

If tropomyosin-influenced actin-actin interactions cause, in significant part, the cooperativity of tropomyosin's binding to actin, the immediate issue is to identify the nature of these interactions. Structural and thermodynamic aspects of subunit-subunit interactions can be presumed to underlie any mechanism. The present difficulty in obtaining such insight (y $\approx$ 100 indicates that the expected effects are quite small, especially since part of this cooperativity involves tropomyosin end-to-end binding), might seem to weaken the plausibility of the overall idea, moving it toward speculation. This weakness is genuine, but not without partial amelioration. By spanning several actins, tropomyosin could hardly fail to order the actin filament, to make it less flexible. This is an experimental observation and more than a contention. Thin filament persistence length is increased two-fold by either smooth muscle or skeletal muscle tropomyosin, increases similar to the effect of phalloidin.[25] Thus, there is no need to propose that tropomyosin changes the conformation of actin in a small, unknown way so as to promote cooperative tropomyosin binding to the thin filament. Rather, the explanation may lie with a less speculative tropomyosin-induced decrease in actin monomer mobility, i.e., a more restrained actin monomer within thin filaments where tropomyosin is attached, corresponding to the decreased flexibility of F-actin in the presence of tropomyosin.

Conclusions

Tropomyosin end-to-end overlap complexes, comprised by the N-terminus of one tropomyosin and the C-terminus of another, facilitate the formation of continuous tropomyosin strands along the actin filament. The overlap complexes vary considerably in size and composition among tropomyosin isoforms, but are uniformly present for all tropomyosins. Correspondingly, a key characteristic of tropomyosin-actin binding is that it is a cooperative process, demonstrable from the shapes of binding isotherms. However, the degree of cooperativity during actin binding does not correlate with the strength of end-to-end binding in solution. The cooperativity of tropomyosin-actin binding likely involves effects on the actin filament lattice, as well as direct contacts between adjacent tropomyosins.

References

1. Phillips GN Jr, Lattman EE, Cummins P et al. Crystal structure and molecular interactions of tropomyosin. Nature 1979; 278:413-417.
2. Whitby FG, Phillips GNJ. Crystal structure of tropomyosin at 7 Angstroms resolution. Proteins 2000; 38:49-59.
3. Drees B, Brown C, Barrell BG et al. Tropomyosin is essential in yeast, yet the TPM1 and TPM2 products perform distinct functions. J Cell Biol 1995; 128:383-392.
4. Strand J, Nili M, Homsher E et al. Modulation of Myosin Function by Isoform-Specific Properties of S. Cerevisiae and Muscle Tropomyosins. J Biol Chem 2001; 276:34832-34839.

5. McGhee JD, von Hippel PH. Theoretical aspects of DNA-protein interactions: cooperative and non-cooperative binding of large ligands to a one-dimensional lattice. J Mol Biol 1974; 86:469-489.
6. Tobacman LS. Structure-function studies of the amino-terminal region of bovine cardiac troponin T. J Biol Chem 1988; 263:2668-2672.
7. Greenfield NJ, Huang YJ, Swapna GV et al. Solution NMR structure of the junction between tropomyosin molecules: implications for actin binding and regulation. J Mol Biol 2006; 364:80-96.
8. Sousa AD, Farah CS. Quantitative analysis of tropomyosin linear polymerization equilibrium as a function of ionic strength. J Biol Chem 2002; 277:2081-2088.
9. Lorenz M, Poole KJV, Popp D et al. An atomic model of the unregulated thin filament obtained by x-ray fiber diffraction on oriented actin-tropomyosin gels. J Mol Biol 1995; 246:108-119.
10. Lehman W, Hatch V, Korman VL et al. Tropomyosin and actin isoforms modulate the localization of tropomyosin strands on actin filaments. J Mol Biol 2000; 302:593-606.
11. Ruiz-Opazo N, Nadal-Ginard B. Alpha-tropomyosin gene organization. Alternative splicing of duplicated isotype-specific exons accounts for the production of smooth and striated muscle isoforms. J Biol Chem 987; 262(10):4755-4765.
12. McLachlan AD, Stewart M. The 14-fold periodicity in α-tropomyosin and the interaction with actin. J Mol Biol 1976; 103:271-298.
13. Vibert P, Craig R, Lehman W. Steric-model for activation of muscle thin filaments. J Mol Biol 1997; 266:8-14.
14. Xu C, Craig R, Tobacman LS et al. Tropomyosin positions in regulated thin filaments revealed by cryoelectron microscopy. Biophys J 1999; 77:985-992.
15. Rosol M, Lehman W, Craig R et al. Three-dimensional reconstruction of thin filaments containing mutant tropomyosin. Biophys J 2000; 78(2):908-917.
16. Brown JH, Zhou Z, Reshetnikova L et al. Structure of the mid-region of tropomyosin: bending and binding sites for actin. Proc Natl Acad Sci USA 2005; 102:18878-18883.
17. Hill LE, Mehegan JP, Butters CA et al. Analysis of troponin-tropomyosin binding to actin. Troponin does not promote interactions between tropomyosin molecules. J Biol Chem 1992; 267:16106-16113.
18. Tsuchiya T, Szabo A. Cooperative binding of n-mers with steric hindrance to finite and infinite one-dimensional lattices. Biopolymers 1982; 21:979-994.
19. Heeley DH, Golosinska K, Smillie LB. The effects of troponin T fragments T1 and T2 on the binding of nonpolymerizable tropomyosin to F-actin in the presence and absence of troponin I and troponin C. J Biol Chem 1987; 262:9971-9978.
20. Cho Y-J, Liu J, Hitchcock-DeGregori SE. The amino terminus of tropomyosin is a major determinant for function. J Biol Chem 1990; 265:538-545.
21. Willadsen KA, Butters CA, Hill LE et al. Effects of the amino-terminal regions of tropomyosin and troponin T on thin filament assembly. J Biol Chem 1992; 267(33):23746-23752.
22. Butters CA, Willadsen KA, Tobacman LS. Cooperative interactions between adjacent troponin-tropomyosin complexes may be transmitted through the thin filament. J Biol Chem 1993; 268:15565-15570.
23. Tobacman LS, Lee R. Isolation and functional comparison of bovine cardiac troponin T isoforms. J Biol Chem 1987; 262:4059-4064.
24. Cabral-Lilly D, Tobacman LS, Mehegan JP et al. Molecular polarity in tropomyosin-troponin T cocrystals. Biophys J 1996; 73:1763-1770.
25. Isambert H, Venier P, Maggs AC et al. Flexibility of actin filaments derived from thermal fluctuations. Effect of bound nucleotide, phalloidin and muscle regulatory proteins. J Biol Chem 1995; 270:11437-11444.

CHAPTER 8

Tropomyosin and the Steric Mechanism of Muscle Regulation

William Lehman* and Roger Craig

Abstract

Contraction in all muscles must be precisely regulated and requisite control systems must be able to adjust to changes in physiological and myopathic stimuli. In this chapter, we outline the structural evidence for a steric mechanism that governs muscle activity. The mechanism involves calcium and myosin induced changes in the position of tropomyosin along actin-based thin filaments. This process either blocks or uncovers myosin crossbridge binding sites on actin and consequently regulates crossbridge cycling on thin filaments, the sliding of thin and thick filaments and muscle shortening and force production.

Introduction

Tropomyosin, a major F-actin binding protein, is found in virtually all eukaryotic cells. By binding alongside actin subunits of thin filaments, elongated tropomyosin molecules buttress F-actin and protect filaments from depolymerization. In skeletal and cardiac muscle, tropomyosin plays an additional specialized role: together with its thin filament partner, troponin, it functions to activate and inhibit actin-myosin interaction in a process that controls muscle shortening and force production. Elucidating the role(s) played by tropomyosin (and troponin) in this on-off switching mechanism is therefore essential for understanding thin filament-linked regulation of muscle contraction. It is known that point mutations in tropomyosin and troponin can lead to inherited cardiomyopathies as well as contribute to the development of hypertension, respiratory and other diseases (see Chapters 10-13). Thus solving the mechanism of thin filament regulation is of especial biomedical significance.

Tropomyosin controls actin—myosin interaction by a steric mechanism that is modulated by the binding of Ca^{2+} to troponin. Explaining the structural basis of steric-regulation requires making brief prefatory remarks outlining characteristics of the protein players involved and the role of Ca^{2+} in the process.

The Interaction of Actin and Myosin with ATP

Contraction in all muscles results from the relative sliding of thick and thin filaments and is driven by myosin-crossbridge heads projecting from thick filaments, which in a cyclic and repetitive process of attachment and detachment advance along the actin molecules of thin filaments. Crossbridge dynamics are a function of the myosin ATPase, which in turn is dependent on the activation of myosin by its binding to actin. The atomic structures of both the "globular" G-actin monomer (Fig. 1A) and the myosin head (subfragment-1 (S1)) have been solved.[1-5] For reviews, see references 6-8. Atomic models of the overall structure of actin filaments (F-actin) and the as-

*Corresponding Author: William Lehman—Department of Physiology and Biophysics, Boston University School of Medicine, 715 Albany Street, Boston, MA 02118, USA.
Email: wlehman@bu.edu

Tropomyosin, edited by Peter Gunning. ©2008 Landes Bioscience and Springer Science+Business Media.

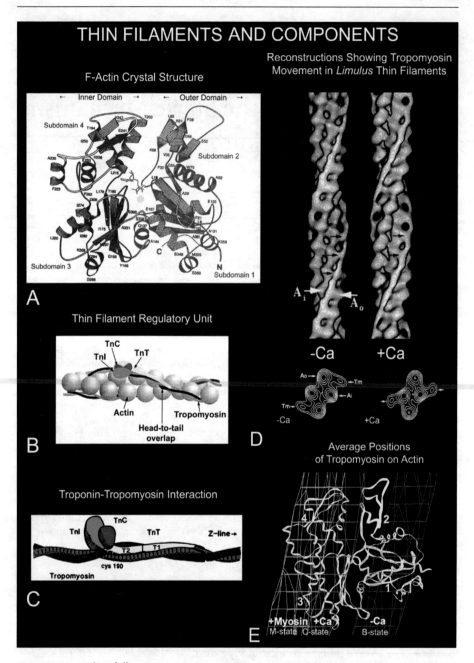

Figure 1. Legend on following page.

Figure 1, viewed on previous page. Images of thin filaments and components. A) Ribbon representation of the atomic structure of the actin molecule. Note the domain structure, and the bound Ca^{2+} and nucleotide in the cleft between subdomains. (Adapted and reprinted with permission from Kabsch W, Mannherz HG, Suck D et al. Atomic structure of actin:DNAase 1 complex. Nature 1990; 347:37-43. ©Nature Publishing Group.) B) A diagram showing the arrangement of troponin, tropomyosin and actin monomers that form "regulatory units" along thin filaments. Troponin subunits (TnC (red), TnT (yellow), and TnI (green)) lie along the tropomyosin coiled-coil (dark brown and orange), which in turn produces helical strands that follow the actin long-pitch helices. Actin monomers (gray) are represented schematically as a double-helical chain of beads. TnC is now known to be oriented obliquely relative to the filament axis[102,113] and the ends of TnT and TnI are intertwined.[25,26] (Reprinted with permission from Gordon AM, Homsher E, Regnier M Regulation of contraction in striated muscle. Physiol Rev 2000; 80:853-924. ©American Physiological Society.) C) A diagram of the tropomyosin-troponin complex (no actin shown). TnI, TnC and the C-terminal part of TnT (T2) localize near Cys190 of tropomyosin. The N-terminal "tail" of TnT (TnT1) extends along the C-terminal half of tropomyosin. (Thus when TnT and tropomyosin are bound to each other, their amino acid sequences run antiparallel.) The polarity of the diagram is such that in a sarcomere the Z-line would be to the right. (Adapted and reprinted with permission from Flicker, PF, Phillips GN, Cohen C. Troponin and its interactions with tropomyosin: An electron microscope study. J Mol Biol 1982; 162:495-501. ©Elsevier.) (D, E) 3D reconstructions of thin filaments showing the positions of tropomyosin in different regulatory states. D) Limulus thin filament reconstructions (Top, surface views; Bottom, helical projections (i.e., projections made to follow the helices of the filament)) showing tropomyosin strands (indicated by black arrows) on the inner edge of the outer domain of actin (A_o) at low Ca^{2+} and on the outer edge of the inner domain of actin (A_i) at high Ca^{2+}. The pointed end of the filament is facing up. (Reprinted with permission from Lehman W, Craig R, Vibert P. Ca^{2+}-induced tropomyosin movement in Limulus thin filaments revealed by three dimensional reconstruction. Nature 1994; 368:65-67. ©Nature Publishing Group.) E) The three-state steric model showing three locations occupied by tropomyosin on the surface of actin. A single actin monomer of the thin filament is represented by the actin crystal structure, depicted as an α-carbon chain (yellow, refer to Fig. 1A) in face-on view (actin subdomains 1 to 4 are indicated; clusters of amino acids on subdomain 1 that are involved in the strong (stereospecific) binding of myosin are highlighted in cyan). The red, magenta and green wire-cages represent the respective B-, C- and M-state regulatory positions of tropomyosin revealed by EM reconstructions. Note that in the absence of Ca^{2+}, B-state tropomyosin, obstructs access to sites of strong myosin binding on actin and that in the Ca^{2+}-induced C-state one cluster of amino acids still remains blocked. The myosin-binding site is only fully open in the myosin-induced M-state. Weak, electrostatic myosin binding to charged amino acids at the N-terminus of actin and the backside of subdomain 1 (amino acids involved highlighted in white) are not obstructed by tropomyosin in any of these states. To obtain this diagram, 3D reconstructions of filaments in their respective regulatory states were aligned and superimposed. The atomic model of F-actin[114] was fitted to the actin density in the reconstructions and substituted for corresponding EM densities. The extra density represented by tropomyosin in each map was then determined and highlighted. (Based on molecular fitting and adapted from figures in Vibert P, Craig R, Lehman W. Steric-model for activation of muscle thin filaments. J Mol Biol 1997; 266:8-14 and made with permission. ©Elsevier.)

sociation of S1 with F-actin also have been constructed by fitting the atomic coordinates of G-actin to X-ray fiber diffraction data from F-actin and by fitting atomic coordinates to EM reconstructions of undecorated and "S1-decorated" F-actin filaments.[7,9-11] Based on this analysis, insightful and elegant molecular models for the crossbridge cycle have been proposed which describe likely intramolecular changes in S1 resulting from ATP hydrolysis and interaction with actin, which is extensively reviewed in references 7, 8, 10, 12-15; also see http://www.mpimf-heidelberg.mpg. de/~holmes/. Moreover, the various crystal structures and the atomic models of F-actin have provided an architectural reference and mechanistic framework for understanding the impact of regulatory proteins on actomyosin interaction.

Ca²⁺—Regulation of the Actin-Myosin Interaction

General Considerations

Following plasma membrane excitation, muscle contraction is initiated by release of Ca^{2+} from the sarcoplasmic reticulum. The increase in cytosolic free Ca^{2+} concentration to micromolar levels leads to binding of Ca^{2+} to troponin. During relaxation, Ca^{2+} levels drop and Ca^{2+} dissociates from troponin.[16,17] While tropomyosin is found on thin filaments in all muscles, in vertebrates, troponin is limited to striated muscle, whereas, in invertebrates, troponin is present in both smooth and striated muscles.[18,19] In vertebrate smooth muscle, where troponin is absent, evidence suggests that thin filament-linked caldesmon and/or calponin may partly substitute for troponin and participate along with tropomyosin (and myosin-phosphorylation) in a complex dual regulatory system (see Chapter 9).

Troponin-Tropomyosin—Based Thin Filament-Linked Regulation

Troponin, the receptor for Ca^{2+}, exerts its influence on F-actin indirectly by acting on tropomyosin, which then controls myosin crossbridge cycling. Troponin is actually a complex of three subunits, one of which, troponin-I (TnI) inhibits actomyosin ATPase; another, troponin-C (TnC), binds Ca^{2+}; and a third, troponin-T (TnT), links the entire complex to tropomyosin.[20-22] In high amounts, TnI alone can inhibit actomyosin ATPase, but at normal stoichiometry the TnI-induced inhibition requires the presence of tropomyosin and is then neutralized by TnC and Ca^{2+}. TnT is more than just a link between troponin subunits and tropomyosin, since it interacts intimately with TnI, augments inhibition in the off-state and, in concert with tropomyosin, potentiates actomyosin ATPase in the on-state.[23-26]

The Structure of Tropomyosin on Actin Filaments

Our present understanding of troponin-tropomyosin action has been achieved to a large degree because of structural studies performed on thin filaments and on isolated troponin and tropomyosin. Tropomyosin is a 40 nm long "coiled-coil" α-helical protein, which lies on thin filaments along the two long-pitch helical strands of actin monomers.[27-29] Tropomyosin itself is a modular molecule and possesses a series of 7 quasi-repeating motifs designed to bind to each of 7 successive actin monomers along filaments.[30-32] Whether all modules bind to actin with equal strength is not known. Tropomyosin molecules associate together in an end-to-end fashion[33,34] to form a continuous helical cable (Fig. 1B), with each tropomyosin spanning 7 successive actin molecules (38 nm). In turn, one troponin complex binds at a specific site on each tropomyosin molecule;[16,35-37] troponin complexes therefore assume the tropomyosin periodicity of 38 nm. Thus, 7 actins, 1 tropomyosin and 1 troponin complex define a repeating "regulatory unit" of the thin filament. A single troponin complex is shorter (26.5 nm) than tropomyosin and extends over about two-thirds of each tropomyosin molecule.[35-37] TnT is a fairly long asymmetric molecule (19 nm long), whereas TnC and TnI are more globular and in the troponin complex bind at the C-terminal end of troponin-T.[38] The TnT "tail" is thought to bind alongside tropomyosin, bridging the head-to-tail joint between adjacent tropomyosin molecules and then extending over and interacting with the C-terminal half of tropomyosin where TnC and TnI localize (Figs. 1B, C). For reviews, see references 24, 39; also see reference 40. The confluence of TnI and TnC at the end of TnT forms the so-called core-domain of troponin, for which crystal structures have been solved.[25,26]

The binding of individual tropomyosin molecules to F-actin is very weak (K_d 0.1-1 mM).[41,42] However, the head-to-tail association of tropomyosin molecules (25 tropomyosin molecules/ micron F-actin) increases the binding because of the collective interactions of the tropomyosin strand on actin. By bridging and presumably reinforcing the end-to-end connection between neighboring tropomyosin molecules on F-actin, TnT and hence whole troponin, enhances tropomyosin binding and stabilizes the tropomyosin strand on thin filaments;[43-45] also see Chapters 5-7. Perturbations in end-to-end connectivity can greatly diminish tropomyosin binding to actin;[46,47] also see Chapters 5-7.

The Steric-Blocking Model

Background

X-ray diffraction studies on intact muscle suggested that the binding of Ca^{2+} to troponin induces changes in the relationship of tropomyosin and actin on thin filaments.[48-50] These studies formed the basis for the well-known steric-blocking model of muscle regulation, originally envisioned by Hanson and Lowy,[51] which holds that tropomyosin strands running along thin filaments block myosin-binding sites on actin in relaxed muscle and expose them when muscle is activated, allowing crossbridge interaction and contraction to proceed. Similar models, incorporating crystallographic data on actin and tropomyosin, are consistent with this view.[52-54] However, while analysis of X-ray patterns could provide models of filament structure, unambiguous interpretation was not possible because phase information was lacking. In contrast, 3D imaging of thin filament electron micrographs, using helical reconstruction methods developed by DeRosier and Klug,[55] offered a means of directly testing the tropomyosin movement model. Over 20 years of attempts to reveal tropomyosin by this approach resulted in an often-confusing literature. For reviews, see references 56-59. Tropomyosin was eventually resolved in EM-reconstructions of S1-decorated filaments[60] but not in undecorated filaments in the inhibited (low Ca^{2+}) state (discussed in ref. 61). Hence, the steric-blocking hypothesis could not be directly tested. Unequivocal observation of tropomyosin in the inhibited state was first achieved in reconstructions of "native" thin filaments isolated from the striated muscles of the horseshoe crab, *Limulus polyphemus* and tropomyosin was seen to move over actin in a manner consistent with the steric model (Fig. 1D).[62] The *Limulus* filament preparations were well suited for study since they retained a full complement of functional tropomyosin and troponin components, even the at low concentrations necessary for EM imaging; the analysis was also aided by new, well-documented programs for helical reconstruction,[63] reference models of F-actin that aided interpretation of the 3D maps[9,60] and computer workstations able to rapidly calculate and average density maps. Later studies showed similar Ca^{2+}-dependent tropomyosin movement in thin filaments isolated from vertebrate skeletal and cardiac muscles, as well as in filaments reconstituted from individual vertebrate components (i.e., F-actin, troponin and tropomyosin).[64,65] The ability to resolve tropomyosin in characteristically distinct positions on actin in both on- and off-states directly validated the hypothesis that tropomyosin does move on thin filaments in a manner compatible with the steric model of regulation.[61,62,64-70] These results quelled the debate about the veracity of the proposed tropomyosin movement (e.g., see discussion in refs. 56, 58, 71). Consistent with the steric model, tropomyosin in the relaxed state was noted to cover the myosin contact site on actin involved in strong stereospecific actomyosin interaction.[62,66] Interestingly, a number of charged amino acid residues on the periphery of actin remained exposed, even at low-Ca^{2+}. These residues may be involved in weak electrostatic interactions between myosin heads and actin made prior to strong binding.[72] Hence tropomyosin at low Ca^{2+} appears to block the transition from an initially weak to a strong crossbridge interaction, thereby inhibiting actomyosin ATPase, crossbridge cycling and force production.

The Three-State Version of the Steric-Blocking Model

EM—reconstructions showed that in the absence of Ca^{2+}, tropomyosin is constrained in a position on the outer domain of actin that covers the known myosin-docking site, resulting in the relaxed "blocked" or B-state (State #1) (Fig. 1E). Full activation by reversal of steric blocking was shown to involve two additional thin filament states (Fig. 1E), requiring successive tropomyosin movements away from the blocked position. Ca^{2+} binding to troponin causes tropomyosin movement towards the "inner domain" of actin, exposing most of the myosin-binding site (referred to as "Ca^{2+}-induced", "closed-" or C-state; State #2). However, even following this change, tropomyosin still covers an essential part of the site. A further tropomyosin shift, promoted by the binding of myosin heads themselves, was shown to expose the entire myosin-binding site, fully activating the filament (referred to as the "myosin-induced", "open-" or M-state; State #3).[61,62,64-67] The concept that the binding of Ca^{2+} to troponin is necessary but not sufficient to trigger muscle activation is supported by biochemical data on tropomyosin's influence on actin-myosin interactions and on the hydrolysis of ATP.[73-75]

Thus, in the three-state version of the steric model, Ca^{2+} binding induces a filament conformational change where tropomyosin unblocks actin. This favors myosin crossbridge binding, which in turn causes further tropomyosin movement fully exposing the myosin binding site and leading to full activity.[24,65,66,73-75] By facilitating tropomyosin movement, myosin appears to act as an effector, cooperatively promoting its own binding during muscle activation, a conclusion also supported by modeling of X-ray diffraction data on intact fibers.[54,70] These studies also indicated that the effect of myosin on tropomyosin position propagates over many actin monomers, suggesting that the tropomyosin molecule moves cooperatively as a relatively stiff cable while adapting well to the surface contours of actin (see Chapter 7). Kinetic data indicated further that the three regulatory states are in rapid equilibrium with one another, where any one state may dominate depending on the influence of troponin and myosin.[74,75]

Thin Filaments Trapped in the "Closed" Ca^{2+}-Induced State

To be consistent with the 3-state model of thin filament regulation in which both Ca^{2+} and myosin-induced movements of tropomyosin are required for activation, tropomyosin in the intermediate Ca^{2+}-induced "closed" C-state should sterically inhibit the binding of myosin crossbridges, although to a lesser extent than in the "blocked" B-state (in the absence of Ca^{2+}). Hence a troponin-tropomyosin complex that permits Ca^{2+}-induced movement but not myosin-induced movement should inhibit myosin cycling.

Filaments with a tropomyosin deletion mutation, D234, which spans 4 instead of 7 actin monomers (engineered so that actin binding pseudo-repeat modules 2, 3 and 4 are missing), appeared to behave as if they were stabilized in the C-state.[76] D234 retains regions of tropomyosin that bind troponin and form end-to-end bonds, while binding to actin. Despite these apparently normal interactions, D234 conferred inhibition on actomyosin ATPase and filament sliding, which Ca^{2+} and troponin did not reverse.[76] EM and 3D reconstruction showed that the mutation did not affect Ca^{2+}-induced tropomyosin movement, which also occurred normally.[77] It was concluded that D234 tropomyosin was unable to shift from the C-state to the completely activated M-state position[77], which supported the view that the Ca^{2+}-induced state is not a fully switched-on configuration of the thin filament. Rather, the Ca^{2+}-state is switched-off by being relatively "closed" to myosin binding. Similarly, work on two yeast tropomyosin molecules that inhibit actomyosin ATPase showed that in one case tropomyosin is strongly biased to the C-state[78] and in the other that it is virtually immobilized in the C-state position.[79] The results as a whole provide strong support for the 3-state model of regulation in which activation is considered to be a stepwise process requiring sequential Ca^{2+}- and myosin-induced transitions to release inhibition.

Refining the Three-State Model

To further characterize the three mean positions occupied by tropomyosin, atomic models of actin, tropomyosin and the actin-crossbridge complex were aligned to respective densities in EM reconstructions of Ca^{2+}-free, Ca^{2+}-treated and S1-decorated thin filaments by least squares fitting.[70] The actin and actin-S1 models were taken from Holmes et al[11] and the tropomyosin coiled-coil was generated to follow the long-pitch actin helix as in Lorenz et al[31] and to match recent crystal structures.[80,81] This process (see Fig. 2A, B) placed tropomyosin over F-actin in virtually identical positions to the ones originally proposed by Vibert et al[66] and Xu et al[61] and discussed above.

This modeling revealed an additional aspect of steric regulation that had not been previously appreciated. When myosin interacts with actin during the crossbridge cycle, a cleft at the tip of the myosin head needs to be shut after strong binding to actin.[7,10] Results of Poole et al[70] showed that in relaxed muscle tropomyosin might act as a molecular gag and prevent the cleft from closing properly (Fig. 2C). Thus, tropomyosin in relaxed muscle may hinder myosin interactions on actin by (1) obstructing the myosin target site on actin and (2) possibly interfering with an obligatory conformation change during the crossbridge cycle.[70]

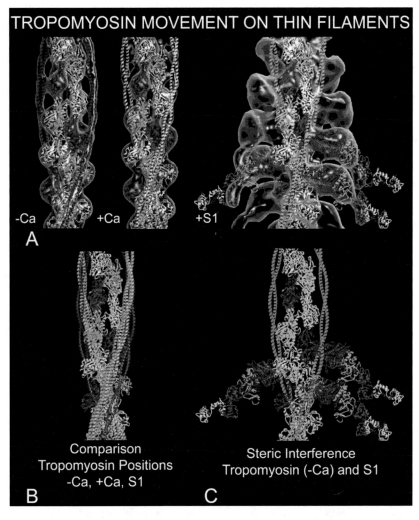

Figure 2. Tropomyosin movement on thin filaments. A) Fitting of atomic models of F-actin (actin subunits: blue, cyan and white), tropomyosin (red, yellow and green) and those of S1-decorated F-actin into 3D reconstructions of Ca^{2+}-free and Ca^{2+}- and S1-treated filaments.[70] Note the angular shift of tropomyosin between the different states. B) The tropomyosin movement is especially evident when the 3 positions of tropomyosin are superimposed to form a composite map.[70] C) The thin filament in the blocked-state clashing with S1 binding (S1 painted here and above as in Rayment et al[5]). Note the steric interference between tropomyosin (salmon) and "50K domain" (red) of the ATP-free "rigor" bound cross-bridge. The actin binding site is split by the tropomyosin, which is positioned between the "upper" and "lower" 50K domains.[70] (Reprinted with permission from Poole KJ, Lorenz M, Evans G et al. A comparison of muscle thin filament models obtained from electron microscopy reconstructions and low-angle X-ray fibre diagrams from non-overlap muscle. J Struct Biol 2006; 155:273-284. ©Elsevier.)

Tropomyosin Flexibility

Schematic models of F-actin are often drawn as two chains of spherical beads wound round each other (as in Fig. 1B). This depiction misrepresents the shape of actin monomers and hence the double helix that they form. Actin molecules are not at all spherical but instead flat.

The simple chain of beads model does not accurately describe tropomyosin movement on actin. If tropomyosin lay on a double helical array of spherical molecules, then azimuthal regulatory movement would require changes in tropomyosin's radial position and therefore its length (contrary to observation). In addition, if the surface over which tropomyosin shifted were uneven, then tropomyosin would need to be additionally flexible to move past obstructions. Indeed, the literature is replete with references to tropomyosin flexibility as an inherent feature of regulatory switching.[34,39,82-86] However, during regulatory movement, tropomyosin does not in fact change radius appreciably as it traverses the flat face of actin and does not encounter obvious steric barriers.[70] Moreover, were actin-bound tropomyosin molecules or end-to-end linked tropomyosin strands very flexible, then the structural effects of Ca^{2+}- or myosin-head binding on tropomyosin position would be dampened out locally, not propagated as observed and cooperative activation of filaments thereby compromised. It is well recognized that the cooperative regulatory unit size of thin filaments is greater than the length of single tropomyosin molecules,[70,87-89] with estimates varying from between 10 to 12 successive actin subunits[87] to the entire length of the thin filament.[70,88] Such long-range effects would be expected to be associated with a rather rigid, not flexible, tropomyosin cable.

Information on the mechanical properties of isolated tropomyosin molecules is limited. Estimates of persistence length, treating tropomyosin as an isotropic rod, range from 50 to 150 nm.[89,90] These values, typical for coiled-coils,[91] suggest that a mechanical deflection at any point along tropomyosin will be sensed over the entire molecule. Additional data reflecting the mechanical behavior of tropomyosin bound to actin also is sparse. Tropomyosin does increase the stiffness of F-actin[92-94] and tends to straighten wavy F-actin filaments (unpublished observations). The surfaces of F-actin and tropomyosin appear to be well adapted to each other judging from measurements quantifying the twist of the F-actin helix in EMs, which show that the 167° angular displacement between adjacent actin monomers along filaments is unaltered by the presence of tropomyosin or troponin-tropomyosin.[95] However, extrapolating from any of these measurements to behavior at the molecular level is difficult. Thus, connecting information on the material properties of tropomyosin and the structural mechanics of thin filaments is premature.

Modeling the Molecular Shape of Tropomyosin

A 3D atomic model of the tropomyosin coiled-coiled coil proposed by the Holmes group[31] and based on fiber diffraction patterns of oriented actin-tropomyosin gels (no troponin) has proven to be very useful in considering the structural mechanics of thin filaments. The analysis suggests that elongated tropomyosin localizes uniformly along F-actin at an approximately 40 Å radius from the filament axis. This places tropomyosin above the surface of actin at a distance that would appear to preclude strong stereospecific interaction. (The closest distance between C^{α} atoms of actin and tropomyosin is approximately 10 to 11 Å.) Further modeling showed that multiple electrostatic interactions between charged side-chains of tropomyosin and actin are likely to dominate the interactions on thin filaments.[31]

The helical contours of the Lorenz/Holmes model[31] of the tropomyosin molecule match remarkably well to corresponding tropomyosin densities in EM reconstructions of Ca^{2+}-free, Ca^{2+}-treated and S-1 decorated filaments.[70] No bending or reconfiguration of the tropomyosin model is needed to obtain a precise fitting to any of these three conformational states (Fig. 2A, B). Examination of the molecular landscape between conformations confirmed that tropomyosin encounters no obvious geometrical obstructions when moving between states and does not change radial position appreciably.[70] Given that one tropomyosin model fits equally well to all states, large-scale flexibility in tropomyosin shape seems unnecessary for regulatory switching. In addition, high-resolution crystal structures of segments of tropomyosin[80,81] fit very well to the Holmes/Lorenz model as well as to the tropomyosin densities in reconstructions (Holmes, personal communication).[80,81,85] The agreement between structural data obtained by widely different methods supports the view that the contours of the tropomyosin coiled-coiled coil match well to the surface of F-actin regardless of regulatory state. In fact, the amino acid sequence of tropomyosin is fairly unique among coiled-coils. Patches of alanine clusters along tropomyosin cause periodic and specific bends that occur along the length of the coiled-coiled coil.[80,81,84] These bends presumably are adaptations that allow tropomyosin to align precisely to the interface of F-actin. Significantly, mutations in the alanine clusters reduce the binding of tropomyosin to F-actin, apparently by disrupting the pairing between the actin and tropomyosin helices.[83,84] The complementarity of tropomyosin and F-actin structures, no doubt, provides the freedom for tropomyosin to move over a relatively flat actin interface and at low energy cost.

Sliding vs Rolling of Tropomyosin on F-Actin

The F-actin helix, formed from successive actin subunits, presents a gently curving "convex" surface over which the concave surface of the tropomyosin helical strand binds precisely (Fig. 2 A, B).[54,70] If, as postulated above, movement of tropomyosin between positional states does not involve significant change in its configuration, then tropomyosin should be capable of sliding from one state to the other. It is difficult to envision it rolling between states, as any significant rolling would diminish complementarity and contact between F-actin and tropomyosin helices.[70] Without high resolution structural maps detailing the interaction sites of tropomyosin on F-actin and specifically defining the changes that tropomyosin undergoes during regulatory movements, it is equally difficult to evaluate alternative hypotheses that invoke a rolling motion of tropomyosin on F-actin.[30,96-98]

Towards a Statistical-Mechanical Understanding of Steric-Regulation

Tropomyosin Position Is Governed by Weak Interactions That Are Easily Perturbed

Evaluating the positions of different tropomyosin isoforms on troponin-free actin has proven to be a valuable way of demonstrating the suppleness of azimuthal positioning of tropomyosin on actin. For any given actin-tropomyosin pair, tropomyosin (no troponin) localizes, on average, in either the B- or the C-state position on actin.[65] This suggests that the binding positions are determined by two sets of interactions defined by respective tropomyosin and actin surfaces (cf. refs. 30, 31, 52). In all cases examined, differences in the equilibrium positions assumed by tropomyosin on actin depended on minor amino acid variation among the isoforms tested. Hence, the energy barrier between tropomyosin states must be small, suggesting that in the absence of troponin or myosin, tropomyosin position on actin is not strongly fixed. These results imply that the regulatory roles of troponin and myosin are to bias and/or stabilize tropomyosin in inhibitory and activating states. Even in smooth muscle, where there is no troponin, myosin binding alone may influence cooperative switching between tropomyosin states and the kinetics of muscle regulation (see Chapter 9).

Categorizing and Sorting Filament Data to Different Regulatory Classes

Structural data demonstrating movement of tropomyosin from one positional state to another provides a time-averaged snapshot of what likely is a dynamic equilibrium. Solution studies, in comparison, suggest that tropomyosin oscillates rapidly between positions at all Ca^{2+} levels and that it is the position of this equilibrium that is controlled by Ca^{2+} and S1 binding.[74,75]

Helical reconstruction, so valuable in revealing different tropomyosin positions on thin filaments, yields the mean position of tropomyosin on the filament, but not the local dynamics of tropomyosin in any one regulatory-state. The method treats actin monomers over a given length of filament as equivalent and therefore averages densities derived from tropomyosin or any other actin-binding protein, as if they were the same on each actin monomer. The method cannot identify local differences and thus, if tropomyosin were in a dynamic equilibrium between positions, favoring but never being truly fixed in one place, then averaging would mask the variability.

Iterative helical real space reconstruction (IHRSR), an adaptation of standard single particle analysis of EMs, is better suited to determining local differences in filament configuration.[99,100]

In the method, filament images are divided computationally into short segments (7 actins and 1 tropomyosin molecule long), which are then treated as "single particles".[68] These can be matched to filament models in which tropomyosin is in the high Ca^{2+} or low Ca^{2+} position. Using this method to sort segments from either Ca^{2+}-free or Ca^{2+}-treated thin filaments showed that most segments fitted as expected to low- and high-Ca^{2+} filament models. However, about 20% of segments from Ca^{2+}-free filaments fitted best to the high-Ca^{2+} model, yielding a corresponding high-Ca^{2+} reconstruction. Conversely, approximately 20% of segments from Ca^{2+}-treated filaments fitted best to the low-Ca^{2+} model and produced a low-Ca^{2+} reconstruction.[68] This structural evidence thus indicates that the position of tropomyosin on actin is not fixed even in the presence of troponin. These results provided direct structural evidence for the equilibration of tropomyosin position in blocked and closed states (as suggested by the solution studies) and for the concept that Ca^{2+} binding to troponin controls the position of this equilibrium. Local oscillation in tropomyosin location centered on a mean position is an additional feature that would allow steric regulation to occur at low energy cost.

The view that that tropomyosin can equilibrate as far as the myosin-induced position, even in the absence of myosin, is also supported by these methods.[68] In addition, strong myosin binding would be expected to trap tropomyosin in the open position, a prediction borne out by results on thin filaments that were either partially or fully decorated with S1 (under "rigor" conditions in the absence of ATP).[66,68] Trapping tropomyosin in the open state, however transient, favors additional myosin binding and cooperatively switches on thin filaments during Ca^{2+}-activation.

The Structural Influence of Troponin on Tropomyosin

Determining the Regulatory Positions of Troponin in Low- and High-Ca^{2+} States

Although the location and regulatory movements of tropomyosin are well defined, the structural organization of troponin on thin filaments has not been determined definitively and molecular models of troponin action remain tentative. The globular end of troponin molecules can be directly visualized in EM images of thin filaments as distinct bulb-like projections accompanying well-defined tropomyosin strands. However, 3D reconstruction of troponin on thin filaments has proven to be very difficult because troponin occurs on only every seventh actin and is therefore averaged out using standard reconstruction methods. At present, structural models developed for troponin on F-actin differ widely and are being actively evaluated.[69,101,102]

The Mobile Domain of TnI

A number of structural studies have defined a specific region of troponin that appears to interact with F-actin in a Ca^{2+}-sensitive manner. At low-Ca^{2+}, this part of troponin extends across actin subdomain 1 on the extreme periphery of actin. Addition of Ca^{2+}, releases this mobile troponin domain from actin.[69,101,103] These results add structural support for the long-held hypothesis that at low-Ca^{2+} troponin constrains tropomyosin on actin's outer domain to inhibit myosin binding.[21,22] Disconnecting the troponin-actin linkage at high Ca^{2+} apparently permits tropomyosin movement to actin's inner domain and consequently myosin interaction with actin and contraction.

These structural observations parallel studies on a series of mutations made in the C-terminal "mobile domain" of TnI by several investigators suggesting that inhibition of muscle contraction at low-Ca^{2+} concentration depends critically on the binding of this region of TnI to actin.[104-109] By latching onto actin at low-Ca^{2+} concentrations, the mobile domain of TnI may position the neighboring TnI "inhibitory peptide" appropriately on actin[110] and/or by being very basic affect the filament surface charge balance to attract tropomyosin to the blocked state.[69] These data are in agreement with studies showing that this region of TnI dissociates from actin at high Ca^{2+} to interact with the N-lobe of TnC and relieve inhibition. Additionally, they are in accord with predictions based on crystal structure studies of the core-domain of troponin[26] and also the modeling and reconstruction of thin filaments.[69,110] Finally, EM reconstructions show that the C-terminal domains of TnI bind to actin subdomain 1 as predicted and in a way that is consistent with this proposed thin filament regulatory scheme.[111] The correspondence between structural changes in troponin and tropomyosin in response to Ca^{2+} and the regulation of actomyosin ATPase and actin-crossbridge is compelling. While we favor a view that the positioning of tropomyosin on actin by TnI directly affects myosin binding by a steric mechanism, others have proposed that troponin and tropomyosin act indirectly by causing an allosteric change in actin that propagates along thin filaments to modulate myosin interaction (e.g., see Chapter 9 and ref. 112).

Perspectives

Our current understanding of the structural changes accompanying steric regulation of muscle contraction is based on diverse X-ray and EM evidence and is amply supported by biochemical data. While our picture of steric regulation is very appealing in its simplicity, a corresponding atomic resolution description of the thin filament, including all its components and detailing filament dynamics completely, is not available. Hence, the complete picture requires refinement of current data and higher resolution structural information about thin filament participants in the regulatory process. Fundamental questions regarding the mechanism of steric regulation remain unresolved, some of which have been highlighted in this chapter. These unanswered questions include:

1. What are the atomic interactions of myosin that are blocked by tropomyosin?
2. What are the chemical interactions between tropomyosin and the surface of F-actin?
3. What are the kinetics of tropomyosin when oscillating on actin between regulatory states and what is the influence of troponin, Ca^{2+} and myosin on these kinetic transitions?
4. How well matched are the contours of the tropomyosin coiled coil-coil and the F-actin surface?
5. How flexible is tropomyosin and does the molecule act mechanically as a uniform isotropic rod?
6. How are the structural mechanics of tropomyosin related to cooperative activation and inhibition of muscle contraction?
7. What are the structure and properties of the end-to-end link between adjacent tropomyosin molecules?
8. Does tropomyosin slide or roll between different regulatory positions?
9. What is the structure of the troponin core domain on actin?
10. How does TnI trap tropomyosin in the blocked state?
11. What is the structural relationship between the TnT tail and tropomyosin and how does this change during tropomyosin movement?

New experimental approaches are within our grasp to answer many of these open questions.

Acknowledgements

We gratefully acknowledge support from the NIH (grants HL36153 and HL86655 to W.L. and AR34711 to R.C.).

We dedicate this paper to the memory of Dr. Setsuro Ebashi, who first showed the regulatory effects of troponin-tropomyosin and was very supportive of our work on the control of muscle contraction.

References

1. Kabsch W, Mannherz HG, Suck D et al. Atomic structure of actin:DNAase 1 complex. Nature 1990; 347:37-43.
2. Holmes KC, Kabsch W. Muscle proteins: actin. Current Opinion Struct Biol 1991; 1:270-280.
3. Otterbein LR, Graceffa P, Dominguez R. The crystal structure of uncomplexed actin in the ADP state. Science 2001; 293:616-618.
4. Rould MA, Wan Q, Joel PB et al. Crystal structures of expressed nonpolymerizable monomeric actin in the ADP and ATP states. J Biol Chem 2006; 281:31909-31919.
5. Rayment I, Rypniewski WR, Schmidt-Bäse K et al. Three-dimensional structure of myosin subfragment-1: A molecular motor. Science 1993a; 261:50-58.

6. Houdusse A, Sweeney HL. Myosin motors: missing structures and hidden springs. Curr Opin Struct Biol 2001; 11:182-194.

7. Geeves MA, Holmes KC. The molecular mechanism of muscle contraction. Adv Protein Chem 2005; 71:161-193.

8. Baghaw CR. Myosin mechanochemistry. Structure 2007; 15:511-512.

9. Holmes KC, Popp D, Gebhard W et al. Atomic model of the actin filament. Nature 1990; 347:44-47.

10. Rayment I, Holden HM, Whittaker M et al. Structure of the actin-myosin complex and its implications for muscle contraction. Science 1993b; 261:58-65.

11. Holmes KC, Angert I, Kull FJ et al. Electron cryo-microscopy shows how strong binding of myosin to actin releases nucleotide. Nature 2003; 425:423-427.

12. Cooke R. The sliding filament model: 1972-2004. J Gen Physiol 2004; 123:643-656.

13. Kull FJ, Endow SA. A new structural state of myosin. Trends Biochem Sci 2004; 29:103-106.

14. Warshaw DM. Lever arms and necks: a common mechanistic theme across the myosin superfamily. J Muscle Res Cell Motil 2004; 25:467-474.

15. Yang Y, Gourinath S, Kovács M et al. Rigor-like structures from muscle myosins reveal key mechanical elements in the transduction pathways of this allosteric motor. Structure 2007; 15:553-564.

16. Ebashi S, Endo M. Calcium ion and muscle contraction. Prog Biophys Mol Biol 1968:28, 123-183.

17. Murray JM, Weber A. Molecular control mechanisms in muscle contraction. Physiol Rev 1973; 53:612-673.

18. Lehman W, Szent-Györgyi AG. Regulation of muscular contraction. Distribution of actin control and myosin control in the animal kingdom. J Gen Physiol 1975; 66:1-30.

19. Lehman W. Thin-filament-linked regulation in molluscan muscles. Biochim Biophys Acta 1981; 668:349-356.

20. Greaser M, Gergely J. Reconstitution of troponin activity from three protein components. J Biol Chem 1971; 246:4226-4233.

21. Hitchcock SE, Huxley HE, Szent-Györgyi AG. Calcium sensitive binding of troponin to actin-tropomyosin: A two-site model for troponin action. J Mol Biol 1973; 80:825-836.

22. Potter JD, Gergely J. Troponin, tropomyosin and actin interactions in the Ca^{2+} regulation of muscle contraction. Biochemistry 1974; 13:2697-2703.

23. Potter JD, Sheng Z, Pan B-S et al. A direct regulatory role for troponin T and a dual role for troponin C in the Ca^{2+} regulation of muscle contraction. J Biol Chem 1995; 270:2557-2562.

24. Tobacman LS. Thin filament-mediated regulation of cardiac contraction. Annu Rev Physiol 1996; 58:447-481.

25. Takeda S, Yamashita A, Maeda K et al. Structure of the core domain of human cardiac troponin in the Ca^{2+}-saturated form. Nature 2003; 424:35-41.

26. Vinogradova MV, Stone DB, Malanina GG et al. Ca^{2+}-regulated structural changes in troponin. Proc Natl Acad Sci USA 2005;102:5038-5043.

27. Moore PB, Huxley HE, DeRosier DJ. Three-dimensional reconstruction of F-actin, thin filaments and decorated thin filaments. J Mol Biol 1970; 50:279-292.

28. O'Brien EJ, Bennett PM, Hanson J. Optical diffraction studies of myofibrillar structure. Philos Trans Roy Soc Lond B 1971; 261:201-208.

29. Spudich JA, Huxley HE, Finch JT. The regulation of skeletal muscle contraction. II. Structural studies of the interaction of the tropomyosin-troponin complex with actin. J Mol Biol 1972; 72:619-632.

30. McLachlan AD, Stewart M. The 14-Fold Periodicity in alpha-tropomyosin and the interaction with actin. J Mol Biol 1976; 103:271-298.

31. Lorenz M, Poole KJV, Popp D et al. An atomic model of the unregulated thin filament obtained by X-ray fiber diffraction on oriented actin-tropomyosin gels. J Mol Biol 1995; 246:108-119.

32. Hitchcock-DeGregori SE, An Y. Integral repeats and continuous coiled coil are required for binding of striated muscle tropomyosin to the regulated actin filament. J Biol Chem 1996; 271:3600-3603.

33. Caspar DLD, Cohen C, Longley, W. Tropomyosin: Crystal structure, polymorphism and molecular interactions. J Mol Biol 1969; 41:87-107.

34. Greenfield NJ, Huang YJ, Swapna GV et al. Solution NMR structure of the junction between tropomyosin molecules: implications for actin binding and regulation. J Mol Biol 2006; 364:80-96.

35. Ohtsuki I, Masaki T, Nonomura Y et al. Periodic distribution of troponin along the thin filament. J Biochem (Tokyo) 1967; 61:817-819.

36. Cohen C, Caspar DLD, Johnson JP et al. Tropomyosin-troponin assembly. Cold Spring Harbor Symp Quant Biol 1972; 37:287-297.

37. Ohtsuki I. Localization of troponin in thin filaments and in tropomyosin paracrystals. J Biochem (Tokyo) 1974; 75:753-765.

38. Flicker PF, Phillips GN, Cohen C. Troponin and its interactions with tropomyosin: An electron microscope study. J Mol Biol 1982; 162:495-501.

39. Gordon AM, Homsher E, Regnier M. Regulation of contraction in striated muscle. Physiol Rev 2000; 80:853-924.
40. Regnier M, Rivera AJ, Wang CK et al. Thin filament near-neighbor regulatory unit interactions affect rabbit skeletal muscle steady-state force-Ca^{2+} relations. J Physiol 2002; 540:485-497.
41. Wegner A. Equilibrium of the actin-tropomyosin interaction. J Mol Biol 1979; 131:839-853.
42. Wegner A. The interaction of alpha, alpha- and alpha , beta-tropomyosin with actin filaments. FEBS Lett 1980; 119:245-248.
43. Wegner A, Walsh TP. Interaction of tropomyosin-troponin with actin filaments. Biochemistry 1981; 20:5633-5642.
44. Heald RW, Hitchcock-DeGregori SE. The structure of the amino terminus of tropomyosin is critical for binding to actin in the absence and presence of troponin. J Biol Chem 1988; 263:5254-5259.
45. Hinkle A, Goranson A, Butters CA et al. Roles for the troponin tail domain in thin filament assembly and regulation. A deletional study of cardiac troponin T. J Biol Chem 1999; 274:7157-7164.
46. Monteiro PB, Lataro RC, Ferro JA et al. Functional alpha-tropomyosin produced in Escherichia coli. A dipeptide extension can substitute the amino-terminal acetyl group. J Biol Chem 1994; 269:10461-10466.
47. Palm T, Greenfield NJ, Hitchcock-DeGregori SE. Tropomyosin ends determine the stability and functionality of overlap and troponin T complexes. Biophys J 2003; 84:3181-3189.
48. Huxley HE Structural changes in actin- and myosin-containing filaments during contraction. Cold Spring Harbor Symp Quant Biol 1972; 37:361-376.
49. Haselgrove JC. X-ray evidence for a conformational change in actin-containing filaments of vertebrate striated muscle. Cold Spring Harbor Symp Quant Biol 1972; 37:341-352.
50. Parry DAD, Squire JM. Structural role of tropomyosin in muscle regulation: Analysis of the X-ray patterns from relaxed and contracting muscles. J Mol Biol 1973; 75:33-55.
51. Hanson J, Lowy J. The structure of actin filaments and the origin of the axial periodicity in the I-substance of vertebrate striated muscle. Proc Royal Soc Lond B 1964; 160:449-460.
52. Phillips GN, Fillers JP, Cohen C. Tropomyosin crystal structure and muscle regulation. J Mol Biol 1986; 192:111-131.
53. Al-Khayat HA, Yagi N, Squire JM. Structural changes in actin-tropomyosin during muscle regulation: Computer modelling of low-angle X-ray diffraction data. J Mol Biol 1995; 252:611-632.
54. Poole KJV, Evans G, Rosenbaum G et al. The effect of crossbridges on the calcium sensitivity of the structural change of the regulated thin filament. Biophys J 1995; 68:A365.
55. DeRosier DJ, Klug A. Reconstruction of three-dimensional structures from electron micrographs. Nature 1968; 217:130-134.
56. Squire JM, Morris E. A new look at thin filament regulation in vertebrate skeletal muscle. FASEB J 1998; 12:761-771.
57. Cohen C, Vibert PJ. Actin filaments: Images and models. In: Squire, JM, Vibert PJ eds. Fibrous Protein Structure. London: Acad. Press, 1987; 283-306.
58. Squire J. Muscle regulation: a decade of steric blocking. Nature 1981; 291:614-615.
59. Lehman W, Craig R. The structure of the vertebrate striated muscle thin filament: a tribute to the contributions of Jean Hanson. J. Muscle Research Cell Motility 2004; 25:455-466.
60. Milligan RA, Whittaker M, Safer D. Molecular structure of F-actin and the location of surface binding sites. Nature 1990; 348:217-221.
61. Xu C, Craig R, Tobacman L et al. Tropomyosin positions in regulated thin filaments revealed by cryo-electron microscopy. J Mol Biol 1999; 77:985-992.
62. Lehman W, Craig R, Vibert P. Ca^{2+}-induced tropomyosin movement in Limulus thin filaments revealed by three dimensional reconstruction. Nature 1994; 368:65-67.
63. Owen C, Morgan DG, DeRosier DJ. Image analysis of helical objects: The Brandeis helical package. J Struct Biol 1996; 116:167-175.
64. Lehman W, Vibert P, Uman P et al. Steric-blocking by tropomyosin visualized in relaxed vertebrate muscle thin filaments. J Mol Biol 1995; 251:191-196.
65. Lehman W, Hatch V, Korman, V et al. Tropomyosin and actin isoforms modulate the localization of tropomyosin strands on actin filaments. J Mol Biol 2000; 302:593-606.
66. Vibert P, Craig R, Lehman W. Steric-model for activation of muscle thin filaments. J Mol Biol 1997; 266:8-14.
67. Craig R, Lehman W. Crossbridge and tropomyosin positions observed in native, interacting thick and thin filaments. J Mol Biol 2001; 311:1027-1036.
68. Pirani A, Xu, C, Hatch V et al. Single particle analysis of relaxed and activated muscle thin filaments. J Mol Biol 2005; 346:761-772.
69. Pirani A, Vinogradova MV, Curmi PMG et al. An atomic model of the thin filament in the relaxed and Ca^{2+}-activated states. J Mol Biol 2006; 357:707-717.

70. Poole KJ, Lorenz M, Evans G et al. A comparison of muscle thin filament models obtained from electron microscopy reconstructions and low-angle X-ray fibre diagrams from non-overlap muscle. J Struct Biol 2006; 155:273-284.

71. Payne MR, Rudnick SE. Regulation of vertebrate striated muscle contraction. Trends Biochem Sci 1989; 14:357-360.

72. Chalovich JM, Chock PB, Eisenberg E. Mechanism of action of troponin:tropomyosin inhibition of actomyosin ATPase activity without inhibition of myosin binding to actin. J Biol Chem 1981; 256: 575-578.

73. Lehrer SS, Morris EP. Dual Effects of tropomyosin and troponin-tropomyosin on actomyosin subfragment 1 ATPase. J Biol Chem 1982; 257:8073-8080.

74. McKillop DFA, Geeves MA. Regulation of the interaction between actin and myosin subfragment 1: Evidence for three states of the thin filament. Biophys J 1993; 65:693-701.

75. Lehrer SS, Geeves MA. The muscle thin filament as a classical cooperative/allosteric regulatory system. J Mol Biol 1998; 277:1081-1089.

76. Landis CA, Bobkova A, Homsher E et al. The active state of the thin filament is destabilized by an internal deletion in tropomyosin. J Biol Chem 1997; 272:14051-14056.

77. Rosol M, Lehman W, Landis C et al. Three-dimensional reconstruction of thin filaments containing mutant tropomyosin, Biophys J 2000; 78:918-926.

78. Kalomoira S, Coulton AT, Lehman W et al. Acetylation regulates tropomyosin function in the fission yeast Schizosaccharomyces pombe. J Cell Sci 2007; 120:1635-1645.

79. Maytum R, Konrad M, Hatch, V et al. Ultra short yeast tropomyosins show novel myosin regulation. 2007 (submitted).

80. Brown JH, Kim KH, Jun G et al. Deciphering the design of the tropomyosin molecule. Proc Natl Acad Sci USA 2001; 98:8496-8501.

81. Brown JH, Zhou Z, Reshetnikova L et al. Structure of the mid-region of tropomyosin: bending and binding sites for actin. Proc Natl Acad Sci USA 2005;102:18878-18883.

82. Chen Y, Lehrer SS. Distances between tropomyosin sites across the muscle thin filament using luminescence resonance energy transfer: evidence for tropomyosin flexibility. Biochemistry 2004; 43:11491-11499.

83. Singh A, Hitchcock-DeGregori SE. Local destabilization of the tropomyosin coiled coil gives the molecular flexibility required for actin binding. Biochemistry 2003; 42:14114-14121.

84. Singh A, Hitchcock-DeGregori SE. Dual requirement for flexibility and specificity for binding of the coiled-coil tropomyosin to its target, actin. Structure 2006; 14:43-50.

85. Brown JH, Cohen C. Regulation of muscle contraction by tropomyosin and troponin: how structure illuminates function. Adv Protein Chem 2005; 71:121-159.

86. Nitanai Y, Minakata S, Maeda K et al. Crystal structures of tropomyosin: flexible coiled-coil. Adv Exp Med Biol 2007; 592:137-151.

87. Geeves MA, Lehrer SS. Dynamics of the muscle thin filament regulatory switch: the size of the cooperative unit. Biophys J 1994; 67:273-282.

88. Brandt PW, Diamond MS, Rutchik JS et al. Co-operative interactions between troponin-tropomyosin units extend the length of the thin filament in skeletal muscle. J Mol Biol 1987; 195:885-896.

89. Phillips GN Jr, Chacko S. Mechanical properties of tropomyosin and implications for muscle regulation. Biopolymers 1996; 38:89-95.

90. Swenson CA, Stellwagen NC. Flexibility of smooth and skeletal tropomyosins. Biopolymers 1989; 28:955-963.

91. Wolgemuth CW, Sun SX. Elasticity of alpha-helical coiled coils. Phys Rev Lett 2006; 97:24810.

92. Isambert H, Venier P, Maggs AC et al. Flexibility of actin filaments derived from thermal fluctuations. Effect of bound nucleotide, phalloidin and muscle regulatory proteins. J Biol Chem 1995; 270:11437-11444.

93. Goldmann WH. Binding of tropomyosin-troponin to actin increases filament bending stiffness. Biochem Biophys Res Commun 2000; 276:1225-1228.

94. Greenberg M, Pant K, Lehman W et al. Mechanical effect of tropomyosin and caldesmon on F-actin. Biophys J 2007 (abstract).

95. Pant K, Poole KJV, Craig R et al. Structural studies on tropomyosin—F-actin interaction. Biophys J 2007 (abstract).

96. Bacchiocchi C, Lehrer SS. Ca^{2+}-induced movement of tropomyosin in skeletal muscle thin filaments observed by multi-site FRET. Biophys J 2002; 82:1524-1536.

97. Bacchiocchi C, Graceffa P, Lehrer SS. Myosin-induced movement of alphaalpha, alphabeta and betabeta smooth muscle tropomyosin on actin observed by multisite FRET. Biophys J 2004; 86:2295-2307.

98. Holthauzen LM, Correa F, Farah CH. Ca^{2+}-induced rolling of tropomyosin in muscle thin filaments: The alpha- and beta-band hypothesis revisited. J Biol Chem 2004; 279:15204-15213.

99. Egelman EH. The iterative helical real space reconstruction method: surmounting the problems posed by real polymers. J Struct Biol 2007; 157:83-94.
100. Egelman EH. A robust algorithm for the reconstruction of helical filaments using single-particle methods. Ultramicroscopy 2000; 85:225-234.
101. Narita A, Yasunaga T, Ishikawa T et al. Ca^{2+}-induced switching of troponin and tropomyosin on actin filaments as revealed by electron cryo-microscopy. J Mol Biol 2001; 308:241-261.
102. Sun YB, Brandmeier B, Irving M. Structural changes in troponin in response to Ca^{2+} and myosin binding to thin filaments during activation of skeletal muscle. Proc Natl Acad Sci 2006;103:17771-17776.
103. Lehman W, Rosol M, Tobacman LS et al. Troponin organization on relaxed and activated thin filaments revealed by electron microscopy and three-dimensional reconstruction. J Mol Biol 2001; 307:739-744.
104. Rarick HM, Tu XH, Solaro RJ et al. The C terminus of cardiac troponin I is essential for full inhibitory activity and Ca^{2+} sensitivity of rat myofibrils. J Biol Chem 1997; 272:26887-26892.
105. Kobayashi T, Solaro RJ. Increased Ca^{2+} affinity of cardiac thin filaments reconstituted with cardiomyopathy-related mutant cardiac troponin. J Biol Chem 2006; 281:13471-13477.
106. Ramos CH. Mapping subdomains in the C-terminal region of troponin I involved in its binding to troponin C and to thin filament. J Biol Chem 1999; 274:18189-18195.
107. Foster DB, Noguchi T, VanBuren P et al. C-terminal truncation of cardiac troponin I causes divergent effects on ATPase and force: implications for the pathophysiology of myocardial stunning. Circ Res 2003; 93:917-924.
108. Luo Y, Leszyk J, Li B et al. Troponin-I interacts with the Met47 region of skeletal muscle actin. Implications for the mechanism of thin filament regulation by calcium. J Mol Biol 2002; 316:429-434.
109. Leek D, Homsher E, Heller M et al. Unexpected functional effects of TnI inhibitory region replacement with a flexible linker. Biophys J 2007 (abstract).
110. Hoffman RM, Blumenschein TM, Sykes BD. An interplay between protein disorder and structure confers the Ca2+ regulation of striated muscle. J Mol Biol 2006; 361:625-633.
111. Galińska-Rakoczy A, Engel P, Tobacman LS et al. Structural basis for the regulation of muscle contraction by troponin and tropomyosin. J Mol Biol 2008; 379(5):929-935.
112. Patchell VB, Gallon CE, Evans JS et al. The regulatory effects of tropomyosin and troponin-I on the interaction of myosin loop regions with F-actin. J Biol Chem 2005; 280:14469-11475.
113. Ferguson RE, Sun Y-B, Mercier P et al. In situ orientations of protein domains: Troponin C in skeletal muscle fibers. Mol Cell 2003; 11:865-874.
114. Lorenz M, Popp D, Holmes KC. Refinement of the F-actin model against X-ray fiber diffraction data by use of a directed mutation algorithm. J Mol Biol 1993; 234:826-836.

CHAPTER 9

Role of Tropomyosin in the Regulation of Contraction in Smooth Muscle

Steve Marston* and M. El-Mezgueldi

Abstract

Smooth muscle contraction is due to the interaction of myosin filaments with thin filaments. Thin filaments are composed of actin, tropomyosin, caldesmon and calmodulin in ratios 14:2:1:1. Tissue specific isoforms of α and β tropomyosin are expressed in smooth muscle. Compared with skeletal muscle tropomyosin, the cooperative activation of actomyosin is enhanced by smooth muscle tropomyosin: cooperative unit size is 10 and the equilibrium between on and off states is shifted towards the on state. The smooth muscle-specific actin-binding protein caldesmon, together with calmodulin regulates the activity of the thin filament in response to Ca^{2+}. Caldesmon and calmodulin control the tropomyosin-mediated transition between on and off activity states.

Introduction

Thin filaments were first extracted from smooth muscle in 1976 and identified as containing actin and tropomyosin,[1] however subsequent experimentation showed that native thin filaments were Ca^{2+}-regulated due to the presence of additional proteins.[2,3] It is now well established that the Ca^{2+}-regulated smooth muscle thin filament is made up of actin, tropomyosin, caldesmon and calmodulin in molar ratios 14:2:1:1.[4-6] Smooth muscle thin filaments and the regulatory role of caldesmon has been reviewed several times;[7-12] in this chapter we will discuss the current state of knowledge of the mechanism of regulation of thin filaments in smooth muscle together with recent evidence that has established a critical role for tropomyosin.

The Components of Smooth Muscle Thin Filaments

Actin

In smooth muscles, actin filaments are major components of both the actin cytoskeleton and the contractile apparatus. These form separate cellular compartments which are linked through the dense bodies, homologous with Z lines, which provide anchorage points for the contractile actin filaments as well as for intermediate filaments of the cytoskeleton.[13,14] The contractile filaments of smooth muscle are made up from smooth muscle α (ACTA2 gene) and γ (ACTAG2 gene) actin whilst the cytoskeletal actin isoforms are cytoplasmic β (ACTB gene) and γ actin (ACTG1 gene). α-actin predominates in visceral and other phasic smooth muscles whilst γ-actin is the main isoform in tonic smooth muscles such as aorta. Actin is a highly conserved protein and all isoforms form filaments that are made up of a right handed helix of actin monomers with two strands that cross over every 36 nm; each crossover unit contains 13 actin monomers[15,16] (see

*Corresponding Author: Steve Marston—Cardiac Medicine, National Heart and Lung Institute, Imperial College London, Dovehouse St., London SW3 6LY, UK. Email: s.marston@imperial.ac.uk

Tropomyosin, edited by Peter Gunning. ©2008 Landes Bioscience and Springer Science+Business Media.

Fig. 1). Although smooth muscles do not form regular arrays of thick and thin filaments like the sarcomeres of striated muscles, contractility is still due to the same sliding filament mechanism powered by myosin crossbridges interacting with actin filaments.[17] Smooth muscle myosin has a much slower rate of crossbridge cycling and a higher duty cycle compared with striated muscle and the thick filaments form side-polar rather than bipolar structures.[18-20] Nevertheless, at the molecular level the crossbridge cycle is essentially the same in smooth and striated muscles.

Tropomyosin

Smooth muscle thin filaments, from both tonic and phasic muscle, contain approximately equal quantities of α-(TPM1) and β-(TPM2) smooth muscle tropomyosin;[21] 90% of tropomyosin is in the form of heterodimers in vivo.[22] The smooth muscle isoforms are produced from the same genes as striated and nonmuscle tropomyosin with tissue-specific alternative splicing. The smooth muscle α-tropomyosin is produced by splicing in exons 2a and 9d in place of exons 2b, 9a and 9b found in striated muscle tropomyosin. In β-tropomyosin exons 6a and 9d are expressed in place of 6b and 9a in skeletal muscle (see Vrhovski and Thiebaud, Chapter 2). The exons expressed in smooth

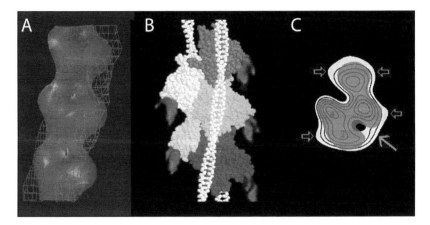

Figure 1. Structure of the smooth muscle thin filament. *A) Helical reconstruction of electron micrograph of smooth muscle thin filaments.* Reproduced from[15]. The location of tropomyosin and caldesmon densities (Red and green cages respectively) is shown superimposed on three actin monomers of one of the long-pitch actin filament helices (the other actin helix is removed for clarity). Tropomyosin is in the C position whilst caldesmon is clearly well separated from tropomyosin with no evidence of interaction. *B) Model of smooth muscle thin filament based on 3D helical reconstruction of actin-tropomyosin containing caldesmon domain 4.* The figure shows the structure of 5 actin molecules from F-actin according to the model of Lorenz et al[98] with tropomyosin in the location found for the inhibited smooth muscle thin filament.[99] These are drawn from atomic coordinates and rendered using RASMOL. The location of extra density due to caldesmon domain 4 seen in difference maps of helical reconstructions of negatively stained em images was fitted to the actin structure manually using Photoshop (purple objects).[100] Caldesmon domain 4 is located over the C-terminus of actin. *C) Transverse section through a helical reconstruction of negatively stained filaments made up of actin-caldesmon domains 3 + 4 superimposed on actin to show the location of caldesmon mass.* Because adjacent actin monomers on either side of the filament axis are staggered by half a subunit, sectioning through the center of subdomains 1 and 3 of one monomer will result in sectioning through subdomains 2 and 4 of the other monomer. The *open bold arrows* indicate regions of significant caldesmon density, most prominent on subdomain 1. The *red arrow* points to the interstrand density, derived from caldesmon domain 3 forming a bridge from actin subdomain 1 to subdomain 3 of the neighboring actin monomer in the other strand.[32]

muscle are thus the same as in nonmuscle tropomyosins, in fact smooth muscle β tropomyosin is identical to the cytoskeletal tropomyosin 1. Thus it is evident that the striated muscle exons are the exceptions and it has been proposed that they are adapted for interaction with troponin T.[23,24]

Exon 9d confers strong end to end interactions on smooth muscle tropomyosin, as a consequence cooperative activation of actin interaction with myosin is enhanced relative to skeletal muscle tropomyosin. The cooperative unit size is 10 compared with 7 for skeletal muscle and the equilibrium between on and off activity states of actin-tropomyosin is shifted towards the on state.[25,26] This is illustrated in Figure 2 which shows greater activation by myosin subfragment 1 compared with skeletal muscle tropomyosin and an increase in filament sliding speed in the in vitro motility assay due to smooth muscle tropomyosin. Tropomyosin is incorporated into smooth muscle thin filaments with a stoichiometry of 1 per 7 actin monomers and is located in a continuous strand along the actin helix. Like skeletal muscle tropomyosin, smooth muscle tropomyosin is able to take up a variety of positions on actin corresponding to the M, C and B states of the thin filament defined by Lehman (see Chapter 8). Actin-smooth muscle tropomyosin is found in the B conformation and the addition of caldesmon or S-1 can move it to the M and C positions respectively.[16,27,28]

Caldesmon

The third most abundant protein of smooth muscle thin filaments is caldesmon (Fig. 3). Caldesmon is an elongated molecule, with 793 amino-acids and a molecular mass of 93 kDa in human. The length of a single caldesmon molecule is 80 nm and it is made up of four structured domains separated by unstructured linkers that are sensitive to proteolysis. The first three domains approximate to a single alpha-helical structure which is stabilised by a repeating motif of acidic and basic side chains that form salt-bridges along the alpha helix. The fourth domain forms a more globular but also very flexible structure with few secondary structural elements. Domain 4

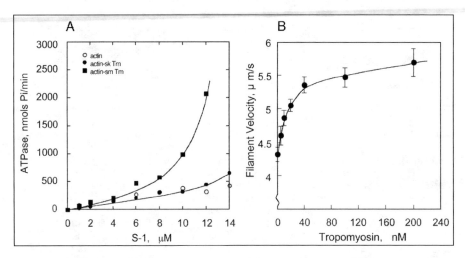

Figure 2. Activation of actomyosin interaction by smooth tropomyosin. *A) Dependence of ATP hydrolysis rate on S-1 concentration at a fixed actin concentration; the effect of different tropomyosin species.* Cooperative activation of ATPase by S-1 (increased slope) is much greater with smooth muscle tropomyosin than skeletal muscle tropomyosin. Conditions: 4 μM actin (Tm:actin 0.4 w/w), 5 mM MgATP, 50 mM KCl, 35 mM Imidazole-HCl, pH 7.4, 4 mM MgCl₂, 1 mM EDTA, 5 mM DTT, 1 mM CaCl₂. *B) The effect of smooth muscle tropomyosin on actin filament velocity at 28°C measured by in vitro motility assay.* Actin-tropomyosin complexes were formed at a range of tropomyosin concentrations in 50 mM KCl, 25 mM Imidazole-HCl pH 7.4, 4 mM MgCl₂, 1 mM EDTA, 5 mM DTT and the velocity of filaments analysed. Data points represent mean velocities with standard errors from 20 filaments.[59]

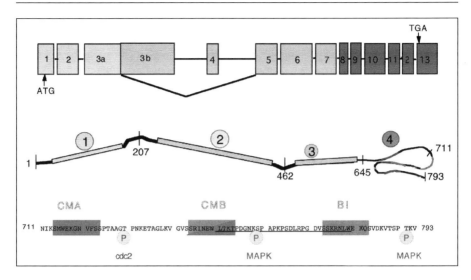

Figure 3. Caldesmon structure. Top) The exon structure of the human caldesmon gene is based on the genomic sequence.[101,102] The nonmuscle isoform message is produced by excluding exons 3b and 4. Centre) The domain structure of human smooth muscle caldesmon in relation to the exon structure. Amino acid numbers, defining the beginning of each domain, refer to the human caldesmon cDNA sequence. Actin binding segments in domain 4 are shown in red, Ca^{2+}-calmodulin binding segments are in green. Phosphorylation sites are in yellow. Bottom) The sequence of the C-terminal regulatory domain 4b, showing the calmodulin (green) and actin (pink) binding motifs and the phosphorylation sites. A color version of this image is available online at www.Eurekah.com.

contains the main actin and Ca^{2+}-calmodulin binding sites and is responsible for the regulatory property of caldesmon.

Caldesmon has been shown to bind to actin, tropomyosin, calmodulin and myosin in vitro.[10] The most important binding interaction is with actin; this binding is strongly influenced by tropomyosin, but this does not necessarily mean that there is a direct binding of tropomyosin to caldesmon in thin filaments. Evidence has been produced for tropomyosin binding to sites in all four domains of caldesmon; however the sites have differing affinities and characteristics (reviewed in ref. 10). Thus the site in caldesmon domain 3 binds to skeletal muscle tropomyosin but not to smooth muscle tropomyosin[29] and the site in domain 2 has only been detected with recombinant fragments and is not detected in the same sequence obtained by proteolysis. Dependence of binding upon salt concentration also varies and a biosensor study has shown that the only site with significant affinity in physiological salt concentrations is in domain 4; this site corresponds to a sequence homology with troponin T.[30,31] X-ray diffraction of Bailey-type tropomyosin crystals containing added caldesmon or caldesmon domain 4 show discrete areas of extra mass along the tropomyosin molecules indicating the presence of a complex.[30]

Despite the evidence for binary actin-tropomyosin binding in vitro there is no direct evidence for caldesmon-tropomyosin contacts in the intact thin filament. In fact, helical reconstructions of smooth muscle thin filaments indicate that caldesmon forms a continuous strand along the actin filament, parallel to tropomyosin but separated by about 90°[15] (Fig. 1A). This is supported by helical reconstructions of actin complexed with domain 4 of caldesmon, which is located at the bottom of actin subdomain 1,[16,32] as far away as possible from the tropomyosin strands (Fig. 1B). NMR analysis of actin-caldesmon binding also places the main contact in subdomain 1 near the actin C-terminus.[33] Interestingly, the location of domain 4 of caldesmon on actin appears to be around the same place where the inhibitory C-terminus of troponin I has been proposed to bind.[34]

Although the structural evidence indicates no contacts between tropomyosin and caldesmon, there is a strong functional interaction. Caldesmon is an inhibitor of actomyosin ATPase and motility and both actin binding and caldesmon inhibition are greatly enhanced in the presence of tropomyosin.[35,36] The converse is also observed: caldesmon enhances the affinity of tropomyosin for actin.[37] Thus tropomyosin and caldesmon behave as allosterically coupled ligands of actin.

Caldesmon interaction with actin is thus central to caldesmon's function in regulating thin filament activity. We have consistently observed biphasic binding curves consisting of a high affinity ($>10^7$ M^{-1}), low stoichiometry component with a stoichiometry of around 1 per 14 actins and a low affinity component (10^6 M^{-1}) which saturates at a total amount bound of 1 caldesmon per actin.[35,38-40] It is the tight binding component that is associated with the inhibition of actin-tropomyosin and this component of binding is completely dependent on tropomyosin. This biphasic binding has also been found for troponin I+C binding to actin-tropomyosin. Zhou et al[41] report 0.14 mols troponin I+C per mol actin binding at 6×10^6 M^{-1} and 0.86 troponin I+C/actin binding at 3×10^5 M^{-1}. It is therefore probable that this biphasic pattern of binding is characteristic of cooperative regulatory actin binding proteins. It should, however, be noted that at physiological ratios of actin to caldesmon or troponin only the tight binding sites can be occupied so the low affinity binding is not physiologically relevant.

It is well established that domain 4, the C-terminal 170 amino acids, contains all the actin binding sites of caldesmon.[42] Extensive structure-function analysis using recombinant peptides derived from various parts of domain 4 have shown that there are three actin-binding segments, each about 9 amino acids long and that they act together since only peptides containing two or more segments have caldesmon-like regulatory properties.[43-45] Figure 3B shows a model of how the peptide chain of domain 4 might be folded when it is bound to actin-tropomyosin. We have proposed that the three regions which contribute to inhibition are positioned to form a single actin binding zone.[43] The placement of the three actin binding sequences close together is supported by nuclear magnetic resonance measurements which showed that amino acids from all three putative inhibitory segments are within 1.5 nm of the unique cysteine 636 that is at the junction between domains 3 and 4.[46] The actin binding sites essential for inhibition are located in the C-terminal half of domain 4 (termed domain 4b) and are designated CMB and B' in Figure 3C. Both sites plus the linking peptide form a minimal actin-binding inhibitory domain.[9,33,39,43,47,48]

Ca²⁺-Binding Protein

Smooth muscle thin filaments contain a Ca^{2+}-binding protein that confers Ca^{2+} dependent regulation on caldesmon inhibition. The Ca^{2+}- binding protein was identified as calmodulin and it binds to caldesmon both in the presence and absence of activating Ca^{2+}.[49,50] Ca^{2+}-calmodulin binds to caldesmon through two short sequences in domain 4b, termed CMA and CMB in Figure 3C.[51-53] It is noteworthy that the binding sequence CMB is shared by Ca^{2+}-calmodulin and actin, therefore it is likely that reversal of caldesmon inhibition is achieved by displacing actin from site CMB .

Kinetic Pathway of Myosin-Thin Filament Interaction and Its Regulation

Smooth muscle contraction results from actin activation of myosin ATPase[54] (Fig. 4A). In the absence of ATP, smooth muscle myosin head binds tightly to actin. ATP binding at the myosin active site weakens the affinity of myosin for actin and dissociates the actomyosin complex. ATP hydrolysis at the active site leads to the formation of a stable myosin.ADP.Pi complex. Actin binding to this complex triggers phosphate and ADP release. The basic ATPase mechanism is similar to that of skeletal muscle myosin, but the product-release steps that determine the overall rate of the ATPase are more than 20 fold slower.[18]

In the presence of caldesmon and tropomyosin, the actomyosin ATPase is strongly inhibited. The inhibition is very limited in the absence of tropomyosin showing that caldesmon inhibition is dependent on tropomyosin.[55] Equilibrium and transient kinetics investigations have shown

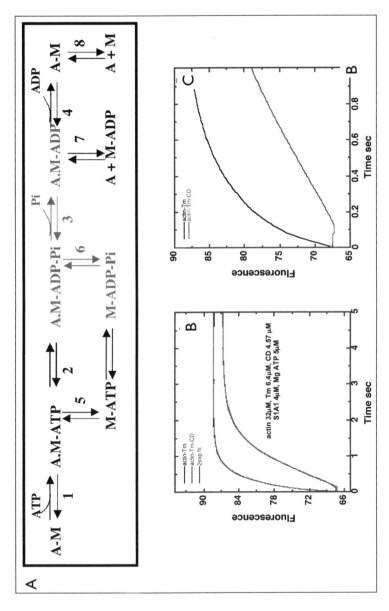

Figure 4. Kinetics of smooth muscle thin filament activation. A) Acto-myosin ATPase cycle. Highlighted in red are the steps involved in phosphate release. B) Shows the time course of Pi release measured by the change in the fluorescence of MDCC-PBP upon mixing 4 μM skeletal muscle S1 with 5μM ATP in a delay line for 1sec and then mixing this solution with an equal volume of 32 μM actin and 7 μM smooth muscle Tm in the absence or presence of 4.6 μM caldesmon. A fit to a double exponential function is superimposed on the experimental traces. C) Shows an expansion of the initial part of the transients. In the presence of caldesmon the transient clearly display a lag of around 150 ms followed by a slow exponential function.

that the caldesmon-tropomyosin complex bound to actin does not affect ATP induced acto-S1 dissociation, S1.ADP.Pi binding to actin or ADP release.[56,57] Caldesmon-tropomyosin, however, drastically inhibits the rate of phosphate release from actin.S1.ADP.Pi. In the presence of caldesmon-tropomyosin, the transient of phosphate release also showed a substantial lag (Fig. 4).[56] The presence of a lag is an indication that a prior slow step on the pathway is taking place and can be simply interpreted by a cooperative equilibrium. In the cooperative-allosteric mechanism (Fig. 6) this step would be the transition between the on and off states. At the start of the reaction the fraction of actin in the on state is very low due to caldesmon binding to the off state but as strong binding complexes are formed they will switch the thin filament to the on state leading to an acceleration of the reaction. In confirmation of this hypothesis, when actin-tropomyosin-caldesmon filaments were incubated with S-1 (1 per 4 actin) to switch on all the thin filaments before starting the reaction, the lag was no longer present.[56]

Regulatory Mechanism of Smooth Muscle Thin Filaments

The Ca^{2+}-sensitive regulation of smooth muscle thin filaments and the requirement of actin, tropomyosin, caldesmon and a Ca^{2+}-binding protein in this regulation is well established[2,3,12] but the mechanism of Ca^{2+}-regulation has been a controversial topic. Like skeletal muscle thin filaments, the thin filaments of smooth muscles are negatively regulated: the function of caldesmon binding to actin-tropomyosin is to inhibit the activity of a constitutively active filament and the function of Ca^{2+} binding to the CaBP is to reverse the inhibition. Caldesmon inhibition is cooperative with up to 14 actins being inhibited by the binding of one caldesmon molecule to actin-tropomyosin; moreover, Ca^{2+} and calmodulin (CaM) interacting with caldesmon potentiate thin filaments to up to 150% of the activity of actin tropomyosin rather than simply neutralising the inhibitory effect of caldesmon[35,49,50] (Fig. 5A,B).

In a series of papers we have given evidence that the only model of regulation that can account for all the observed regulatory characteristics is a cooperative allosteric mechanism[9,12,49,55,57-59] (Fig. 6). In this model actin-tropomyosin exists in two activity states, on and off that are linked by a concerted cooperative equilibrium. Caldesmon acts as an allosteric inhibitor by preferentially binding to actin-tropomyosin in the off state whilst at activating Ca^{2+} concentration the Ca^{2+}-CaM-Caldesmon complex acts as an activator of actin-tropomyosin activity by preferentially binding to the on state.[60,61] This mechanism is very similar to that established for troponin-tropomyosin as recently described by Lehrer and Geeves:[62] caldesmon is equivalent to troponin I or troponin in the absence of Ca^{2+} and Ca^{2+}-CaM-Caldesmon is equivalent to troponin in the presence of activating Ca^{2+}. Alternative models have been proposed that include a role for mutually exclusive competitive binding of caldesmon or myosin heads to actin-tropomyosin in determining thin filament interaction with myosin. The original model of Sobue[63] proposed a purely competitive "flip-flop" mechanism which was ruled out by measurements showing that caldesmon and S-1.ADP.Pi could bind simultaneously to actin-tropomyosin.[58] However several studies appeared to show a relationship between caldesmon inhibition and S1.ADP.Pi displacement.[64-69]

Recently we have reported direct and unambiguous evidence for the cooperative-allosteric mechanism. We made measurements of the effects of caldesmon and Ca^{2+}-CaM-Caldesmon on the actin-tropomyosin on-off transition using pyrene-conjugated tropomyosin. The excimer fluorescence of pyrene-tropomyosin is sensitive to the activity state of actin-tropomyosin[70] (Fig. 5 C,D).

The changes in actin-tropomyosin state as monitored by excimer fluorescence correspond to the changes in thin filament activity as determined from measurements of activation of S-1 ATPase activity (Fig. 5). Fluorescence and ATPase are reduced by low concentrations of caldesmon relative to actin-tropomyosin similar to the physiological ratio found in native thin filaments (1:16)[71] and increased by similar concentrations of Ca^{2+}-calmodulin. Ca^{2+}-calmodulin increased ATPase and fluorescence to 18-30% above the levels for actin tropomyosin alone in accord with our earlier measurements.[35,49,50]

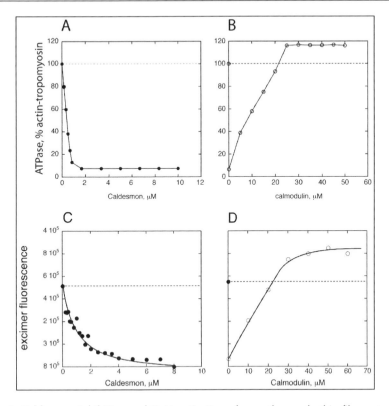

Figure 5. Caldesmon inhibition and CaM activation of smooth muscle thin filaments. *A, B) Control of actin-tropomyosin ATPase activation of S-1 ATPase by caldesmon and Ca²⁺-calmodulin.* Actin-tropomyosin activation of skeletal muscle myosin S-1 MgATPase activity was measured at 37°C. Conditions: 2 μM skeletal muscle S1, 12 μM skeletal muscle actin, 4 μM smooth muscle tropomyosin, in 120 mM KCl, 2.4 mM MgCl₂, 5 mM PIPES.K₂, pH 7.1, 1 mM NaN₃, 1 mM DTT, reaction initiated with 5 mM MgATP. Results expressed as percent of uninhibited ATPase activity. Mean uninhibited ATPase was 0.35 sec⁻¹. A) Inhibition of ATPase activity by 0-10 μM caldesmon, full inhibition is obtained at less than 0.2 caldesmon per actin. B) Ca²⁺-calmodulin re-activation of ATPase activity in the presence of 0.8 μM caldesmon. ATPase is enhanced to 118% of uninhibited activity. *C, D) Caldesmon and calmodulin control the thin filament on-off equilibrium.* The on-off equilibrium was detected by changes in pyrene-tropomyosin excimer fluorescence. Change is actin-tropomyosin state correlates with change in actin-tropomyosin-activated ATPase. C) Caldesmon switches actin-tropomyosin to off state (low excimer fluorescence). 12 μM actin, 2 μM pyrene-labelled tropomyosin, 0-8 μM caldesmon. D) Ca²⁺-calmodulin switches thin filaments to the on state (high excimer fluorescence). 12 μM actin, 2 μM pyrene-labelled tropomyosin, 8 μM caldesmon, 0-60 μM calmodulin.

The direct evidence for caldesmon regulation by a troponin-like mechanism is supported by measurements of how S1 and caldesmon binding to smooth muscle thin filaments depends on the on-off equilibrium. Weak binding (S1.ADP.Pi) binding to actin-tropomyosin is not affected by the binding of inhibitory concentrations of caldesmon, indicating that on and off states have equal affinities for S1.ADP.Pi[58,72] whilst the binding of strong binding complexes (S1.ADP, S1.AMP. PNP) is inhibited by caldesmon and becomes cooperative:[57] this effect parallels troponin-inhibited actin-tropomyosin[73] and is due to strong binding complexes having a much higher affinity for the on state than the off state leading to cooperative switching on of thin filaments[62,74] (Fig. 6).

The basis of cooperative inhibition is that the inhibitory ligand has a higher affinity for the off state than the on state. In vitro, Caldesmon binding to actin-tropomyosin in the on state is weakened at least 20-fold and becomes cooperative, whilst caldesmon binding to actin-tropomyosin in the off state is similar to binding to actin-tropomyosin alone, indicating that caldesmon preferentially binds to the off state as expected.[61] The activating effect of Ca^{2+}.CaM.CaD produces the opposite effect on affinity for actin-tropomyosin: Ca^{2+}.CaM.CaD binding to actin-tropomyosin in the on state is similar to binding to actin-tropomyosin alone, but Ca^{2+}.CaM.CaD binding to actin-tropomyosin in the off state is weakened about 20x and is now cooperative, indicating that the activated complex binds preferentially to the on state as predicted by the cooperative-allosteric model. Finally, as already described, the time course of the Pi release step (Fig. 4) of actin-tropomyosin ATPase inhibited by caldesmon can only be accounted for by the cooperative allosteric mechanism.

The role of tropomyosin in caldesmon inhibition remains controversial and seems to depend critically on ionic conditions. Whilst every laboratory reports a consistently low caldesmon:actin stoichiometry for inhibition in the presence of tropomyosin (see Fig. 5), inhibition in the absence of tropomyosin seems to be rather variable. At one extreme no caldesmon inhibition in the absence of tropomyosin was reported,[35] others reported full inhibition required 1 caldesmon per actin and several papers show less than 1 caldesmon per actin is required.[9,36,58,65,67,75-77] At the other extreme we have found that at very low ionic strength fully cooperative caldesmon inhibition can be obtained in the complete absence of tropomyosin.[78]

If thin filaments can be cooperatively regulated without tropomyosin in the absence of added KCl, what is the function of tropomyosin in native thin filaments? Tropomyosin is not a typical protein ligand. It is located at a radius of 3.8 nm from the actin filament axis and appears to make only a few contacts with actin.[79] Individual tropomyosin molecules have a very low affinity for actin (10^4 M^{-1}) and binding affinity only becomes high when tropomyosin molecules are joined end to end.[80] Charge plays a large role in binding since the affinity of tropomyosin for actin is optimal

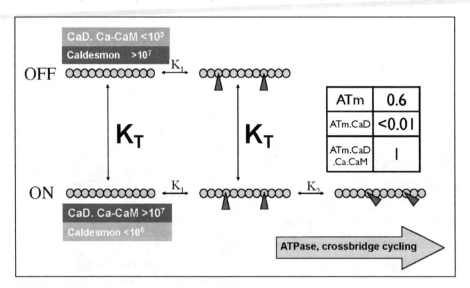

Figure 6. Cooperative allosteric mechanism for Ca^{2+}-regulation of smooth muscle thin filaments. Adapted from Lehrer and Geeves.[62] The thin filament is a cooperative two-state (on-off) system. Myosin ADP.Pi can bind equally to either state (K_1) but the transition to the strong binding state that is associated with crossbridge movement and force generation, K_2, can only take place from the on state. The population of the on state is controlled by caldesmon and calmodulin. Caldesmon binds strongly to the off state and so shifts the equilibrium K_T from 0.6 to <0.01. CaD.Ca^{2+}-CaM binds strongly to the on state and so shifts K_T from 0.6 to 1.

around physiological ionic strength and very low at both low and high ionic strengths.[81,82] Holmes et al[83] have proposed a model in which the negatively charged tropomyosin strand 'floats' over a bed of positively charged residues on the surface of actin with its position being determined by the pattern of surface charges on actin (itself defined by the allosteric ligands that bind to actin). Thus the evidence from the study of the actin-tropomyosin-caldesmon interaction suggests that the fundamental cooperative interactions takes place directly from actin to actin, predominantly via charge—charge interactions and that the function of tropomyosin is to shield the actin surface from the solvent so that these interactions could take place in physiological conditions. In this hypothesis the different positions of tropomyosin associated with different activity states are a consequence of allosteric transitions in actin rather than their cause.[78]

Caldesmon Phosphorylation and the Molecular Mechanism of Thin Filament Regulation

Phosphorylation of caldesmon may be an alternative mechanism that would relieve caldesmon inhibition at low Ca^{2+}. Three sites have been identified in the regulatory domain 4b at threonine 730, serine 759 and serine 789 in the human sequence (Fig. 3).[84,85] Interestingly, the phosphorylation sites are in the middle of linking peptides, 10-14 amino-acids downstream from the tryptophan at the core of the regulatory segments CMA, CMB and B' respectively. In mammalian smooth muscle serines 759 and 789 are substrates of MAP kinase and threonine 730 does not get phosphorylated. Phosphorylation at either or both of these sites leads to loss of inhibition and a reduction in actin-tropomyosin binding affinity.[86] The structural effects of phosphorylation were studied in detail in a minimally inhibitory peptide (LW30, underlined in Fig. 3) using NMR spectroscopy.[87] The peptide linking the sites CMB and B' forms a structured turn which is hypothesised to position the two sites for docking onto actin in the switched off conformation.[33] The effect of phosphorylation (or mutation of the serine to aspartic acid) at serine 759, which is close to the turn, is to destroy its structure and hence eliminate two-sited binding.[32,87]

The concept of obligatory two-site binding for caldesmon inhibition unites structural and functional studies on caldesmon (Fig. 7).[89,90] We propose that the CMB-peptide-B' segment of domain 4 forms a structure which binds to actin—tropomyosin only in the off state, thus caldesmon inhibits actin-tropomyosin activity. Inhibition may be relieved either by Ca^{2+}-calmodulin binding to sites CMA and CMB, thus displacing site CMB from actin, or by phosphorylation of serines 759 and/or 789 that disrupts the structure necessary for two-site binding to actin-tropomyosin. Caldesmon is not dissociated from actin by Ca^{2+}-calmodulin or phosphorylation because there is an additional actin binding site, C, in the N-terminal half of domain 4 (Fig. 3B) and Ca^{2+}-free calmodulin can remain bound to caldesmon through site CMA. To account for the activating effect of Ca^{2+}-calmodulin, we presume that caldesmon. Ca^{2+}-CaM complex binds through site C to actin

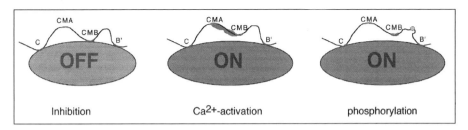

Figure 7. 2 site binding model for caldesmon regulation of actin-tropomyosin. Inhibition of actin-tropomyosin is due to two-site docking of caldesmon sites CMB and B' specifically onto actin in the off state. Inhibition may be released by Ca^{2+}-CaM (green) binding to CMA and CMB thus displacing caldesmon from CMB, which abolishes two-site binding, or by phosphorylation that destabilises the linker peptide, also preventing two-site docking. Site C tethers actin to caldesmon in activating conditions and site CMA tethers calmodulin to caldesmon in relaxing conditions.

preferentially in the on state. This model is supported by studies of a caldesmon peptide, named H2 (683-767), containing sites C, CMA and CMB but lacking site B' necessary for inhibition. H2 is a tropomyosin-dependent activator of ATPase and has been shown to switch the filament to a state resembling the switched on state obtained with rigor crossbridges.[43,91]

Conclusions

Tropomyosin plays an essential part in the regulation of smooth muscle thin filament activity by the troponin-like concerted cooperative mechanism but the physiological role of this regulation is yet to be fully clarified. Compared with troponin, caldesmon has a lower affinity for actin-tropomyosin in all activity states and the calculated cooperative unit size is reduced by the binding of caldesmon, whereas it is increased by binding troponin;[92] these properties mean that caldesmon is not able to switch activity in the same way as troponin does. Smooth muscle is a dual regulated muscle and the primary mechanism of Ca^{2+}-regulation is via the activation of myosin by phosphorylation of the regulatory light chain by Ca^{2+}-CaM dependent myosin light chain kinase. Ca^{2+}-dependent caldesmon inhibition seems to play a secondary role in modulating Ca^{2+}-sensitivity[93] by accelerating relaxation[94,95] and in maintaining basal relaxation.[96,97]

Acknowledgements

Supported by a Research Career Development Fellowship grant from the Wellcome Trust (to M.E.) and by Grants from the British Heart Foundation (to S.B.M.).

References

1. Sobieszek A, Small JV. Myosin-linked calcium regulation in vertebrate smooth muscle. J Mol Biol 1976; 101:75-92.
2. Marston SB, Trevett RM, Walters M. Calcium ion-regulated thin filaments from vascular smooth muscle. Biochem J 1980; 185(2):355-365.
3. Marston SB, Smith CWJ. Purification and properties of Ca^{2+}-regulated thin filaments and f-actin from sheep aorta smooth muscle. J Musc Res Cell Motil 1984; 5:559-575.
4. Smith CWJ, Marston SB. Disasembly and reconstitution of the Ca^{2+}-sensitive thin filaments of vascular smooth muscle. FEBS Lett 1985; 184:115-119.
5. Marston SB, Lehman W. Caldesmon is a Ca^{2+}-regulatory component of native smooth-muscle thin filaments. Biochem J 1985; 231:517-522.
6. Lehman W, Denault D, Marston SB. Caldesmon content of vertebrate smooth muscles. Biochim Biophys Acta 1993; 1203:53-59.
7. EL-Mezgueldi M, Marston SB. Caldesmon. In: Creighton TE, ed. Wiley encyclopedia of molecular medicine. Vol 5. New York: John Wiley and Sons Inc, 2001:428-430.
8. Huber PAJ, Marston SB, Hodgkinson JL et al. Caldesmon. In: Kreis T, Vale R, eds. Guidebook to the Cytoskeletal and Motor Proteins. 2 ed. Oxford: A Sambrook and Tooze Oxford University Press, 1999:52-57.
9. Marston S, Burton D, Copeland O et al. Structural interactions between actin, tropomyosin, caldesmon and calcium binding protein and the regulation of smooth muscle thin filaments. Acta Physiol Scand 1998; 164:401-414.
10. Marston SB, Huber PAJ. Caldesmon. In: Barany M, Barany K, eds. Biochemistry of Smooth Muscle Contraction. San Diego: Academic Press, 1996:77-90.
11. Marston SB, Redwood CS. The molecular anatomy of caldesmon. Biochem J 1991; 279:1-16.
12. Marston SB, Smith CWJ. The thin filaments of smooth muscles. J Musc Res Cell Motil 1985; 6:669-708.
13. Small JV, Gimona M. The cytoskeleton of the vertebrate smooth muscle cell. Acta Physiol Scand 1998; 164(4):341-348.
14. North AJ, Gimona M, Lando Z et al. Actin isoform compartments in chicken gizzard smooth muscle cells. J Cell Sci 1994; 107:445-455.
15. Lehman W, Vibert P, Craig R. Visualisation of caldesmon on smooth muscle thin filaments. J Mol Biol 1997; 274:310-317.
16. Hodgkinson JL, Marston SB, Craig R et al. 3D image reconstruction of reconstituted smooth muscle thin filaments: effects of caldesmon. Biophys J 1997; 72:2398-2404.
17. Hodgkinson JL, Newman TM, Marston SB et al. The structure of the contractile apparatus in ultra-rapidly frozen smooth muscle: freeze-fracture, deep etch and freeze-substitution studies. J Struct Biol 1995; 114:93-104.

18. Marston SB, Taylor EW. Comparison of the myosin and actomyosin ATPase mechanisms of the four types of vertebrate muscles. J Mol Biol 1980; 139:573-600.
19. VanBuren P, Guilford WH, Kennedy G et al. Smooth muscle myosin: a high force-generating molecular motor. Biophys J 1995; 68:256s-259s.
20. Xu JQ, Harder BA, Uman P et al. Myosin filament structure in vertebrate smooth muscle. J Cell Biol 1996; 134(1):53-66.
21. Szymanski PT, Chacko TK, Rovner AS et al. Differences in contractile protein content and isoforms in phasic and tonic smooth muscles. Am J Physiol 1998; 275(3 Pt 1):C684-692.
22. Jancso A, Graceffa P. Smooth muscle tropomyosin coiled-coil dimers. Subunit composition, assembly and end-to-end interaction. J Biol Chem 1991; 266(9):5891-5897.
23. Colote S, Widada JS, Ferraz C et al. Evolution of tropomyosin functional domains: differential splicing and genomic constraints. J Mol Evol 1988; 27:228-235.
24. Maytum R, Bathe F, Konrad M et al. Tropomyosin exon 6b is troponin specific and required for correct acto-myosin regulation. J Biol Chem 2004.
25. Lehrer SS, Morris EP. Comparison of the effects of smooth and skeletal tropomyosin on skeletal acto-myosin subfragment 1 ATPase. J Biol Chem 1984; 259:2070-2072.
26. Williams DL, Greene LE, Eisenberg E. Comparison of the effects of smooth and skeletal tropomyosins on interactions of actin and subfragment 1. Biochemistry 1984; 23:4150-4155.
27. Moody C, Lehman W, Craig R. Caldesmon and the structure of smooth muscle thin filaments: electron microscopy of isolated thin filaments. J Muscle Res Cell Motil 1990; 11:176-185.
28. Lehman W, Hatch V, Korman V et al. Tropomyosin and actin isoforms modulate the localization of tropomyosin strands on actin filaments. J Mol Biol 2000; 302(3):593-606.
29. Huber PAJ, Fraser IDC, Marston SB. Location of smooth muscle myosin and tropomyosin binding sites in the C-terminal 288 residues of human caldesmon. Biochem J 1995; 312:617-625.
30. Hnath EJ, Wang C-LA, Huber PAJ et al. Affinity and structure of complexes of tropomyosin and caldesmon domains. Biophys J 1996; 71:1920-1933.
31. Hayashi K, Yamada S, Kanda K et al. 35 kDa fragment of h-caldesmon conserves two consensus sequences of the tropomyosin binding domain of troponin T. Biochem Biophys Res Commun 1989; 161:38-45.
32. Foster DB, Huang R, Hatch V et al. Modes of caldesmon binding to actin: sites of caldesmon contact and modulation of interactions by phosphorylation. J Biol Chem 2004; 279(51):53387-53394.
33. Gao Y, Patchell VB, Huber PAJ et al. The interface between caldesmon domain 4b and subdomain 1 of actin studied by nuclear magnetic resonance spectroscopy. Biochemistry 1999; 38:15459-15469.
34. Pirani A, Vinogradova MV, Curmi PM et al. An Atomic Model of the Thin Filament in the Relaxed and Ca(2+)-Activated States. J Mol Biol 2006; 357(3):707-717.
35. Smith CW, Pritchard K, Marston SB. The mechanism of Ca^{2+} regulation of vascular smooth muscle thin filaments by caldesmon and calmodulin. J Biol Chem 1987; 262:116-122.
36. Dabrowska R, Goch A, Galazkiewicz B et al. The influence of caldesmon on ATPase activity of the skeletal muscle actomyosin and bundling of actin filaments. Biochim Biophys Acta 1985; 842:70-75.
37. Yamashiro-Matsumura S, Matsumura F. Characterization of 83-kilodalton nonmuscle caldesmon from cultured rat cells: stimulation of actin binding of nonmuscle tropomyosin and periodic localization along microfilaments like tropomyosin. J Cell Biol 1988; 106:1973-1983.
38. Redwood CS, Marston SB, Bryan J et al. The functional properties of full length and mutant chicken gizzard smooth muscle caldesmon expressed in E. Coli. FEBS Lett 1990; 270:53-56.
39. Redwood CS, Marston SB. Binding and regulatory properties of expressed functional domains of chicken gizzard smooth muscle caldesmon. J Biol Chem 1993; 268:10969-10976.
40. Yamashiro S, Yamakita Y, Yoshida K et al. Characterization of the COOH terminus of nonmuscle caldesmon mutants lacking mitosis-specific phosphorylation sites. J Biol Chem 1995; 270:4023-4030.
41. Zhou X, Morris EP, Lehrer SS. Binding of troponin I and the troponin I-troponin C complex to actin-tropomyosin. Dissociation by myosin subfragment 1. Biochemistry 2000; 39(5):1128-1132.
42. Szpacenko A, Dabrowska R. Functional domain of caldesmon. FEBS Lett 1986; 202:182-186.
43. Fraser IDC, Copeland O, Wu B et al. The inhibitory complex of smooth muscle caldesmon with actin and tropomyosin involves three interacting segments of the C-terminal domain 4. Biochemistry 1997; 36:5483-5492.
44. Wang Z, Chacko S. Mutagenesis analysis of functionally important domains within the C-terminal end of smooth muscle caldesmon. J Biol Chem 1996; 271:25707-25714.
45. El-Mezgueldi M, Copeland O, Fraser IDC et al. Characterisation of the functional properties of smooth muscle caldesmon domain 4a: Evidence for an independant inhibitory actin-tropomyosin binding domain. Biochem J 1998; 332:395-401.
46. Mornet D, Bonet-Kerrache A, Strasburg GM et al. The binding of distinct segments of actin to multiple sites in the C-terminus of caldesmon: comparative aspects of actin interaction with troponin-I and caldesmon. Biochemistry 1995; 34:1893-1901.

47. EL-Mezgueldi M, Derancourt J, Callas B et al. Precise identification of the regulatory F-actin and calmodulin binding sequences in the 10 kDa carboxyl terminal domain of caldesmon. J Biol Chem 1994; 269:12824-12832.

48. Huber PAJ, Gao Y, Fraser IDC et al. Structure-activity studies of the regulatory interaction of the 10 Kilodalton C-terminal fragment of caldesmon with actin and the effect of mutation of caldesmon residues 691-696. Biochemistry 1998; 37:2314-2326.

49. Notarianni G, Gusev NB, Lafitte D et al. A novel Ca^{2+} binding protein associated with caldesmon in Ca^{2+}-regulated smooth muscle thin filaments: evidence for a structurally altered form of calmodulin. J Musc Res Cell Motil 2000; 21:537-549.

50. Pritchard K, Marston SB. Ca^{2+}-calmodulin binding to caldesmon and the caldesmon-actin- tropomyosin complex. Its role in Ca^{2+} regulation of the activity of synthetic smooth-muscle thin filaments. Biochem J 1989; 257:839-843.

51. Marston SB, Fraser IDC, Huber PAJ et al. Location of two contact sites between human caldesmon and Ca^{2+} calmodulin. J Biol Chem 1994; 269:8134-8139.

52. Huber PAJ, EL-Mezgueldi M, Grabarek Z et al. Multiple sited interaction of caldesmon with Ca^{2+} calmodulin. Biochem J 1996; 316:413-420.

53. Huber PAJ, Levine BA, Copeland O et al. Characterisation of the effects of mutation of the caldesmon sequence 691glu-trp-leu-thr-lys-thr696 to pro-gly-his-tyr-asn-asn on caldesmon-calmodulin interaction. FEBS Letters 1998; 423:93-97.

54. Arner A, Malmqvist U. Cross-bridge cycling in smooth muscle: a short review. Acta Physiol Scand 1998; 164(4):363-372.

55. Marston SB, Redwood CS. The essential role of tropomyosin in cooperative regulation of smooth muscle thin filament activity by caldesmon. J Biol Chem 1993; 268:12317-12320.

56. Alahyan M, Webb MR, Marston SB et al. The mechanism of smooth muscle caldesmon-tropomyosin inhibition of the elementary steps of the actomyosin ATPase. J Biol Chem 2006; 281(28):19433-19448.

57. Marston SB, Fraser IDC, Huber PAJ. Smooth muscle caldesmon controls the strong binding interactions between actin-tropomyosin and myosin. J Biol Chem 1994; 269:32104-32109.

58. Marston SB, Redwood CS. Inhibition of actin-tropomyosin activation of myosin MgATPase activity by the smooth muscle regulatory protein caldesmon. J Biol Chem 1992; 267:16796-16800.

59. Fraser IDC, Marston SB. In vitro motility analysis of smooth muscle caldesmon control of actin-tropomyosin filament movement. J Biol Chem 1995; 270:19688-19693.

60. Changeux J-P, Edelstein SJ. Allosteric mechanisms of signal transduction. Science 2005; 308:1424-1428.

61. Ansari SN, Marston S, et al. Role of caldesmon in the Ca^{2+}-regulation of smooth muscle thin filaments: Evidence for a cooperative switching mechanism. J Biol Chem 2007; 10: 1074.

62. Lehrer SS, Geeves MA. The muscle thin filament as a classical cooperative/allosteric regulatory system. J Mol Biol 1998; 277:1081-1089.

63. Sobue K, Morimoto K, Inui M et al. Control of actin-myosin interaction of gizzard smooth muscle by calmodulin and caldesmon-linked flip-flop mechanism. Biomed Res 1982; 3:188-196.

64. Hemric ME, Chalovich JM. Effect of caldesmon on the ATPase activity and the binding of smooth and skeletal myosin subfragments to actin. J Biol Chem 1988; 263:1878-1885.

65. Velaz L, Hemric ME, Benson CE et al. The binding of caldesmon to actin and its effect on the ATPase activity of soluble myosin subfragments in the presence and absence of tropomyosin. J Biol Chem 1989; 264:9602-9610.

66. Chalovich JM, Hemric ME, Velaz L. Regulation of ATP hydrolysis By caldesmon. A novel change in the interaction of myosin with actin. Ann NY Acad Sci 1990; 599:85-99.

67. Velaz L, Ingraham RH, Chalovich JM. Dissociation of the effect of caldesmon on the ATPase activity and on the binding of smooth heavy meromyosin to actin by partial digestion of caldesmon. J Biol Chem 1990; 265:2929-2934.

68. Fredricksen S, Cai A, Gafurov B et al. Influence of ionic strength, actin state and caldesmon construct size on the number of actin monomers in a caldesmon binding site. Biochemistry 2003; 42(20):6136-6148.

69. Chalovich JM, Sen A, Resetar A et al. Caldesmon: binding to actin and myosin and effects on elementary steps in the ATPase cycle. Acta Physiol Scand 1998; 164:427-435.

70. Ischii Y, Lehrer SS. Fluorescence probe studies of the state of tropomyosin in reconstituted muscle thin filaments. Biochemistry 1987; 26:4922-4925.

71. Marston SB. Stoichiometry and stability of caldesmon in native thin filaments from sheep aorta smooth muscle. Biochem J 1990; 272:305-310.

72. Chalovich JM, Eisenberg E. Inhibition of actomyosin ATPase activity by troponin-tropomyosin without blocking the binding of myosin to actin. J Biol Chem 1982; 257:2432-2437.

73. Greene LE, Eisenberg E. Cooperative binding of myosin subfragment-1 to the actin-troponin-tropomyosin complex. Proc Natl Acad Sci USA 1980; 77:2616-2620.

74. Hill TL, Eisenberg E, Greene LE. Theoretical model for the cooperative equilibrium binding of myosin subfragment 1 to the actin-troponin-tropomyosin complex. Proc Natl Acad Sci USA 1980; 77:3186-3190.

75. Chalovich JM. Caldesmon and thin-filament regulation of muscle contraction. Cell Biophys 1988; 12:73-85.

76. Horiuchi KY, Chacko S. Caldesmon inhibits the cooperative turning-on of the smooth muscle heavy meromyosin by tropomyosin-actin. Biochemistry 1989; 28:9111-9116.

77. Ngai PK, Walsh MP. Inhibition of smooth muscle actin-activated Myosin Mg^{2+} ATPase activity by caldesmon. J Biol Chem 1984; 259:13656-13659.

78. Ansari SN, EL-Mezgueldi M, Marston SB. Cooperative inhibition of actin filaments in the absence of tropomyosin. J Musc Res Cell motil 2003; 24(8):513-520.

79. Xu C, Craig R, Tobacman L et al. Tropomyosin positions in regulated thin filaments revealed by cryoelectron microscopy. Biophys J 1999; 77(2):985-992.

80. Vilfan A. The binding dynamics of tropomyosin on actin. Biophys J 2001; 81:3146-3155.

81. Perry SV. Vertebrate tropomyosin: distribution, properties and function. J Musc Res Cell motil 2001; 22(1):5-49.

82. Perry SV. What is the role of tropomyosin in the regulation of muscle contraction? J Musc Res Cell motil 2003; 24:593-596.

83. Holmes KC. The actomyosin interaction and its control by tropomyosin. Biophys J 1995; 68:2s-7s.

84. Shirinsky VP, Vorotnikov AV, Gusev NB. Caldesmon phosphorylation and smooth muscle contraction. Molecular mechanisms and their disorder in smooth muscle contraction. Georgetown, TX: LANDES Bioscience, 1998.

85. Vorotnikov AV, Krymsky MA, Shirinsky VP. Signal transduction and protein phosphorylation in smooth muscle contraction. Biochemistry (Mosc) 2002; 67(12):1309-1328.

86. Redwood CS, Marston SB, Gusev NK. The functional effects of mutants thr^{673*}>asp and ser^{702*}>asp at the pro directed kinase phosphorylation sites in the C terminus of chicken gizzard caldesmon. FEBS Lett 1993; 327:85-89.

87. Patchell VB, Vorotnikov AV, Gao Y et al. Phosphorylation of the minimal inhibitory region at the C-terminal of Caldesmon alters its structural and actin binding properties. Biochim Biophys Acta 2002; 1596(1):121-130.

88. Gao WD, Atar D, Liu Y et al. Role of troponin I proteolysis in the pathogenesis of stunned myocardium. Circ Res 1997; 80(3):393-399.

89. Marston SB, Levine BA, Gao Y et al *MAP kinase phosphorylation at serine 702 alters structural and actin binding properties of caldesmon. Biophys J 2001; 80(1):69a.

90. Marston S, Copeland O, Patchell VB et al. *Multipoint binding of caldesmon to actin is essential for cooperative inhibition. J Musc Res Cell Motil 2002; 23(1):38.

91. Borovikov Yu S, Avrova SV, Vikhoreva NN et al. C-terminal actin binding sites of smooth muscle caldesmon switch actin between conformational states. Int J Biochem Cell Biol 2001; 33(12):1151-1159.

92. Geeves MA, Lehrer SS. Dynamics of the muscle thin filament regulatory switch: the size of the cooperative unit. Biophys J 1994; 67:273-282.

93. Malmqvist U, Arner A, Makuch R et al. The effects of caldesmon extraction on mechanical properties of skinned smooth muscle fibre preparations. Pflugers Archiv 1996; 432:241-247.

94. Barany M, Barany K. Dissociation of relaxation and myosin light chain dephosphorylation in porcine uterine muscle. Arch Biochem Biophys 1993; 305:202-204.

95. Barany M, Barany K. Protein phosphorylation during contraction and relaxation. In: Barany M, ed. Biochemistry of smooth muscle contraction. San Diego: Academic Press Inc, 1996:321-339.

96. Katsuyama H, Wang C-LA, Morgan KG. Regulation of vascular smooth muscle tone by caldesmon. J Biol Chem 1992; 267:14555-14558.

97. Earley JJ, Su X, Moreland RS. Caldesmon inhibits active crossbridges in unstimulated vascular smooth muscle: an antisense oligodeoxynucleotide approach. Circ Res 1998; 83(6):661-667.

98. Lorenz M, Poole KJV, Popp D et al. An atomic model of the unregulated thin filament obtained by x-ray diffraction on orientated actin-tropomyosin gels. J Mol Biol 1995; 246:108-119.

99. Vibert P, Craig R, Lehman W. Three-dimensional reconstruction of caldesmon-containing smooth muscle thin filaments. J Cell Biol 1993; 20:57-10.

100. Hodgkinson JL, EL-Mezgueldi M, Craig R et al. 3-D image reconstuction of reconstituted smooth muscle thin filaments containing calponin: visualisation of interactions between F-actin and calponin. J Mol Biol 1997; 273:150-159.

101. Hayashi K, Yano H, Hashida T et al. Genomic structure of the human caldesmon gene. Proc Natl Acad Sci USA 1992; 89:12122-12126.

102. Humphrey MB, Herrera-Sosa H, Gonzalez G et al. Molecular cloning of human caldesmons. Gene 1992; 112:197-205.

CHAPTER 10

Tropomyosin as a Regulator of Cancer Cell Transformation

David M. Helfman,* Patrick Flynn, Protiti Khan and Ali Saeed

Abstract

Tropomyosins (Tms) are among the most studied structural proteins of the actin cytoskeleton that are implicated in neoplastic-specific alterations in actin filament organization. Decreased expression of specific nonmuscle Tm isoforms is commonly associated with the transformed phenotype. These changes in Tm expression appear to contribute to the rearrangement of microfilament bundles and morphological alterations, increased cell motility and oncogenic signaling properties of transformed cells. Below we review aspects of Tm biology as it specifically relates to transformation and cancer including its expression in culture models of transformed cells and human tumors, mechanisms that regulate Tm expression and the role of Tm in oncogenic signaling.

Introduction

Over thirty years ago cell biologists made the seminal observation that transformed cells exhibit loss of actin filament bundles, also called stress fibers.[1-5] Since then subsequent studies have shown that alterations in the actin-based cytoskeleton are an established characteristic of transformed cells. It is now known that oncogenic signaling pathways directly target the actin cytoskeleton including the expression of actin-binding proteins, as well as pathways that regulate cytoskeleton dynamics. Oncogene-mediated disruption of stress fibers and associated adhesive structures are responsible for enhanced motility and invasiveness of tumor cells. In addition to changes in cell morphology and motility, transformation is also associated with abnormal growth control of cells in culture including the ability to grow in low serum, grow on soft agar and to escape apoptosis. The first clue suggesting that the actin cytoskeleton directly participates in growth control came from early studies showing that changes in microfilament structure were correlated with anchorage-independent growth and cellular tumorigenicity.[6] There is a well-developed body of knowledge that suggests changes in the cytoskeleton are causally associated with activation of oncogenic signaling pathways because ectopic expression of specific actin filament stabilizing proteins in transformed cells not only restores microfilament bundles and focal adhesions, but revereses the ability of transformed cells to grow in low serum, grow on soft agar, escape apoptosis and form tumors in mice. These observations raise the intriguing hypothesis that the actin cytoskeleton plays a direct role in oncogenic signaling. However, the mechanism(s) by which oncogene-mediated changes in the actin cytoskeleton contribute to aberrant signaling events and thereby provide a tumor cell with a selective growth advantage, remain to be discovered. Once we understand how the actin cytoskeleton

*Corresponding Author: David M. Helfman—Department of Cell Biology and Anatomy, Sylvester Comprehensive Cancer Center, Leonard M. Miller School of Medicine, Papanicolaou Building, Room 317, 1550 NW 10th Avenue (M-877), Miami, Florida 33136, USA. Email: dhelfman@med.miami.edu

Tropomyosin, edited by Peter Gunning. ©2008 Landes Bioscience and Springer Science+Business Media.

functions in oncogenic signaling, it will be possible to develop new therapeutic strategies that target signaling pathways dependent on the cytoskeleton.

As described above, transformed cells have characteristic changes in the expression of actin filament associated proteins. Tropomyosins (Tms) are among the most studied structural proteins of the actin cytoskeleton that are implicated in alterations of actin filament organization in transformed cells. Decreased expression of nonmuscle tropomyosins is commonly associated with the transformed phenotype. The changes in Tm expression appear to correlate well with the rearrangement of microfilament bundles and morphological alterations observed in transformed cells. The decrease in Tm synthesis has been reported to occur in cells transformed by a variety of agents including chemical carcinogens, UV radiation, DNA and RNA tumor viruses and various oncogenes. In addition, the changes in Tm expression following transformation occur in cells of all species examined including chicken, rodents (mouse and rat) and human, indicating that alterations of Tm expression is a common feature of the transformed phenotype and that Tm gene expression may represent a target for oncogene action. Below we review aspects of Tm biology as it specifically relates to transformation and cancer including its expression in transformed cells and human tumors, mechanisms that regulate Tm expression and the role of Tm in oncogenic signaling.

Tm Expression in Transformed Cells and Human Tumors

Tms are a family of actin-filament binding proteins that bind to actin filaments and stabilize actin filaments. They are expressed from a multigene family comprised of four genes via alternative promoters and alternative RNA splicing, giving rise to approximately 40 different isoforms (See chapters 2 and 16). Nonmuscle cells express both HMW (high molecular weight. 284 amino acids) and LMW low molecular weight (LMW, 248 amino acids) Tms, termed HMW Tm1, Tm2, Tm3 and Tm6 and LMW isoforms LMW Tm-4, TM-5(NM1), Tm-5a and Tm-5b (see Chapter 2). In untransformed cells Tm-1, Tm-2 and Tm-3 are the major HMW Tms and Tm-4 is the major LMW Tm. Although nonmuscle cells express multiple forms of both HMW and LMW Tms, the expression of only HMW TM isoforms are decreased during oncogenic transformation. Since the first observations by Hal Weintraub's lab in the early 1980s, alterations in Tm expression have been reported in a variety of transformed cell lines.[7-15] Perturbations in Tm synthesis have been reported to occur in cells transformed by a variety of agents including chemical carcinogens, UV radiation, DNA and RNA tumor viruses and various oncogenes including Ras, raf, Src, fes, fms, mos, myc, c-Jun, raf and erbB2 (reviewed in Stehn et al[16]). In addition, the changes in Tm expression following transformation occur in cells of all species examined including chicken, rodents (mouse and rat) and human, indicating that modulations in Tm expression is a common feature of the transformed phenotype and that Tm gene expression may represent a target for oncogene action. Decreased expression of HMW Tms is associated with the disruption of stress fibers in transformed cells. As described below, HMW Tms protect actin filaments from severing proteins better than LMW Tms, consistent with their absence leading to a loss of stress fibers following transformation.

The importance of Tms in human cancer is highlighted by several studies indicating that changes in Tm expression are found in a variety of human tumors. Studies of breast tumors demonstrate that HMW Tms are decreased in malignant breast lesions when compared to benign or normal tissue.[17-19] Down regulation of HMW Tm1, Tm2 and Tm3 were found in transitional cell carcinoma of the urinary bladder.[20] Studies of tumors associated with the central nervous system revealed that low-grade astrocytic tumors express HMW Tms, while highly malignant CNS tumors did not, suggesting a correlation between HMW Tm expression and tumor grade.[21] Studies of astrocytomas show an increase in HMW Tms in neoplastic astrocytes, as compared to normal astrocytes.[22] Interestingly, studies by Lin and colleagues identified a novel LMW Tm isoform preferentially associated with colon cancer.[23] It is possible that differences are due to cell-type specific differences in the patterns of Tm expression observed in malignancies associated with different tissues. These studies using human tumor tissues demonstrate that alterations in the expression of Tms observed in transformed cells are likely not simply the result of in vitro culture conditions. Clearly more studies will be required that characterize other tumor types to gain a better understanding of the changes in Tm expression in human tumors. These results suggest that altered Tm expression is an important aspect of tumor biology. As described below, studies using culture models suggest that loss of Tm contributes to increased cell motility and metatstasis, alterations in cell signaling and resistance to apoptotic signals. Further studies will be required to determine how changes in Tm expression contribute to tumor growth and if Tm expression will be a useful diagnostic, prognostic and therapeutic target.[16]

Regulation of Tm Expression in Transformed Cells

The mechanism by which Tm expression is regulated in transformed cells is still poorly understood. Cellular transformation by oncogenic Ras and Src leads to down-regulation of HMW Tms.[8,9] This has led researchers to determine which oncogenic signaling pathways regulate Tm expression. Ras is known to activate multiple pathways including the MAP kinase pathway, phosphatidylinositol 3-kinase (PI 3-K) and the RalGDS family of guanine nucleotide exchange factors for Ral GTPases.[24] A major task is to discern which effector pathway contributes to which aspect of the transformed phenotype.[25] Studies of oncogenic Ras have suggested a role for components of the Ras-Raf-MEK-ERK pathway in down-regulating the expression of HMW Tms. In one series of studies, the ras-induced downregulation of Tm was found to be Raf-mediated, but MEK-independent because treatment with the MEK1 inhibitor PD98059 or had little effect on Tm levels, suggesting that a novel pathway exists downstream of Raf which may play an important role in the regulation of Tm expression.[26-28] In a study of c-Jun transformed cells, however, the downregulation of Tm was reversed following treatment of cells with the MEK1 inhibitor PD98059.[29] Similarly, studies of Ras-transformed RIE-1 cells demonstrated that treatment with the UO126 or PD98059 MEK inhibitors did partially restore the expression of HMW Tms.[30] Likewise studies of T24 bladder carcinoma cells, which contain activated H-Ras, show that treatment with UO126 resulted in up-regulation of Tm1, Tm2 and Tm3.[20] Interestingly, TGF-beta induction of HMW Tm and stress fibers are significantly inhibited by Ras-ERK signaling in the metastatic breast cancer cell line MDA-MB-231, but inhibition of the Ras-ERK pathway using UO126 restores TGF-beta induction of HMW Tms and stress fibers.[31] Thus, components of the Ras-Raf-MEK-ERK pathway contribute to the downregulation of HMW Tm expression in various systems.

In addition to being targeted by oncogenic signaling pathways, down-regulation of Tm expression is also mediated by DNA methylation and microRNA.[19,32,33] Studies in breast cancer cell lines revealed that HMW Tm1 is down-regulated due to promoter methylation because combined treatment with 5-aza-2′-deoxycytodine (AZA) and trichostatin A (TSA) resulted in detectable expression of Tm1, but not that of other isoforms.[32] The upregulation of Tm-1 following treatment with AZA plus TSA paralleled the emergence of Tm1 containing microfilaments and restored anchorage-dependent cell growth.[32] The authors also demonstrated that ectopic expression of Tm1 also resulted in formation of stress fibers and anchorage-dependence, further showing an important role for Tm1 expression in reversal of the transformed phenotype. These data demonstrate that hypermethylation of DNA and chromatin remodeling is involved in the mechanism by which Tm1 expression is downregulated in breast cancer. Subsequent studies showed that silencing of the HMW Tm1 and Tm3 gene by DNA methylation is responsible for the inability of TGF-beta to induce expression of these HMW Tms in breast cancer cells.[19] These authors also provide direct evidence that DNA sequences within the Tm1 gene are methylated. Further support for a role of DBA methylation come from studies in Ras-transformed RIE-1, HT1080 and DLD-1 cells, showing treatment of cells with azadeoxycytidine restored Tm expression.[30] Another genetic mechanism involving microRNAs has been reported to be involved in silencing Tm1 expression in breast cancer.[33] HMW Tm1 was silenced by microRNA-21 (mir-21). Mir-21 has been suggested to function as an oncogene because it is overexpressed in many types of tumors.[34-36] Suppression of mir-21 by antisense oligonucleotides inhibits tumor growth.[34,36] Interestingly, overexpression of TM1 in breast cancer cells expressing mir-21 suppressed anchorage independent growth further suggesting that downregulation of HMW TMs by this microRNA is an essential part of the transformed phenotype, contributing to alterations in cell morphology, cytoarchitecture, motility and abnormal signaling.

Finally, nonmuscle HMW Tms have been reported to be subject to phosphorylation.[37-39] Phosphorylation of HMW Tm by PI(3)K was found to play a role in regulating endocytosis.[37] DAP kinase 1 was found to phosphorylate Tm-1 downstream of the ERK pathway leading to stress fiber formation.[39] Since both the PI(3)K and ERK signaling pathways are often times hyperactivated in cancer, further studies will be required to determine if phosphorylation of Tms following activation of these pathways mediate any of the properties associated with the transformed phenotype.

The Role of Tropomyosin Expression in Tumor Cell Motility, Invasion and Metastasis

The down-regulation of HMW Tm expression in transformed cells appears to be causally related to the disruption of stress fibers and focal adhesions. Support for this idea comes from studies demonstrating that ectopic expression of HMW Tms in Ras and Src transformed fibroblasts restores stress fibers and significantly reduces cell motility.[40-45] These studies also demonstrated that forced-expression of Tm also suppressed the ability of cells to form tumors in nude mice.[40,43,45] Further evidence for a role of Tm in tumorigenicity comes from studies of Lewis lung carcinoma and melanoma cells.[14,46] In addition, the importance of Tms in the control of tumor invasion and metastasis is highlighted by several studies indicating that high-grade tumors of breast, prostate, bladder and brain express significantly lower levels of Tms than that of normal tissues.[17,18,20,21,47] Not all studies have demonstrated that ectopic expression of TM reverses the transformation-associated changes in the actin cytoskeleton. Shields et al[30] were unable to demonstrate any affects of stable expression of HMW Tms in transformed RIE-1 epithelial cells. Likewise exogenous expression of Tm1 in neuroblastoma cells failed to alter cell morphology or organization of the actin cytoskeleton.[48] These latter two studies suggest that other factors are involved in these cell systems.

The loss of HMW Tms in transformed cells is thought to contribute to the improper assembly of microfilaments and adhesive structures, thereby contributing to the invasive and metastatic properties of cancer cells. Support for a role for Tms in microfilament dynamics come from biochemical studies that demonstrate that HMW Tms protect actin filaments from severing proteins gelsolin and cofilin better than LMW Tms, consistent with their absence leading to a loss of stable actin filaments following transformation. Thus, Tms bound to filamentous actin prevent access of ADF/cofilins or gelsolin to actin filaments thereby stabilizing actin filaments and reducing actin dynamics (see Chapter 17 and 18).

In addition to the down-regulation of HMW Tms, down-regulation of RhoA/ROCK/ Lim-kinase/cofilin pathway also contributes to the disruption of stress fibers in transformed cells.[49-53] The RhoA/ROCK/LIM-kinase/cofilin pathway regulates stress fiber formation by regulating myosin II phosphorylation[54,55] and the actin depolymerizing activity of ADF/cofilin.[56] The loss of Tms in transformed cells likely contributes to the loss of stress fibers by allowing cofilin to sever actin filaments. Thus, Tms may compensate or substitute for the loss the ROCK/LIMK/ cofilin by blocking ADF/cofilins and gelsolin from binding to actin filaments. While much attention has been focused on the role of Tms in modulating the activities of severing proteins, it is also possible that Tms play a role by modulating the function and activity of myosin II. Myosin II is essential for formation of stress fibers and focal adhesions. Inhibition of the Rho/ROCK pathway in transformed cells also contributes to the loss of stress fibers by decreasing the levels of phosphorylated myosin light chain. How different nonmuscle Tms will affect the actions of myosin II is not fully understood. Studies of smooth muscle and skeletal muscle Tms demonstrate they differ in their ability to activate the MgATPase of myosin II (See Chapter 20). Smooth muscle Tms can activate myosin II, whereas, skeletal muscle Tms are inhibitory. Importantly, in preliminary experiments we found that nonmuscle HMW Tms activate myosin II. It will be interesting to determine if HMW Tm can antagonize the suppression of the Rho/ROCK pathway in Ras transformed cells by protecting actin filaments from severing proteins and activating myosin II through actin-activated ATPase function. Therefore, suppression of HMW Tms might represent

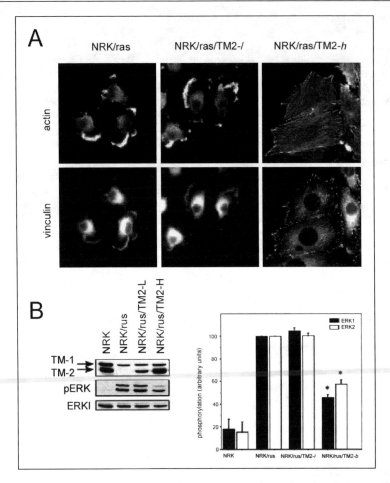

Figure 1. Restoration of microfilament assembly and decreased ERK phosphorylation in NRK/Ras cells expressing Tropomyosin 2. A) NRK/Ras, NRK/Ras/TM2-*l* and NRK/ras/TM2-*h* cells grown on glass coverslips were stained with Oregon green-conjugated phalloidin and anti-vinculin mAb, followed by Cy3-conjugated anti-mouse antibody. Note the reappearance of actin bundles and vinculin-containing focal adhesions in NRK/ras/TM2-*h* cells. B) Exponentially growing cells were harvested and protein extracts analyzed by Western blotting for expression of Tropomyosins (TM-1 and TM-2 isoforms) and phospho-ERK, Graph on the right shows the average ERK phosphorylation from 3 independent experiments.y axis is in arbitrary units *, *P* value of <0.001, as determined by Student's *t* test. (From Helfman and Pawla.[62])

critical cellular targets that can act independently, or synergistically, with repression of the Rho/ ROCK pathway, to facilitate transformation mediated disruption of the actin cytoskeleton, leading to enhanced motility.

Tm and the Actin Cytoskeleton in the Regulation of Oncogenic Signaling

Several studies have suggested that specific isoforms of HMW Tms may possess tumor suppressor activity and HMW Tm isoforms can be classified as a class II tumor suppressor.[57] Consistent with this hypothesis is the observation that forced-expression of HMW TMs into transformed cells exhibiting a loss of these isoforms not only reverts the transformation associated changes in cytoarchitecture, but also several aspects of the transformed phenotype, including a reversal of the ability to grow in low serum, grow on soft agar, escape apoptosis and form tumors in mice.[43-45,58-60] In addition antisense expression of Tm1 in untransformed cells resulted in properties associated with transformation including anchorage independent cell growth.[61] Collectively these results raise the intriguing hypothesis that the loss of Tms plays a direct role in oncogenic signaling. Once we understand how the actin cytoskeleton functions in oncogenic signaling it will be possible to develop new therapeutic strategies that target signaling pathways dependent on the cytoskeleton.

How loss of Tm is mechanistically linked to changes in oncogenic signaling is not well understood. As discussed in the previous section, although it is established that these changes in the actin cytoskeleton play a critical role in pathways linked to increased motility and metastasis of tumor cells, it is not known how the cytoskeleton functions in growth control. One clue comes from studies showing that ectopic expression of Tm2 in Ras transformed cells led to a decrease in ERK activation.[62] They previously reported that forced expression of HMW Tm2 in Ras transformed fibroblasts restores microfilament organization and concomitantly restores the requirement for growth factors of these cells.[44] The extent of ERK inhibition is correlated with the degree of Tm2 over-expression, which, in turn, is associated with a well-spread morphology and less membrane ruffling (see Fig. 1). Interestingly, in the same studies the authors report that Ras signaling to ERK is dependent on myosin II, under the control of myosin light chain kinase (MLCK).[62] This has lead us to hypothesize a previously uncharacterized role for Tm, the actin cytoskeleton and myosin II, MLCK in ERK signaling in Ras-transformed cells. Because oncogenic Ras can profoundly affect microfilament organization it is also possible that Ras might remodel the actin cytoskeleton into structures required for efficient signaling to ERK. The mechanism remains to be determined, but it is possible that stress fibers act to sequester molecules involved in oncogenic signaling and oncogene-mediated disruption of stress fibers frees molecules to promote aberrant signaling. In addition to their role in stress fiber formation, HMW Tms have been reported to function in intracellular vesicle trafficking.[37] Since some oncogenic signaling involve endocytic trafficking, it is possible that Tms participate in regulating signaling events dependent on intracellular trafficking. In the future it will be important to delineate how Tm participates in oncogenic signaling events. This knowledge about TMs and regulation of signaling pathways will advance the cytoskeletal field and related areas of study. In addition, it is possible that this information will be useful for identifying potential molecular targets for the development of novel, more effective cancer therapies.

Conclusions

The studies discussed above demonstrate that Tms are targets of oncogenic signaling and also can function as regulators of oncogenic signaling. Further studies will be required to determine the mechanisms by which Tms participate in properties associated with the transformed phenotype. As we obtain more information about the roles of Tm in cancer it is possible that in the future Tms might serve as diagnostic and prognostic biomarkers. Finally, it has been suggested that Tms might be potential chemotherapeutic targets (reviewed in Stehn et al[16]). Understanding the role of this family of actin filament binding proteins has enormous implications for undertanding human cancers.

References

1. Pollack R, Osborn M, Weber K. Patterns of organization of actin and myosin in normal and transformed cultured cells. Proc Natl Acad Sci USA 1975; 72:994-998.
2. Goldman RD, Yerna MI, Schloss IA. Localization and organization of microfilaments and related proteins in normal and virus-transformed cells. J Supramolecular Struct 1976; 5:155-183.
3. Wang H, Goldberg AR. Changes in microfilament organization and surface topography upon transformation of chick embryo fibroblasts with rous sarcoma virus. Proc Natl Acad Sci USA 1976; 73:4065-4069.
4. Edelman G, Yahara I. Temperature-sensitive changes in surface modulating assemblies of fibroblasts transformed by mutants of Rous sarcoma virus. Proc Natl Acad Sci USA 1976; 73:2047-2051.

5. Vollett JJ, Brugge JS, Noonan CA et al. The role of SV40 gene A in the alteration of microfilaments in transformed cells. Exp Cell Res 1977; 105:119-126.
6. Shin S, Freedman VH, Risser R et al. Tumorigenicty of virus-transformed cells in nude mice is correlated specifically with anchorage independent growth in vitro. Proc Natl Acad Sci USA 1975; 72:4435-4439.
7. Hendricks M, Weintraub H. Tropomyosin is decreased in transformed cells. Proc Natl Acad Sci USA 1981; 78:5633-5637.
8. Hendicks M, Weintraub H. Multiple tropomyosin polypeptides in chicken embryo fibroblasts: differential repression of transcription by Rous sarcoma virus transformation. Mol Cell Biol 1984; 4:1823-1833.
9. Leonardi CL, Warren RH, Rubin RW. Lack of tropomyosin correlates with the absence of stress fibers in transformed rat kidney cells. Biochem Biophys Acta 1982; 720:154-162.
10. Matsumura F, Lin JJC, Yamashiro-Matsumura S et al. Differential expression of tropomyosin froms in the micro-filaments isolated from normal and transformed rat cultured cells. J Biol Chem 1983; 258:13954-13964.
11. Cooper HL, Feuerstain N, Noda M et al. Suppression of tropomyosin synthesis, a common biochemical feature of oncogenesis by structurally diverse retroviral oncogenes. Mol Cell Biol 1985; 5:972-983.
12. Lin JHC, Helfman DM, Hughes SH et al. Tropomyosin isoforms in chicken embryo fibroblasts: purification, characterization and changes in Rous sarcoma virus-transformed cells. J Cell Biol 1985; 100:692-703.
13. Leavitt I, Latter G, Lutomski L et al. Tropomyosin isoforms switching in tumorigenic human fibroblasts Mol Cell Biol 1986; 6:2721-2726.
14. Takenaga K, Nakamura Y, Sakiyama S. Differential expression of a tropomyosin isoforms in low- and high-metastatic Lewis lung carcinoma cells. Mol cell Biol 1988; 8:3934-3937.
15. Takenaga K, Nakamura Y, Sayiyama S. Suppresion of synthesis of tropomyosin isoforms 2 in metastatic v-Ha-ras-transformed NIH 3T3 cells. Biochem Biophys Res Commun 1988; 157:1111-1116.
16. Stehn JR, Schevzov G, O'Neill GM et al. Specialisation of the tropomyosin composition of actin filaments provides new potential targets for chemotherapy. Current Cancer Drug Targets 2006; 6:245-256.
17. Franzen B, Linder S, Uryu K et al. Expression of tropomyosin isosforms in benign and malignant human breast lesions. Brit J Cancer 1996; 73:909-913.
18. Raval GN, Bharadwaj S, Levine EA et al. Loss of expression of tropomyosin-1, a novel class II tumor suppressor that induces anoikis, in primary breast tumors. Oncogene 2003; 22:6194-6203.
19. Varga AE, Stourman NV, Zheng Q et al. Silencing of the tropomyosin-1 gene by DNA methylation alters tumor suppressor function of TGF-beta. Oncogene 2005; 24:5043-5052.
20. Pawlak G, McGarvey TW, Nguyen TB et al. Alterations in tropomyosin isoform expression in human transitional cell carcinoma of the urinary bladder. Int J Cancer 2004; 110:368-373.
21. Hughes JA, Cook-Yarborough CM, Chadwick NC et al. High-molecular-weight tropomyosins localize to the contractile rings of dividing CNS cells but are absent from malignant pedoatric and adult CNS tumors. Glia 2003; 42:25-35.
22. Galloway PG, Likavec MJ, Perry G. Tropomyosin isoforms expression in normal and neoplastic astrocytes. Lab Invest 1990; 62:163-170.
23. Lin JL, Geng X, Bhattacharya SD et al. Isolation and sequencing of a novel tropomyosin isoforms preferentially associated with colon cancer. Gastroenterology 2002; 123:152-162.
24. Katz ME, McCormick F. Signal transduction from multiple Ras effectors. Curr Opin Genet Dev 1997; 7:75-79.
25. Shields JM, Pruitt K, McFall A et al. Understanding Ras: it ain't over 'til it's over. Trends Cell Biol 2000; 10:147-154.
26. Janssen RAJ, Veenstra KG, Jonasch P et al. Ras- and Raf-induced down-modulation of nonmuscle tropomyosin are MEK-independent. J Biol Chem 1998; 273:32182-32186.
27. Kim PN, Jonasch E, Mosterman BC et al. Radicicol suppresses transformation and restores tropomyosin-2 expression in both ras- and MEK-transformed cells without inhibiting the Raf/MEK/ERK signaling cascade. Cell Growth Differ 2001; 12:543-550.
28. Janssen RAJ, Kim PN, Mier JW et al. Overexpression of kinase suppressor of Ras upregulates the high-molecular weight tropomyosin isoforms in ras-transformed NIH 3T3 fibroblasts. Mol Cell Biol 2003; 23:1786-1797.
29. Ljungdahl S, Linder S, Franzen B et al. Down-regulation of tropomyosin-2 expression in c-Jun-transformed rat fibroblasts involves induction of a MEK-1 dependent autocrine loop. Cell Growth Differ 1998; 9:565-573.
30. Shields JM, Mehta H, Pruitt K et al. Opposing roles of the extracellular signal-regulated kinase and p38 mitogen-activated protein kinase cascades in Ras-mediated downregulation of tropomyosin. Mol Cell Biol 2002; 22:2304-2317.
31. Bakin AV, Rinehart C, Safina A et al. A critical role of tropomyosins in TGF-β regulation of the actin cytoskeleton and cell motility in epithelial cells. Mol Biol Cell 2004; 15:4682-4694.
32. Bharadwaj S, Prasad GL. Tropomyosin-1, a novel suppressor of cellular transformation is downregulated by promoter methylation in cancer cells. Cancer Lett 2002; 183:205-213.
33. Zhu S, Si ML, Wu H et al. MicroRNA-21 targets the tumor suppressor gene tropomyosin 1 (TPM1) J Biol Chem 2007; 282:14328-14336.

34. Chan JA, Krichevsky AM, Kosik KS. MicroRNA-21 is an antiapoptotic factor in human glioblastoma cells. Cancer Res 2005; 65:6029-6033.

35. Roldo C, Missiaglia E, Hagan JP et al. MicroRNA expression abnormalities in pancreatic endocrine and acinar tumors are associated with distinctive pathologic features and clinical behavior. J Clin Oncol 2006; 24:4677-4684.

36. Si ML, Zhu S, Wu H et al. miR-21-mdiated tumor growth Oncogene 2007; 26:2799-2803.

37. Prasad SVN, Jayatilleke A, Madamanchi A et al. Protein kinase activity of phosphoinositide 3-kinase regulates beta-adrenergic receptor endocytosis. Nature Cell Biol 2005; 7:785-796.

38. Houle F, Rousseau S, Morrice N et al. Extracellular signal-regulated kinase mediates phosphorylation of tropomyosin-1 to promote cytoskeleton remodeling in response to oxidative stress: impact on membrane blebbing. Mol Biol Cell 2003; 14:1418-1432.

39. Houle F, Poirer A, Dumaresq et al. DAP kinase mediates the phosphorylation of tropomyosin-1 downstream of the ERK pathway, which regulates the formation of stress fibers in response to oxidative stress. J Cell Sci 2007; 120:3666-3677.

40. Prasad GL, Fuldner RA, Cooper HL. Expression of transduced tropomyosin 1 cDNA suppresses neoplastic growth of cells transformed by the ras oncogene. Proc Natl Acad Sci USA 1993; 90:7039-7043.

41. Prasad GL, Masuelli L, Raj MH et al. Suppression of src-induced transformed phenotype by expression of tropomyosin-1. Oncogene 1999; 18:2027-2031.

42. Takenaga K, Masuda A. Restoration of microfilament bundle organization in v-raf-transformed NRK cells after transduction with tropomyosin 2 cDNA. Cancer Lett 1994; 87:47-53.

43. Braverman RH, Cooper HL, Lee HS et al. Anti-oncogenic effects of tropomyosin: isoform specificity and importance of protein coding sequences. Oncogene 1996; 13:537-545.

44. Gimona M, Kazzaz J, Helfman DM. Forced expression of tropomyosin 2 or 3 in vi-Ki-ras-transformed fibroblasts results in distinct phenotypic effects. Proc Natl Acad Sci USA 1996; 93:9618-9623.

45. Janssen RAJ, Mier JW. Tropomyosin-2 cDNA lacking the 3' untranslated region riboregulator induces growth inhibition of v-Ki-ras-transformed fibroblasts. Mol Biol Cell 1997; 8:897-908.

46. Hashimoto Y, Shindo-Okada N, Tani M et al. Identification of genes differentially expressed in association with metastatic potential of K-1735 murine melanoma by messenger RNA differential display. Cancer Res 1996; 56:5266-5271.

47. Wang FL, Wang Y, Wong WK et al. Two differentially expressed genes in normal human prostate tissue and in carcinoma. Cancer Res 1996; 56:3634-3637.

48. Yager ML, Hughes JAI, Lovicu FJ et al. British J Cancer 2003; 89:860-863.

49. Pawlak G, Helfman DM. Posttranscriptional down-regulation of ROCKI/Rho-kinase through an MEK-dependent pathway leads to cytoskeleton disruption in Ras-transformed fibroblasts. Mol Biol Cell 2002a; 13(1):336-347.

50. Pawlak G, Helfman DM. MEK Mediates v-Src-induced disruption of the actin cytoskeleton via inactivation of the Rho-ROCK-LIM kinase pathway. J Biol Chem 2002b; 277:26927-26933.

51. Lee S, Helfman DM. Cytoplasmic p21Cip1 is involved in Ras-induced inhibition of the ROCK/LIMK/cofilin pathway. J Biol Chem 2004; 279:1885-1891.

52. Sahai E, Olson MF, Marshall CJ. Cross-talk between ras and rho signalling pathways in transformation favors proliferation and increased motility. EMBO J 2001; 20:755-766.

53. Vial E, Sahai E, Marshall CJ. ERK-MAPK signaling coordinately regulates activity of Rac1 and RhoA for tumor cell motility. Cancer Cell 2003; 4:67-79.

54. Amano M, Ito M, Kimura K et al. Phosphorylation and activation of myosin by Rho-associated kinase (Rho-kinase). J Biol Chem 1996; 271:20246-20249.

55. Kimura K, Ito M, Amano M et al. Regulation of myosin phosphatase by Rho and Rho-associated kinase (Rho-kinase). Science 1996; 273:245-248.

56. Bamburg JR. Proteins of the ADF/cofilin family:essential regulators of actin dynamics. Annu Rev Cell Dev Biol 1999; 15:185-230.

57. Lee SW, Tomasetto C, Sager R. Positive selection of candidate tumor-suppressor genes by subtractive hybridization. Proc Natl Acad Sci USA 1991; 88:2825-2829.

58. Shah V, Bharadwaj S, Kaibuchi K et al. Cytoskeletal organization in tropomyosin-mediated reversion of ras-transformation: evidence for Rho kinase pathway. Oncogene 2001; 20:2112-2121.

59. Bharadwaj S, Thanawala R, Bon G et al. Resensitization of breast cancer cells to anoikis by tropomyosin1: role of Rho-kinase-dependent cytoskeleton and adhesion. Oncogene 2005; 24:8291-8303.

60. Mahadev K, Raval G, Bharadwaj S et al. Suppression of the transformed phenotype of breast cancer by tropomyosin-1. Exp Cell Res 2002; 279:40-51.

61. Boyd J, Risinger JI, Wiseman RW et al. Regulation of microfilament organization and anchorage-independent growth by tropomyosin 1. Proc Natl Acad Sci USA 1996; 92:11534-11538.

62. Helfman DM, Pawlak G. Myosin light chain kinase and acto-myosin contractility modulate activation of the ERK cascade downstream of oncogenic Ras. J Cell Biochem 2005; 95:1069-1080.

CHAPTER 11

The Role of Tropomyosin in Heart Disease

David F. Wieczorek,* Ganapathy Jagatheesan and Sudarsan Rajan

The Role of Tropomyosin in Heart Disease

Cardiovascular disease is the number one cause of mortality in the Western world, with heart failure representing one of the fastest growing subgroups over the past decade. Heart failure, the progressive loss of cardiac contractile performance resulting in an inability to pump an adequate supply of systemic blood, affects an estimated 5 million Americans with estimated medical costs of $21-$50 billion per year.[1] A number of common disease stimuli can induce heart failure, including hypertension, myocardial infarction, ischemia associated with coronary artery disease, congenital malformation, familial hypertrophic and dilated cardiomyopathies and diabetic cardiomyopathy. Systolic and diastolic dysfunction is common in patients suffering from coronary artery disease and hypertension and is a main cause of heart failure. Hypertrophic growth of cardiomyocytes also occurs in many forms of heart failure and may contribute to the pathogenesis of the failure state.[2]

Tissue and Developmental Specific Expression of Tropomyosin Isoforms in the Heart

To understand the role of tropomyosin (Tm) in the heart, it is first necessary to define Tm isoform specific expression in this tissue. Studies by Cummins and Perry[3] and Izumo et al[4] found that the myocardium of adult small mammals express the striated α-Tm isoform, while fetal heart tissue expresses both α- and β-Tm isoforms. Previous studies on chicken primitive cardiomyocytes show Tm antibodies react with stress fiber-like structures within these cells.[5] To more fully examine Tm isoform expression during mammalian development, we analyzed the expression of various Tm genes during murine embryogenesis and in developing embryonic stem cells, with a particular emphasis on the developing myocardium.[6] Results show that the Tm genes (α, β, γ and δ) are expressed in differentiated embryoid bodies, with the striated muscle-specific β-Tm isoform being constitutively expressed in the embryoid bodies and during murine embryogenesis in utero. In contrast, the striated α-Tm isoform is not present until the day 5 embryoid body and the day 7.5 post coitus embryo. Further analyses show that both the striated muscle α- and β-Tm isoforms are expressed during cardiogenesis (day 11-19 embryonic hearts), with the α-Tm transcripts becoming the predominant Tm isoform in the adult heart[6]; the ratio of striated α- to β-Tm mRNAs changes from 5:1 to 60:1 during the embryonic to adult transition.

To address whether the striated β-Tm isoform could substitute for α-Tm in the heart, we generated transgenic mice that express the striated muscle β-Tm specifically in the myocardium.[7] There is an 86% amino acid identity exhibited between α- and β-Tm with 39 amino acid differences distributed

*Corresponding Author: David F. Wieczorek—Department of Molecular Genetics, Biochemistry and Microbiology, University of Cincinnati Medical Center, Cincinnati, OH 45267-0524, U.S.A. Email: david.wieczorek@uc.edu

Tropomyosin, edited by Peter Gunning. ©2008 Landes Bioscience and Springer Science+Business Media.

throughout the entire molecule; 25 of the 39 changes are located in the carboxy terminus of Tm. These differences may indicate an isoform specific response occurs to calcium activation through the troponin (Tn) complex. By conducting the β-Tm transgenic mouse experiments, we would address whether there are functional differences between α- and β-Tm in the sarcomere. Cardiac specific expression was achieved through use of the α-myosin heavy chain promoter which drove the β-Tm cDNA; we could readily distinguish the amount of β-Tm expression in these transgenic mice since endogenous β-Tm protein expression is less than 2% in the adult mouse heart.

Multiple β-Tm transgenic lines were generated which showed a 150-fold increase in β-Tm mRNA expression in the heart, along with a 34-fold increase in the associated protein.[7] As expected, we found that expression of the transgene was restricted to the cardiac compartment. With the increase in β-Tm mRNA and protein in the transgenic hearts, there was a concomitant decrease in the levels of α-Tm transcripts and their associated protein. This ability of the α- and β-Tm genes to "cross-talk" and modulate the mRNA and proteins levels of striated muscle Tm isoforms so that there is no net increase in Tm production appears to be a regulatory mechanism utilized by striated muscle to control Tm isoform production as this process also occurs with other Tm transgenic models.[8-12] Interestingly, this regulatory mechanism does not appear to operate with cytoskeletal Tm isoforms (Gunning, personal communication).

Morphological and physiological analyses were conducted on these β-Tm transgenic hearts.[7] We found that when there was 55-60% β-Tm protein expressed in the myocardium, there were no structural changes in the hearts or in the sarcomeres. Physiological analyses revealed that functional parameters associated with myocardial contractility appear normal; however, there is a significant delay in the time of relaxation and a decrease in the maximum rate of relaxation in these hearts. We also found that the myofilaments containing β-Tm demonstrated an increase in the activation of the thin filament by strongly bound cross-bridges, an increase in calcium sensitivity of steady state force and a decrease in the rightward shift of the calcium-force relation induced by cAMP-dependent phosphorylation.[13] When isolated cardiomyocytes were studied, we found the β-Tm transgenic cells exhibited significantly reduced maximal rates of contraction and relaxation with no change in the extent of shortening.[14] Additional results show that the Tm isoform population modulates the dynamics of contraction and relaxation of single myocytes by a mechanism that does not alter the rate-limiting step of crossbridge detachment.

To explore further the significance of altering the α- to β-Tm isoform ratio in murine myocardium, we generated transgenic mice which express β-Tm at high levels in the heart (80% β-Tm and 20% α-Tm). Our results show that higher levels of β-Tm expression are lethal with death ensuing between 10-14 days postnatally. A detailed histological analysis demonstrates that the hearts of these mice exhibit severe pathological abnormalities, including thrombus formation in the lumen of atria and ventricles, atrial enlargement and fibrosis. Physiological analyses reveal that there is severe systolic and diastolic dysfunction. Thus, there are essential differences in Tm isoform function in physiologically regulating cardiac performance.

The fact that cardiac structure and function can be dramatically altered with different Tm isoforms is interesting. When we examined Tm isoform expression in murine skeletal muscle, we found that β-Tm mRNA is the predominant isoform in embryonic and neonatal skeletal muscles and in adult slow twitch muscle (i.e., soleus).[15] In addition to β-Tm expression, striated muscle γ-Tm is also expressed in significant levels in slow twitch musculature. The γ-Tm isoform exhibits a 93% amino acid identity with α-Tm. At the protein level, all three striated Tm isoforms are expressed in abundance in slow twitch muscle, with α-Tm being predominant in adult fast twitch musculature. Interestingly, there is no endogenous γ-Tm expression in murine hearts. When we generated transgenic mice that express the γ-Tm isoform in the heart (40-60% γ-Tm protein), physiological results show a hyperdynamic effect on systolic and diastolic function, coupled with a decreased sensitivity to calcium in cardiac fiber bundles;[16] there are no morphological or pathological alterations in cardiac structure in these transgenic hearts. Thus, the cumulative results from differential expression of Tm isoforms in the heart demonstrate that sarcomere performance is "context dependent"—that is, cardiac specific isoforms for the contractile proteins of the sarcomere play an essential role in the regulation of physiological performance of the heart. These isoforms cannot be substituted without affecting the function of the heart as exemplified by the transgenic models that express β- or γ-Tm. We hypothesize that cardiac TnT, cardiac TnI, cardiac TnC and cardiac actin, proteins which interact either directly or indirectly with Tm, possess specific domains that are required for normal cardiac function. However, during pathological or physiological hypertrophy, the heart maintains the capability to express embryonic contractile protein isoforms (i.e., β-Tm) to be able to meet new performance requirements.

Involvement of Tm in Familial Hypertrophic Cardiomyopathy

The significance of sarcomeric contractile proteins in human cardiac disease was first demonstrated by Drs. J. and C. Seidman's laboratories who found that missense mutations in myosin heavy chain correlate with familial hypertrophic cardiomyopathy (FHC).[17] FHC is inherited as a Mendelian autosomal dominant trait and is caused by mutations in any one of ten genes, each encoding protein components of the cardiac sarcomere. Mutations in cardiac α- and β-myosin heavy chain, myosin binding protein C, cardiac TnT, regulatory and essential myosin light chains, titin, α-Tm, α-actin and cardiac TnI are associated with hypertrophic cardiomyopathy. This genetic diversity is compounded by intragenic heterogeneity with about 200 mutations now identified; most of these are missense mutations with a single amino acid residue substitution.[18,19] The incidence of this disease is 1 out of 500 people; fortunately, many of these individuals exhibit very mild symptoms only with a late onset in life. The FHC phenotype in humans is characterized by left and/or right ventricular hypertrophy in the absence of an increased external load, left ventricular or asymmetrical septal hypertrophy, myocyte disarray, fibrosis, increased calcium sensitivity of myofilaments and cardiac arrhythmias that may lead to premature sudden death and/or heart failure.

The association of FHC with the α-Tm gene was initially reported by the Seidman laboratory.[20,21] In the United States population, the Tm associated FHC cases are relatively few, accounting for less than 5% of all FHC patients.[22] These patients exhibit relatively benign symptoms, with mild hypertrophy that is often not manifest until the later years in life. In Japan, the number of Tm-associated FHC cases is still relatively few in number, however, the pathological symptoms of these individuals is much more severe than in the United States population.[23,24] Interestingly, in Finland, Tm associated cases are the most prevalent of all of the contractile proteins involved in causing FHC with an incidence of 11%[25]; this is most likely due to a "founders" effect of the Tm mutations, especially the Asp175Asn amino acid substitution, in the population. The pathology of the disease is quite severe in the Finnish population with a majority of patients exhibiting a dramatic phenotype. The variability of the incidence and the phenotype associated with the Tm cases in different populations most likely reflects the ability of the environment and "modifier genes" in altering the onset and pathological symptoms of FHC.

Eleven mutations have been defined in α-Tm that lead to FHC. Six of the mutations occur in the troponin-T binding region (Ile172Thr; Asp175Asn; Glu180Gly; Glu180Val; Leu185Arg; Glu192Lys); three mutations lie near the amino end of the Tm molecule (Glu62Gln; Ala63Val; Lys70Thr); one mutation lies in the middle (Val95Ala) and one at the carboxyl end of the molecule (Met281Thr)[18,23,26-28] (Seidman—http://genetics.med.harvard.edu/~seidman/cg3/) (Fig. 1). Five of these mutations are the result of a point mutation that leads to a change in the charge of the original amino acid. Since Tm is a 100% alpha-helical coiled-coil protein that dimerizes with itself, the charge of each specific amino acid residue can play a critical role in both its own structure and how it interacts with its associated proteins of actin and troponin. For alpha-helical coiled-coil proteins, there is a highly conserved heptad motif or repeating seven amino acid unit (a-b-c-d-e-f-g); structural and molecular modeling studies suggest that the fifth and seventh position (e and g) amino acid side-chains that are typically of opposite charge can contribute to the stability of the coiled-coil through formation of salt bridges.[29] With mutations in Tm amino acid residues that alter their charge or size, the normal interactions with troponin and actin can be disrupted leading to altered sarcomeric structure and physiological performance. Supporting evidence for altered Tm-actin interactions was found by Kremneva et al[30] with results showing

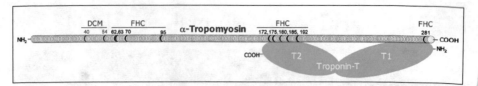

Figure 1. Mutations in α-tropomyosin that are linked to cardiovascular disease. Diagramed in the figure is α-TM and the regions where TnT binds Tm. The numbers above the Tm molecule represent the amino acid residues where mutations have been found that cause either DCM (dilated cardiomyopathy) or FHC (familial hypertrophic cardiomyopathy).

that actin-induced stabilization of the FHC Tm Glu180Gly is significantly less than for wild type α-Tm. Also, at least five of the FHC Tm mutations confer an increased calcium sensitivity of the myofilaments and decreased systolic and diastolic cardiac function which may be causative for the development of the FHC phenotype.[8,9,31-34]

Studies by Bottinelli et al[35] demonstrate that in human patients carrying the Asp175Asn mutation, aberrant Tm is expressed and that its expression most likely contributes to alteration in sarcomeric performance, rather than a null allele or decrease in total amount of Tm that produced. Further studies by this group also show that myofibers from these patients exhibit increased sensitivity to calcium when compared with control fibers.

In an attempt to understand the process whereby specific point mutations in contractile protei can lead to hypertrophic cardiomyopathy, investigators have developed animal models of FH Most of these studies have employed the usage of transgenic or knock-in mice. Our laborate was the first to develop in vivo transgenic model systems to examine the effects of FHC Tm mu tions. Initially, we investigated the substitution of asparagine for aspartic acid at amino acid 1 (Asp175Asn) and substitution of glycine for glutamic acid at amino acid 180 (Glu180Gly). A consistent feature with transgenic expression of Tm is that as an exogenous Tm construct expressed, there is a reciprocal decrease in the endogenous Tm protein expression so that total amount of Tm protein remains unchanged in the heart.[7,16] A similar scenario exists with transgenic mice expressing the FHC Tm Asp175Asn and FHC Tm Glu180Gly mutant prot where expression of the FHC mutant proteins in the various transgenic mouse hearts are associ with a concomitant decrease in expression of the endogenous wild type α-Tm protein. Histolo analyses show the FHC Tm Asp175Asn hearts exhibit a mild hypertrophic response, affecting ~5% of the myocardium; in contrast, the FHC Tm Glu180Gly hearts develop a severe conce hypertrophy with significant ventricular fibrosis and atrial enlargement that progressively incr from 2.5 months and results in death between 4.5 and 6 months (Fig. 2). In vivo physiolc analyses show severe impairment of both contractility and relaxation in hearts of both FHC n models. Both the rates of contraction and relaxation are significantly depressed in these mi addition, myofilaments that contain the mutant FHC protein demonstrate an increased activ of the thin filament through enhanced calcium sensitivity of steady-state force[8,9,36]; this incre myofiber calcium sensitivity is a common feature of many of the FHC associated Tm muta We also found a correlation between an increase in myofiber calcium sensitivity with a de in relaxation rate and a blunted response to β-adrenergic stimulation.[37] Isolated cardiomy from transgenic FHC Tm Glu180Gly mice exhibit an increase in calcium sensitivity of production.[36] Thus, it is apparent that the FHC associated Tm proteins alter cardiac perfor in the individual myocytes that collectively cause the aberrant function of the entire heart l to hypertrophic cardiomyopathy.

In vitro analyses have provided invaluable information on the functional properties mutant FHC proteins. Using wild type and mutant Tm proteins expressed in *E. coli*, studie that binding to actin is much weaker with the Glu180Gly protein than either the wild Asp175Asn proteins;[38,39] these results are supported by the structural analyses on Tm-acti ing conducted by Kremneva et al.[30] In vitro motility assays show that filaments contain

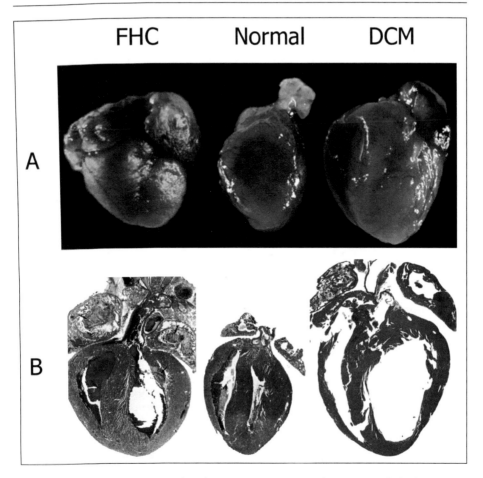

Figure 2. FHC α-Tm180, normal and DCM α-Tm54 mouse hearts. A) Whole hearts at 5 months of age. B) Histopathology of longitudinal sections of these hearts with hematoxylin and eosin staining. Note the increased size of the FHC and DCM hearts. The FHC hearts show increased size of the atria, thickened walls of the ventricle and thrombi/mineralization within the atria. The DCM hearts show increased size of the ventricular cavities, coupled with thin ventricular walls.

Glu180Gly and Asp175Asn Tm missense mutations exhibit an increased sensitivity to calcium, but similar filament velocities and similar numbers of motile filaments with respect to wild type TM.[38,40] The FHC mutant Tms result in an alteration in the interaction of Tm with skeletal troponin, leading to an increase in filament velocity in the presence of calcium that is much higher than found with wild type Tm;[38] when cardiac troponin is used, however, there is no difference in the velocity increase.[40] These results indicate that the cardiac and skeletal muscle troponin isoforms have differential effects in their interactions with Tm.

Investigations on the α-Tm FHC missense mutation Val95Ala has led to similar findings regarding the physiological effects of this mutation on sarcomeric performance. This mutation results in a mild hypertrophic phenotype, but with a poor prognosis.[28] Both myosin cycling and calcium binding are affected by this mutation, with myofilaments demonstrating an increased sensitivity to calcium and a decreased MgATPase rate.[28] There is also a slight decrease in sliding speed in the presence of calcium when assayed with the in vitro motility assay.

It is worth considering why the FHC mutations which are autosomal dominant mutations cause such a dramatic pathological phenotype in the heart with significantly altered cardiac performance, whereas there are no noticeable alterations in skeletal muscle morphology or function. These Tm mutations occur in α-Tm which is expressed almost exclusively in the heart, but is also a predominant isoform in skeletal muscle. We believe that the reason for this compensation in skeletal muscle is due to three reasons: (1) the fact that Tm can form homo- and heterodimers; (2) the extent of diversity in Tm expression in skeletal muscle; and (3) expression of skeletal versus cardiac isoform thin filament contractile proteins. With respect to dimer formation, in the heart virtually all Tm is a homodimer since α-Tm is expressed at 98% of all Tm. As such, an FHC mutation in one allele would be expected to affect 50% of all Tm that is expressed, leading to a significant production of mutant homo- and heterodimers. The situation is much different in skeletal muscle where α-, β- and γ-Tm are all expressed abundantly at the protein level.[15] An FHC mutation in α-Tm could still form homodimers; however, there is an increased probability for heterodimer formation with either β- or γ-TM. In fact, in most skeletal muscle, there is an increased tendency for Tm heterodimer formation.[41] Since our transgenic models of β- and γ-Tm demonstrate that sarcomere function is altered with their expression, the functional effects of the FHC (and DCM) Tm mutations may be blunted in this more heterogenous system. In a similar manner, the diversity of Tm expression would increase the number of sarcomeric units that are comprised of Tm homo- and heterodimers (i.e., α/α-Tm; β/β-Tm; γ/γ-Tm; α/β-Tm α/γ-Tm, β/γ-Tm). The ratio of these different Tm dimers would differ depending upon the specific muscle and its contractile speed. Thus, the effects of a specific Tm FHC mutation on muscle performance may be minimized. With respect to cardiac versus skeletal isoform contractile protein expression, the thin filament proteins in skeletal muscle are also much more divergent than expressed in the heart, with both fast and slow skeletal isoforms being common for many proteins (i.e., TnT, TnI, myosin heavy chain). This isoform diversity may also serve to negate the physiological effects of a FHC or DCM mutation. Thus, this lack of a myopathy in skeletal muscle for the FHC and DCM mutations appears to be one of dimer formation, increased diversity of Tm expression and the "context" of where the mutant Tm is expressed, namely skeletal muscle versus the heart.

Involvement of Tm in Dilated Cardiomyopathy

Dilated cardiomyopathy (DCM), a disease often associated with congestive heart failure, is characterized by depressed systolic function, cardiomegaly and ventricular dilation. DCM is a relatively common disease with an incidence of 36.5 out of 100,000 people.[42] The causes of DCM may be idiopathic, viral/immune, alcoholic/toxic, associated with other cardiovascular disease, or familial. Mutations associated with DCM have been associated with proteins of the sarcomere, cytoskeleton and the sarcolemma. With respect to muscle proteins, mutations that lead to DCM have been identified in β-myosin heavy chain, myosin binding protein C, actin, Tm, troponin T, I and C, titin, T-cap, desmin, vinculin and muscle LIM protein.[42]

To date, there are 3 known DCM mutations associated with Tm: Glu40Lys, Glu54Lys and Glu180Val[29,43] (Fig. 1). These amino acid changes are positioned in the inner regions of the Tm coiled-coil dimer where the electrostatic charge interactions between specific amino acids may alter the Tm dimerization and/or binding to actin. The 2-Å crystal structure of Tm indicates that Glu54 is linked to Lys49 and Glu40 is linked to Arg35[44] which are hypothesized to contribute to the stability of the coiled-coil through formation of salt bridges.[29] Disruption of a salt bridge by a DCM mutation could alter the Tm stability or Tm-actin interactions, thus compromising thin filament integrity or function. As such, a defect in force transmission has been attributed to be a cause of DCM.[29]

To investigate the functional consequences of the α-Tm mutations associated with DCM, we generated transgenic mice that express the DCM Tm Glu54Lys mutation.[12] This was the first mouse model in which a mutation in a sarcomeric thin filament protein, specifically Tm, leads to DCM. As with the transgenic FHC mice that were generated, the increase in transgenic Tm protein expression led to a reciprocal decrease in endogenous wild type α-Tm levels, with total myofilament Tm protein levels remaining unaltered. Histological and morphological analyses revealed development of DCM (Fig. 2) with progression to heart failure and frequently death by 6 months. There is often myocyte hypertrophy, coupled with diffuse hyalinization of the myocyte cytoplasm. The cytoplasmic alterations also include loss of striations and a homogenous, ground-glass appearance. Dilation is seen in both ventricles and there is an increased heart weight/body weight ratio. The increase in body weight may be attributable to peripheral edema which is often associated with heart failure.

To assess whether functional alterations in cardiac performance occur in DCM mice, we conducted physiological analyses including echocardiography, a work-performing heart model and calcium-force measurements. Doppler echocardiographic analyses of these DCM mice demonstrated increased left ventricular diastolic and systolic chamber diameter, in addition to a significant reduction in the left ventricular fractional shortening. The cardiac output was also significantly reduced, but the heart rate was not affected. The work-performing heart model was used to obtain an ex vivo assessment of cardiac performance.[12] Results show there is significant impairment of systolic and diastolic function, coupled with a concomitant increase in time to peak pressure and half-time to relaxation. End-diastolic and diastolic pressures were significantly increased, whereas the systolic pressure was significantly decreased, demonstrating their systolic and diastolic dysfunction.

To examine the correlation between physiological results from the whole heart to the sarcomere, we conducted experiments using skinned fiber bundles. These experiments were conducted to compare the relation between calcium and tension developed by myofilaments obtained from the left ventricles of control versus DCM α-Tm Gly54Lys hearts. Results show there is a significant reduction in the maximum tension that is developed by the mutant myofilaments and a decrease in the calcium sensitivity of the mutant myofilaments. These studies correlate with our finding of depressed cardiac function as determined by echocardiography and the isolated working hearts.

Tm mutations associated with DCM have also been studied with in vitro biochemical analyses. Using reconstituted thin filaments with biochemically exchanged Tm encoding the DCM mutations, it has been shown that these filaments decrease their calcium sensitivity.[45] Also, with the DCM α-Tm Glu40Lys mutation, there is a decrease in the maximum velocity of actin-Tm activated S-1 ATPase. Similar results were found with in vitro motility assays.[45] These results are in agreement with the in vivo results using myofilments from DCM transgenic mice. Additional structural studies show that the DCM mutations decrease Tm flexibility and decrease Tm-actin binding.[12,46]

Two points that are worth considering center around the encoding of the FHC and DCM mutations within Tm isoforms and the distribution of these mutations throughout the entire Tm molecule. Close inspection of the specific amino acid involvement of the FHC and DCM mutations shows that all of the known mutations (with the exception of the Met281Thr) would be incorporated into both striated muscle and cytoskeletal Tm isoforms. To date, virtually all of the mutations associated with FHC are associated with cardiac sarcomeric proteins. In fact, Tm is the only sarcomeric protein that could possibly incorporate these mutations in cytoskeletal proteins, which would occur through the alternative splicing process. The potential involvement of cytoskeletal proteins in the development of FHC has not been addressed by the research community to date. In a similar manner, the DCM mutations would also be expected to be incorporated into cytoskeletal isoforms to potentially cause this cardiac phenotype. Since other cytoskeletal proteins, such as desmin and vinculin, have been associated with the DCM phenotype, involvement of cytoskeletal Tm is quite possible. Thus, DCM mutations in Tm would affect both sarcomeric and cytoskeletal isoforms and potentially could cause this pathological phenotype through different structural and/or signaling pathways.

The fact that the FHC and DCM causing mutations occur over the entire Tm molecule suggests that these disease phenotypes can result from a variety of sarcomeric structural and/or physiological defects. For the FHC Tm mutations, there is a cluster of mutations in the amino acid 172-192 region which may disrupt Tm-TnT binding and calcium signaling. Mutations in the amino end of the protein for both DCM and FHC (residues 40-95) may alter Tm-actin interactions which may disrupt propagation of contractile force along the length of the sarcomere. The lone mutation at the carboxyl end of Tm (amino acid 281) may alter Tm-TnT interactions and Tm-Tm overlap, thereby affecting the interaction of these proteins, their function and the cooperativity of force transmission within sarcomeres. We should not consider it surprising that multiple mutations in Tm result in either FHC or DCM considering that there are multiple proteins in the sarcomere that cause these disease phenotypes when they undergo specific mutations. Thus, it appears that the heart remodels itself to respond to alterations in functional performance by either of two primary processes: hypertrophy or dilation.

Repairing TM Associated Cardiomyopathies

The ultimate goal of research involving transgenic animals is to design animal model systems that mimic the human pathogenic process. When successful, these model systems can be utilized to design therapeutic trials/experiments with the hope of rescuing the animal from the disease and provide future information for human trials. With respect to Tm associated cardiomyopathies, recent studies have led investigators to explore various methods and drugs to repair hearts that encode Tm-associated FHC mutations. In our work, we determined that myofilaments from FHC α-Tm Glu180Gly transgenic mouse hearts exhibit an increased sensitivity to calcium. This increased sensitivity to calcium of the myofilaments is a common feature of many FHC associated cardiomyopathies.

Recent studies demonstrate that modifying calcium cycling and direct changes in the myofilaments can alter the pathophysiology of FHC and DCM. In our FHC α-Tm Glu180Gly transgenic mouse model, we tested the hypothesis that an attenuation of the increased myofilament's calcium sensitivity would improve the pathology associated with this FHC mutation. We cross-bred the FHC mice with a mouse expressing a chimeric α-/β-Tm protein that induces a desensitization of the sarcomere to calcium.[10,47] The resulting double transgenic mice were rescued, showing a normal heart size and morphology, significantly improved cardiac function and normal myofilament calcium sensitivity. Also, preliminary studies demonstrate that hypertrophy and cardiac dysfunction are prevented in the FHC α-Tm Glu180Gly mice crossed with phospholamban knock-out mice.[48] In addition, cardiac hypertrophy and hemodynamic performance are improved by gene transfer of SERCA2a into FHC α-Tm Glu180Gly neonates.[49] With another model of the FHC α-Tm Glu180Gly mice, another research group has shown that cardiac relaxation abnormalities can be corrected when the FHC mice are genetically crossed to transgenic mice expressing parvalbumin, a calcium buffer.[50]

With DCM, there is often a decreased sensitivity to calcium exhibited by myofilaments. This was found in both animal models and in vitro motility assays where a mutation in Tm is associated with DCM.[12,45] Pimobendan, a phosphodiesterase II inhibitor and calcium sensitizer, increases the response of skinned fiber bundles to calcium by enhancing binding of calcium to troponin C.[51] This drug has been successfully used in a TnT mouse model of DCM where its usage prolonged survival, reduced end diastolic and systolic dimensions and significantly increased the ejection fraction.[52] This agent has not yet been used to rescue DCM mice that encode Tm mutations; but, it would be interesting to determine whether the pathological phenotype could be improved through a drug agent that is known to affect calcium binding to troponin C, that would then modify the functional effects of the Tm mutation on the thin filament. In conclusion, the rescue of mice with FHC and DCM through direct modification of sarcomeric proteins and/or therapeutics that alter their sarcomeric performance provides hope for the development of rational and successful therapies for the treatment of human cardiomyopathies and heart failure.

Conclusions

As cited above, Tm plays a major role in cardiovascular disease. Understanding how Tm mutations contribute to aberrant sarcomeric performance and resulting pathologies is essential for understanding the normal function of Tm, both as an integral component of the thin filament, but also as a potential component of a signaling complex to the cell when its function is abnormal and triggers a cascade of events culminating in myocyte hypertrophy or dilation. Potential molecular targets of gene therapy to correct Tm-associated cardiomyopathies will need to be identified. As we demonstrated in a microarray analysis of two FHC mouse models,[53] numerous genes are transcriptionally altered with an early onset of the heart disease phenotype. An area of future investigation will be to focus on identifying and modifying the expression of those genes, which are the signaling agents for the development of cardiac hypertrophy and heart failure.

References

1. Klein L, O'Connor CM, Gattis WA et al. Pharmacologic therapy for patients with chronic heart failure and reduced systolic function: review of trials and practical considerations. Am J Cardiol 2003; 91(9A):18F-40F.
2. Rothermel BA, Berenji K, Tannous P et al. Differential activation of stress-response signaling in load-induced cardiac hypertrophy and failure. Physiol Genomics 2005; 23(1):18-27.
3. Cummins P, Perry SV. Chemical and immunochemical characteristics of tropomyosins from striated and smooth muscle. Biochem J 1974; 141(1):43-49.
4. Izumo S, Nadal-Ginard B, Mahdavi V. Protooncogene induction and reprogramming of cardiac gene expression produced by pressure overload. Proc Natl Acad Sci USA 1988; 85(2):339-343.
5. Wang SM, Greaser ML, Schultz E et al. Studies on cardiac myofibrillogenesis with antibodies to titin, actin, tropomyosin and myosin. J Cell Biol 1988; 107(3):1075-1083.
6. Muthuchamy M, Pajak L, Howles P et al. Developmental analysis of tropomyosin gene expression in embryonic stem cells and mouse embryos. Mol Cell Biol 1993; 13(6):3311-3323.
7. Muthuchamy M, Grupp IL, Grupp G et al. Molecular and physiological effects of overexpressing striated muscle beta-tropomyosin in the adult murine heart. J Biol Chem 1995; 270(51):30593-30603.
8. Muthuchamy M, Pieples K, Rethinasamy P et al. Mouse model of a familial hypertrophic cardiomyopathy mutation in alpha-tropomyosin manifests cardiac dysfunction. Circ Res 1999; 85(1):47-56.
9. Prabhakar R, Boivin GP, Grupp IL et al. A familial hypertrophic cardiomyopathy alpha-tropomyosin mutation causes severe cardiac hypertrophy and death in mice. J Mol Cell Cardiol 2001; 33(10):1815-1828.
10. Jagatheesan G, Rajan S, Petrashevskaya N et al. Functional importance of the carboxyl-terminal region of striated muscle tropomyosin. J Biol Chem 2003; 278(25):23204-23211.
11. Jagatheesan G, Rajan S, Petrashevskaya N et al. Physiological significance of troponin T binding domains in striated muscle tropomyosin. Am J Physiol Heart Circ Physiol 2004; 287(4):H1484-1494.
12. Rajan S, Ahmed RP, Jagatheesan G et al. Dilated cardiomyopathy mutant tropomyosin mice develop cardiac dysfunction with significantly decreased fractional shortening and myofilament calcium sensitivity. Circ Res 2007; 101(2):205-214.
13. Palmiter KA, Kitada Y, Muthuchamy M et al. Exchange of beta- for alpha-tropomyosin in hearts of transgenic mice induces changes in thin filament response to Ca2+, strong cross-bridge binding and protein phosphorylation. J Biol Chem 1996; 271(20):11611-11614.
14. Wolska BM, Keller RS, Evans CC et al. Correlation between myofilament response to Ca2+ and altered dynamics of contraction and relaxation in transgenic cardiac cells that express beta-tropomyosin. Circ Res 1999; 84(7):745-751.
15. Pieples K, Wieczorek DF. Tropomyosin 3 increases striated muscle isoform diversity. Biochemistry 2000; 39(28):8291-8297.
16. Pieples K, Arteaga G, Solaro RJ et al. Tropomyosin 3 expression leads to hypercontractility and attenuates myofilament length-dependent Ca(2+) activation. Am J Physiol Heart Circ Physiol 2002; 283(4):H1344-1353.
17. Geisterfer-Lowrance AA, Kass S, Tanigawa G et al. A molecular basis for familial hypertrophic cardiomyopathy: a beta cardiac myosin heavy chain gene missense mutation. Cell 1990; 62(5):999-1006.
18. Maron BJ. Hypertrophic cardiomyopathy: a systematic review. JAMA 2002; 287(10):1308-1320.
19. Seidman JG, Seidman C. The genetic basis for cardiomyopathy: from mutation identification to mechanistic paradigms. Cell 2001; 104(4):557-567.
20. Watkins H, MacRae C, Thierfelder L et al. A disease locus for familial hypertrophic cardiomyopathy maps to chromosome 1q3. Nat Genet 1993; 3(4):333-337.
21. Thierfelder L, Watkins H, MacRae C et al. Alpha-tropomyosin and cardiac troponin T mutations cause familial hypertrophic cardiomyopathy: a disease of the sarcomere. Cell 1994; 77(5):701-712.
22. Tardiff JC. Sarcomeric proteins and familial hypertrophic cardiomyopathy: linking mutations in structural proteins to complex cardiovascular phenotypes. Heart Fail Rev 2005; 10(3):237-248.
23. Nakajima-Taniguchi C, Matsui H, Nagata S et al. Novel missense mutation in alpha-tropomyosin gene found in Japanese patients with hypertrophic cardiomyopathy. J Mol Cell Cardiol 1995; 27(9):2053-2058.

24. Yamauchi-Takihara K, Nakajima-Taniguchi C, Matsui H et al. Clinical implications of hypertrophic cardiomyopathy associated with mutations in the alpha-tropomyosin gene. Heart 1996; 76(1):63-65.
25. Jaaskelainen P, Soranta M, Miettinen R et al. The cardiac beta-myosin heavy chain gene is not the predominant gene for hypertrophic cardiomyopathy in the Finnish population. J Am Coll Cardiol 1998; 32(6):1709-1716.
26. Coviello DA, Maron BJ, Spirito P et al. Clinical features of hypertrophic cardiomyopathy caused by mutation of a "hot spot" in the alpha-tropomyosin gene. J Am Coll Cardiol 1997; 29(3):635-640.
27. Jongbloed RJ, Marcelis CL, Doevendans PA et al. Variable clinical manifestation of a novel missense mutation in the alpha-tropomyosin (TPM1) gene in familial hypertrophic cardiomyopathy. J Am Coll Cardiol 2003; 41(6):981-986.
28. Karibe A, Tobacman LS, Strand J et al. Hypertrophic cardiomyopathy caused by a novel alpha-tropomyosin mutation (V95A) is associated with mild cardiac phenotype, abnormal calcium binding to troponin, abnormal myosin cycling and poor prognosis. Circulation 2001; 103(1):65-71.
29. Olson TM, Kishimoto NY, Whitby FG et al. Mutations that alter the surface charge of alpha-tropomyosin are associated with dilated cardiomyopathy. J Mol Cell Cardiol 2001; 33(4):723-732.
30. Kremneva E, Boussouf S, Nikolaeva O et al. Effects of two familial hypertrophic cardiomyopathy mutations in alpha-tropomyosin, Asp175Asn and Glu180Gly, on the thermal unfolding of actin-bound tropomyosin. Biophys J 2004; 87(6):3922-3933.
31. Hernandez OM, Housmans PR, Potter JD. Invited Review: pathophysiology of cardiac muscle contraction and relaxation as a result of alterations in thin filament regulation. J Appl Physiol 2001; 90(3):1125-1136.
32. Michele DE, Albayya FP, Metzger JM. Direct, convergent hypersensitivity of calcium-activated force generation produced by hypertrophic cardiomyopathy mutant alpha-tropomyosins in adult cardiac myocytes. Nat Med 1999; 5(12):1413-1417.
33. Prabhakar R, Petrashevskaya N, Schwartz A et al. A mouse model of familial hypertrophic cardiomyopathy caused by a alpha-tropomyosin mutation. Mol Cell Biochem 2003; 251(1-2):33-42.
34. Westfall MV, Borton AR, Albayya FP et al. Myofilament calcium sensitivity and cardiac disease: insights from troponin I isoforms and mutants. Circ Res 2002; 91(6):525-531.
35. Bottinelli R, Coviello DA, Redwood CS et al. A mutant tropomyosin that causes hypertrophic cardiomyopathy is expressed in vivo and associated with an increased calcium sensitivity. Circ Res 1998; 82(1):106-115.
36. Michele DE, Gomez CA, Hong KE et al. Cardiac dysfunction in hypertrophic cardiomyopathy mutant tropomyosin mice is transgene-dependent, hypertrophy-independent and improved by beta-blockade. Circ Res 2002; 91(3):255-262.
37. Evans CC, Pena JR, Phillips RM et al. Altered hemodynamics in transgenic mice harboring mutant tropomyosin linked to hypertrophic cardiomyopathy. Am J Physiol Heart Circ Physiol 2000; 279(5): H2414-2423.
38. Bing W, Redwood CS, Purcell IF et al. Effects of two hypertrophic cardiomyopathy mutations in alpha-tropomyosin, Asp175Asn and Glu180Gly, on Ca2+ regulation of thin filament motility. Biochem Biophys Res Commun 1997; 236(3):760-764.
39. Golitsina N, An Y, Greenfield NJ et al. Effects of two familial hypertrophic cardiomyopathy-causing mutations on alpha-tropomyosin structure and function. Biochemistry 1997; 36(15):4637-4642.
40. Bing W, Knott A, Redwood C et al. Effect of hypertrophic cardiomyopathy mutations in human cardiac muscle alpha -tropomyosin (Asp175Asn and Glu180Gly) on the regulatory properties of human cardiac troponin determined by in vitro motility assay. J Mol Cell Cardiol 2000; 32(8):1489-1498.
41. Schachat FH, Bronson DD, McDonald OB. Heterogeneity of contractile proteins. A continuum of troponin-tropomyosin expression in mammalian skeletal muscle. J Biol Chem 1985; 260(2):1108-1113.
42. Chang AN, Potter JD. Sarcomeric protein mutations in dilated cardiomyopathy. Heart Fail Rev 2005; 10(3):225-235.
43. Regitz-Zagrosek V, Erdmann J, Wellnhofer E et al. Novel mutation in the alpha-tropomyosin gene and transition from hypertrophic to hypocontractile dilated cardiomyopathy. Circulation 2000; 102(17): E112-116.
44. Brown JH, Kim KH, Jun G et al. Deciphering the design of the tropomyosin molecule. Proc Natl Acad Sci USA 2001; 98(15):8496-8501.
45. Mirza M, Marston S, Willott R et al. Dilated cardiomyopathy mutations in three thin filament regulatory proteins result in a common functional phenotype. J Biol Chem 2005; 280(31):28498-28506.
46. Mirza M, Robinson P, Kremneva E et al. The effect of mutations in alpha-tropomyosin (E40K and E54K) that cause familial dilated cardiomyopathy on the regulatory mechanism of cardiac muscle thin filaments. J Biol Chem 2007; 282(18):13487-13497.

47. Jagatheesan G, Rajan S, Petrashevskaya N et al. Rescue of tropomyosin-induced familial hypertrophic cardiomyopathy mice by transgenesis. Am J Physiol Heart Circ Physiol 2007; 293(2):H949-958.
48. Pena J, Urboniene D, Goldspink P et al. Phospholamban knockout prevents the development of hypertrophy and cardiac dysfunction in a FHC alpha-tropomyosin (Glu180Gly) mouse model. Paper presented at: Keystone Symposia: Molecular Biology of Cardiac Diseases and Regeneration 2005; Steamboat Springs, CO.
49. Pena JR, Goldspink PH, Prabhakar R et al. Neonatal Gene Transfer of SERCA2a Improves the Response to ß-Adrenergic Stimulation in the -Tropomyosin (Glu180Gly) MouseModel of Familial Hypertrophic Cardiomyopathy. Paper presented at: Scientific Conference on Molecular Mechanisms of Growth, Death and Regeneration in the Myocardium: Basic Biology and Insights Into Ischemic Heart Disease and Heart Failure 2003; Snowbird Conference Center, Snowbird, Utah.
50. Coutu P, Bennett CN, Favre EG et al. Parvalbumin corrects slowed relaxation in adult cardiac myocytes expressing hypertrophic cardiomyopathy-linked alpha-tropomyosin mutations. Circ Res 2004; 94(9):1235-1241.
51. Fujino K, Sperelakis N, Solaro RJ. Sensitization of dog and guinea pig heart myofilaments to Ca2+ activation and the inotropic effect of pimobendan: comparison with milrinone. Circ Res 1988; 63(5):911-922.
52. Du CK, Morimoto S, Nishii K et al. Knock-in mouse model of dilated cardiomyopathy caused by troponin mutation. Circ Res 2007; 101(2):185-194.
53. Rajan S, Williams SS, Jagatheesan G et al. Microarray analysis of gene expression during early stages of mild and severe cardiac hypertrophy. Physiol Genomics 2006; 27(3):309-317.

CHAPTER 12

Tropomyosins in Skeletal Muscle Diseases

Anthony J. Kee and Edna C. Hardeman*

Abstract

A number of congenital muscle diseases and disorders are caused by mutations in genes that encode the proteins present in or associated with the thin filaments of the muscle sarcomere.[1] These genes include α-skeletal actin (*ACTA1*), β-tropomyosin (*TPM2*), α-tropomyosin slow (*TPM3*), nebulin (*NEB*), troponin I fast (*TNNI2*), troponin T slow (*TNNT1*), troponin T fast (*TNNT3*) and cofilin (*CFL2*). Mutations in two of the four tropomyosin (Tm) genes, *TPM2* and *TPM3*, result in at least three different skeletal muscle diseases and one disorder as distinguished by the presence of specific clinical features and/or structural abnormalities—nemaline myopathy (*TPM2* and *TPM3*),[2,3] distal arthrogryposis (*TPM2*),[4] cap disease (*TPM2*)[5] and congenital fiber type disproportion (*TPM3*).[6] These diseases have overlapping clinical features and pathologies and there are cases of family members who have the same mutation, but different diseases (Table 1). The relatively recent discovery of nonmuscle or cytoskeletal Tms in skeletal muscle[7] adds to this complexity since it is now possible that a disease-causing mutation could be in a striated isoform and a cytoskeletal isoform both present in muscle.

Tropomyosins in Skeletal Muscle

In order to try to understand the pathophysiology of the Tm-based congenital disorders, it is necessary to review the expression of Tms in skeletal muscle. Transcripts for four striated muscle-specific Tms have been reported in mammalian skeletal muscles and proteins corresponding to three of these Tm species have been detected.[8] Two of the Tm transcript species, α-Tm$_{fast}$ (encoded by the α*Tm* gene; *TPM1*) and α-Tm$_{slow}$ (encoded by the γ*Tm* gene; *TPM3*) are expressed in specific types of muscle fibers, fast and slow twitch, respectively. The other two Tm transcript species, β-Tm (encoded by the β*Tm* gene; *TPM2*) and Tm4 (encoded by the δ*Tm* gene; *TPM4*) are expressed in both fast and slow twitch fibers. α-Tm$_{fast}$, α-Tm$_{slow}$ and β-Tm proteins have been detected in skeletal muscles, but not Tm4 which may be due to its relative low abundance (less than 5% α-Tm$_{fast}$ or α-Tm$_{slow}$). Therefore, within each muscle fiber at least two striated Tms are expressed, either α-Tm$_{fast}$ and β-Tm or α-Tm$_{slow}$ and β-Tm so that heterodimers of these combinations as well as homodimers of α-Tm$_{fast}$ or α-Tm$_{slow}$ constitute the thin filaments. β-Tm appears to be preferentially expressed in oxidative fibers[9,10] and therefore would be more abundant in type 1 (slow, oxidative) and type 2A (fast, oxidative) than type 2B (fast, glycolytic) fibers. While α-Tm$_{fast}$ is the predominant isoform expressed in the human heart, α-Tm$_{slow}$ is also present raising the possibility that myopathy-causing mutations in it could also affect cardiac function.

Recently, we discovered that filaments comprised of the cytoskeletal Tm isoforms Tm5NM1 (encoded by the γ*Tm* gene) and Tm4 are present in skeletal muscle fibers.[7] These filaments are

*Corresponding Author: Edna C. Hardeman—Department of Anatomy School of Medical Sciences, Faculty of Medicine, University of New South Wales, Sydney NSW 2052, Australia. Email: e.hardeman@unsw.edu.au

Tropomyosin, edited by Peter Gunning. ©2008 Landes Bioscience and Springer Science+Business Media.

Table 1. Reported cases of topomyosin-based congenital myopathies

Mutation	Inheritance	Clinical Features	Potential Impact on Tm Function
Nemaline Myopathy (NM)			
TPM3[3] heterozygous Met9Arg (exon 1a)	Autosomal dominant	**Mild, childhood onset (<10 yrs)**: feet affected first, slow progression of muscle weakness, lower limb and proximal arm muscle involvement, progressive wasting of lower limbs, dysphagia. **Pathologies**: rods in type 1 fibers, fiber diameter variability, type 1 fiber predominance	Mutation in position a of heptapeptide repeat. Reduced activation of actomyosin ATPase activity in the presence of Ca²⁺[68]; increased relaxation kinetics[54]; altered Tm dimer preference[50]
TPM3[43] homozygous Gln31Stop (exon 1a)	Autosomal recessive	**Severe infantile**: died at 21 months of age, extremely delayed and impaired motor development, extremely hypotonic, immobile, no head control. **Pathologies**: rods in type 1 fibers, type 1 fiber atrophy/hypotrophy, mild type 2 fiber predominance, fibers with central nuclei	**Predicted**: no TPM3 product is made or truncated protein is made and prevents dimer formation or disrupts α-helical coiled-coil
TPM3[44] compound heterozygous Stop285Ser (exon 9b) c.855-1G>A (intron 9a)	Autosomal sporadic	**Father (Stop285Ser)**. No clinical features or pathologies. **Son (compound heterozygote). Intermediate**. Hypotonic at birth, walked at 17 months, wheel-chair bound at 6 years. **Pathologies**: rods in type 1 fibers, type 1 fiber predominance, occasional fibers with central nuclei, fibrosis	Stop285Ser. **Predicted**: extensive disruption to α-helical coiled-coil prevents dimerization. c.855-1G>A. **Predicted**: alters interaction with actin. Reduces βTm protein that may alter Tm dimer preference as with TPM3(Met9Arg)?
TPM3[45,46] heterozygous Arg168His (exon 5) Same mutation causes CFTD (see next page)	[45]Autosomal de novo	**Mild, childhood onset. Atypical**. Mild hypotonia at birth, delayed motor milestones, mild proximal weakness in upper limbs in childhood; distal limb and axial muscle involvement, mild atrophy of shoulder girdle muscles, waddling gait, high-arched palate and myopathic facies, progressive kyphoscoliosis. **Pathologies**: rods in type 1 fibers, type 1 fiber atrophy/hypotrophy and predominance, fiber diameter variability	**Predicted**: change in position f of heptapeptide repeat alters charge in α-helical coiled-coil and thermodynamics of helix formation

continued on next page

Table 1. Continued

Mutation	Inheritance	Clinical Features	Potential Impact on Tm Function
[46]Autosomal dominant		**Mild, childhood onset.** Normal to delayed motor milestones, poor physical performance; hypotonia throughout life, slender build, impaired respiratory function, distal and proximal limb, axial and spinal muscle involvement, high-arched palate, myopathic facies, occasional scoliosis. **Pathologies:** rods in type 1 fibers, type 1 fiber atrophy/hypotrophy and predominance, fiber diameter variability, occasional fibers with central nuclei, fat infiltration and/or fibrosis	**Predicted:** mutation in the first aa of the fifth heptapeptide repeat may alter troponin T binding and/or Ca^{2+} activation
$TPM2^2$ heterozygous Gln147Pro (exon 4)	Autosomal De novo	**Mild, childhood onset. Atypical.** Difficulty walking at 12 years; asymmetrical limb muscle involvement, mild facial and neck muscle weakness in adulthood; wheelchair-bound at 48 years; died from respiratory causes at 51 years. **Pathologies:** rods in small fibers (fiber type not established), type 1 fiber atrophy/hypotrophy and predominance	**Predicted:** neutral, polar to neutral, hydrophobic residue change at position g of heptapeptide repeat disrupts α-helical coiled-coil and interaction with actin
$TPM2^2$ heterozygous Glu117Lys (exon 3)	Autosomal dominant	**Atypical. Mother.** never able to run, asymmetric limb involvement, weak neck flexors, myopathic facies, high-arched palate. **Pathologies:** no biopsy available; suspected case of NM. **Son:** Severe hypotonia at birth; feeding difficulties, delayed motor milestones, achieved ambulation, mild facial weakness, ankle contractures. **Pathologies:** type 1 fiber predominance, fiber diameter variability, no definite nemaline rods, broad Z-lines; suspected case of NM. CFTD?	**Predicted:** acidic to basic residue change at position e of heptapeptide repeat disrupts α-helical coiled-coil and interaction with actin

Nemaline Myopathy and/or Congenital Fiber Type Disproportion (CFTD)

Mutation	Inheritance	Clinical Features	Potential Impact on Tm Function
$TPM3^6$ heterozygous Arg168His (exon 5)	Autosomal dominant	**Mild, childhood onset (Family 6, Patient 10).** Hypotonia at birth, walking at 18 months; can run, mild proximal limb girdle, neck and abdomen muscle involvement, mild scoliosis. Other family member has CFTD (see below). **Pathologies:** nemaline rods in small, type 1 fibers (1.8% of fibers), type 1 fiber atrophy/hypotrophy and predominance, type 2 fiber hypertrophy, occasional fibers with central nuclei	**Predicted:** conservative aa change in position f of heptapeptide repeat alters actin interaction

continued on next page

Table 1. *Continued*

Mutation	Inheritance	Clinical Features	Potential Impact on Tm Function
Nemaline Myopathy and/or Cap Myopathy			
$TPM2^{61}$ heterozygous Glu41Lys (exon 2)	Autosomal De novo	**Mother.** Neonatal respiratory insufficiency, delayed motor milestones; slow progressive weakness; impaired respiratory function, moderate weakness in proximal, neck, facial and foot muscles progressing to moderate muscle weakness in proximal and distal muscles, long narrow face, high arched palate, difficulty swallowing, lumbar hyperlordosis. **Pathologies:** fiber diameter variability, but no rods or other inclusions at 32 years; type 1 fiber predominance, fiber diameter variation, cap-like structures in type 1 fibers, nemaline rods, ragged red fibers at 57 years. **Daughter.** Neonatal hypotonia, feeding difficulties; adult clinical features, muscle involvement and progression similar to mother. **Pathologies:** type 1 fiber atrophy/hypotrophy and predominance, fiber diameter variation, cap-like structures in type 1 fibers, no inclusions, no rods at 26 years	None suggested
$TPM2^5$ heterozygous Glu139del (exon 4)	Autosomal De novo	Mild hypotonia at birth, delayed motor milestones; never able to run, nonprogressive, general muscle weakness, small muscle bulk in limbs, impaired respiratory function, moderate muscle weakness in distal muscles of upper limbs, proximal and distal muscles of lower limbs, myopathic facies, high-arched palate. **Pathologies:** type 1 fiber atrophy/hypotrophy and predominance, type 2 fiber hypertrophy, cap-like structures predominantly in type 1 fibers	**Predicted:** deletion in position *f* of the heptapeptide repeat mildly disrupts coiled-coil and dimer formation; reduced interaction with actin through removal of surface acidic residue
Distal Arthrogryposis (DA1)			
$TPM2^4$ heterozygous Arg91Gly (exon 3)	Autosomal dominant	Peripheral contractures, no neurological abnormalities. **Pathologies:** no pathological features, notably no nemaline rods	**Predicted:** nonconservative amino acid substitution of invariant residue causes a local reduction in surface charge, may alter local conformation of the α-helical coiled-coil increasing flexibility and affecting interaction with actin

continued on next page

Table 1. *Continued*

Mutation	Inheritance	Clinical Features	Potential Impact on Tm Function
Congenital Fiber Type Disproportion			
TPM3^6 heterozygous Arg245Gly (exon 8)	Autosomal dominant de novo	Delayed milestones, impaired respiratory function; moderate proximal > distal muscle, scapular and neck muscle weakness, mild ptosis, lumbar lordosis. **Pathologies:** type 1 fiber atrophy/hypotrophy and predominance, type 2 fiber hypertrophy = typical CFTD	**Predicted:** mutation in position *f* of heptapeptide repeat may influence interaction with actin
TPM3^6 heterozygous Arg168Cys (exon 5)	Autosomal dominant de novo	Poor head control; impaired respiratory function, cannot run, moderate proximal = distal muscle and neck muscle weakness, mild ptosis, severe kyphoscoliosis. **Pathologies:** typical CFTD	**Predicted:** mutation in position *f* of heptapeptide repeat alters interactions with actin filament
TPM3^6 heterozygous Lys169Glu (exon 5)	Autosomal dominant de novo	Hypotonia at birth; moderate proximal > distal muscle, facial and neck muscle weakness, mild ptosis, lumbar lordosis. **Pathologies:** typical CFTD	**Predicted:** mutation in position *g* of heptapeptide repeat alters interactions with actin filament
TPM3^6 heterozygous Arg168Gly (exon 5)	Autosomal dominant de novo (?)	Slow running, impaired respiratory function, mild proximal, facial and neck flexor muscle weakness, mild ptosis, lumbar lordosis. **Pathologies:** typical CFTD	**Predicted:** mutation in position *f* of heptapeptide repeat alters interactions with actin filament
TPM3^6 Heterozygous Arg168His (exon 5)	Autosomal dominant	Hypotonia at birth, delayed motor milestones; range of abilities from slow walk to run, impaired respiratory function, moderate distal > proximal muscle weakness, scoliosis to lumbar lordosis. **Pathologies:** typical CFTD + fibers with internal nuclei, infrequent fibers with nemaline rods in one family member	**Predicted:** mutation in position *f* of heptapeptide repeat alters interactions with actin filament
TPM3^6 heterozygous Leu100Met (exon 3)	Autosomal dominant	Hypotonia, delayed milestones to reduced activity from birth to 2 years; range of abilities from slow walk to run, difficulty climbing stairs to playing sport, impaired respiratory function, moderate proximal ≥ distal muscle and scapular muscle weakness, mild ptosis, mild to no scoliosis. **Pathologies:** typical CFTD + fibers with internal nuclei	**Predicted:** mutation in position *a* of heptapeptide repeat alters dimer preference

located adjacent to the Z-line and run perpendicular to the striated Tm-decorated thin filaments. In addition, Tm4-defined filaments orientated parallel with the muscle fiber are present in myofibers undergoing repair/remodeling.[11] These cytoskeletal Tm isoforms were detected with isoform-specific antibodies which raises the possibility that more isoforms in myofibers will be identified once the means to distinguish them is available. The striated and cytoskeletal Tms in myofibers sort to different filaments and perturbation of the cytoskeletal Tm filaments can cause dystrophic features in muscles.[7] Taken together it is possible that mutations in exons shared by muscle and cytoskeletal isoforms will disrupt different functions within the myofiber which may contribute different clinical features.

Nemaline Myopathy (NM)

The first mutation identified in a Tm gene that causes a congenital myopathy/disorder was in a missense mutation Met9Arg in the *TPM3* gene that causes nemaline myopathy (NM).[3] NM is the best characterized of the congenital myopathies and is readily diagnosed, having a distinct pathognomonic feature—the nemaline rod. NM is a hereditary disease of skeletal muscle, presenting at birth or in early childhood as hypotonia and muscle weakness. It is the most common of the congenital myopathies, with an incidence estimated to be 1 in 50,000 live births. A defining feature of this condition is the presence of electron dense rod-shaped structures in the cytoplasm and/or nuclei of myofibers termed nemaline rods. Rods appear to be extensions of the Z-line, the structure in the contractile unit or sarcomere of striated muscle cells that anchors the actin thin filaments. NM was first described by Conen et al[12] and Shy et al[13] in 1963 and its name reflects the thread-like appearance of the rod structures (*nema* being Classical Greek for thread). So far six genes with NM-causing mutations in humans have been identified: α-skeletal actin (*ACTA1*), β-tropomyosin (*TPM2* or β-*Tm*), α-tropomyosin$_{slow}$ (*TPM3* or γ-*Tm*), nebulin (*NEB*), troponin T slow (*TNNT1*) and very recently cofilin-2 (*CFL2*).

Even though mutations in *TPM3* have been identified in a relatively small number of patients with NM (1-2% of all NM), the first disease-causing mutation *TPM3*(Met9Arg) has been studied extensively both biochemically and physiologically. The only mouse model for a congenital myopathy is modeled on this mutation and it has proven to be a particularly valuable tool in understanding the pathophysiology of the disease. Data on this mouse will be discussed in some detail. For information on other forms of the disease the reader is referred to more comprehensive reviews.[14-16]

Clinical Presentation of NM

There is a wide range of clinical presentations of this disease spanning from neonatal-lethal to late onset slowly progressive forms. Physical features common in NM are hypotonia and muscle weakness, a lean body, bulbar weakness reflected in a high, arched palate, proximal muscles more affected than distal muscles and joint deformities or contractures. To aid in defining phenotype-genotype relationships NM has been classified by the ENMC International Consortium on Nemaline Myopathy into six clinical subtypes based on age of onset and severity of weakness: (1) severe congenital, (2) typical, (3) intermediate, (4) mild form of childhood- or juvenile onset, (5) adult onset and (6) other.[15,17,18] Severe NM presents at birth with profound muscle weakness particularly of the respiratory muscles which results in respiratory insufficiency. These patients usually require ventilatory support and death often occurs in the first months of life. The most common form of NM, the typical form, presents as peripheral and respiratory muscle weakness and hypotonia at birth or in early infancy. In these patients, the weakness is static or slowly progressive and the patients can usually lead an active life. In the mild form, patients have similar clinical and pathological features to the typical cases, but with childhood onset of symptoms. The adult-onset condition is a clinically heterogeneous group of patients with onset in the third to sixth decade of life. There is usually no family history or early symptoms in these cases. The pattern of inheritance varies depending on the nature of the mutation and includes autosomal recessive, autosomal dominant and sporadic de novo mutations.[15] There is a poor relationship between the gene affected or the position of the mutation in the protein and the severity of the disease.[19-21] The most common feature is likely to be failure of the actin thin filament in skeletal muscle.

Muscle Pathologies in NM

The defining feature of NM is the presence of nemaline rods within muscle fibers. In most cases they are present in the cytoplasm, but in rare cases can be found in the myofiber nuclei.[23-26] The proportion of fibers containing rods can vary widely and does not correlate with the degree of muscle weakness.[15,26,27] Changes in fiber type proportion and size is a common feature of the disease. In many cases, there is a predominance of slow oxidative (type 1) fibers and often the rod-containing fibers are atrophic.[28] Rods can be present in all fiber types, but often they are preferentially in either type 1 or type 2 fibers.

When examined by electron microscopy, the rods have a characteristic defining structure. The rods are electron dense and have a similar lattice structure to the Z-lines.[29] They are thought to largely contain Z-line proteins, mainly α-actinin, but other Z-line associated proteins have been detected including α-actin,[30,31] myotilin,[32] desmin and vinculin.[33] This has led to the hypothesis that rods form through an unchecked expansion of the Z-line.[29] The mechanism of rod formation is unknown, but the fact that all of the genes in which NM-causing mutations have been identified encode proteins of or associated with the thin filament system suggests it is a consequence of altered thin filament function. However, rod-like structures are not restricted to NM. Rod-like bodies have been observed during myofiber regeneration,[34] in tenotomized muscle,[35] in muscles from patients with HIV myopathy[37] and mitochondrial myopathy,[36] in normal extra-ocular muscle, in muscle under constant contractile stress[38] and during prolonged (7 months) immobilization.[39] Thus, rod formation rather than being a specific consequence of mutations in thin filament genes is probably a common response to certain types of mechanical and pathological stresses. This is emphasized in a recent study on the *TPM3*(Met9Arg) mouse model where immobilization of a hindlimb muscle in a shortened position resulted in an increase in the number of rods per myofiber.[40]

Recent gene profiling studies on nemaline patients and the *TPM3*(Met9Arg) transgenic mouse model have shown that chronic repair is a previously unrecognized feature of NM. Sanoudou and colleagues examined the expression patterns of >21,000 genes (Affymetric oligonucleotide arrays) in muscles from a heterogeneous group (i.e., various mutations) of patients with NM.[41] They found increased expression of genes associated with proliferating myoblasts and satellite cells (*NCAM1* and *CDK4*). This was confirmed immunohistochemically using a satellite cell-specific marker, Pax7, where there was a 10-fold increase in satellite cell abundance in the nemaline patient samples compared to normal healthy muscle. This is consistent with data from the mouse model where markers of satellite cell number, activated satellite cells and immature fibers (M-cadherin, MyoD, desmin, Pax7 and Myf6) were elevated as determined by Western-blot and immunohistochemical analyses.[42] This study showed direct evidence of focal muscle repair in a number of muscles from the nemaline mouse as identified by segmental regeneration with centrally-located myofiber nuclei. In keeping with ongoing repair, there was an increase in the number of fibers with centralized nuclei compared to wild-type mice. The number of central nucleated fibers was rather low (7-12%) compared to diseases characterized by overt regeneration (e.g., muscular dystrophies), which may explain why this feature had not been reported previously for NM. In addition, muscles from nemaline patients and from the mouse model have elevated levels of the tropomyosin isoform Tm4 which is indicative of muscle repair.[11] Taken together, these studies demonstrate that there is a process of ongoing repair in nemaline muscle. This repair is distinct from the classical form of muscle regeneration that occurs in the muscular dystrophies where there is myonecrosis and extensive numbers of regenerating myofibers with centralized nuclei. The focal repair in NM may be specific to diseases of the sarcomeric thin filament and are distinct from sarcolemmal repair in muscular dystrophy.

Genetics of NM

The protein composition of rods and their thin filament association suggest that candidate genes for NM are likely to be involved in the thin filament network. Indeed, all of the disease-associated mutations to date occur in genes that encode proteins that form part of or are closely associated with the sarcomeric thin filaments. Mutations in a particular gene cannot predict the form of inheritance or the severity of the disease and the wide range of clinical presentation has made phenotype-genotype correlations difficult (Table 1). It has been estimated that mutations in the *NEB* (nebulin) gene are responsible for 50% of NM cases, with *ACTA1* the next most commonly mutated gene (25% of cases) and the other identified genes accounting for 5-10% of cases.[17,21] It is expected that mutations in other thin filament associated genes will be identified with time.

TPM3 (α-Tropomyosin Slow) and NM

The first NM-causing mutation described was a missense mutation (Met9Arg) in the *TPM3* gene in a single Australian family resulting in a late onset form of NM.[3] Since there have been only four other case reports of NM caused by *TPM3* mutations (Table 1).[43-46] One homozygous nonsense mutation (Gln31Stop) was identified in a sporadic severe infantile case[43] and two *TPM3* mutations (Stop285Ser and a mutation leading to an inappropriate splice between exons 9a and 9d) were found in a compound heterozygous patient with intermediate NM.[45] Recently Penisson-Besnier et al[46] identified an autosomal dominant mutation (Arg167His) in a four generation family with a mild classical form of the disease. This mutation had been reported previously in a sporadic case presenting with atypical NM.[44] The clinical phenotype of *TPM3*-based NM patients is quite variable, although of the reported cases the autosomal recessive mutations appear to be more severe than the dominant mutations. The homozygous patient (Gln31Stop mutation) had extremely delayed motor development and died at 21 months of age[43] while the compound heterozygous patient was hypotonic at birth, was able to walk at 17 months, but became wheelchair bound at 6 years of age.[44] In contrast, the patients with the dominant mutations showed childhood onset and slow disease progression.[3,46] It is important to note that the Arg168His mutation is present in all cytoskeletal isoforms and the Stop285Ser mutation is present in six cytoskeletal Tm isoforms.[47] A number of these cytoskeletal Tms are expressed in all nonmuscle cells as well as skeletal muscle. This raises the question of whether any of the observed features in these patients are due to dysfunction of these cytoskeletal Tms in nonmuscle as well as muscle tissues.

The TPM3(Met9Arg) Mouse Model of NM

We generated a transgenic mouse model of NM by expressing the dominant negative TPM3(Met9Arg) mutant in skeletal muscle.[48] This mutation results in a mild childhood-onset form of the disease (Table 1).[3] This mouse model has all features of the human disease including lean body mass, the presence of nemaline rods in skeletal muscle, an increase in slow/oxidative fibers and fast fiber hypertrophy. The hypertrophy of glycolytic fast fibers was apparent at 2 months of age, but this hypertrophy declined as the mice aged coincident with muscle weakness beyond 5-6 months of age. This mimics the late-onset of the disease of patients with this mutation and suggests that the hypertrophy of fast fibers is a compensatory mechanism to reduce muscle dysfunction.[49] There was also an increase in the number of slow/oxidative fibers at 1 month of age and this was maintained through adulthood, indicating disruption of the early postnatal maturation of the different fiber types. As has been observed in muscles of a human nemaline patient,[26] the number of rod-containing fibers in different muscles varied significantly in the mouse and was not dependent on the level of mutant protein expression. In some muscles (e.g., soleus and gastrocnemius) there was little evidence of disruption to the thin filaments suggesting that the presence of the Met9Arg mutation per se does not alter the normal formation of the sarcomeric thin filament. The mutant protein appeared to incorporate correctly into the sarcomere of the myofibers in the mouse[48,50] which agrees with data obtained when ectopic TPM3(Met9Arg) protein was expressed in cultured cardiomyocytes.[51]

Mechanisms of Muscle Weakness in NM—Information from TPM3(Met9Arg)

There is much debate about the precise involvement of nemaline rods and other nemaline pathologies in the development of muscle weakness. For example, in a number of studies the number of rod-containing fibers has been shown to correlate poorly with age of presentation and severity of disease.[26,52,53] The results in the nemaline mice concur with this as in early life (<5-6 months of age) these mice are not grossly weak and yet there are many rod-affected fibers in the diaphragm and many forearm and hindlimb muscles.[48] However, in humans the more severe forms of NM tend to be associated with more extensive sarcomeric disruption[26] and the greater number of rods in the diaphragm is associated with ventilatory insufficiency.[26,27] It seems reasonable that a threshold level of rods per fiber or rod density has to be exceeded before sarcomere disruption becomes extensive enough to result in clinical signs of muscle weakness. Below this threshold, compensatory mechanisms such as fast fiber hypertrophy and slow fiber predominance may be able to effectively combat the functional defects of the mutated protein.

Metzger and coworkers expressed the TPM3(Met9Arg) protein in primary cardiomyocytes to investigate the mechanisms for muscle weakness in NM.[51,54] Expression of the TPM3(Met9Arg) protein leads to a decrease in sensitivity of the thin filament to Ca^{2+} and more rapid muscle relaxation following a muscle stimulus. These alterations predict a reduction in muscle strength. However, extrapolation from studies in which a mutant Tm is expressed in the inappropriate cell type to disease features is problematic. The same Tm mutation expressed in both heart and skeletal muscle may only elicit a phenotype in one of these tissues. In addition, expression of a mutant protein in skeletal muscles does not elicit the same pathologies or degree of muscle weakness in all muscles. These observations tell us that the effect of the mutant protein on muscle function is context dependent (see Chapter 11).

De Haan and colleagues measured the contractile properties of muscle from the TPM3(Met9Arg) mouse model to try and understand the mechanism for muscle weakness.[56] Analysis of muscle contractile properties in these mice failed to detect muscle weakness when measured at optimum muscle length. However, isometric force was found to be decreased at lengths below optimum which may indicate compromised thin filament function. The relatively mild alterations to contractile function observed in this study speaks to the relatively benign nature of the Met9Arg mutation and the fact that measurements were made on a muscle (gastrocnemius) that has few rods (< 5% of fibers) and from mice of an age when they are not overtly weak.[48]

A study in the TPM3(Met9Arg) mouse suggests that the mutant Tm elicits an alteration to tropomyosin dimer formation which could result in muscle weakness.[50] In normal muscle, the αβ Tm heterodimers are the predominant dimer species. A preferential decrease in expression of β-Tm occurs in muscles of the TPM3(Met9Arg) mouse and in patients with this mutation. This was evident even in the early stages of postnatal development in the mouse model (1-2 weeks after birth). A decrease in β-Tm was also observed in the compound heterozygous patient with intermediate NM (discussed above),[53] indicating that this may be a common feature of TPM3-associated NM and a useful diagnostic marker for this form of the disease. In vitro studies using recombinant proteins or sarcomeric extracts from the mouse model showed that the presence of the mutated α-Tm$_{slow}$ protein promotes the formation of αα dimers rather than the normal αβ dimer pair.[50] As the ββ Tm dimer species has poor actin binding properties, it is proposed that the Met9Arg mutation promotes the preferential incorporation of the αα dimer into the thin filament (see Chapter 6). The change in composition of the actin filament rather than the presence of the mutated protein per se may be the primary cause of the contractile dysfunction and muscle weakness in this form of NM.

Potential Treatments for NM

Since so many different mutations in different genes result in NM, therapies for NM have focused on treatments that are not mutation specific, but rather that can alleviate general pathologies and clinical conditions such as muscle weakness.

Exercise

There is some debate about the use of exercise as a treatment modality for muscle weakness in the myopathies. This has largely stemmed from the fact that the dystrophies are characterized by increased susceptibility to exercise-induced damage. However, there is good anecdotal evidence that patients with NM who are able to exercise can increase their muscle strength and endurance capabilities. We examined in detail the exercise capabilities of the *TPM3*(Met9Arg) mice.[56] Nemaline mice were put through an intensive 4 week treadmill training program. The mice successfully completed the 4 week treadmill exercise program with no evidence of increased pathology.

Patients with NM experience prolonged muscle weakness following periods of immobility.[29,53] Having shown that the *TPM3*(Met9Arg) mutation can engage in exercise without adverse effects, we examined endurance exercise as a means of improving recovery following muscle inactivity in the transgenic mouse model.[40] Physical inactivity, mimicked using a hind-limb immobilization protocol, resulted in fiber atrophy and severe muscle weakness. Following immobilization, the NM remained weak for prolonged periods with just cage rest, but with 4 weeks of exercise training were able to completely regain whole body strength. These exercise studies on the mice clearly suggest that exercise may be a useful treatment option for muscle weakness in nemaline patients who are able to perform some form of exercise.

Enhancing Hypertrophy

Hypertrophy-promoting therapies, such as overexpression of insulin-like growth factor-I (IGF-I) and application of myostatin antagonists (antibodies), have been shown to be beneficial in mouse models of muscular dystrophy presumably by increasing muscle strength.[57,58] Compensatory hypertrophy is a common feature of NM and may contribute to the mild phenotype of the *TPM3*(Met9Arg) mouse and patients with this mutation. Thus, the use of these hypertrophy promoting therapies may be particularly effective in treating muscle weakness in NM. The *TPM3*(Met9Arg) mouse and other models with greater disease severity will be extremely useful in evaluating the effectiveness of these molecules to alleviate muscle dysfunction in NM.

Dietary L-Tyrosine

In one reported case, an 11-year-old boy with NM was treated with L-tyrosine and this led to an improvement in muscle strength, appetite and weight gain.[59] Of particular note was that there was a substantial decline in pharyngeal secretions and drooling within 48 hours of commencement of treatment. This prompted a study involving a small number of patients that suggests that oral administration of L-tyrosine may lead to clinical improvement in patients with NM.[60] L-Tyrosine is a non-essential amino acid that is the precursor for the synthesis of the catecholamines dopamine, norepinephrine and epinephrine. These compounds are important neurotransmitters involved in the regulation of motor co-ordination, behaviour, learning, memory, sleep—wake cycle regulation and endocrine functions. In healthy subjects, L-tyrosine administration appears to improve cognition and performance and perhaps the stamina and strength in weight lifters and in sprint athletes. A reduction in patient drooling may reflect increased central dopaminergic activity.

TPM2 (β-Tropomyosin), NM and Cap Myopathy

Skeletal muscle diseases associated with mutations in *TPM2* are rare with only 4 cases reported to date (Table 1).[2,5,61] Donner et al[2] reported two cases that were diagnosed at presentation with NM; however, rods were not confirmed in the second case. The first case was a patient with a heterozygous mutation (Gln147Pro) who had a mild, atypical form of NM with diagnostic rods, but died at age 51 from respiratory causes. The second case was of a mother and son with a heterozygous mutation (Glu117Lys). The son was originally diagnosed with NM because he had typical physical features, type 1 fiber predominance, type 1 fiber hypotrophy and broad Z-lines thought to be rods. However, upon closer inspection rods were not confirmed. Therefore, in the absence of a diagnostic pathology, the disease features appear to be more reminiscent of congenital fiber type disproportion (CFTD) (see below). Both the Gln147Pro and Glu117Lys mutations are in exons shared with the cytoskeletal Tm encoded by *TPM2*, Tm1. However, it is not clear that Tm1 is expressed in skeletal muscle fibers and therefore it is unlikely that the clinical features in the patients are due to dysfunction of the cytoskeletal Tm filaments.

Tajsharghi et al[61] reported a mother (66 years old) and daughter (35 years old) with a missense mutation (Glu41Lys) in *TPM2* who both had proximal and distal muscle weakness and the typical facial features of NM, hypotonia and type 1 fiber predominance. However, only the mother had nemaline rods as confirmed by Gomori-Trichrome and EM analysis. Interestingly, the mother had an earlier biopsy at 32 years of age with no evidence of nemaline or other lesions. However, only limited histology was carried out and only one muscle was examined. Since nemaline rod abundance can vary significantly between muscles of an individual patient,[27] an observation confirmed in the *TPM3*(Met9Arg) mouse model,[48] it is possible that the rods were present in other muscles of the mother at the earlier age and are present in other muscles of the daughter. Interestingly, both mother and daughter had cap-like structures in their muscle (see 'cap myopathies' below). Therefore, this family provides an example of a single mutation in a *TPM* gene that elicits distinctive pathologies characteristic of different myopathies. Cap myopathy with mild nemaline rod involvement was also reported in a patient with a deletion of a single glutamate residue (p.Glu39del) in *TPM2*, the first reported identification of mutation that causes cap myopathy.[5]

Cap myopathy is a congenital myopathy where the diagnostic feature is a "cap" structure at the periphery of myofibers. Caps manifest as disorganized myofibrils comprised primarily of thin filaments with enlarged Z-lines and accumulations of mitochondria and glycogen, and that lack thick filaments and the associated ATPase activity. In caps, thin filament and thin filament-associated material consists of desmin, actin, SERCA2, tropomyosin, troponin, nebulin and myotilin. Each of these features can be found in NM myofibers with the distinction that they are not organized in distinctive 'caps'. Therefore, cap myopathy has many similarities to NM suggesting similar underlying mechanisms for the pathophysiology of the two conditions. Indeed, cap myopathy may be a variant or early form of NM since as mentioned previously, members of the same family carrying the same mutation can have either cap myopathy or NM or both (Table 1).[61,62] As in NM, patients with cap myopathy can have hypotonia and relatively nonprogressive muscle weakness, predominant involvement of the proximal muscles, bulbar weakness, hypotrophy (incomplete growth) or atrophy of type 1 and hypertrophy of type 2 fibers, and predominance of type 1 fibers.

Taken together, these cases suggest that the physical and clinical features of patients with mutations in *TPM2* will be similar to those with NM and that the pathologies may be characteristic of NM, cap myopathy and/or CFTD. In addition, pathologies may vary among family members and NM inclusions may be relatively rare.

TPM2 and Distal Arthrogryposis Type 1 (DA1)

Distal athrogryposis type 1 (DA1) is an autosomal dominant congenital disorder characterized by distal contractures such as camptodactyly (permanent flexion of fingers) and clubfoot. Sung et al[4] identified a missense mutation Arg91Gly in *TPM2* that causes DA1 and they state that there was no evidence of neurological abnormalities and no nemaline rods were found in biopsy sections. Therefore, the clinical features elicited by this mutation are very distinct from those that cause NM and cap disease. They propose that the mutation may cause an irregularity in the coiled coil disrupting actin-Tm interaction. Mutations in *TNNI2* that encodes troponin I fast and *TNNT3* that encodes troponin T fast have been identified that cause a more severe form of distal arthrogryposis DA2B. Troponins I, T and C form the troponin complex that is the sensor of intracellular calcium in muscle fibers and therefore a key regulator of muscle contraction. Troponin T interacts with Tm of the thin filament to transfer the calcium binding signal from TnC through to the actin filament, affecting the engagement of the myosin head with actin. Therefore, it is tempting to speculate that mutations in *TPM2* that result in DA1 affect Tms interaction with the troponin complex.

The mutations identified to date in *TPM2* are expected to alter the cytoskeletal tropomyosin Tm1. Tm1 is present in very low amounts in the skeletal muscle bed and may not be present in muscle fibers. The lack of an overt effect of these mutations in Tm1 in other cell types may reflect isoform compensation by other cytoskeletal Tm isoforms present. Sarcomeric Tm isoforms preferentially form heterodimers; whereas, cytoskeletal Tms exclusively form homodimers and this property may 'save' nonmuscle cells from the poisoning effect of mutations in one isoform (Chapter 6).

TPM3 and Congenital Fiber Type Disproportion (CFTD)

Congenital fiber type disproportion is characterized by the absence of any pathological features with the exception of a predominance of uniformly small type 1 fibers. As such, this defining disease feature is common to other myopathies with thin filament gene involvement and is diagnosed based on the exclusion of other distinct pathologies. Mutations have been identified in three genes to date that give rise to this disorder: *ACTA1*,[63] *SEPN1*,[64] *TPM3*.[6] Missense mutations in *TPM3* currently are the most common cause of CFTD and the clinical features fit in the spectrum described for NM (Table 1). Presentation is early, typically within the first year with marked head and neck muscle weakness. Muscle function improves through to adolescence and stabilizes or declines slowly and respiratory problems can occur. Contractures are common predominantly in the neck and in association with kyphoscoliosis. Individuals are slender with proximal muscle weakness especially in the legs. Z-line distortion is common however, rods are not. The mutation *TPM3*(Arg168His) causes both NM and CFTD and this can occur within a family suggesting that the Z-line distortions typical of CFTD may be precursors of rods.

All but one of the mutations in *TPM3* that cause CFTD occur in positions *f* or *g* of the α helix and alter polar basic residues. It is predicted that these mutations will alter interaction with sarcomeric actin.[6] One mutation (Leu100Met) occurs in the *a* position of the α helix which is a conservative change. It is postulated that this may affect Tm dimer formation since we have shown that this occurs with another conservative mutation in the *a* position, His40Tyr, which causes NM.[50]

All of the mutations in *TPM3* that cause CFTD mutations are present in all of the cytoskeletal isoforms encoded by the gene again raising the possibility that some features of this disease may be due to mutations in the cytoskeletal isoforms rather than or in addition to the mutant skeletal muscle isoform.

Cardiac Involvement in *TPM*-Based Myopathies

In all forms of NM, cardiac involvement is rare; however, in those cases where nemaline rods have been detected in the heart, the result is dilated cardiomyopathy.[33,65] The mutations in patients that present with NM with cardiac involvement have not been identified. It is assumed that the rarity of cardiac involvement in the majority of nemaline patients is due to the fact that most of the genes that have been identified as causing NM do not encode major isoforms expressed in the heart (α-skeletal actin, β-Tm, α-Tm$_{slow}$, nebulin, troponin T slow).[66,67] However, a CFTD patient with the *TPM3*(Arg168His) mutation has a mild left ventricular hypertrophy[6] which suggests that the mutations in even minor isoforms can affect heart function, but that this clinical feature may not be sufficiently overt to detect.

Mutations in both *TPM1* and *TPM2* are known to cause cardiomyopathy (see Chapter 11). However, while the *TPM1* gene is expressed in both skeletal muscle and cardiac muscle, patients with cardiomyopathy-causing mutations in *TPM1* do not appear to have skeletal myopathy. In contrast, patients with cardiomyopathy with *TPM2* mutations often develop central core disease. It is unclear why cardiomyopathy mutations in *TPM1* do not produce overt skeletal muscle abnormalities. However, a compelling argument is made in Chapter 11 that more sarcomeric Tm species are expressed in skeletal muscle than in heart and the presence of both hetero- and homodimers in skeletal muscle in comparison with the reliance on Tm homodimers in the heart, may help to mask the deleterious effect of a mutation in skeletal muscle. In addition, the point is made that the context of the mutation, i.e., heart or skeletal muscle, may significantly impact on clinical features due to the differences in functional demand and associated proteins, e.g., *TPM3*(Met9Arg) results in NM with no apparent impact in the heart.

Conclusions and Perspectives

The discoveries that mutations in Tms encoded by *TPM2* and *TPM3* cause at least four diseases of skeletal muscle are relatively recent findings. At present it isn't understood how different mutations in these genes can give rise to such a range of different pathologies, why specific muscles are affected and why pathologies are not present in all muscles where the mutant protein is expressed. In addition, it is currently unclear how mutations in thin filament genes lead to the formation of rods and other pathophysiological features. Although it is apparent that mutations in sarcomeric Tms impact on the structure and function of the actin thin filament, it is unclear whether these mutations alter specific aspects of muscle contraction or are the result of alterations to the structural integrity of the actin filaments. To date, the only mechanistic dysfunction that has been identified is the alteration to preference for heterodimer formation by the *TPM3*(Met9Arg) mutation that could result in thin filament weakness in NM. Although, there remain many questions to answer, there are emerging trends that in time will provide insight into potential mechanisms of Tm dysfunction as well as lead to important insights into actin thin filament structure and function. Three of the diseases, NM, cap disease and CFTD share a number of clinical features including hypotonia, non or slowly progressive muscle weakness, slender build, predominant involvement of the proximal muscles, bulbar muscle weakness, type 1 fiber hypotrophy and predominance and hypertrophy of type 2 fibers. However, since these features are shared with myopathies caused by mutations in a number of thin filament-associated genes, it is possible that the subtle differences in disease pathologies amongst the *TPM* diseases, i.e., 'caps', Z-line distortion vs rods, type 1 fiber hypotrophy in the absence of filament disruptions, etc., may ultimately provide insight into the function of different Tms and different regions of Tm proteins. An important concept that has come to light is that muscle context affects the impact of a mutant Tm—skeletal vs cardiac muscle, distal vs proximal muscles. Clearly, the function of a muscle and the differences in Tm-associated proteins in different muscles will impact on the read-out of the mutant protein. Finally, the discovery that myopathy-causing mutations may also reside in cytoskeletal Tms present in muscle adds another level of complexity to the assignment of disease features to underlying mechanisms.

References

1. Laing NG. Congenital myopathies. Curr Opin Neurol 2007; 20(5):583-9.
2. Donner K, Ollikainen M, Ridanpaa M et al. Mutations in the beta-tropomyosin (TPM2) gene—a rare cause of nemaline myopathy. Neuromuscul Disord 2002; 12:151-158.
3. Laing NG, Wilton SD, Akkari PA et al. A mutation in the alpha tropomyosin gene TPM3 associated with autosomal dominant nemaline myopathy. Nat Genet 1995; 9:75-79.
4. Sung SS, Brassington AME, Grannatt K et al. Mutations in genes encoding fast-twitch contractile proteins cause distal arthrogryposis syndromes. Am J Hum Genet 2003; 72:681-690.
5. Lehtokari VL, Ceuterick-de Groote C, de Jonghe P et al. Cap disease caused by heterozygous deletion of the beta-tropomyosin gene TPM2. Neuromuscul Disord 2007; 17:433-442.
6. Clarke NF, Kolski H, Dye DE et al. Mutations in TPM3 are a common cause of congenital fiber type disproportion. Ann Neurol 2008; 63 in press.
7. Kee AJ, Schevzov G, Nair-Shalliker V et al. Sorting of a nonmuscle tropomyosin to a novel cytoskeletal compartment in skeletal muscle results in muscular dystrophy. J Cell Biol 2004; 166(5):685-96.
8. Gunning P, Gordon M, Wade R et al. Differential control of tropomyosin mRNA levels during myogenesis suggests the existence of an isoform competition-autoregulatory compensation control mechanism. Dev Biol 1990; 138(2):443-53.
9. Cummins P, Perry SV. Chemical and immunochemical characteristics of tropomyosin from striated and smooth muscle. Biochem J 1974; 141:43-49.
10. Salviati G, Betto R, Betto D. Polymorphism of myofibrillar proteins of rabbit skeletal muscle fibers: An electrophoretic study of single myofibers. Biochem J 1982; 207:261-272.
11. Vlahovich V, Schevzov G, Nair-Shaliker V et al. Tropomyosin 4 defines novel filaments in skeletal muscle associated with muscle remodelling/regeneration in normal and diseased muscle. Cell Motil Cytoskeleton 2008; 65(1):73-85.
12. Conen PE, Murphy EG, Donohue WL. Light and electron microscopic studies of 'myogranules' in a child with hypotonia and muscle weakness. Can Med Assoc J 1963; 89:983-6.
13. Shy GM, Engel WK, Somers JE et al. Nemaline myopathy. A new congenital myopathy. Brain 1963; 86:793-810.
14. Clarkson E, Costa CF, Machesky LM. Congenital myopathies: diseases of the actin cytoskeleton. J Pathol 2004; 204:407-417.
15. Sanoudou D, Beggs AH. Clinical and genetic heterogeneity in nemaline myopathy—a disease of skeletal muscle thin filaments. Trends Mol Med 2001; 7:362-368.

16. Wallgren-Pettersson C, Laing NG. 138th ENMC Workshop: nemaline myopathy, Naarden, The Netherlands. Neuromuscul Disord 2006; 16:54-60.
17. Wallgren-Pettersson C, Beggs AH, Laing NG. 51st ENMC International Workshop: Nemaline Myopathy. Naarden, The Netherlands. Neuromuscul Disord 1998; 8:53-56.
18. Wallgren-Pettersson C, Laing NG. Report of the 83rd ENMC International Workshop: 4th Workshop on Nemaline Myopathy, Naarden, The Netherlands. Neuromuscul Disord 2001; 11:589-595.
19. Agrawal PB, Strickland CD, Midgett C et al. Heterogeneity of nemaline myopathy cases with skeletal muscle alpha-actin gene mutations. Ann Neurol 2004; 56:86-96.
20. Sparrow JC, Nowak KJ, Durling HJ et al. Muscle disease caused by mutations in the skeletal muscle alpha-actin gene (ACTA1). Neuromuscul Disord 2003; 13:519-531.
21. Wallgren-Pettersson C, Pelin K, Nowak KJ et al. Genotype-phenotype correlations in nemaline myopathy caused by mutations in the genes for nebulin and skeletal muscle alpha-actin. Neuromuscul Disord 2004; 14:461-470.
22. Goebel HH, Piirsoo A, Warlo I et al. Infantile intranuclear rod myopathy. J Child Neurol 1997; 12(1):22-30.
23. Goebel HH, Warlo I. Nemaline myopathy with intranuclear rods—Intranuclear rod myopathy. Neuromuscul Disord 1997; 7(1):13-19.
24. Paulus W, Peiffer J, Becker I et al. Adult-onset rod disease with abundant intranuclear rods. J Neurol 1988; 235:343-347.
25. Rifai Z, Kazee AM, Kamp C et al. Intranuclear rods in severe congenital nemaline myopathy. Neurology 1993; 43:2372-2377.
26. Ryan MM, Ilkovski B, Strickland CD et al. Clinical course correlates poorly with muscle pathology in nemaline myopathy. Neurology 2003; 60:665-673.
27. Shafiq SA, Dubowitz V, Peterson HC et al. Nemaline myopathy: report of a fatal case, with histochemical and electron microscopic studies. Brain 1967; 90:817-828.
28. North KN, Laing NG, Wallgren-Pettersson C. Nemaline myopathy: current concepts. The ENMC international consortium and nemaline myopathy. J Med Genet 1997; 34:705-713.
29. Morris EP, Nneji G, Squire JM. The three-dimensional structure of the nemaline rod Z-band. J Cell Biol 1990; 111:2961-2978.
30. Yamaguchi M, Robson RM, Stromer MH et al. Actin filaments form the backbone of nemaline myopathy rods. Nature 1978; 271:265-267.
31. Yamaguchi M, Robson RM, Stromer MH et al. Nemaline myopathy rod bodies. Structure and composition. J Neurol Sci 1982; 56:35-56.
32. Schroder R, Reimann J, Salmikangas P et al. Beyond LGMD1A: myotilin is a component of central core lesions and nemaline rods. Neuromuscul Disord 2003; 13:451-455.
33. Muller-Hocker J, Schafer S, Mendel B et al. Nemaline cardiomyopathy in a young adult: an ultraimmunohistochemical study and review of the literature. Ultrastruct Pathol 2000; 24:407-416.
34. Engel AG, Banker BQ. Ultrastructural changes in diseased muscle. In: Engel AG, Franzini-Armstrong C Ed. Myology: Basic and Clinical. New York: McGraw Hill, Inc., 1994; 889-1017.
35. Karpati G, Carpenter S, Eisen AA. Experimental core-like lesions and nemaline rods. A correlative morphological and physiological study. Arch Neurol 1972; 27:237-251.
36. Feinberg DM, Spiro AJ, Weidenheim KM. Distinct light microscopic changes in human immunodeficiency virus-associated nemaline myopathy. Neurology 1998; 50:529-531.
37. Fukunaga H, Osame M, Arimura Y et al. A case of nemaline myopathy with ophthalmoplegia and mitochondrial abnormalities (author's transl). Rinsho Shinkeigaku 1978; 18:35-43.
38. Fukuhara N, Yuasa T, Tsubaki T et al. Nemaline myopathy: Histological, histochemical and ultrastructural studies. Acta Neuropathol (Berl) 1978; 42:33-41.
39. Baranska B. Formation of the nemaline structures in soleus muscle of rats subjected to long-lasting immobilization. Folia Morphol (Warsz) 1999; 58:207-214.
40. Joya JE, Kee AJ, Nair-Shalliker V et al. Muscle weakness in a mouse model of nemaline myopathy can be reversed with exercise and reveals a novel myofiber repair mechanism. Hum Mol Genet 2004; 13:2633-2645.
41. Sanoudou D, Haslett JN, Kho AT et al. Expression profiling reveals altered satellite cell numbers and glycolytic enzyme transcription in nemaline myopathy muscle. Proc Natl Acad Sci USA 2003; 100:4666-4671.
42. Sanoudou D, Corbett MA, Han M et al. Skeletal muscle repair in a mouse model of nemaline myopathy. Hum Mol Genet 2006; 15:2603-2612.
43. Tan P, Briner J, Boltshauser E et al. Homozygosity for a nonsense mutation in the alpha-tropomyosin slow gene TPM3 in a patient with severe infantile nemaline myopathy. Neuromuscul Disord 1999; 9:573-579.

44. Durling HJ, Reilich P, Muller-Hocker J et al. De novo missense mutation in a constitutively expressed exon of the slow alpha-tropomyosin gene TPM3 associated with an atypical, sporadic case of nemaline myopathy. Neuromuscul Disord 2002; 12:947-951.
45. Pénisson-Besnier I, Monnier N, Toutain A et al. A second pedigree with autosomal dominant nemaline myopathy caused by TPM3 mutation: a clinical and pathological study. Neuromuscul Disord 2007; 17:330-337.
46. Wattanasirichaigoon D, Swoboda KJ, Takada F et al. Mutations of the slow muscle alpha-tropomyosin gene, TPM3, are a rare cause of nemaline myopathy. Neurology 2002; 59:613-617.
47. Gunning P, O'Neill G, Hardeman E. Tropomyosin-based regulation of the actin cytoskeleton in time and space. Physiol Rev 2008; 88(1):1-35.
48. Corbett MA, Robinson CS, Dunglison GF et al. A mutation in alpha-tropomyosin(slow) affects muscle strength, maturation and hypertrophy in a mouse model for nemaline myopathy. Hum Mol Genet 2001; 10:317-328.
49. Wallgren-Pettersson C. Congenital nemaline myopathy. A clinical follow-up of twelve patients. J Neurol Sci 1989; 89:1-14.
50. Corbett MA, Akkari PA, Domazetovska A et al. An alpha-tropomyosin mutation alters dimer preference in nemaline myopathy. Ann Neurol 2005; 57:42-49.
51. Michele DE, Albayya FP, Metzger JM. A nemaline myopathy mutation in alpha-tropomyosin causes defective regulation of striated muscle force production. J Clin Invest 1999; 104:1575-1581.
52. Shimomura C, Nonaka I. Nemaline myopathy: comparative muscle histochemistry in the severe neonatal, moderate congenital and adult-onset forms. Pediatr Neurol 1989; 5:25-31.
53. Wallgren-Pettersson C, Rapola J, Donner M. Pathology of congenital nemaline myopathy. A follow-up study. J Neurol Sci 1988; 83:243-257.
54. Michele DE, Coutu P, Metzger JM. Divergent abnormal muscle relaxation by hypertrophic cardiomyopathy and nemaline myopathy mutant tropomyosins. Physiol Genomics 2002; 9:103-111.
55. de Haan V, Gommans IM, Hardeman EC et al. Skeletal muscle of mice with a mutation in slow alpha-tropomyosin is weaker at lower lengths. Neuromuscul Disord 2002; 12:952-957.
56. Nair-Shalliker V, Kee AJ, Joya JE et al. Myofiber adaptational response to exercise in a mouse model of nemaline myopathy. Muscle Nerve 2004; 30:470-480.
57. Patel K, Macharia R, Amthor H. Molecular mechanisms involving IGF-1 and myostatin to induce muscle hypertrophy as a therapeutic strategy for Duchenne muscular dystrophy. Acta Myol 2005; 24:230-241.
58. Shavlakadze T, White J, Hoh JF et al. Targeted expression of insulin-like growth factor-I reduces early myofiber necrosis in dystrophic mdx mice. Mol Ther 2004; 10:829-843.
59. Kalita D. A new treatment for congenital nonprogressive nemaline myopathy. J Orthomol Med 1989; 4:70-74.
60. Ryan MM, Sy C, Rudge S et al. Dietary L-Tyrosine supplementation in nemaline myopathy. J Child Neurol 2008; 23(6):609-613.
61. Tajsharghi H, Ohlsson M, Lindberg C et al. Congenital myopathy with nemaline rods and cap structures caused by a mutation in the β-tropomyosin gene (TPM2). Arch Neurol 2007; 64:1334-1338.
62. Cuisset JM, Maurage CA, Pellissier JF et al. 'Cap myopathy': case report of a family. Neuromuscul Disord 2006; 16(4):277-81.
63. Laing NG, Clarke NF, Dye DE et al. Actin mutations are one cause of congenital fiber type disproportion. Ann Neurol 2004; 56:689-694.
64. Clarke NF, Kidson W, Quijano-Roy S et al. SEPN1: associated with congenital fiber-type disproportion and insulin resistance. Ann Neurol 2005; 59:546-552.
65. Ishibashi-Ueda H, Imakita M, Yutani C et al. Congenital nemaline myopathy with dilated cardiomyopathy: an autopsy study. Hum Pathol 1990; 21:77-82.
66. Ilkovski B, Clement S, Sewry C et al. Defining alpha-skeletal and alpha-cardiac actin expression in human heart and skeletal muscle explains the absence of cardiac involvement in ACTA1 nemaline myopathy. Neuromuscul Disord 2005; 15:829-835.
67. Michele DE, Metzger JM. Physiological consequences of tropomyosin mutations associated with cardiac and skeletal myopathies. J Mol Med 2000; 78:543-553.
68. Moraczewska J, Greenfield NJ, Liu Y et al. Alteration of tropomyosin function and folding by a nemaline myopathy-causing mutation. Biophysics J 2000; 79:3217-3225.

CHAPTER 13

Tropomyosins in Human Diseases:
Ulcerative Colitis

Kiron M. Das* and Manisha Bajpai

Abstract

Ulcerative colitis (UC) is a form of chronic inflammatory bowel disease (IBD) that almost always affects the rectal mucosa and variable length of the colon in continuity and at times mucosa of the entire colon. It is not caused by any specific pathogen. Genetics, environmental factors and altered immune responses to dietary macromolecules, colonic bacteria and cellular proteins have been implicated in the pathogenesis of UC. Autoimmune response against cytoskeletal, microfilament protein tropomyosin (Tm) seems to play an important role in the pathogenesis of UC. The predominant colonic epithelial Tm isoform, hTm5, can induce both humoral (B-cells) and cellular (T-cells) response in patients with UC. Such responses are not seen in normal subjects and disease control subjects, such as patients with Crohn's disease (CD, another type of IBD) and patients with lupus. A novel observation that hTm5 is expressed on colon epithelial cell surface but not on small intestinal epithelial cells provides evidence for presentation to immune effector cells. This surface expression of hTm5 seems to be facilitated by a colon epithelial cell membrane associated protein, CEP, that acts as a chaperone for the trans-migration of hTm5 to the surface and both hTm5 and CEP are then released outside the cell. Both CEP and hTm5 expression are increased with pro-inflammatory cytokine, such as γ-interferon. hTm5 expression in UC mucosa is also significantly increased compared to normal. Finally, autoantibodies against hTm5 observed both in circulation and in the colon mucosa of patients with UC are pathogenic causing colon epithelial cell destruction by antibody and complement mediated cytolysis.

Introduction

IBD is a general term for a group of chronic inflammatory disorders of unknown etiology involving the gastrointestinal tract. UC is a form of IBD primarily associated with chronic inflammation of the large intestine (colon mucosa) starting from the rectum proximally up to the variable length of the colon. The other form of IBD is known as CD that involves the entire thickness of the bowel and can affect both small and large intestines. Symptoms of ulcerative colitis include rectal bleeding, mucus discharge and diarrhea. Depending on the state of the disease, endoscopy reveals reddening of the mucosa, increased friability, mucosal bleeding, ulcerations, pseudopolyps, granularity and loss of vascular architecture. UC is usually associated with recurrent attacks or flares with complete remission of symptoms in the interim. Drugs-Corticosteroids, aminosalicylates, immunomodulators and anti-TNFα preparations interacting at various levels along the immune and inflammatory cascades are available for the treatment of UC. They effectively induce remission and some of them are largely used to prevent disease recurrence.

*Corresponding Autor: Kiron M. Das—Division of Gastroenterology and Hepatology, Department of Medicine, Crohn's and Colitis Center of New Jersey, UMDNJ-Robert Wood Johnson Medical School, New Brunswick, NJ, 08903, U.S.A. Email: daskm@umdnj.edu

Tropomyosin, edited by Peter Gunning. ©2008 Landes Bioscience and Springer Science+Business Media.

In patients with IBD, the immune system seems to be abnormally activated in genetically susceptible host by an unknown antigen (dietary, bacterial and colon epithelial) in the GI tract. Although UC and CD share several common anatomical locations such as colon and clinical features, the mucosal immune response in UC differs from that occurring in CD. A T-cell driven immune response indeed predominates in CD and most of the pathophysiological changes in CD inflamed tissue can be related to the effects of T helper cell type 1 (Th1) cytokines.[1-3] Differently in UC, characteristics of pathological changes, including the epithelial damage, the occurrence of multiple (auto)antibodies and evidences from several immunopathological studies suggest that in UC an enhanced humoral immunity predominates. In UC also there is an increased number and state of activation of lamina propria mononuclear cells (LPMC) in the involved gut that gives rise to an increased mucosal release of soluble mediators. Although the cytokine profile in UC is less defined that for CD, the role of IL-5 in UC is of interest as this cytokine contributes to the development of a humoral-mediated immune response.[3] The continued abnormal activation of the immune system results in chronic inflammation. UC is, however, a systemic disease that can affect other parts of the body outside the intestine, involving joints, skin, eyes and the bile ducts in up to 20% of the patients.

Epidemiology

The disease is frequently seen among young adults in their twenties or thirties. It is more common in Caucasians than in Blacks or Orientals with an increased incidence (three to six folds) in Jewish ethnicity. Both sexes are equally affected. In Western Europe and in the USA, UC has an incidence of approximately 6 to 8 cases per 100,000 populations and an estimated prevalence of approximately 70 to 150 per 100,000 populations.

Factors Involved in the Pathogenesis of UC

Extrinsic Factors

Diet

No specific dietary factor has been shown to be involved in the pathogenesis of UC. Lactose intolerance, causing diarrhea, is a common problem in almost half of the world's adult population with some ethnic variation. It does not directly affect UC except that it can increase diarrhea.

Bacterial Infection

The bacteria that normal live in the colon also have an important role in the development of the disease, since animals at risk for developing colitis do not develop it when raised in a bacteria-free environment.[4] Patients who are susceptible for UC may develop the chronic disease following an attack of bacterial colitis.

Environmental Factors

Cigarette smoking prevents flare-ups of colitis, particularly among the past smokers. The mechanism of this protection is unclear.

Stress

While stress can aggravate the symptoms, it does not cause the disease.

Intrinsic Factors

Genetic Susceptibility

Various factors are suspected of triggering UC in people who have a genetic susceptibility. However, no single factor has been consistently proven to be the primary trigger. In contrast to the identification of a definite susceptibility gene NOD/CARD15 in Crohn's disease no specific gene has yet been linked to UC. There is compelling evidence that ulcerative colitis tends to run in families, suggesting that genetics does have a role in this disease. About 10 to 25 percent of affected people have a first-degree relative (either sibling or parent) with inflammatory bowel disease (either ulcerative colitis or CD). Linkage studies have associated colitis with the HLA classII alleles on chromosome 6P.[6,7] Other gene families with potential yet differing population association are Interleukin 1 family of genes on chromosome 2q13[6,7] and the multidrug resistance gene (MDR1) on chromosome 7.[6]

Autoimmune Etiology of Ulcerative Colitis

Autoimmunity has been emphasized in the pathogenesis of UC.[9] Broberger and Perlmann (1959), from Sweden, were the first to report that ulcerative colitis might be an autoimmune disease. Using a phenol-water extract of fetal colon as antigen, they demonstrated high-titer haemagglutinating antibodies to an unknown colon antigen in children with ulcerative colitis.[10] Using the indirect immunofluorescent technique, they showed that those antibodies reacted with colonic epithelial cells. Autoantibodies against colonic epithelial components have been subsequently confirmed by many other investigators.[11]

Patients with UC appear to have a disturbance in oral tolerance. Peripheral blood lymphocytes (PBL), as well as lamina propria lymphocytes (LPL)-T-cells from patients with UC, are cytotoxic in vitro specifically for human colonic, including autologous, epithelial cells.[12] In an animal model of chronic colitis with trinitrobenzene sulfonic acid (TNBS), oral tolerance was demonstrated by feeding total colon extract as well as colon epithelial cell extract to the animals.[13] Such tolerance lacked with small intestinal extract, suggesting organ specificity of the autoimmune process.

That a colon epithelial antigen is crucial in organ-specific inflammation in UC, is strongly supported by a model of UC in mice, transgenic for the human CD3e gene (Tge26), which displays early arrest in T-cell development.[14] It appears that T-cells selected in an aberrant thymic micro environment contain a population of cells that can induce severe colitis, but that this can be prevented by T-cells that have undergone normal thymic development. Inoue et al[15] reported that B-cell lines, established from LPL and PBL of UC patients that produce anti-colon epithelial cell antibody, expressed a restricted V_H3 family usage, strongly suggesting that a particular antigenic stimulus from colon epithelial cell contributed to the pathogenesis of UC.[15]

Tropomyosin (Tm) as an Autoantigen in UC

Humoral Response to Tm, Particularly to hTm5, in UC

We reported a disease specific IgG antibody bound to colon mucosa (colitis colon bound IgG antibody or CCA-IgG) in UC and not in CD.[16] Using the CCA-IgG, by Western blot assay we identified a 40 kDa protein termed "p40" that is present in colon mucosal extract and specifically binds with CCA-IgG.[17] IgG antibodies in UC, capable of binding to colon epithelial cell targets and causing antibody dependent cell mediated cytolysis (ADCC) and a significant increase in IgG1 producing cells in the mucosa was found in UC when compared to CD, where all IgG subclasses (particularly IgG2) predominated.[18,19] Furthermore, in UC and not in CD, this IgG1 deposition on colonic epithelium was associated with C_3b and terminal complement complex deposition against the "p40".[20]

P40 was subsequently purified to homogeneity and sequence analysis demonstrated 93-100% identity with Tm.[21] Tms are cytoskeletal microfilament-associated proteins present in all eukaryotic cells, with organ specific isoform(s) (molecular weight ranging from Mr 30 to 40K) and with distinct functions (see chapters 4,15 and 16).[22] hTm5 cooresponds to the mammalian isoform Tm5nm1 (see chapters 2 and 16). The majority of UC sera, as well as IgG (mostly IgG1) synthesized in vitro by lamina propria lymphocytes (LPL)-B-cells from UC, but not from CD, recognized hTms, particularly isoform 5 (hTm5),[23] the isoform most abundant in colon epithelial cells.[24] Plasma cells isolated from the involved intestinal mucosa of both UC and CD patients produce high immunoglobulins G (IgG) levels. However, up to 42% of mucosal B-cells in UC were found to be committed to produce IgG antibody against hTm5.[25] Such an anti-hTm5 immune response was absent in CD, suggesting disease specificity of hTm5 as an autoantigen in UC. While in CD mucosa the IgG1/IgG2 subclass ratio is similar to controls, in UC-diseased gut there is a marked increase of IgG1 subclass antibodies, capable of complement activation.[26]

IgG antibodies against Tm isoform 5 (Tm5) and to a lesser extent hTm1 have been shown to be spontaneously released by LPMC infiltrating UC tissues.[23,24] The major hTm isoforms present in colonic and jejunal epithelial cells are hTm5 and hTm4, whereas intestinal smooth muscles contain hTm1, hTm2 and hTm3 isoforms.[24] IgG, particularly IgG1, synthesized in vivo by LPMCs from UC recognized hTm5 and hTm1, more significantly ($p < 0.04$ and $p < 0.001$) when compared with CD and controls, IgG produced by LPMCs from CD did not show such anti-hTm reactivity. In UC non IBD colon epithelium, deposits of activated complement and IgG1 antibodies have been detected by immunofluorescence analysis to be colocalized with the expression of "p40" antigen that was subsequently found to be hTm5.[20,21] These observations suggest that in UC colon, the in situ immune-recognition of a putative autoantigen "p40", by specific IgG1 antibodies, is followed by complement activation causing cell destruction. This mechanism of cytolysis of colon epithelial cells may represent one of the important pathogenic processes capable of amplifying and perpetuating the acute and chronic inflammatory process in UC.

Cellular Immune Response to hTm5 in UC

Subsequently, we further demonstrated that hTm5 can induce T-cell response with release of γ-IFN in UC.[27] Such response was not seen in CD, indicating disease specificity. This study demonstrated, for the first time, that a defined colon epithelial cell antigen, hTm5, is capable of inducing a significant T-cell response in UC but not in CD.[27]

Other Studies Supporting the Role of Tm in UC

In an independent study from Japan, the anti-Tm antibody was detected frequently in UC but not in CD.[28] Furthermore, antibody dependent cell mediated cytolystic (ADCC) activity of UC sera was associated with the antibody against a synthetic Tm peptide.[28]

Mizoguchi el al[29] demonstrated IgG antibodies against Tm in the animal model of TCRα[-/-] mice that develop spontaneous colitis. They further reported a positive correlation of anti-Tm antibody titer to severity of colitis.[30] That Tm has potent antigenic potential is supported by a structural analysis of 109 autoantigens involved in various autoimmune diseases that showed a majority of antigenic peptides have significantly charged coiled-coiled helices. Interestingly, α-Tm has the highest potential as an autoantigen.[31] Autoimmunity to alpha-tropomyosin was also found in Behcet's syndrome and Tm was found to be pathogenic as Tm induced lesions in the uveal tract and skin with features of Behcet's disease.[32] It has been shown that Tm extracted from human cardiac muscle has immunogenic epitopes that cross react with group A streptococcal M protein that causes autoimmune myocarditis.[33]

Family Study

Using a large number of IBD patients and their first degree blood relatives, Biancone, et al reported that in UC, anti-hTm5 IgG was higher in sera from UC probands were more frequently seropositive for hTm5 IgG, while sera from UC relatives were more frequently seropositive against both hTm1 and hTm5, suggesting genetic susceptibility to immune recognition of hTm isoforms in UC.[34]

Surface Expression of hTm5 in Colon Epithelial Cells

We further demonstrated a novel observation that hTm5 physically binds with a colon epithelial membrane associated glycoprotein (Mr > 200K), termed CEP that reacts with the monoclonal antibody 7E12H12.[35,36] CEP acts as a chaperone and appears to form CEP+hTm5 complex and both are expressed on cell surface and spontaneously released from the cells in the environment.[36] CEP is expressed specifically in colon epithelial cells and not with any other parts of the gastrointestinal tract, including small intestine.[35] This may explain why hTm5 is not expressed on the surface of small intestinal enterocytes.[37] The novel observation, that hTm5 is expressed on colon epithelial cell surface and not on small intestinal enterocytes, provides the possibility that the putative autoantigen may be accessible to the hyper-responsive mucosal immune effector cells, both humoral and cellular response. This may also be important to explain why UC is restricted to colon. In a colon cancer cell line model, we observed that both hTm5 and CEP expression on the surface is increased when cultured with interferon-γ.[38,39] Expression of hTm5 in the colonic mucosa is significantly increased in patients with UC.[40,41]

Extraintestinal Manifestations of UC

Up to 20% of patients with UC demonstrate extraintestinal inflammation including the biliary epithelium (primary sclerosing cholangitis), skin (Pyoderma gangrenosum), eyes (uveitis) and joints (arthritis). As mentioned above, CEP is specific to colon epithelial cells, however, the corresponding epitope reactive to the 7E12H12 mAb has been detected in biliary epithelium, keratinocytes, the nonpigmented ciliary epithelium of the eyes and chondrocytes.[42,43] More recently, hTm5 has also been localized at these extraintestinal sites where CEP is also expressed (Fig. 1).[37] Such a selective reactivity matches well with established extracolonic complications in UC involving the eyes, skin, joints and biliary epithelium.[44]

The pathogenesis of UC and of the most common extraintestinal manifestations such as primary sclerosing cholangitis is also immunologically mediated and appears to be mainly due to an autoimmune-related process.[28,45-47] Antibodies against biliary epithelial cells (BEC) have been reported in patients with PSC.[45,28] The anti-hTm autoantibody was found in 100% of patients with primary sclerosing cholangitis.[28] Furthermore, the specific IgG antibodies to BEC were capable of initiating ERK1/2 signaling and up-regulation of TLR and production of cytokines and chemokines leading to recruitment of inflammatory cells.[45] These results suggest that in PSC the BECs are not only targets of the immune attack, but may also act as inflammatory mediators.

Aberrant homing of mucosal T-cells has also been suggested to be responsible for extraintestinal manifestations of IBD.[46] Various inflammatory cytokines also have an important role in the recruitment of inflammatory cells and tissue damage. The autoimmune basis of extraintestinal manifestations is also supported by several clinical observations including a higher prevalence of autoimmune disease among patients with UC with extraintestinal inflammations compared to control populations,[48] improvement of disease activity following immunomodulator and anti-TNF therapies. Pyoderma gangrenosum was remarkably improved with anti-TNF treatment.[49]

A reasonable hypothesis is that a central process to the occurrence of extraintestinal manifestations is the development of self-reactive B-cells, which are triggered to produce IgG autoantibodies directed against self antigen(s) such as hTm5+CEP related epitopes in UC that is present in the target colon epithelial cells and biliary epithelial cells.[20,24,28,37,47] The specific antibodies are capable of inducing inflammatory response.[45,50] This process is facilitated by CD4+ T-cells, which may cause enhanced antigen presentation, aberrant homing in various organs,[46] thereby facilitating an immune response, particularly in genetically susceptible individuals. In addition, autoreactive T-cells (CD4+ or CD8+) may be primed by microbial antigens that are crossreactive to autoantigens restricted to specific extracolonic organs, the concentrations of which are normally too low to permit recognition by naïve T-cells.[51]

Differential Expression of "P40 (Tm)" in the Colon Mucosa and Influence of Cytokines on hTm5 Expression

Using two- and three-color immunofluorescence assay, Halstensen et al reported colocalization of IgG1 autoantibody with p40, along with activated complement products, in UC and not in CD.[20] They further reported that the distribution of "p40" in the colon was intriguing, with increasing expression caudally from cecum to left colon and the rectum showing intense staining of all colonocytes. Such an expression correlates with the clinical distribution of UC. These results may explain the location of the disease, severity of disease and why the rectum is the last site to heal following treatment. Expression of hTm5 has been recently shown to be upregulated in the colon epithelium of patients with UC.[41]

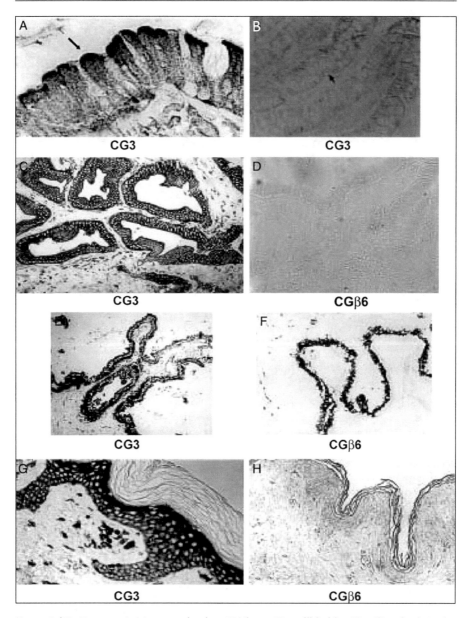

Figure 1. hTm5 expression in normal colon (A), ileum (B), gallbladder (C), ciliary body in the eye (E) and skin (G).37 hTm5 expression in the colonic mucosa is intense and cytoplasmic, with even stronger reactivity (dense bandlike) evident along the brush border area (arrow) and basal areas. The reactivity in the ileum is faint cytoplasmic and no reactivity is evident along the brush border (arrow). Strong reactivity with CG3 monoclonal antibody (anti-hTm5) is evident in the biliary epithelium from a gallbladder mucosa, nonpigmented ciliary epithelium (outer layer) in the eye and keratinocytes in the skin. CGβ6 (anti-hTm2/3) reacted with neither the epithelium of the colon and ileum (not shown) nor gallbladder (D), eye (F) and skin (H). Pigmented layer (inner layer) of ciliary process is seen in both (E) and (F).

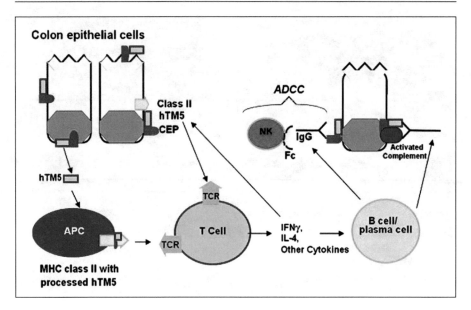

Figure 2. On the basis of current information, this is a model for colon epithelial cell destruction in UC through an autoimmune response to human tropomyosin isoform 5 (hTm5).[50] The hTm5 is closely associated with colonic epithelial cell protein (CEP) and is presented to T- cells through MHC Class II. The T-cells, stimulated by hTm5, produce cytokines, such as IFNγ which up-regulates expression of hTm5 and MHC Class II on the epithelial cells. T-cells may produce B-cell stimulatory factors that promote the production of hTm5-specific antibodies. These antibodies may induce disease by triggering antibody-dependent cellular cytotoxicity (ADCC) and complement mediated lysis.

Expression of hTm5 in Pouchitis

Patients with UC who do not respond to medical therapy may need to undergo surgery. The common operation that is performed is total colectomy and ileo-anal pull through operation to create an artificial rectum (pouch) prepared from the distal ileum. Twenty to 40% of these patients develop pouchitis with similar symptoms as in UC. In these patients with pouchitis, the ileal epithelium in the pouch expresses hTm5 although in normal ileal epithelium and in the absence of pouchitis, hTm5 can hardly be detected except in occasional goblet cells. There was a significant correlation between pouchitis disease activity index and hTm5 score.[52]

Cytoskeletal Proteins Involved in the Immune Responses to Bacteria-Host Interactions

The involvement of cytoskeletal proteins (including Tms, vinculin, actin, villin) in the mucosal immune response in UC gut is also supported by recent evidences showing a rearrangement of the cytoskeletal protein expression in human enterocytes induced by apoptosis and bacteria-host interactions. Cytoskeletal proteins include a number of proteins (α-actinin, talin, vinculin, villin myosin II, ezrin, calpactin, gelsolin, laminin, tropomyosin) which modulate cells structure, shape and motility.[53] Evidences indicate that bacterial-host interactions and apoptosis may induce the expression of cryptic cytoskeletal proteins on the cells surface.[54] The Enteropathogenetic Escherichia Coli (EPEC) may indeed bind to enterocytes by injecting a Translocated Intimin Receptor (TIR) in the host cells membrane, linking to the intimin receptor of the bacterium itself. This mechanism is followed by a rearrangement of the cytoskeletal proteins present in the cytoplasm of the enterocytes (α-actinin, talin, ezrin, villin, F-actin, myosin II, tropomyosin), thus forming pedestals linking the bacterium to colonic epithelial cells.[54] Vinculin, a cytoskeletal protein which modulates the extracellular matrix interactions may be expressed "ex novo" on the surface of apoptotic cells, thus leading to tolerance or autoimmunity.[55] These observations suggest that several mechanisms may induce the expression of cryptic cytoskeletal proteins on the cells surface, with possible development of specific local immune response, both humoral and cellular, towards these antigens.

Autoantibodies against hTm5 Are Pathogenic

That anti-hTm5 auto-antibodies are pathogenic in UC has recently been reported for the first time to cause antibody mediated and complement mediated cytolysis.[50] Auto-antibody against a specific hTm peptide that causes ADCC was reported in UC sera.[28] The antibody titer in the sera against the hTm correlated with ADCC. With more recent data using recombinant hTm5, we demonstrated that colon epithelial cell lysis mediated by autoantibody present in UC could be blocked by hTm5.[50] This further confirms a direct role of hTm in this pathogenic process. Figure 2 shows the model for colon epithelial cell destruction in UC through an autoimmune response to hTm5.[50]

Conclusion

Many studies, during the last 4 decades since the original landmark paper by Broberger and Perlmann,[10] confirmed autoimmunity as a major pathogenetic mechanism in UC. More recent studies provide evidence that hTm5, the dominant hTm5 isoform in colon epithelium, is an important cellular autoantigen that mount humoral and cellular immune responses in UC. Furthermore, surface expression of hTm5 on colon epithelial cells allows the binding of anti-hTm5 autoantibodies present in UC. These autoantibodies are pathogenic to colon epithelium and can cause cell destruction by ADCC and complement mediated lysis, as summarized in Figure 2.[50] Future studies of mapping the specific peptide(s) of hTm5 involved in the immune responses in UC and extraintestinal manifestations of UC, may provide both diagnostic and therapeutic possibilities in UC.

References

1. Fiocchi C. Inflammatory bowel disease: etiology and pathogenesis. Gastroenterology 1998; 115:182-205.
2. MacDonald TT, Monteleone G. Immunity, inflammation and allergy in the gut. Science 2005; 307:1920-1925.
3. Fuss IJ, Neurath M, Boirivant M et al. Disparate CD4+ lamina propria (LP) lymphokine secretion profiles in inflammatory bowel disease. Crohn's disease LP cells manifest increased secretion of IFN-γ, whereas ulcerative colitis LP cells manifest increased secretion of IL-5. J Immunol 1996; 157:1261-1270.
4. Sartor RB. Therapeutic manipulation of the enteric microflora in inflammatory bowel diseases: antibiotics, probiotics and prebiotics. Gastroenterology 2004; 126:1620-1633.
5. Ahmad T, Marshall S, Jewell D. Genotype-based phenotyping heralds a new taxonomy for inflammatory bowel disease. Curr Opin Gastroenterol 2003; 19:327-335.
6. Bonen DK, Cho JH. The genetics of inflammatory bowel disease. Gastroenterology 2003; 124:521-536.
7. Satsangi J, Morecroft J, Shah NB et al. Genetics of inflammatory bowel disease: scientific and clinical implications. Best Pract Res Clin Gastroenterol 2003; 17:3-18.
8. Schwab M, Schaeffeler E, Marx C et al. Association between the C3435T MDRI gene polymorphism and susceptibility for ulcerative colitis. Gastroenterology 2003; 124:26-33.
9. Brandtzaeg P. Autoimmunity and ulcerative colitis: Can two enigmas make sense together? Gastroenterology 1995; 109:3007-312.
10. Broberger O, Perlmann P. Autoantibodies in human ulcerative colitis. J Exp Med 1959; 110:657-674.
11. Fiocchi C, Roche JK, Michener WM. High prevalence of antibodies to intestinal epithelial antigens in patients with inflammatory bowel disease and their relatives. Ann Intern Med 1989; 110:786-794.
12. Yonamine Y, Watanabe M, Kinjo F et al. Generation of MHC class 1-restricted cytotoxic T-cell lines and clones against colonic epithelial cells from ulcerative colitis. J Clin Immunol 1999; 110:786-794.
13. Dasgupta A, Ramaswamy K, Giraldo J et al. Colon epithelial cellular protein induces oral tolerance in the experimental model of colitis by trinitrobenzene sulfonic acid. J Lab and Clin 2001; 138:257-269.
14. Hollander GA, Simpson SJ, Mozoguchi E et al. Severe colitis in mice with aberrant thymic selection. Immunity 1995; 3:27-38.

15. Inoue N, Watanabe M, Sato T et al. Restricted V_H gene usage in lamina propria B-cells producing anticolon antibody from patients with ulcerative colitis. Gastroenterology 2001; 121:15-23.
16. Das KM, Dubin R, Nagai T. Isolation and characterization of colonic tissue bound antibodies from patients with idiopathic ulcerative colitis. Proc Natl Acad Sci (USA) 1978; 75:4528-4532.
17. Takahashi F, Das KM. Isolation and characterization of a colonic autoantigen specifically recognized by colon tissue-bound IgG from idiopathic ulcerative colitis. J Clin Invest 1985; 76:311-318.
18. Halstensen TS, Mollnes TE, Barred P et al. Surface epithelium-related activation of complement differs in Crohn's disease and ulcerative colitis. Gut 1992; 33:902-908.
19. Halstensen TS, Mollnes TE, Garred P et al. Epithelial deposition of immunoglobulin G1 and activated complement (C3b and terminal complement complex) in ulcerative colitis. Gastroenterology 1990; 98:1264-1271.
20. Halstensen TS, Das KM, Brandtzaeg P. Epithelial deposits of immunoglobulin G1 and activated complement colocalize with the Mr 40K colonic autoantigen in ulcerative colitis. Gut 1993; 34:650-657.
21. Das KM, Dasgupta A, Mandal A et al. Autoimmunity to cytoskeletal protein tropomyosin. A clue to the pathogenetic mechanism for ulcerative colitis. J Immunol 1993; 150:2487-2493.
22. Lin JJC, Warren KS, Wamboldt DD. Tropomyosin isoforms in nonmuscle cells. Int Rev Cytol 1997; 170:1-38.
23. Biancone L, Mandal A, Yang H et al. Production of immunoglobulin G and G1 antibodies to cytoskeletal protein by lamina propria cells in ulcerative colitis. Gastroenterology 1995; 109:3-12.
24. Geng X, Biancone L, Dai HH et al. Tropomyosin isoform in intestinal mucosa: production of autoantibodies to tropomyosin isoform in ulcerative colitis. Gastroenterology 1998; 114:912-922.
25. Onuma EK, Amenta PS, Ramaswamy K et al. Autoimmunity in ulcerative colitis (UC): a predominant colonic mucosal B-cell response against human tropomyosin isoform 5. Clin Exp Immunol 2000; 121:466-471.
26. Kett K, Tognum TO, Brandtzaeg P. Mucosal subclass distribution of immunoglobulin G-producing cells is different in ulcerative colitis and Crohn's disease of the colon. Gastroenterology 1987; 93:919-924.
27. Taniguchi M, Geng X, Glazier KD et al. Cellular immune response against tropomyosin isoform 5 in ulcerative colitis. Clin Immunol 2001; 101:1-7.
28. Sakamaki S, Takayanagi N, Yoshizaki N et al. Autoantibodies against the specific epitope of human tropomyosin(s) detected by patients with ulcerative colitis show antibody dependent cell-mediated cytotoxicity against HLA-DPw9 transfected L-cell. Gut 2000; 47:236-241.
29. Mizoguchi A, Mizoguchi E, Chiba C et al. Cytoskeletal imbalance and autoantibody production in T-cell receptor-α mutant mice with inflammatory bowel disease. J Exp Med 1996; 183:847-856.
30. Mizoguchi A, Mozoguchi E, Chiba C et al. Role of the appendix in the development of inflammatory bowel disease in TCR alpha mutant mice. J Exp Med 1996; 184:707-715.
31. Dohlman JG, Lupas A, Carson M. Long charge-rich α-helices in systemic autoantigens. Biochem Biophys Res Immunol 2001; 195:686-696.
32. Mor F, Weinberger A, Cohen IR. Identification of alpha-tropomyosin as a target self-antigen in Behcet's syndrome. Eur J Immunol 2002; 32:356-365.
33. Fenderson PG, Fischetti VA, Cunningham MW. Tropomyosin shares immunologic epitopes with group A streptococcal M proteins. J Immunol 1989; 142:2475-2481.
34. Biancone L, Monteleone G, Marasco R et al. Autoimmunity to tropomyosin isoforms in ulcerative colitis (UC) patients and unaffected relatives. Clin Exp Immunol 1998; 113:198-205.
35. Das KM, Sakamaki S, Vecchi M et al. The production and characterization of monoclonal antibodies to a human colonic antigen associated with ulcerative colitis: cellular localization of the antigen using the monoclonal antibody. J Immunol 1987; 139:77-84.
36. Kesari KV, Yoshizaki N, Geng X et al. Externalization of tropomyosin isoform 5 in colon epithelial cells. Clin Exp Immunol 1999; 118:219-227.
37. Mirza ZK, Sastri B, Lin JJ-C et al. Autoimmunity against human tropomyosin isoforms (hTms) in ulcerative colitis: localization of specific hTms in the intestine and extraintestinal organs. Inflamm Bowel Dis 2006; 12:1036-1043.
38. Das KM, Squillante L, Robertson F. An increased expression of the Mr 40,000 colonic epithelial protein in DLD-1 colon cancer cells in response to gamma interferon (γ-IFN) and tumor necrosis factor (TNF). Gastroenterology 1989; 96:A111.
39. Geng X, Liu J, Lin JJ-C et al. Gamma interferon increases surface expression and externalization of human tropomyosin isoform 5 (hTm5) in colon epithelial cells. Gastroenterology 2003; 124:A157.
40. Tatar E, Cohen HD, Geng X et al. Human tropomyosin isoform 5 (hTm5) expression is increased in the colonic mucosa from patients with active ulcerative colitis. Gastroenterology 2002; 122:A531.
41. Yantiss RK, Das KM, Farraye F et al. Alterations in the immunohistochemical expression of Das-1 and CG-3 in colonic mucosal biopsy specimens help distinguish ulcerative colitis from Crohn's disease and from other forms of colitis. Am J Surg Pathol, In Press.

42. Das KM, Vecchi M, Sakamaki S. A shared and unique epitope(s) on human colon, skin and biliary epithelium detected by a monoclonal antibody. Gastroenterology 1990; 98:464-469.
43. Bhagat S, Das KM. A shared and unique peptide in human colon, eye and joint detected by a novel monoclonal antibody. Gastroenterology 1994; 107:103-108.
44. Das KM. Relationships of extracolonic involvement in inflammatory bowel disease: New insights into autoimmune pathogenesis. Dig Dis Sci 1999; 44:1-13.
45. Karrar A, Broome U, Sodergren T et al. Biliary epithelial cell antibodies link adaptive and innate immune responses in primary sclerosing cholangitis. Gastroenterology 2007; 132:1504-1514.
46. Adams DH, Eksteen B. Aberrant homing of mucosal T-cells and extraintestinal manifestations of inflammatory bowel disease. Nat Rev Immunol 2006; 6:244-251.
47. Mandal A, Dasgupta A, Jeffers L et al. Autoantibodies in sclerosing cholangitis against a shared epitope in biliary and colon epithelium. Gastroenterology 1994; 106:185-192.
48. Monsen U, Sorstad J, Hellers G et al. Extracolonic diagnoses in ulcerative colitis: An epidemiological study. Am J Gastroenterol 1990; 85:711-716.
49. Botros N, Pickover L, Das KM. Image of the month. Gastroenterology 2000; 118:654.
50. Ebert EC, Geng X, Lin J et al. Autoantibodies against human tropomyosin isoform 5 in ulcerative colitis destroys colonic epithelial cells through antibody and complement-mediated lysis. Cell Immunol 2006; 244:43-49.
51. Elson CJ, Barker RN, Thompson SJ et al. Immunologically ignorant autoreactive T-cells, epitope spreading and repertoire limitation. Immunol Today 1995; 16:71-76.
52. Biancone L, Palmieri G, Lombardi A et al. Tropomyosin expression in the ileal pouch: a relationship with the development of pouchitis in ulcerative colitis. Am J Gastroenterol 2003; 98:2719-2726.
53. Luo Y, Frey EA, Pfuztzner RA et al. Crystal structure of enteropathogenetic Escherichia Coli. Intimin-receptor complex. Nature 2000; 405:1077-1077.
54. Vallance BA, Finlay BB. Exploitation of host cells by enteropathogenic Escherichia Coli. Proc Natl Acad Sci USA 2000; 97:8799-8806.
55. Propato A, Cutrona G, Francavilla V et al. Apoptotic cells overexpress vinculin and induce vinculin-specific cytotoxic T-cell cross priming. Nat Med 2001; 7:807-813.

CHAPTER 14

Tropomyosin Function in Yeast

David Pruyne*

Abstract

Tropomyosins were discovered as regulators of actomyosin contractility in muscle cells, making yeasts and other fungi seem unlikely to harbor such proteins. Fungal cells are encased in a rigid cell wall and do not engage in the same sorts of contractile shape changes of animal cells. However, discovery of actin and myosin in yeast raised the possibility for a role for tropomyosin in regulating their interaction.[1,2] Through a biochemical search, fungal tropomyosins were identified with strong similarities to their animal counterparts in terms of protein structure and physical properties. Two particular fungi, the budding yeast *Saccharomyces cerevisiae* and the fission yeast *Schizosaccharomyces pombe*, have provided powerful genetic systems for studying tropomyosins in nonmetazoans. In these yeasts, tropomyosins associate with subsets of actin filamentous structures. Mutational studies of tropomyosin genes and biochemical assays of purified proteins point to roles for these proteins as factors that stabilize actin filaments, promote actin-based structures of particular architecture and help maintain distinct biochemical identities among different filament populations. Tropomyosin-enriched filaments are the cytoskeletal structures that promote the major cell shape changes of these organisms: polarized growth and cell division.

Conserved Biochemical and Sequence Features of Fungal Tropomyosins

Unlike many other protein families, identification of tropomyosins in fungi is not possible through simple BLAST homology searches using animal protein templates.[3] Tropomyosins are almost exclusively α-helical proteins and such homology searches yield coiled-coil proteins of many sorts.[4] Instead, the first nonmetazoan tropomyosin was discovered through biochemical purification by subjecting budding yeast extracts to a protocol for isolating nonmuscle tropomyosin.[5] A recovered yeast protein resembled other tropomyosins in being heat-stable and associating with actin filaments in a Mg^{2+}-dependent, high salt-sensitive manner. The protein was also highly elongated, exhibited an anomalously high apparent molecular weight in SDS gels and had an acidic isoelectric point (pI = 4.5).

Further studies have found other key biochemical features conserved in yeast tropomyosins. Yeast tropomyosins are fully α-helical, form dimers, associate with actin filaments cooperatively and stabilize filaments.[6-8] Budding and fission yeast tropomyosins are NH_2-terminally acetylated, a modification that enhances the head-to-tail interaction between tropomyosin dimers and increases their affinity for actin filaments.[6,9] Budding yeast mutants lacking the acetyltransferase have reduced association of tropomyosin with actin in vivo, causing phenotypes similar to loss of tropomyosin function (described below).[10-13] Acetylated budding and fission yeast tropomyosins regulate the interaction between actin and myosin subfragment 1 (S1) in a manner similar to animal tropomyosins (see Chapters 8, 9). That is, linear chains of tropomyosin dimers occupy the closed state on actin filaments, obscuring the myosin binding site, but these chains will shift to the

*David Pruyne—Department of Molecular Biology & Genetics, Cornell University, Ithaca, New York, USA Email: dwp3@cornell.edu

Tropomyosin, edited by Peter Gunning. ©2008 Landes Bioscience and Springer Science+Business Media.

open position with increasing concentrations of S1, resulting in cooperative myosin binding.[9-14] One surprising feature of the fission yeast tropomyosin is that the acetylated protein interacts in a head-to-tail manner so strongly that tropomyosin filaments form even in the absence of actin, a property so far undescribed for any other tropomyosin.[9]

The first fungal tropomyosin gene, *tropomyosin 1* (*TPM1*), was identified through screening an expression library of budding yeast genes using antiserum raised against the putative yeast tropomyosin.[15] With availability of this fungal tropomyosin sequence, a fission yeast gene responsible for *cell division cycle* defects, *cdc8*, was recognized to encode a tropomyosin, as was a second budding yeast gene, *TPM2*.[8-16] (By convention, budding yeast gene names are capitalized and italicized while fission yeast genes are written in lowercase italicized letters.) Using these fungal sequences as starting templates rather than animal sequences, BLAST searches of complete fungal genomes at the NCBI (http://www.ncbi.nih.gov/), the *Saccharomyces* Genome Database (http://www.yeastgenome.org/) and the Fungal Genome Initiative (www.broad.mit.edu/annotation/fungi/fgi/) now show tropomyosins are widespread among fungi, with homologs detected in four of six major phyla (Fig. 1A, B).[17,18] Tropomyosins have not yet been found in eukaryotes more distant from animals and fungi, but this likely reflects the weak sequence identity among homologs. For example, despite the absence of a candidate slime mold tropomyosin based on sequence similarity, high salt, heat-stable extracts of *Physarum polycephalum* contain a F-actin-binding protein recognized by antiserum raised against the yeast *TPM1* product (Tpm1p).[5] Protein purifications based on the unique biochemical properties of tropomyosins may therefore be the best method to identify homologs in other eukaryotes.

In addition to weak sequence identity, fungal tropomyosins are consistently shorter that animal homologs, but they share the characteristic feature of quasirepeats along their length (Fig. 1C).[8,15,16] Among animal tropomyosins, these repeats are low-affinity actin-binding sites (see Chapters 2, 5 and 7).[19,20] The short fungal tropomyosins result from fewer repeats, with the budding yeast Tpm2p and fission yeast Cdc8p comprising four repeats and Tpm1p comprising five, compared to animal tropomyosins with six or seven repeats.[8,15,16,21] As such, the fungal proteins span fewer actin subunits along a filament, with Tpm1p binding at an approximate stoichiometry of five actin subunits per tropomyosin dimer and Tpm2p binding four subunits per dimer, as compared to a ratio of six or seven for animal proteins.[8]

The presence of multiple tropomyosin genes among fungi appears specific to *Saccharomyces cerevisiae* and closely related species (Fig. 1B). Genomic analyses show that an ancestor to this group experienced an entire genome duplication, possibly through the accidental fusion of two diploid yeast cells.[22] All yeast species with evidence of this ancestral duplication bear two tropomyosin genes, while more distant budding yeasts, other members of the Ascomycota and representatives of Basidiomycota, Chytridiomycota and Zygomycota exhibit no genomic duplication and encode a single isoform. Variation of tropomyosin size also appears limited to *Saccharomyces*-related yeasts, suggesting the variation arose in one gene either before or just after genome duplication (Fig. 2A). In this one tropomyosin gene, a tandem duplication of thirty-eight residues lengthened the protein and generated an extra actin-binding repeat (Fig. 1C, 2B). Thus, *Saccharomyces*-related yeasts encode a five-repeat and a four-repeat tropomyosin, while other fungi harbor a single four-repeat isoform.

The consequence of having two tropomyosin genes is unclear, since other budding yeasts such as *Candida albicans* survive with one. In *S. cerevisiae*, Tpm1p and Tpm2p share similar subcellular localizations and when expression levels are matched, either alone performs essential tropomyosin-dependent functions.[8,23] However, the two have some distinct properties, with Tpm2p expressed at lower levels but having a higher affinity for actin filaments than Tpm1p and Tpm2p specifically inhibiting yeast myosin II in gliding assays.[7,8,14,24] Whether the two isoforms have unique functions and how these isoform differences might be utilized by *S. cerevisiae* and related species remains to be seen. Also unknown is whether alternative splicing might generate multiple isoforms from the single tropomyosin gene of other fungal species.

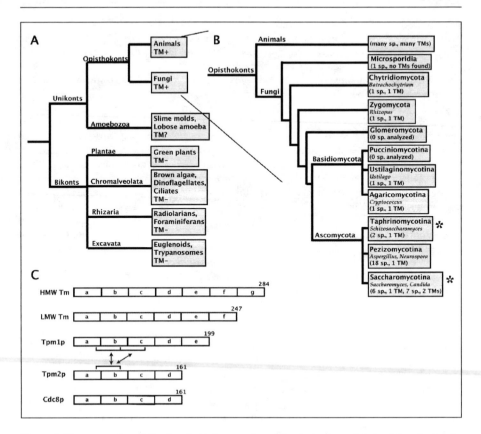

Figure 1. Tropomyosins of the fungi. A) Among the major branches of the eukaryotic family tree, tropomyosins have been identified among animals and fungi (TM+). Biochemical evidence suggests the slime molds of Amoebazoa may harbor tropomyosin-like proteins (TM?), but homologs among other eukaryotes have not yet been described (TM-). B) Tropomyosins are widespread among fungi. A tree expanding on the opisthokont group in (A) shows a simplified phylogeny of the fungi, including major phyla and subphyla and common sample genera.[18] For groups with tropomyosins present, the number of species (sp.) whose genome was analyzed by BLAST and the number of tropomyosin isoforms (TM) detected in each genome are indicated. The subphyla containing the *Schizosaccharomyces* fission yeasts and *Saccharomyces* budding yeasts are indicated (*). C) Animal and fungal tropomyosins exhibit quasirepeats. Models of the primary sequence of high and low molecular weight (HMW and LMW) vertebrate tropomyosins, budding yeast Tpm1p and Tpm2p and fission yeast Cdc8p show overall length in amino acids and approximate boundaries between predicted actin binding repeats (a, b, c, etc.). The region of duplication within Tpm1p and its corresponding region within Tpm2p are shown (double arrows).

Establishment of Filament Identity

Actin filaments in many fungi, including the yeasts, are organized into a few stereotypical types of structures: ~150 nm-wide membrane-associated cortical patches, ~5 μm long bundles called actin cables and a circumferential bundle of filaments that forms a contractile cytokinetic ring (Fig. 3A).[25-28] Of these, tropomyosins associate only with actin cables and the contractile ring (Fig. 3B).[9,15,16,23-29] The mode of actin filament assembly for these structures may play a key role in this segregation.

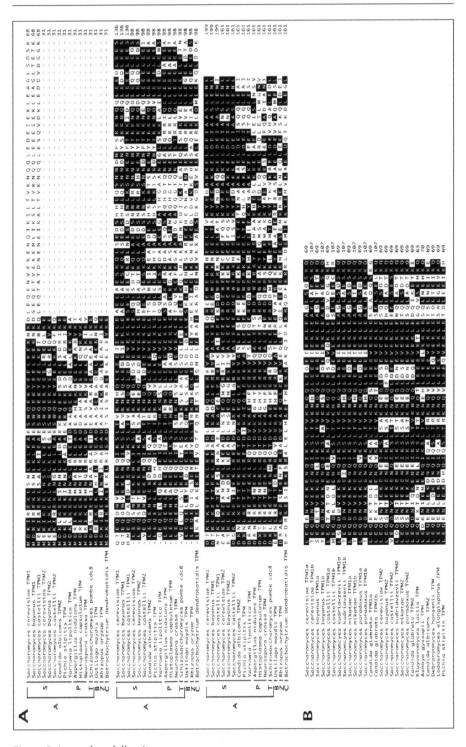

Figure 2. Legend on following page.

Figure 2, viewed on previous page. Fungal tropomyosin sequences. A) Tropomyosins from diverse fungal species show strong sequence similarity. Aligned tropomyosin protein sequences from member species of Basidiomycota (B), Zygomycota (Z), Chytridiomycota (C) and the subphyla Saccharomycotina (S), Pezizomycotina (P) and Taphrinomycotina (T) of Ascomycota (A) are shown with identical residues shaded. B) The duplicated regions of *Saccharomyces*-related *TPM1* homologs (labeled TPM1a and TPM1b) show strong sequence identity to each other and to a corresponding region of *TPM2* homologs from the same fungi, as well as to the single tropomyosin of six other Saccharomycetaceae fungi. Alignments were generated using MegAlign 5.52 (DNASTAR Inc.) and sequences were obtained from the NCBI (http://www.ncbi.nih.gov/), the *Saccharomyces* Genome Database (http://www.yeastgenome.org/) and the Fungal Genome Initiative (www.broad.mit.edu/annotation/fungi/fgi/).

Two classes of actin nucleating factors direct filament assembly in yeasts, the actin-related proteins 2 and 3 (Arp2/3)-complex and the formin family proteins. The Arp2/3-complex is recruited to patches at the cell cortex to stimulate localized filament assembly and in its absence actin-staining patches are lost.[30-36] The formins direct the assembly of filaments composing the actin cables and contractile ring. In the budding yeast, two partially redundant formins (Bni1p, Bnr1p) share these functions, while three fission yeast formins are specialized to assemble the filaments of the actin cables (For3p), the contractile ring (Cdc12p), or structures specific to mating (Fus1p).[12,37-43]

The Arp2/3-complex and the formins nucleate actin filaments by distinct mechanisms and this may be the basis for segregating tropomyosin to particular filament populations. The Arp2/3-complex docks onto the side of a pre-existing filament and shifts its actin-related protein subunits to mimic a filament end, nucleating new filaments that sprout from the sides of old (Fig. 4A).[44] Purified budding yeast cortical patches observed by electron microscopy show tight filament networks, with branches sprouting every 25 to 35 nm along filaments.[45] Such branching is incompatible with tropomyosin association, disrupting the cooperative head-to-tail interactions made between tropomyosin dimers along a filament (Fig. 4B).[46] In contrast, formins stimulate filament assembly free of preformed filaments.[47,48] A 500-amino acid region called the formin homology-2 (FH2) domain dimerizes into a flexible ring that wraps around and stabilizes nuclei of actin dimers (Fig. 4C).[49-51] The FH2 domains remain associated with filament barbed ends while these ends elongate, leaving lateral surfaces clear for tropomyosin association (Fig. 4D).[48,52-55] In turn, tropomyosin may reinforce the segregation of nucleating factors. Some vertebrate tropomyosins physically interact with the FH2 domains of several vertebrate formins and stimulate actin assembly at the formin-bound barbed end, but inhibit lateral docking of the Arp2/3-complex.[56,57] These interactions have not all been demonstrated for yeast homologs, but they suggest that mutual exclusion between tropomyosin/formin- and Arp2/3-dependent systems may maintain the distinction between different actin-containing structures.

Filament Stabilization and Morphogenesis of Actin-Containing Structures

Studies of yeast bearing conditional tropomyosin mutations show that one essential function of these proteins is to stabilize actin filaments. The clearest demonstration is in the budding yeast. Its two tropomyosins are semi-redundant, but cells that lack both are inviable.[8,15,58] Yeast cells lacking one isoform and bearing a temperature-sensitive mutation of the other are viable at room temperature with a normal actin cytoskeleton. But at elevated temperatures, the actin cables and the contractile ring disassemble within one minute while tropomyosin-free structures (the cortical patches) are unaffected.[23,37] When shifted back to cooler temperatures, tropomyosin reassembles with actin to form cables within one minute. Similarly, a temperature-sensitive tropomyosin mutation in fission yeast destabilizes actin cables and the contractile ring within minutes at an elevated temperature, yet cortical patches are retained.[29,59-61]

Tropomyosins can stabilize filaments by enhancing interactions between actin subunits and inhibiting disassembly from the pointed ends, but their importance in yeast is to protect against

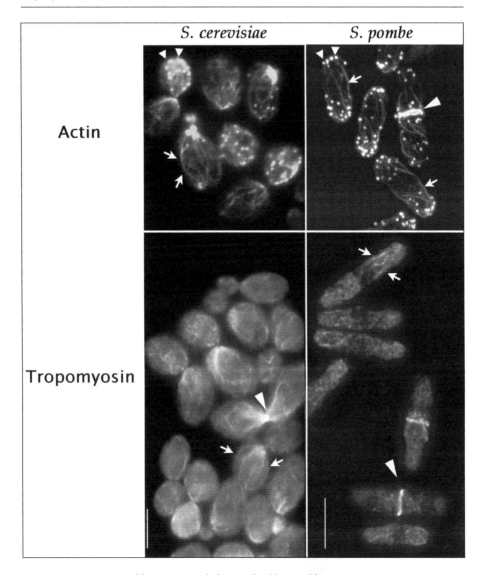

Figure 3. Organization of the actin cytoskeleton in budding and fission yeasts. *Top)* Actin staining of budding (*S. cerevisiae*) and fission yeast (*S. pombe*) shows three types of actin-containing structures. Cortical patches containing actin filaments (small arrowheads) cluster beneath the regions of cell growth, the bud in *S. cerevisiae* and the tips of elongating *S. pombe* cells. Elongated cables of actin filaments (arrows) extend along the length of both types of yeast cells. During mitosis, a cytokinetic actomyosin ring (large arrowhead, shown in *S. pombe* only) assembles at the site of cell division, the bud neck for *S. cerevisiae* and the cell equator for *S. pombe*. During cytokinesis, the ring constricts and actin cables are reorganized from the division site to radiate into the two nascent daughter cells. *Bottom)* Tropomyosin associates with only the actin cables (arrows) and the contractile ring (arrowhead). Bar for *S. cerevisiae*, 5 μm. For *S. pombe*, 10 μm. *S. pombe* F-actin fluorescence courtesy of S. Martin, University of Luasanne and F. Chang, Columbia University. *S. pombe* tropomyosin immunofluorescence courtesy of D. East and D. Mulvilhill, University of Kent.

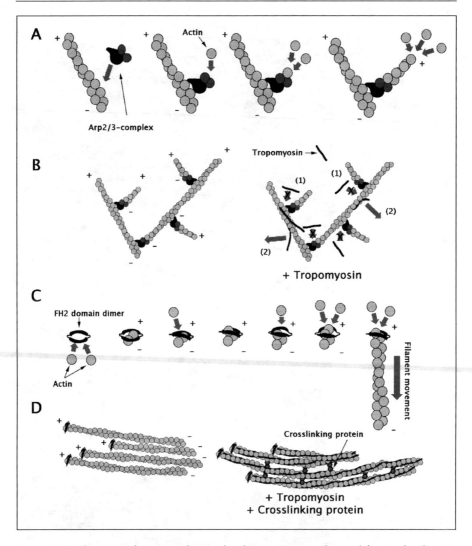

Figure 4. Mechanisms of actin nucleation by the Arp2/3-complex and formin family proteins. A) Arp2/3-dependent nucleation results in branched filaments. The Arp2/3-complex binds to the sides of pre-existing actin filaments. The Arp2p and Arp3p subunits (dark ovals) act as templates for nucleation of a new filament that elongates at its free barbed end. B) Branching in Arp2/3-assembled networks blocks binding of tropomyosin at branch sites (1), disrupting the cooperativity among tropomyosin dimers and reducing overall affinity (2). C). Formin-dependent nucleation results in unbranched filaments. Formin FH2 domains dimerize to form a flexible ring. The FH2 dimer nucleates actin filaments and then processively caps the barbed end, undergoing conformational shifts to permit continued insertion of actin subunits. D) Formin-assembled filaments have free lateral surfaces, permitting cooperative binding by tropomyosin and tight bundling by actin crosslinking proteins. Barbed ends (+), pointed ends (−).

disassembly by actin depolymerization factor (ADF)/cofilin.[7,62-63] ADF/cofilin family proteins, together with a cofactor called Aip1p, bind and twist actin filaments to the point of severing and enhance pointed-end disassembly.[64-66] Tropomyosins and ADF/cofilin bind actin competitively (see Chapter 18) and with the loss of tropomyosin function, cable and ring filaments are exposed as substrates for rapid disassembly.[67] In cells with reduced ADF/cofilin or Aip1p activity, well-bundled cables and contractile rings persist at reduced levels of tropomyosin.[68,69] In the wild-type condition, ADF/cofilin and Aip1p promote the normal turnover of cable and ring filaments, though their transient association with cables is seen only when filament disassembly is slowed.[65,68-70]

The extended, bundled forms of actin cables and the contractile ring depend in part on antagonism of tropomyosin for the Arp2/3-complex and ADF/cofilin. Absence of Arp2/3-dependent filament branching facilitates tight bundling that is possibly mediated by actin cross-linking fimbrin and α-actinin homologs, while filament stabilization contributes to the length of constituent filaments, estimated to range into the hundreds of nanometers for actin cables, or even above 1 μm for the fission yeast ring filaments, but only approximately 40 nm for patch filaments.[45,71-77] Consistent with this, when formin-dependent filament assembly outpaces tropomyosin levels in budding yeast, either by partial reduction of tropomyosin levels or by formin overexpression, only truncated cables are formed.[12,23]

What properties might be expected for elongated tropomyosin-rich structures, as opposed to the compact branched networks of cortical patches? Based solely on their geometry, branched networks have been predicted to be useful in generating compressive force, while long bundles would have tensile strength suitable to resist the pull of motors.[78] Consistent with this, filament assembly in cortical patches pushes associated endocytic vesicles away from the plasma membrane, while the functions of actin cables and contractile rings as myosin substrates are discussed below.[32-33,79]

Actin Cables and Polarized Cell Growth

Budding and fission yeast exhibit distinct patterns of polarized growth (Fig. 5). In budding yeast, cortical expansion begins at a single point called the nascent bud site. A rigid collar limits the growing region of the cortex, which results in an expanding bud joined by a narrow neck to the mother cell. Growth terminates when the bud reaches a size similar to the mother cell, triggering passage through mitosis and cell division. In fission yeast, polarized growth occurs by cell elongation, beginning first at one end of an oblong cell, then occurring at both ends after a growth transition called new end take-off (NETO). Again, polarized growth terminates during mitosis, which is followed by cell division.

For yeasts, the driving force for cell growth is turgor pressure.[80] Yeast cytoplasm is hyperosmotic relative to the environment, such that cells draw in water and push against their rigid cell wall. Growth occurs by remodeling the cell wall to permit expansion. Localized secretion of wall-modifying enzymes controls the direction of growth. Secretory vesicles carry these enzymes from Golgi elements distributed throughout the cell to discrete sites at the cell cortex (Fig. 5).[81,82] Defects in polarized vesicle transport depolarize growth, leaving cells to swell into spherical shapes with no subsequent cell replication.

Polarity is established by molecular cues at the cell cortex, delivered by microtubules in fission yeast or inherited from previous growth cycles in budding yeast, which in turn recruit formins.[83] The formins direct the assembly of actin filaments that acquire tropomyosin and bundle into actin cables (Fig. 5, 6A). These cables continually elongate into the cell body while remaining attached to the formin-rich cortex with their growing barbed ends oriented toward their anchor site, possibly through association with the formin FH2 domains.[23,61,71,84] Once established, actin cables are sufficient to maintain polarity in both yeast species; other cytoskeletal elements such as cortical patches and microtubules are not required.[36,85-86]

Class V myosins guide secretory vesicles along these cables (Fig. 6A). Myosin Vs are optimized for cargo transport, comprising twelve light chains associated with two heavy chains that each have a NH$_2$-terminal actin-binding motor and a COOH-terminal globular tail.[87] For both yeasts, one of their two myosin V heavy chain isoforms mediates vesicle transport for polarized growth:

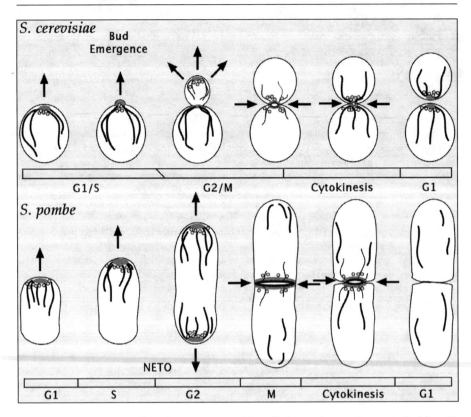

Figure 5. Tropomyosin-rich actin structures guide cell shape changes in yeast. Budding (*S. cerevisiae*) and fission (*S. pombe*) yeast follow stereotypical patterns of polarized growth and cell division (arrows). Actin cables (black lines) radiate from formin-rich regions of the cell cortex (grey) and align along the growth axis. Polarized growth results from the guidance of secretory vesicles (small circles) along actin cables. With bud emergence and NETO, secondary formin-rich sites of cable assembly develop at the bud neck (*S. cerevisiae*) and the second pole (*S. pombe*). Cell division depends on both actin cables and a contractile ring (black ring) assembled by formins at the cell cortex (grey). Actin cables guide vesicles to the division site while the contractile ring marks the leading edge of the ingression furrow.

Myo2p in budding yeast and Myo52p in fission yeast.[61,88-90] Myosin V motor activity propels the protein along actin cables and vesicles are dragged along bound to the globular tail, moving 3 μm/sec in the case of budding yeast.[23,61,91-93] Orientation of the barbed ends of cable filaments toward growth sites directs transport there. Consequently, loss of actin cables from either tropomyosin or formin mutations disperses myosin V and secretory vesicles within minutes, while defects in the myosin V motor prevent the myosin and vesicles from moving along cables and defects in the myosin V tail prevent the polarized myosin from recruiting vesicles to growth sites (Fig. 6B). For budding yeast, cable-dependent transport is essential and loss of actin cables or myosin V function completely depolarizes growth.[12,23,38,88,89-91] In fission yeast, the loss of cables or myosin V only partially depolarizes growth, resulting in cells with swollen ends.[29,40,61,90] The basis for the remaining growth polarity is not clear, but might be vesicle transport along microtubules, or some vesicle-capturing mechanism at the cortex.

Organelle segregation across the narrow bud neck of *S. cerevisiae* also requires active transport. Its two myosin V isoforms share transport of vacuolar membranes (yeast lysosomes), peroxisomes, late Golgi elements, ER membranes and specific mRNAs along actin cables into the bud.[94-99] Even

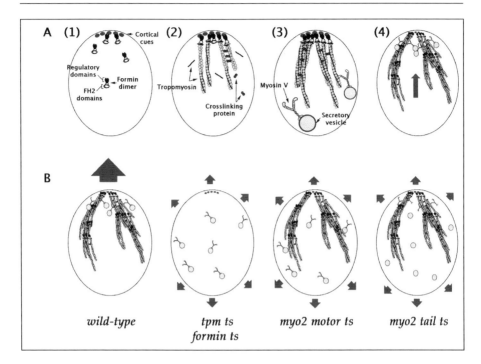

Figure 6. A simplified model for actin cable assembly and function. A) Establishment of polarity occurs by (1) recruitment of formins to growth sites, (2) actin filament nucleation by formins, stabilization by tropomyosin, bundling by crosslinking proteins and (3) association of myosin Vs with secretory vesicles and actin cables. (4) Migration of myosin Vs along cables (grey arrows) results in vesicle accumulation near filament barbed ends anchored at the cortex by formins. B) Budding yeast mutants with defects in growth polarity (grey arrows) helped reveal the order of this pathway. Yeast with temperature-sensitive (Ts) tropomyosin or formin mutations lose actin cables at elevated temperatures and have depolarized myosin V and secretory vesicles. Ts mutations in the myosin V motor domain result in normal actin cables but delocalized myosin V and secretory vesicles. Ts mutations in the myosin V cargo-binding domain result in normal actin cables and myosin V localization, but delocalized secretory vesicles.

microtubules interact with this system, with microtubule tips drawn along actin cables to orient the microtubule cytoskeleton early in the cell cycle.[100-103] The sole known exceptions are mitochondria, which migrate along cables by a nonmyosin actin polymerization-driven mechanism and the microtubule-dependent entry of the nucleus into the bud during anaphase.[100,104-105] The myosin Vs of fission yeast also move nonvesicular cargoes, maintaining vacuoles in a distributed state throughout the cell and guiding astral microtubules along actin cables to align the mitotic spindle.[106-107] How these myosins discriminate between so many cargoes is an area of active research. Distinct myosin V-receptors have been identified for many and structural analysis of the budding yeast Myo2p tail shows receptors can interact with the tail in distinct ways.[99,101,108-118] Selection of cargo may thus reflect a combination of regulation of the different receptors and of their distinct binding sites on the myosin tail.

It is unclear whether stabilization of actin cables is the sole contribution of tropomyosin to myosin V-dependent transport. For example, the two budding yeast class V myosins exhibit nonprocessive motor activity against purified actin filaments, but whether tropomyosin might alter this activity is unknown.[119] In cofilin/Aip1 mutant yeast with tropomyosin-poor cables, polarized secretion and organelle segregation continue, but whether myosin V-dependent transport is as efficient or rapid as in wild-type strains is also unexplored.[68,69]

The Contractile Ring and Cell Division

After completion of growth, cells divide (Fig. 5). While internal pressure is used to expand the cell during growth, cell division must oppose this pressure to draw cell boundaries inward. Both yeasts use a combination of mechanisms for this: polarized secretion to insert new membrane for furrow ingression, assembly of a septum between nascent cells and closure of a contractile ring to spatially guide these.[120-121]

As with establishment of polarized growth sites, cortical cues define where cell division begins and the two yeasts differ in how these cues are placed. In budding yeast, the division site is established as polarized growth begins. Prior to bud emergence, septin filaments are laid down at the nascent bud site so that when the bud emerges, the septins remain as a collar around the neck, defining the future site of cell division.[122-124] In fission yeast, the plane of division is defined prior to mitosis by diffusion of an anillin homolog from the nucleus to the plasma membrane (Fig. 7A). Since the nucleus generally resides near the cell center, a diffuse ring around the equator becomes marked.[41,125] Despite differences in the molecular identity of the initial cues, the final complement of cytokinetic machinery is similar between the two organisms, including cytokinesis-specific components such as septins, anillins, class II myosins, IQGAP and pombe-cdc15-homology (PCH)-proteins, as well as proteins more generally involved in polarized growth, including actin, formins, tropomyosin, myosin Vs and various actin crosslinkers.[120-121]

Localized membrane insertion during cell division is identical to that during polarized growth. During mitosis, formins redistribute from growing cell tips to the sites of cell division and assemble tropomyosin-stabilized cables, which are utilized by myosin Vs to deliver vesicles (Fig. 5). Vesicle delivery coincides with the end of mitosis, providing additional membrane just prior to constriction of the contractile ring and supplying the enzymes that synthesize the septum laid down between the separating cells.[61,90,92,126-127] The loss of cables in tropomyosin or formin mutants or loss of motor activity or cargo-binding in myosin V mutants abolishes proper polarized delivery to the division site, just as for growth sites.[12,23,38,40,61,91,92] In budding yeast, the narrow bud neck facilitates cell division, such that some *S. cerevisiae* strains do not require a contractile ring and membrane insertion and septum assembly are sufficient.[128-129] However, this mode of cell division results in multiple misaligned septa, indicating that the contractile ring guides normal septum assembly.[130-131] For fission yeast, the cylindrical cell presents a much wider cross sectional area that requires spatial guidance by the contractile ring.

The activity of the contractile ring is to cinch inward while contacting the plasma membrane. Its filaments are also nucleated by formins and stabilized and bundled by tropomyosin and crosslinking proteins (Fig. 7B). Rather than utilizing cargo-bearing myosin Vs, the ring filaments function with class II myosins, whose heavy chains assemble into bipolar filaments to promote filament sliding.[39,132-136] Myosin II and a F-actin-binding IQGAP homolog are recruited to the division site in an actin-independent manner and cooperate to guide the actin/tropomyosin filaments into a tight loop around the division site (Fig. 7C).[39,132,133,137-141] Without these factors, actin cables still associate with the division site, but a properly organized ring never assembles.

Just as with actin cables, loss of tropomyosin function destabilizes the actin ring filaments and results in either aberrant (budding yeast) or failed (fission yeast) cytokinesis.[29,37,59-61] It is less clear whether tropomyosin also plays a role in regulating interactions between the ring filaments and myosin II or IQGAP. In fission yeast bearing mutations in both tropomyosin (a filament destabilizing mutation) and cofilin (a filament stabilizing mutation), a bundled ring of actin filaments still forms at the appropriate point of the cell cycle and myosin II still associates with the filaments, but the filaments form an aberrant, wavy loop around the cell equator, indicating some sort of defect.[68] As yet, the ability of these loops to undergo constriction has not been examined.

Once assembled, the ring remains poised to constrict until activation of a signaling cascade, termed the mitotic exit network (MEN) in budding yeast or septation initiation network (SIN)

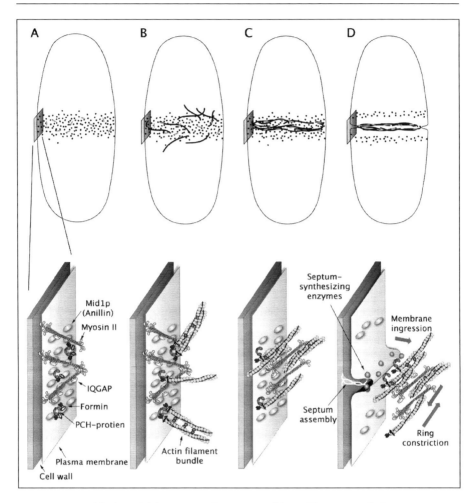

Figure 7. A simplified model for contractile ring assembly and function in fission yeast. Events are shown at the level of the cell (top) and at the molecular level at the cell cortex (bottom). A) An anillin homolog Mid1p defines a broad zone at the cell equator as the future division site. Myosin II, formin, IQGAP and a PCH-family protein are recruited to this zone. B) The formin nucleates actin filaments that are stabilized by tropomyosin and bundled by actin crosslinking proteins, but form an unordered network at the cell equator. C) The actin-binding activity of myosin II and IQGAP orient the actin filaments into a ring around the equator. D) Septins and anillins are released from the immediate vicinity of the actin ring and the ring begins to contract and the plasma membrane ingresses. Contraction is coupled to assembly of the septum by septum-synthesizing transmembrane enzymes associated with the ingression furrow.

in fission yeast.[120,121] The mechanism for activating contraction is unclear. Myosin II is required for contractile ring assembly, particularly in fission yeast, making further actomyosin activation seem unlikely as the mechanism to initiate ring closure. One suggested alternative is that the cortex is regulated.[121] Anillin and septin polymers at the division site cortex might physically block ingression of the plasma membrane. At the time of MEN/SIN signaling, these proteins disperse from the membrane immediately overlying the contractile ring, freeing the plasma membrane to ingress with the contractile ring and exposing surfaces for vesicle fusion (Fig. 7D).

Contraction of the ring is spatially coordinated with assembly of the septum through the embedding of septum-synthesizing enzymes in the plasma membrane of the ingression furrow (Fig. 7D).[127,142] The assembling septum stabilizes the ingression furrow and in its absence, the contractile ring will destabilize.[127-130] The molecular link between the contracting ring and the ingression furrow is unknown, but PCH-proteins are attractive candidates, bearing a membrane-binding NH$_2$-terminal F-BAR domain and a formin-binding COOH-terminal SH3 domain and PCH-protein mutations in yeast can also cause ring destabilization.[143-148] With contraction, actin filaments and other ring components gradually disassemble.[68,148,149] In this, tropomyosin is antagonistic, with overexpression in fission yeast resulting in large aberrant whorls of actin filament bundles.[68] The final abscission occurs by unknown mechanisms, but in budding yeast, actin is not essential for this step.[39,150] The separation of two nascent yeast cells requires further modification of the newly assembled septum, a process dependent on the collection of enzymes previously delivered by the actin cable/myosin V system.[121]

Conclusions

Tropomyosins are now recognized as widespread among fungi and are likely present in other eukaryotes, though poor sequence conservation makes their identification difficult. Biochemically, fungal tropomyosins share a range of structural features and F-actin binding properties with their animal homologs. Among yeasts, tropomyosins associate exclusively with filaments nucleated by formin family proteins, possibly as a consequence of incompatibility between tropomyosin binding and filament branching by the alternative Arp2/3-dependent nucleation. In vivo, yeast tropomyosins shield actin filaments against destabilization by ADF/cofilin, contributing to the formation of elongated actin cables and contractile ring filaments.

Studies of the budding yeast *S. cerevisiae* and the fission yeast *S. pombe* have been extremely useful in establishing the functions of tropomyosin-rich structures. The actin cables are filament bundles that sprout from formin-rich regions of the cell cortex and radiate through the cell. They serve as tracks guiding class V myosins and their secretory vesicle cargo toward growth sites, directing polarized growth of the yeasts. The contractile ring is a closed loop of filaments assembled and organized through cooperation of formins, class II myosins, IQGAP homologs and PCH-family proteins. Constriction of this ring guides ingression of the plasma membrane and the assembly of a septum between dividing cells.

It is unclear whether tropomyosins play roles in these structures beyond stabilization. One important question is whether they regulate access of other proteins. For example, class II and class V myosins cooperate with tropomyosin-rich filaments while class I do not.[151] Is this a consequence of tropomyosin? And do tropomyosins alter the activity of myosins II or V? In vitro, yeast tropomyosins influence the closed/open state of the myosin II binding site on actin filaments, but whether this property is regulated in vivo is unclear.[9,14] In animals, the tropomyosin-binding protein troponin allows for an additional highly-regulated level of actin/myosin inhibition by tropomyosin (see Chapter 8). Might there be yeast proteins that function in a similar manner? For that matter, how is the activity of yeast tropomyosin regulated at all? Tropomyosin protein levels have not been seen to fluctuate, yet actin cables and contractile rings gradually disassemble.[9,23,68,69,148,149] Is there a dynamic regulation of the affinity of tropomyosin for actin, or might the antagonistic ADF/cofilin activity be upregulated, or does disassembly simply occur through stochastic competition between stabilizing and destabilizing forces?

Probing the details of actin cable and contractile ring function remains a robust area of research. Mechanisms of formin function and regulation remain unknown for both structures. For myosin V-dependent trafficking along cables, how the myosin recycles after transport along actin cables is also unknown. Does the motor become inactive and passively ride on actin cables as they elongate back into the cell body?[84] Or as for animal myosin Vs, does the freed myosin globular tail bind the motor and inhibit actin-binding, allowing diffusion back into the cell?[152-153] Basic questions remain regarding the contractile ring as well, such as how the ring associates with the cortex or how the various ring components interact. The powerful genetics of the yeasts and the increasing sophistication of microscopic imaging are helping to answer these questions with a high level of detail on the causative molecular events.

Acknowledgements

I would like to thank Anthony Bretscher and Damien Gabett at Cornell University for critical reading of this review. I also would like to thank Dan East and Dan Mulvihill at the University of Kent, Sophie Martin at the University of Lausanne and Fred Chang at Columbia University for kindly providing fluorescence images of *S. pombe*.

References

1. Koteliansky VE, Glukhova MA, Bejanian MV et al. Isolation and characterization of actin-like protein from yeast Saccharomyces cerevisiae. FEBS Lett 1979; 102(1):55-58.
2. Watts FZ, Miller DM, Orr E. Identification of myosin heavy chain in Saccharomyces cerevisiae. Nature 1985; 316(6023):83-85.
3. Altschul SF, Gish W, Miller W et al. Basic local alignment search tool. J Mol Biol 1990; 215(3):403-410.
4. Phillips GN Jr, Lattman EE, Cummins P et al. Crystal structure and molecular interactions of tropomyosin. Nature 1979; 278(5703):413-417.
5. Liu HP, Bretscher A. Purification of tropomyosin from Saccharomyces cerevisiae and identification of related proteins in Schizosaccharomyces and Physarum. Proc Natl Acad Sci USA 1989; 86(1):90-93.
6. Maytum R, Geeves MA, Konrad M. Actomyosin regulatory properties of yeast tropomyosin are dependent upon N-terminal modification. Biochemistry 2000; 39(39):11913-11920.
7. Wen KK, Kuang B, Rubenstein PA. Tropomyosin-dependent filament formation by a polymerization-defective mutant yeast actin (V266G,L267G). J Biol Chem 2000; 275(51):40594-40600.
8. Drees B, Brown C, Barrell BG et al. Tropomyosin is essential in yeast, yet the TPM1 and TPM2 products perform distinct functions. J Cell Biol 1995; 128(3):383-392.
9. Skoumpla K, Coulton AT, Lehman W et al. Acetylation regulates tropomyosin function in the fission yeast Schizosaccharomyces pombe. J Cell Sci 2007; 120(Pt 9):1635-1645.
10. Hermann GJ, King EJ, Shaw JM. The yeast gene, MDM20, is necessary for mitochondrial inheritance and organization of the actin cytoskeleton. J Cell Biol 1997; 137(1):141-153.
11. Singer JM, Shaw JM. Mdm20 protein functions with Nat3 protein to acetylate Tpm1 protein and regulate tropomyosin-actin interactions in budding yeast. Proc Natl Acad Sci USA 2003; 100(13):7644-7649.
12. Evangelista M, Pruyne D, Amberg DC et al. Formins direct Arp2/3-independent actin filament assembly to polarize cell growth in yeast. Nat Cell Biol 2002; 4(3):260-269.
13. Polevoda B, Cardillo TS, Doyle TC et al. Nat3p and Mdm20p are required for function of yeast NatB Nalpha-terminal acetyltransferase and of actin and tropomyosin. J Biol Chem 2003; 278(33):30686-30697.
14. Maytum R, Konrad M, Lehrer SS et al. Regulatory properties of tropomyosin effects of length, isoform and N-terminal sequence. Biochemistry 2001; 40(24):7334-7341.
15. Liu HP, Bretscher A. Disruption of the single tropomyosin gene in yeast results in the disappearance of actin cables from the cytoskeleton. Cell 1989; 57(2):233-242.
16. Balasubramanian MK, Helfman DM, Hemmingsen SM. A new tropomyosin essential for cytokinesis in the fission yeast S. pombe. Nature 1992; 360(6399):84-87.
17. Cummings L, Riley L, Black L et al. Genomic BLAST: custom-defined virtual databases for complete and unfinished genomes. FEMS Microbiol Lett 2002; 216(2):133-138.
18. James TY, Kauff F, Schoch CL et al. Reconstructing the early evolution of Fungi using a six-gene phylogeny. Nature 2006; 443(7113):818-822.
19. Hitchcock-DeGregori SE, An Y. Integral repeats and a continuous coiled coil are required for binding of striated muscle tropomyosin to the regulated actin filament. J Biol Chem 1996; 271(7):3600-3603.
20. Hitchcock-DeGregori SE, Varnell TA. Tropomyosin has discrete actin-binding sites with sevenfold and fourteenfold periodicities. J Mol Biol 1990; 214(4):885-896.
21. Gunning PW, Schevzov G, Kee AJ et al. Tropomyosin isoforms: divining rods for actin cytoskeleton function. Trends Cell Biol 2005; 15(6):333-341.
22. Wolfe KH, Shields DC. Molecular evidence for an ancient duplication of the entire yeast genome. Nature 1997; 387(6634):708-713.
23. Pruyne DW, Schott DH, Bretscher A. Tropomyosin-containing actin cables direct the Myo2p-dependent polarized delivery of secretory vesicles in budding yeast. J Cell Biol 1998; 143(7):1931-1945.
24. Huckaba TM, Lipkin T, Pon LA. Roles of type II myosin and a tropomyosin isoform in retrograde actin flow in budding yeast. J Cell Biol 2006; 175(6):957-969.

25. Chant J, Mischke M, Mitchell E et al. Role of Bud3p in producing the axial budding pattern of yeast. J Cell Biol 1995; 129(3):767-778.
26. Marks J, Hyams J. Localization of F-actin through the cell division cycle of Schizosaccharomyces pombe. Eur J Cell Biol 1985; 39:27-32.
27. Adams AE, Pringle JR. Relationship of actin and tubulin distribution to bud growth in wild-type and morphogenetic-mutant Saccharomyces cerevisiae. J Cell Biol 1984; 98(3):934-945.
28. Mulholland J, Preuss D, Moon A et al. Ultrastructure of the yeast actin cytoskeleton and its association with the plasma membrane. J Cell Biol 1994; 125(2):381-391.
29. Arai R, Nakano K, Mabuchi I. Subcellular localization and possible function of actin, tropomyosin and actin-related protein 3 (Arp3) in the fission yeast Schizosaccharomyces pombe. Eur J Cell Biol 1998; 76(4):288-295.
30. Sirotkin V, Beltzner CC, Marchand JB et al. Interactions of WASp, myosin-I and verprolin with Arp2/3 complex during actin patch assembly in fission yeast. J Cell Biol 2005; 170(4):637-648.
31. Moreau V, Madania A, Martin RP et al. The Saccharomyces cerevisiae actin-related protein Arp2 is involved in the actin cytoskeleton. J Cell Biol 1996; 134(1):117-132.
32. Kaksonen M, Toret CP, Drubin DG. A modular design for the clathrin- and actin-mediated endocytosis machinery. Cell 2005; 123(2):305-320.
33. Kaksonen M, Sun Y, Drubin DG. A pathway for association of receptors, adaptors and actin during endocytic internalization. Cell 2003; 115(4):475-487.
34. Winter D, Podtelejnikov AV, Mann M et al. The complex containing actin-related proteins Arp2 and Arp3 is required for the motility and integrity of yeast actin patches. Curr Biol 1997; 7(7):519-529.
35. McCollum D, Feoktistova A, Morphew M et al. The Schizosaccharomyces pombe actin-related protein, Arp3, is a component of the cortical actin cytoskeleton and interacts with profilin. EMBO J 1996; 15(23):6438-6446.
36. Winter DC, Choe EY, Li R. Genetic dissection of the budding yeast Arp2/3 complex: a comparison of the in vivo and structural roles of individual subunits. Proc Natl Acad Sci USA 1999; 96(13):7288-7293.
37. Tolliday N, VerPlank L, Li R. Rho1 directs formin-mediated actin ring assembly during budding yeast cytokinesis. Curr Biol 2002; 12(21):1864-1870.
38. Sagot I, Klee SK, Pellman D. Yeast formins regulate cell polarity by controlling the assembly of actin cables. Nat Cell Biol 2002; 4(1):42-50.
39. Bi E, Maddox P, Lew DJ et al. Involvement of an actomyosin contractile ring in Saccharomyces cerevisiae cytokinesis. J Cell Biol 1998; 142(5):1301-1312.
40. Feierbach B, Chang F. Roles of the fission yeast formin for3p in cell polarity, actin cable formation and symmetric cell division. Curr Biol 2001; 11(21):1656-1665.
41. Chang F, Woollard A, Nurse P. Isolation and characterization of fission yeast mutants defective in the assembly and placement of the contractile actin ring. J Cell Sci 1996; 109 (Pt 1):131-142.
42. Chang F, Drubin D, Nurse P. cdc12p, a protein required for cytokinesis in fission yeast, is a component of the cell division ring and interacts with profilin. J Cell Biol 1997; 137(1):169-182.
43. Petersen J, Nielsen O, Egel R et al. FH3, a domain found in formins, targets the fission yeast formin Fus1 to the projection tip during conjugation. J Cell Biol 1998; 141(5):1217-1228.
44. Volkmann N, Amann KJ, Stoilova-McPhie S et al. Structure of Arp2/3 complex in its activated state and in actin filament branch junctions. Science 2001; 293(5539):2456-2459.
45. Young ME, Cooper JA, Bridgman PC. Yeast actin patches are networks of branched actin filaments. J Cell Biol 2004; 166(5):629-635.
46. Lehrer SS, Golitsina NL, Geeves MA. Actin-tropomyosin activation of myosin subfragment 1 ATPase and thin filament cooperativity. The role of tropomyosin flexibility and end-to-end interactions. Biochemistry 1997; 36(44):13449-13454.
47. Sagot I, Rodal AA, Moseley J et al. An actin nucleation mechanism mediated by Bni1 and profilin. Nat Cell Biol 2002; 4(8):626-631.
48. Pruyne D, Evangelista M, Yang C et al. Role of formins in actin assembly: nucleation and barbed-end association. Science 2002; 297(5581):612-615.
49. Xu Y, Moseley JB, Sagot I et al. Crystal structures of a Formin Homology-2 domain reveal a tethered dimer architecture. Cell 2004; 116(5):711-723.
50. Otomo T, Tomchick DR, Otomo C et al. Structural basis of actin filament nucleation and processive capping by a formin homology 2 domain. Nature 2005; 433(7025):488-494.
51. Pring M, Evangelista M, Boone C et al. Mechanism of formin-induced nucleation of actin filaments. Biochemistry 2003; 42(2):486-496.
52. Zigmond SH, Evangelista M, Boone C et al. Formin leaky cap allows elongation in the presence of tight capping proteins. Curr Biol 2003; 13(20):1820-1823.
53. Kovar DR, Kuhn JR, Tichy AL et al. The fission yeast cytokinesis formin Cdc12p is a barbed end actin filament capping protein gated by profilin. J Cell Biol 2003; 161(5):875-887.

54. Moseley JB, Sagot I, Manning AL et al. A conserved mechanism for Bni1- and mDia1-induced actin assembly and dual regulation of Bni1 by Bud6 and profilin. Mol Biol Cell 2004; 15(2):896-907.
55. Kovar DR, Pollard TD. Insertional assembly of actin filament barbed ends in association with formins produces piconewton forces. Proc Natl Acad Sci USA 2004; 101(41):14725-14730.
56. Wawro B, Greenfield NJ, Wear MA et al. Tropomyosin Regulates Elongation by Formin at the Fast-Growing End of the Actin Filament. Biochemistry 2007; 46(27):8146-8155.
57. Blanchoin L, Pollard TD, Hitchcock-DeGregori SE. Inhibition of the Arp2/3 complex-nucleated actin polymerization and branch formation by tropomyosin. Curr Biol 2001; 11(16):1300-1304.
58. Liu H, Bretscher A. Characterization of TPM1 disrupted yeast cells indicates an involvement of tropomyosin in directed vesicular transport. J Cell Biol 1992; 118(2):285-299.
59. Nurse P, Thuriaux P, Nasmyth K. Genetic control of the cell division cycle in the fission yeast Schizosaccharomyces pombe. Mol Gen Genet 1976; 146(2):167-178.
60. Pelham RJ Jr, Chang F. Role of actin polymerization and actin cables in actin-patch movement in Schizosaccharomyces pombe. Nat Cell Biol 2001; 3(3):235-244.
61. Motegi F, Arai R, Mabuchi I. Identification of two type V myosins in fission yeast, one of which functions in polarized cell growth and moves rapidly in the cell. Mol Biol Cell 2001; 12(5):1367-1380.
62. Broschat KO. Tropomyosin prevents depolymerization of actin filaments from the pointed end. J Biol Chem 1990; 265(34):21323-21329.
63. Broschat KO, Weber A, Burgess DR. Tropomyosin stabilizes the pointed end of actin filaments by slowing depolymerization. Biochemistry 1989; 28(21):8501-8506.
64. Maciver SK. How ADF/cofilin depolymerizes actin filaments. Curr Opin Cell Biol 1998; 10(1):140-144.
65. Rodal AA, Tetreault JW, Lappalainen P et al. Aip1p interacts with cofilin to disassemble actin filaments. J Cell Biol 1999; 145(6):1251-1264.
66. Okada K, Obinata T, Abe H. XAIP1: a Xenopus homologue of yeast actin interacting protein 1 (AIP1), which induces disassembly of actin filaments cooperatively with ADF/cofilin family proteins. J Cell Sci 1999; 112 (Pt 10):1553-1565.
67. Cooper JA. Actin dynamics: tropomyosin provides stability. Curr Biol 2002; 12(15):R523-525.
68. Nakano K, Mabuchi I. Actin-depolymerizing protein Adf1 is required for formation and maintenance of the contractile ring during cytokinesis in fission yeast. Mol Biol Cell 2006; 17(4):1933-1945.
69. Okada K, Ravi H, Smith EM et al. Aip1 and cofilin promote rapid turnover of yeast actin patches and cables: a coordinated mechanism for severing and capping filaments. Mol Biol Cell 2006; 17(7):2855-2868.
70. Belmont LD, Drubin DG. The yeast V159N actin mutant reveals roles for actin dynamics in vivo. J Cell Biol 1998; 142(5):1289-1299.
71. Kamasaki T, Arai R, Osumi M et al. Directionality of F-actin cables changes during the fission yeast cell cycle. Nat Cell Biol 2005; 7(9):916-917.
72. Adams AE, Botstein D, Drubin DG. Requirement of yeast fimbrin for actin organization and morphogenesis in vivo. Nature 1991; 354(6352):404-408.
73. Drubin DG, Miller KG, Botstein D. Yeast actin-binding proteins: evidence for a role in morphogenesis. J Cell Biol 1988; 107(6 Pt 2):2551-2561.
74. Asakura T, Sasaki T, Nagano F et al. Isolation and characterization of a novel actin filament-binding protein from Saccharomyces cerevisiae. Oncogene 1998; 16(1):121-130.
75. Wu JQ, Bahler J, Pringle JR. Roles of a fimbrin and an alpha-actinin-like protein in fission yeast cell polarization and cytokinesis. Mol Biol Cell 2001; 12(4):1061-1077.
76. Wu JQ, Pollard TD. Counting cytokinesis proteins globally and locally in fission yeast. Science 2005; 310(5746):310-314.
77. Karpova TS, McNally JG, Moltz SL et al. Assembly and function of the actin cytoskeleton of yeast: relationships between cables and patches. J Cell Biol 1998; 142(6):1501-1517.
78. Zigmond SH. Formin-induced nucleation of actin filaments. Curr Opin Cell Biol 2004; 16(1):99-105.
79. Huckaba TM, Gay AC, Pantalena LF et al. Live cell imaging of the assembly, disassembly and actin cable-dependent movement of endosomes and actin patches in the budding yeast, Saccharomyces cerevisiae. J Cell Biol 2004; 167(3):519-530.
80. Harold FM. Force and compliance: rethinking morphogenesis in walled cells. Fungal Genet Biol 2002; 37(3):271-282.
81. Chappell TG, Warren G. A galactosyltransferase from the fission yeast Schizosaccharomyces pombe. J Cell Biol 1989; 109(6 Pt 1):2693-2702.
82. Preuss D, Mulholland J, Franzusoff A et al. Characterization of the Saccharomyces Golgi complex through the cell cycle by immunoelectron microscopy. Mol Biol Cell 1992; 3(7):789-803.
83. Chang F, Peter M. Yeasts make their mark. Nat Cell Biol 2003; 5(4):294-299.

84. Yang HC, Pon LA. Actin cable dynamics in budding yeast. Proc Natl Acad Sci USA 2002; 99(2):751-756.
85. Huffaker TC, Thomas JH, Botstein D. Diverse effects of beta-tubulin mutations on microtubule formation and function. J Cell Biol 1988; 106(6):1997-2010.
86. Sawin KE, Snaith HA. Role of microtubules and tea1p in establishment and maintenance of fission yeast cell polarity. J Cell Sci 2004; 117(Pt 5):689-700.
87. Sellers JR, Veigel C. Walking with myosin V. Curr Opin Cell Biol 2006; 18(1):68-73.
88. Johnston GC, Prendergast JA, Singer RA. The Saccharomyces cerevisiae MYO2 gene encodes an essential myosin for vectorial transport of vesicles. J Cell Biol 1991; 113(3):539-551.
89. Govindan B, Bowser R, Novick P. The role of Myo2, a yeast class V myosin, in vesicular transport. J Cell Biol 1995; 128(6):1055-1068.
90. Win TZ, Gachet Y, Mulvihill DP et al. Two type V myosins with non-overlapping functions in the fission yeast Schizosaccharomyces pombe: Myo52 is concerned with growth polarity and cytokinesis, Myo51 is a component of the cytokinetic actin ring. J Cell Sci 2001; 114(Pt 1):69-79.
91. Schott D, Ho J, Pruyne D et al. The COOH-terminal domain of Myo2p, a yeast myosin V, has a direct role in secretory vesicle targeting. J Cell Biol 1999; 147(4):791-808.
92. Mulvihill DP, Edwards SR, Hyams JS. A critical role for the type V myosin, Myo52, in septum deposition and cell fission during cytokinesis in Schizosaccharomyces pombe. Cell Motil Cytoskeleton 2006; 63(3):149-161.
93. Schott DH, Collins RN, Bretscher A. Secretory vesicle transport velocity in living cells depends on the myosin-V lever arm length. J Cell Biol 2002; 156(1):35-39.
94. Hill KL, Catlett NL, Weisman LS. Actin and myosin function in directed vacuole movement during cell division in Saccharomyces cerevisiae. J Cell Biol 1996; 135(6 Pt 1):1535-1549.
95. Takizawa PA, Sil A, Swedlow JR et al. Actin-dependent localization of an RNA encoding a cell-fate determinant in yeast. Nature 1997; 389(6646):90-93.
96. Long RM, Singer RH, Meng X et al. Mating type switching in yeast controlled by asymmetric localization of ASH1 mRNA. Science 1997; 277(5324):383-387.
97. Rossanese OW, Reinke CA, Bevis BJ et al. A role for actin, Cdc1p and Myo2p in the inheritance of late Golgi elements in Saccharomyces cerevisiae. J Cell Biol 2001; 153(1):47-62.
98. Hoepfner D, van den Berg M, Philippsen P et al. A role for Vps1p, actin and the Myo2p motor in peroxisome abundance and inheritance in Saccharomyces cerevisiae. J Cell Biol 2001; 155(6):979-990.
99. Estrada P, Kim J, Coleman J et al. Myo4p and She3p are required for cortical ER inheritance in Saccharomyces cerevisiae. J Cell Biol 2003; 163(6):1255-1266.
100. Theesfeld CL, Irazoqui JE, Bloom K et al. The role of actin in spindle orientation changes during the Saccharomyces cerevisiae cell cycle. J Cell Biol 1999; 146(5):1019-1032.
101. Yin H, Pruyne D, Huffaker TC et al. Myosin V orientates the mitotic spindle in yeast. Nature 2000; 406(6799):1013-1015.
102. Beach DL, Thibodeaux J, Maddox P et al. The role of the proteins Kar9 and Myo2 in orienting the mitotic spindle of budding yeast. Curr Biol 2000; 10(23):1497-1506.
103. Hwang E, Kusch J, Barral Y et al. Spindle orientation in Saccharomyces cerevisiae depends on the transport of microtubule ends along polarized actin cables. J Cell Biol 2003; 161(3):483-488.
104. Simon VR, Karmon SL, Pon LA. Mitochondrial inheritance: cell cycle and actin cable dependence of polarized mitochondrial movements in Saccharomyces cerevisiae. Cell Motil Cytoskeleton 1997; 37(3):199-210.
105. Boldogh IR, Yang HC, Nowakowski WD et al. Arp2/3 complex and actin dynamics are required for actin-based mitochondrial motility in yeast. Proc Natl Acad Sci USA 2001; 98(6):3162-3167.
106. Mulvihill DP, Pollard PJ, Win TZ et al. Myosin V-mediated vacuole distribution and fusion in fission yeast. Curr Biol 2001; 11(14):1124-1127.
107. Gachet Y, Tournier S, Millar JB et al. Mechanism controlling perpendicular alignment of the spindle to the axis of cell division in fission yeast. EMBO J 2004; 23(6):1289-1300.
108. Catlett NL, Duex JE, Tang F et al. Two distinct regions in a yeast myosin-V tail domain are required for the movement of different cargoes. J Cell Biol 2000; 150(3):513-526.
109. Takizawa PA, Vale RD. The myosin motor, Myo4p, binds Ash1 mRNA via the adapter protein, She3p. Proc Natl Acad Sci USA 2000; 97(10):5273-5278.
110. Bohl F, Kruse C, Frank A et al. She2p, a novel RNA-binding protein tethers ASH1 mRNA to the Myo4p myosin motor via She3p. EMBO J 2000; 19(20):5514-5524.
111. Itoh T, Watabe A, Toh EA et al. Complex formation with Ypt11p, a rab-type small GTPase, is essential to facilitate the function of Myo2p, a class V myosin, in mitochondrial distribution in Saccharomyces cerevisiae. Mol Cell Biol 2002; 22(22):7744-7757.
112. Ishikawa K, Catlett NL, Novak JL et al. Identification of an organelle-specific myosin V receptor. J Cell Biol 2003; 160(6):887-897.

113. Tang F, Kauffman EJ, Novak JL et al. Regulated degradation of a class V myosin receptor directs movement of the yeast vacuole. Nature 2003; 422(6927):87-92.

114. Itoh T, Toh EA, Matsui Y. Mmr1p is a mitochondrial factor for Myo2p-dependent inheritance of mitochondria in the budding yeast. EMBO J 2004; 23(13):2520-2530.

115. Pashkova N, Catlett NL, Novak JL et al. Myosin V attachment to cargo requires the tight association of two functional subdomains. J Cell Biol 2005; 168(3):359-364.

116. Pashkova N, Catlett NL, Novak JL et al. A point mutation in the cargo-binding domain of myosin V affects its interaction with multiple cargoes. Eukaryot Cell 2005; 4(4):787-798.

117. Pashkova N, Jin Y, Ramaswamy S et al. Structural basis for myosin V discrimination between distinct cargoes. EMBO J 2006; 25(4):693-700.

118. Fagarasanu A, Fagarasanu M, Eitzen GA et al. The peroxisomal membrane protein Inp2p is the peroxisome-specific receptor for the myosin V motor Myo2p of Saccharomyces cerevisiae. Dev Cell 2006; 10(5):587-600.

119. Reck-Peterson SL, Tyska MJ, Novick PJ et al. The yeast class V myosins, Myo2p and Myo4p, are nonprocessive actin-based motors. J Cell Biol 2001; 153(5):1121-1126.

120. Balasubramanian MK, Bi E, Glotzer M. Comparative analysis of cytokinesis in budding yeast, fission yeast and animal cells. Curr Biol 2004; 14(18):R806-818.

121. Wolfe BA, Gould KL. Split decisions: coordinating cytokinesis in yeast. Trends Cell Biol 2005; 15(1):10-18.

122. Faty M, Fink M, Barral Y. Septins: a ring to part mother and daughter. Curr Genet 2002; 41(3):123-131.

123. Longtine MS, Bi E. Regulation of septin organization and function in yeast. Trends Cell Biol 2003; 13(8):403-409.

124. Versele M, Thorner J. Some assembly required: yeast septins provide the instruction manual. Trends Cell Biol 2005; 15(8):414-424.

125. Sohrmann M, Fankhauser C, Brodbeck C et al. The dmf1/mid1 gene is essential for correct positioning of the division septum in fission yeast. Genes Dev 1996; 10(21):2707-2719.

126. Santos B, Snyder M. Targeting of chitin synthase 3 to polarized growth sites in yeast requires Chs5p and Myo2p. J Cell Biol 1997; 136(1):95-110.

127. VerPlank L, Li R. Cell cycle-regulated trafficking of Chs2 controls actomyosin ring stability during cytokinesis. Mol Biol Cell 2005; 16(5):2529-2543.

128. Watts FZ, Shiels G, Orr E. The yeast MYO1 gene encoding a myosin-like protein Srrequired for cell division. EMBO J 1987; 6(11):3499-3505.

129. Rodriguez JR, Paterson BM. Yeast myosin heavy chain mutant: maintenance of the cell type specific budding pattern and the normal deposition of chitin and cell wall components requires an intact myosin heavy chain gene. Cell Motil Cytoskeleton 1990; 17(4):301-308.

130. Schmidt M, Bowers B, Varma A et al. In budding yeast, contraction of the actomyosin ring and formation of the primary septum at cytokinesis depend on each other. J Cell Sci 2002; 115(Pt 2):293-302.

131. Tolliday N, Pitcher M, Li R. Direct evidence for a critical role of myosin II in budding yeast cytokinesis and the evolvability of new cytokinetic mechanisms in the absence of myosin II. Mol Biol Cell 2003; 14(2):798-809.

132. Lippincott J, Li R. Sequential assembly of myosin II, an IQGAP-like protein and filamentous actin to a ring structure involved in budding yeast cytokinesis. J Cell Biol 1998; 140(2):355-366.

133. Kitayama C, Sugimoto A, Yamamoto M. Type II myosin heavy chain encoded by the myo2 gene composes the contractile ring during cytokinesis in Schizosaccharomyces pombe. J Cell Biol 1997; 137(6):1309-1319.

134. May KM, Watts FZ, Jones N et al. Type II myosin involved in cytokinesis in the fission yeast, Schizosaccharomyces pombe. Cell Motil Cytoskeleton 1997; 38(4):385-396.

135. Motegi F, Nakano K, Kitayama C et al. Identification of Myo3, a second type-II myosin heavy chain in the fission yeast Schizosaccharomyces pombe. FEBS Lett 1997; 420(2-3):161-166.

136. Bezanilla M, Forsburg SL, Pollard TD. Identification of a second myosin-II in Schizosaccharomyces pombe: Myp2p is conditionally required for cytokinesis. Mol Biol Cell 1997; 8(12):2693-2705.

137. McCollum D, Balasubramanian MK, Pelcher LE et al. Schizosaccharomyces pombe cdc4+ gene encodes a novel EF-hand protein essential for cytokinesis. J Cell Biol 1995; 130(3):651-660.

138. Epp JA, Chant J. An IQGAP-related protein controls actin-ring formation and cytokinesis in yeast. Curr Biol 1997; 7(12):921-929.

139. Eng K, Naqvi NI, Wong KC et al. Rng2p, a protein required for cytokinesis in fission yeast, is a component of the actomyosin ring and the spindle pole body. Curr Biol 1998; 8(11):611-621.

140. Naqvi NI, Eng K, Gould KL et al. Evidence for F-actin-dependent and -independent mechanisms involved in assembly and stability of the medial actomyosin ring in fission yeast. EMBO J 1999; 18(4):854-862.

141. Shannon KB, Li R. The multiple roles of Cyk1p in the assembly and function of the actomyosin ring in budding yeast. Mol Biol Cell 1999; 10(2):283-296.
142. Liu J, Tang X, Wang H et al. The localization of the integral membrane protein Cps1p to the cell division site is dependent on the actomyosin ring and the septation-inducing network in Schizosaccharomyces pombe. Mol Biol Cell 2002; 13(3):989-1000.
143. Itoh T, Erdmann KS, Roux A et al. Dynamin and the actin cytoskeleton cooperatively regulate plasma membrane invagination by BAR and F-BAR proteins. Dev Cell 2005; 9(6):791-804.
144. Tsujita K, Suetsugu S, Sasaki N et al. Coordination between the actin cytoskeleton and membrane deformation by a novel membrane tubulation domain of PCH proteins is involved in endocytosis. J Cell Biol 2006; 172(2):269-279.
145. Carnahan RH, Gould KL. The PCH family protein, Cdc15p, recruits two F-actin nucleation pathways to coordinate cytokinetic actin ring formation in Schizosaccharomyces pombe. J Cell Biol 2003; 162(5):851-862.
146. Kamei T, Tanaka K, Hihara T et al. Interaction of Bnr1p with a novel Src homology 3 domain-containing Hof1p. Implication in cytokinesis in Saccharomyces cerevisiae. J Biol Chem 1998; 273(43):28341-28345.
147. Wachtler V, Huang Y, Karagiannis J et al. Cell cycle-dependent roles for the FCH-domain protein Cdc15p in formation of the actomyosin ring in Schizosaccharomyces pombe. Mol Biol Cell 2006; 17(7):3254-3266.
148. Lippincott J, Li R. Dual function of Cyk2, a cdc15/PSTPIP family protein, in regulating actomyosin ring dynamics and septin distribution J Cell Biol 1998; 143(7):1947-1960.
149. Wu JQ, Kuhn JR, Kovar DR et al. Spatial and temporal pathway for assembly and constriction of the contractile ring in fission yeast cytokinesis. Dev Cell 2003; 5(5):723-734.
150. Ayscough KR, Stryker J, Pokala N et al. High rates of actin filament turnover in budding yeast and roles for actin in establishment and maintenance of cell polarity revealed using the actin inhibitor latrunculin-A. J Cell Biol 1997; 137(2):399-416.
151. Moseley JB, Goode BL. The yeast actin cytoskeleton: from cellular function to biochemical mechanism. Microbiol Mol Biol Rev 2006; 70(3):605-645.
152. Liu J, Taylor DW, Krementsova EB et al. Three-dimensional structure of the myosin V inhibited state by cryoelectron tomography. Nature 2006; 442(7099):208-211.
153. Thirumurugan K, Sakamoto T, Hammer JA 3rd et al. The cargo-binding domain regulates structure and activity of myosin 5. Nature 2006; 442(7099):212-215.

CHAPTER 15

Isoform Sorting of Tropomyosins

Claire Martin and Peter Gunning*

Abstract

Cytoskeletal tropomyosin (Tm) isoforms show extensive intracellular sorting, resulting in spatially distinct actin-filament populations. Sorting of Tm isoforms has been observed in a number of cell types, including fibroblasts, epithelial cells, osteoclasts, neurons and muscle cells. Different Tm isoforms have differential impact on the activity of a number of actin-binding proteins and can therefore differentially regulate actin filament function. Functionally distinct sub-populations of actin filaments can therefore be defined on the basis of the Tm isoforms associated with the filaments. The mechanisms that underlie Tm sorting are not yet well understood, but it is clear that Tm sorting is a very fluid and dynamic process, with changes in sorting occurring throughout development and cell differentiation. For this reason, it is unlikely that Tm localization is determined by an intrinsic sorting signal that directs particular isoforms to a single geographical location. Rather, a molecular sink model where isoforms accumulate in actin-based structures where they have the highest affinity, is most consistent with current data. This model would predict Tm sorting to be influenced by changes to actin filament dynamics and organization and collaboration with other actin-binding proteins.

Introduction

Mammalian tropomyosins (Tms) are encoded by four genes α, β, γ and δ. These genes undergo extensive alternative splicing to give rise to a large number of isoforms. These isoforms can be divided into two broad classes consisting of high molecular weight (HMW) and low molecular weight (LMW) isoforms through the use of alternative promoters (for more details, see Chapter 2). Tm isoforms have distinct expression patterns in various tissues and throughout development (see Chapter 4) and also show distinct patterns of subcellular localisation. Differential sorting of Tm isoforms was first observed in the 1980's and since then numerous examples of intracellular sorting of nonmuscle Tms have been described in a number of cell types. It is now clear that different Tm isoforms are able to specifically sort to distinct actin structures and subcompartments of cells. With the development of new anti-Tm antibodies and tagged constructs, more and more intracellular compartments defined by Tms are being identified and the functional consequences of this sorting is becoming better understood. The mechanisms that underlie this sorting process, however, are not well understood. In this review we will outline the sorting patterns of Tm isoforms in different cell types, examine how this sorting relates to specific cell functions and review the potential mechanisms that may account for Tm sorting.

*Corresponding Author: Peter Gunning—Oncology Research Unit, Department of Pharmacology, School of Medical Sciences, University of New South Wales, Sydney, NSW 2052, Australia. Email:p.gunning@unsw.edu.au.

Tropomyosin, edited by Peter Gunning. ©2008 Landes Bioscience and Springer Science+Business Media.

Sorting of Tm Isoforms in Specific Cell Types

Fibroblasts

The first direct evidence of differential Tm sorting in cells was obtained using double-label immunofluorescence in fibroblasts.[1] In chicken embryo fibroblast cells, both HMW isoforms of the α gene and LMW isoforms of the γ gene localize to stress fibres, whereas only LMW isoforms also sort to ruffling membrane regions. A similar pattern is seen in human EJ (bladder carcinoma) cells, with HMW isoforms again excluded from the ruffling membrane regions.[1] Cultured mouse embryonic fibroblasts also appear to exclude HMW isoforms from the cell periphery (Fig. 1).[2]

Tm isoforms can also sort to distinct actin structures in NIH 3T3 cells. Synchronised replated cells show differential sorting of isoforms 1h after replating, with γTm isoforms sorting to a peri-nuclear region and αTm isoforms sorting to peripheral stress fibres.[3] This difference in sorting becomes less distinct as cells progress through the G1 phase of the cell cycle, with both sets of isoforms localizing to stress fibres by 5h after replating. There are still some differences, however, with enrichment of the αTm isoforms at the cell periphery compared to γTm. Further studies in NIH 3T3 cells have indicated distinct sorting patterns for the γTm isoforms Tm5NM1 and Tm5NM2. While Tm5NM1 localizes to stress fibres, the WS5/9d antibody which preferentially recognises Tm5NM2 indicates Tm5MN2 sorts to perinuclear actin structures associated with the Golgi complex.[4]

In contrast to earlier studies, microinjection of labelled recombinant αTm isoforms into rat fibroblasts showed no differences in sorting between HMW isoforms and LMW isoforms.[5] All isoforms were incorporated into microfilaments and extended to the edges of the cells. Co-injection of HMW and LMW isoforms (e.g., Tm2 and Tm5a) showed no difference in localization. Tm5b did show fainter staining in microfilaments than the other isoforms, indicating this isoform is less able to incorporate into microfilaments, most likely a result of its lower affinity for actin. The lack of sorting identified in this study may be a result of bacterially-produced proteins which lack posttranslational modifications such as acetylation, or due to an over-abundance of the exogenous protein which is therefore not mimicking the endogenous sorting pattern.[5]

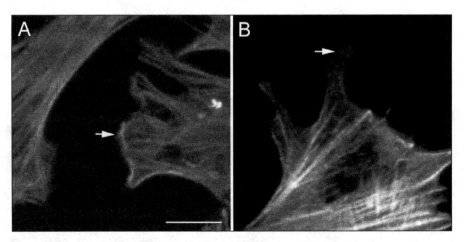

Figure 1. Tm isoforms are differentially sorted in fibroblasts. Mouse embryonic fibroblasts show differential sorting between LMW and HMW isoforms as shown by the antibodies αf9d which recognises isoforms 6, 1, 2, 3, 5a and 5b (A) and Tm311 which recognises isoforms 6, 1, 2 and 3 (B) HMW but not LMW (i.e., Tm5a/5b) isoforms appear to be excluded from the cell periphery. Scale bar, 20 μm.

Epithelial Cells

Distinct Tm sorting patterns have also been observed in epithelial cells. In T84 epithelial monolayers, the LMW isoforms Tm5a and Tm5b show enrichment at the apical membrane, while γTm isoforms and the HMW αTm isoforms are distributed throughout the cytoplasm.[6] This polarization of LMW Tm isoforms becomes more distinct with increasing differentiation. Apical/basal sorting also occurs in vivo, with human colon epithelial cells showing enrichment of HMW Tms at the basolateral surface and enrichment of Tm5NM1/2 at the apical surface.[3]

Differences in Tm localization have been observed in adhesion belts and stress fibres in LLC-PK1 epithelial cells. The LMW Tm5a/5b localize to both stress fibres and adhesion belts, while the HMW αTms localize to stress fibres only.[7] Products of the γ gene also localize to adhesion belts. When exogenous isoforms are transfected into the cells, HMW isoforms are again restricted to the stress fibres, while Tm5a/5b localize to both stress fibres and adhesion belts. Like the HMW αTm isoforms, Tm4 is excluded from adhesion belts, however this isoform binds only weakly to stress fibres.[7]

Studies of *Cryptosporidium parvum* invasion in epithelial cells have shown specific rearrangement and localization of Tm isoforms in response to invasion. In HCT-8 cells infected with *C. parvum*, γTm isoforms accumulate at the infection sites, but Tm4 does not.[8] This localization of γTm is associated with an accumulation of actin filaments at the infection sites. In CHO cells, γTm again specifically localizes to infection sites, as does Tm4 in some cases. A similar pattern of γTm accumulation is also seen in *C. parvum* infected mice in vivo. A CHO cell line stably overexpressing hTm5NM1 is more readily infected by the parasite than a line expressing a hTm5/3 mutant. This data, taken together, suggests that the functional Tm5NM1 isoform may enhance bacterial invasion.[8]

Osteoclasts

Another type of adhesion structure is seen in bone-resorbing osteoclasts. These cells show distinct sorting of Tm isoforms to the podosome attachment structure. Tm4 and the LMW isoforms Tm5a/5b are enriched in the podosomes, whereas Tm5NM1 and the HMW isoforms Tm2/3 are relatively excluded from these structures.[9] Within the podosome structure there is more specific sorting, with Tm4 being enriched at the upper surface and less so at the ventral plasma membrane, while Tm5a/5b encircle the podosomes at the base of the cell and are enriched in the upper and outer edges of the actin ring. While both Tm5NM1 and Tm2/3 are present in the cell interior, there is little colocalization between these isoforms.[9] Thus, at least four isoform specific structures are present in osteoclasts.

Neurons

Distinct and tightly regulated sorting patterns have been observed in neurons and Tm sorting in these cells has therefore been extensively studied. Intracellular localization of Tm in neurons was first studied by Burgoyne and Norman[10] who found an antibody to chicken gizzard Tm showed enriched staining in cell bodies and dendrites compared to axons. Further studies in chromaffin cells showed that a specific Tm is associated with chromaffin granule membranes.[11]

Neurons show temporally-regulated patterns of Tm localization (Fig. 2). In early cortical neurons Tm4 is localized to cell bodies and also strongly enriched in growth cones.[12] TmBr1/3 is not observed significantly in cell bodies or growth cones at this time, however appears after several days in culture[12] and is localized to the axon and presynaptic bouton in the adult neuron.[13] Tm5NM1/2 localize to the axon but not cell bodies and dendrites in early neurons in vivo, but are lost from the axon and appear in the cell body between embryonic days 15-17 in the rat.[13] This is the same time at which TmBr1/3 appear in axons, indicating that isoform "switching" has occurred. In the adult brain Tm5NM1/2 appear to have a somatodendritic localization.[13] Tm5a/5b are also temporally regulated in neurons, being present in growth cones of early neurons in culture, but not in older cultures.[14]

In 14.5 day embryonic cortical neurons an antibody that preferentially detects Tm5NM2 shows staining in the cell body and neurites, but not the growth cone. CG3, which recognises all

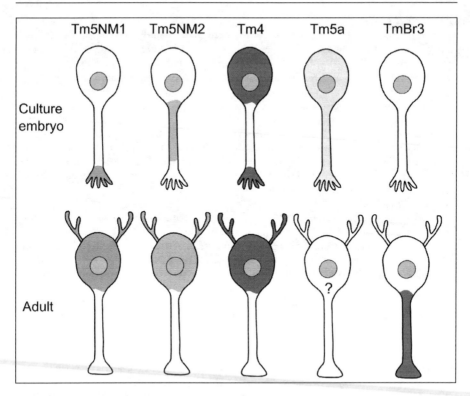

Figure 2. Tm isoform sorting in neurons is developmentally regulated. In the embryonic neuron, Tm5NM1/2, Tm4 and Tm5a show different sorting patterns. These sorting patterns are altered in mature neurons, with Tm5NM1/2 and Tm4 relocating to a somatodendritic compartment and TmBr3 replacing them in the adult axon. Figure adapted from reference 47.

isoforms from the γ gene, does stain growth cones, indicating that other γTm isoforms are present.[14] The γ/9d antibody shows Tm5NM1 is localized to growth cones in embryonic neurons.[15] Finally, in transgenic mice expressing the human Tm5NM1, this Tm shows specific localization to the growth cones and not the cell body or neurites.[15] Tm5NM2 is therefore likely to be the γ9d-containing isoform in the axons of developing neurons. The localization of γTm isoforms with different C- termini has been examined in the adult brain using antibodies specific for exons 9a, 9c and 9d. In adult neurons γ/9d appears to stain cell bodies and dendrites but not axons, whereas γ/9a and γ/9c stain cell bodies, dendrites and axons.[16]

Muscle

Muscle fibres contain three muscle-specific 9a-containing Tm isoforms which form part of the thin filament. These isoforms appear to be restricted to the thin filament, where they act as a regulatory switch to regulate contraction (see Chapter 8).[17] Despite the abundance of these muscle-specific Tms, muscle fibres also contain a number of cytoskeletal Tm isoforms. These cytoskeletal isoforms are not localized to the thin filament, but rather have specific sorting patterns within the myofibril. The γTm isoform Tm5NM1 is specifically sorted to a γ-actin based filament network adjacent to the Z-line and also to a subsarcolemmal actin-filament system at the periphery of the myofibril.[18] The Tm4 isoform is also present in a γ-actin filament system associated with the Z-line and unlike Tm5NM1, Tm4 is also present in longitudinal filaments that run perpendicular to the Z-line.[19] These longitudinal structures are associated with repair and remodelling of the myofibril. Expression of ectopic Tm3 in transgenic mouse muscle leads to accumulation of this isoform in Z-line-adjacent filaments, but also results in a muscular-dystrophy-like phenotype, indicating the normal cytoskeletal network may be disrupted when Tms are expressed in inappropriate locations.[18]

Functional Consequences of Tm Sorting

The sorting of particular Tm isoforms to specific compartments in cells is consistent with specific functional roles for these isoforms. A number of studies have identified links between a particular Tm sorting pattern and functional consequences of this sorting.

Golgi

The localization of Tm5NM2 to a perinuclear compartment in NIH 3T3 cells indicates an association of this isoform with the Golgi complex.[4] This association has been investigated further by immunogold labelling of Tm5NM2 using both CG3 and WS5/9d antibodies. These studies confirm an interaction of γTm isoforms with short Golgi-associated microfilaments and the surface of coated vesicles derived from the Golgi.[4] Earlier studies have also shown that one or more γTm isoforms are associated with selected Golgi-derived vesicles, but Tms from the α and β genes are not.[20]

The Golgi apparatus is closely associated with an actin-based microfilament system, as well a microtubule system[21] and intermediate filaments.[22] Actin microfilaments play an important role in maintaining the shape of the Golgi structure as well as correct functioning of vesicle budding and fission.[23] The localization of specific Tms to these filaments is likely to help modulate actin function in this region, allowing finer regulation of these microfilaments.

Lamellapodia

Lamellapodia are motile structures located at the leading edges of cells. They are characterized by a dynamic actin network comprised of short branched actin filaments which are rapidly turned over. DesMarais et al[24] reported that Tm, while present in lamellapodia, is relatively absent from the leading edge of the cell where the F-actin concentration is high, indicating a tropomyosin-free compartment in the most dynamic region of the lamellapodium. Hillberg et al[25] demonstrated endogenous HMW Tms extend out to the very edge of the lamella in MTLn3 cells, although staining is weaker within 0.1-0.2 μm of the leading edge. Likewise, HMW Tms also extend into the lamella of migrating human fibroblasts, with disorganized Tm structures in the 1-4 μm region transitioning to actin-filament associated Tm further in. These results were confirmed via expression of exogenous Tms. Both HA-tagged and GFP-tagged Tms extend to the edges of the lamellapodia. GFP-tagged Tms show a weaker signal very close to the leading edge, indicating a lower concentration of tagged Tm in this region. HA-tagged Tm4 and Tm5, both LMW, appear to be present at the leading edges of the lamella at higher concentrations than the HMW Tm1 and Tm2, confirming observations in fibroblasts that HMW isoforms are less abundant at the periphery of cells.[1,2] Localization of these tagged Tms appears to be punctate close to the leading edge, becoming more organized further into the lamella until they are integrated into actin stress fibres.[25]

Many other actin-binding and remodelling proteins are enriched in this leading edge, especially Arp2/3 and ADF/cofilin. These proteins are involved in the rapid turnover of actin filaments in this region, which leads to the highly dynamic properties of the leading edge. As Tm isoforms have been shown to inhibit the activity of these proteins, the relatively lower concentration of Tm at the leading edge may allow this rapid remodelling to occur.[25]

CFTR

The cystic fibrosis transmembrane conductance regulator (CFTR) transports chloride ions across the apical surface of epithelial cells. In T84 epithelial cells the LMW Tm5a/5b have a specific apical localization, in contrast to HMW isoforms which are more basally localized.[6] Tm5a/5b specifically localize to regions of the membrane where the CFTR receptor is inserted, indicating these isoforms may have a functional role in regulating membrane levels of this protein. Knockdown of these isoforms using antisense oligonucleotides leads to an increase in CFTR surface expression, confirming a role for Tm5a/5b in regulating the CFTR levels in the plasma membrane.[6]

Neurons

Neurons are highly differentiated cells, which show distinct changes in Tm sorting throughout development. These changes in localization indicate that certain Tm isoforms may have specific roles at various stages of development. The Tm5NM1/2 isoforms for example are highly enriched in the developing axon, but not the mature axon, indicating a possible functional role in axonal development and outgrowth.[13] Sorting of Tm5NM1/2 occurs very early in differentiation and sorting of Tm5NM1/2 mRNA to the axonal pole may occur prior to differentiation, in cells that do not yet have processes. Tm5NM1/2 is therefore an early marker for the development of neural polarity.[26]

Both Tm5NM1/2 and Tm4 are highly enriched in the early growth cone, indicating a role for these isoforms in neurite outgrowth during development.[12,15] Tm4 is also enriched in postsynaptic terminals of neurons in the rat cerebellum, specifically in the post synaptic densities.[12] This indicates a potential role for Tm4 in synaptic function. In contrast, TmBr3 is present at presynaptic sites, indicating this isoform is likely to have a different role in synaptic function to Tm4.[12]

Mechanisms of Tm Sorting

The sorting of Tm isoforms appears to be tightly regulated, both spatially and temporally. While specific locations of Tm isoforms have been described for many cell types and changes in sorting throughout maturation, differentiation and the cell cycle have also been described, the mechanisms which control this sorting are yet to be fully understood. There are a number of potential mechanisms which may be involved and the complexity of Tm sorting indicates that there is likely to be more than one mechanism contributing to the sorting of these molecules.

mRNA Sorting

One way in which proteins can be sorted to intracellular compartments is by sorting mRNA, resulting in localized synthesis which ensures the protein is only expressed where it is required. A number of cytoskeletal proteins show localized mRNA, including actin.[27] In developing neurons in situ, Tm5NM1/2 mRNA is localized within cell bodies and enriched at the axonal pole and in the proximal region of the developing axon.[26] This correlates with an axonal localization for Tm5NM isoforms in early neurons.[13] In mature neurons the Tm5NM1/2 mRNA appears to be distributed more evenly throughout the cell body,[26] again correlating with known protein localization.[13] TmBr2 mRNA is distributed evenly throughout the cell body but excluded from the axonal pole.[26] In cultured neurons, Tm5NM1/2 but not TmBr2 mRNA again appears to have a polarized distribution , with Tm5NM1/2 mRNA present in axons and cell bodies in differentiated cells.[26] TmBr3 mRNA shows a cell body distribution in mature neurons with enrichment near the axon,[28] correlating with the known axonal distribution of the protein.[12,13]

Localization of mRNA does not perfectly correspond to protein localization, however. The protein localization is broader in neurons than the mRNA localization. Tm4 mRNA shows the same localization as Tm5NM1/2 mRNA, being enriched in the axonal pole of the cell body and the proximal axon,[28] but the Tm4 protein is widely distributed in neurons, present in cell bodies, dendrites and axons. So while these two proteins again show similar mRNA localization, their protein localization is different, indicating additional mechanisms must be involved. It may be that mRNA localization can be used to regulate sites of protein synthesis and assembly and other mechanisms are then used to direct the protein to its final location.

Exogenous Tm5NM1 lacking the 3' UTR shows identical sorting to the endogenous protein, localizing to the growth cone in neurons (Fig. 3), while another exogenous isoform not normally expressed in neurons, Tm3, localizes much more broadly to the cell bodies, neurites and growth cones.[15] In fibroblasts, exogenous Tm5NM1 with and without the 3' UTR show identical sorting to that seen for the endogenous protein.[29] These studies therefore indicate that the coding sequence alone is enough to direct sorting of Tm isoforms and the 3' UTR is not essential.

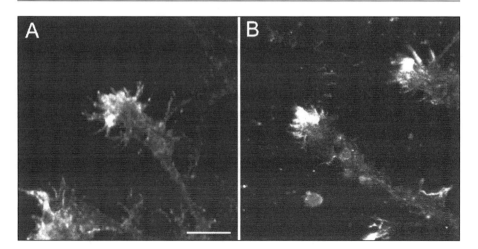

Figure 3. Exogenous Tm in transgenic mice sorts to the same compartment as endogenous Tm. Both endogenous Tm5NM1 as observed by the γ9d antibody (A) and exogenous Tm5NM1 as observed by the LC1 antibody (B) show enrichment in growth cones of mouse cortical neurons in 5 day cultures.[15] Scale bar, 10 μm.

Actin Structures

Tm sorting may be influenced by the actin isoform present in filaments, as it appears as though there are preferred associations between particular actin and Tm isoforms. Overexpression of γ-actin in myoblasts results in reduced sorting of Tm2 but not Tm5 into stress fibres,[30] suggesting competition of isoforms for inclusion into structures may play a role in sorting.

The role of actin structures in sorting of Tm isoforms has been studied using pharmacological agents that can disrupt the actin microfilament system. Treatment of neurons with cytochalasin B results in loss of specific sorting by the γTm isoforms. Washout of the drug leads to relocation of isoforms to their original locations.[14] These studies therefore indicate that an intact microfilament system is required for sorting of Tm isoforms. Intact actin structures also appear to be required for the polarized distribution of Tm5a/5b in epithelial cells. Treatment of these cells with the actin-disrupting drug cytochalasin D eliminates the polarized distribution of these isoforms.[6] Treatment with nocodazole, a microtubule-disrupting drug, does not eliminate polarized staining of Tm5a/5b, indicating that intact microtubules are not required for the polarization of Tms in epithelial cells.[6]

Microtubules form a separate cytoskeletal system from the actin microfilaments and are a major structural component of the axon. Treatment of neurons with nocodozole leads to redistribution of isoforms and a loss of Tm5a/5b and Tm5NM1/2 colocalization in axons,[14] indicating the microtubule system is involved in the maintenance of Tm sorting in neurons.

Isoforms from the γTm and αTm genes both sort to stress fibres in fibroblasts. Treatment with the drug cytochalasin D leads to loss of actin stress fibres, however stress fibres containing γTm isoforms are more resistant to cytochalasin D than those containing αTm and βTm isoforms.[3] It therefore appears that these two groups of isoforms may not bind to the same individual actin filament, but are instead associated with distinct filaments bundled together in the same stress fibre. The concept of homopolymers of Tm isoforms is also supported by the observation of isoform sorting per se. The very fact that Tm isoforms are segregated indicates individual populations of actin filaments contain primarily one isoform.

Isoform Specific Actin Affinities

There is evidence that alternative exon choice is capable of directing alternative sorting. Choice of an alternative N-terminus in the α gene (1a and 2b for HMW isoforms or 1b for LMW isoforms) can send these isoforms to different compartments in fibroblasts[2] and epithelial cells.[6] The choice of an alternative C-terminus in the γ gene can influence sorting in the brain. Isoforms with the 9d terminus are excluded from axons in adult neurons,[13] while 9a and 9c containing isoforms are present in axons, as well as cell bodies and dendrites.[16] An alternative splice choice has also been shown to direct alternative sorting in fibroblasts, with the 6a-containing Tm5NM1 sorting to stress fibres and the 6b-containing Tm5NM2 sorting to a perinuclear compartment.[4] Similarly, Tm5NM2 is targeted to the axon shaft in neurons whereas Tm5NM1 is localised to the growth cone.[15]

Exon 6 has been shown to be important for actin affinity in αTm. The 6a9d-containing isoform binds actin more strongly than the 6b9d-containing isoform and deletion of exon 6 results in loss of actin affinity, indicating that this region of the molecule is required for binding to actin.[31] This loss of actin affinity is more pronounced in isoforms containing the 9d C-terminus than in isoforms containing the 9a C-terminus, indicating that other exons can have a modulating effect and actin affinity does not depend on a single region of the protein. Note that in contrast, the choice of exon 6a or 6b in βTm does not appear to alter actin affinity, although the choice of exon 9a or 9d can.[32] This indicates that the effect on actin affinity of choosing one exon over another is not necessarily conserved between genes. It appears as though sorting of Tms in general is more conserved within genes, than between isoforms of similar exon structure from different genes. For example, a γ9c-containing isoform shows more similar sorting to γ9a-containing isoforms than to a 9c isoform from the α gene.[33] In addition, whereas Tm5b and Tm5NM1 share the same exon structure, containing the exons 1b, 6a and 9d, they show very different sorting patterns in epithelial cells.[6] All Tms exist as dimers when bound to actin and the formation of homo- or hetero-dimers can also alter actin affinity. The information for dimerization is contained within the Tm molecule and can be influenced by alternatively spliced exons (see Chapter 6).[34]

Unlike other proteins that may have a geographical targeting signal included within the alternatively-spliced region, Tm isoforms do not appear to contain an intrinsic targeting sequence that directs them to a particular compartment. Although alternative exon choice can influence sorting, as described above, this sorting is cell-type specific and also changes with development and differentiation, indicating that the process of Tm sorting is flexible and dynamic. This argues against a specific targeting signal in the manner of nuclear targeting or membrane localization signals. Rather, it appears as though multiple regions of the protein and perhaps the molecule as a whole is responsible for sorting. The differences in sorting for isoforms containing different exons may be explained by these exons influencing changes in flexibility and actin affinity, interactions with other proteins and modulation by signalling pathways.

Signalling

Organisation of the actin cytoskeleton is regulated by a number of signalling pathways. These are likely to contribute to Tm sorting by altering the composition of actin filaments in particular regions of the cell, therefore leading to changes in Tm accumulation at these sites. Members of the Rho pathway are involved in reorganisation of the cytoskeleton, with different members involved in promoting formation of different types of structures. Rho is involved in assembly of stress fibres,[35] Rac in formation of lamellipodia and membrane ruffles and Cdc42 in formation of filopodia.[36] Rac and Cdc42 alter actin polymerisation at the cell periphery through activation of the Arp2/3 complex through WAVE and WASP proteins respectively and Rho stimulates actin polymerisation to promote stress fibres through formins and can also promote myosin II actin-filament cross-linking activity through increased phosphorylation of myosin light chain.[37] Rho kinase (ROCK) is the downstream target of Rho and ROCK can also activate the downstream effector LIM kinase (LIMK). LIMK can directly regulate actin polymerisation via phosphorylation and inactivation of the actin-severing proteins ADF/cofilin and has also been implicated as a regulator of microtubule assembly/disassembly. As well as activation by phosphorylation via ROCK, LIMK can also be activated by p21-activated kinase.[38]

Although there is no evidence of a direct link between the Rho and LIM pathways and Tm, there is some evidence that Tm can be phosphorylated. Phosphorylation is a very common post-translational modification that can not only alter protein activity, but can also alter the localization of many proteins. Tropomyosin-1 can be phosphorylated in endothelial cells in response to oxidative stress. This phosphorylation is associated with reorganisation of the actin cytoskeleton and recruitment of Tm1 into stress fibres, indicating that phosphorylation of Tm may be able to alter its localization.[39] It has been proposed that phosphorylation of Tm1 may be a major factor in actin bundling, assembly of focal contacts and generation of cellular tension.[39,40] Phosphorylation of Tm1 occurs downstream of ERK (extracellular signal-regulated kinase), although the kinase that is responsible for this phosphorylation has not yet been identified.

Lessons from Other Cytoskeletal Proteins

Many other cytoskeletal proteins show differential isoform sorting and these may provide models by which the mechanisms of Tm sorting may be understood. Sorting of cytoskeletal actin isoforms has been observed in neurons,[13] muscle[41] and other cell types,[42] although the mechanisms by which this sorting occurs have not been extensively studied. More is understood about the sorting mechanisms of myosin isoforms which, like Tms, comprise a large multigene family. These studies indicate that multiple mechanisms can contribute to the sorting of myosin isoforms.

Myosin IIA and IIB show spatial sorting within migrating endothelial cells, with myosin IIA enriched at the leading edge and IIB enriched at the trailing edge.[43] Injection of fluorescent analogues of these isoforms indicate that sorting is intrinsic to the proteins themselves and timelapse studies indicate that the different isoforms have different rates of incorporation into structures, which may explain their differential localizations. Myosin IIA is incorporated into new structures more quickly than myosin IIB and is also lost more rapidly when structures are disassembled, consistent with the presence of this isoform at the leading, but not the trailing edges of cells.[43]

Phosphorylation of myosins can alter their localization. Myosin II requires de-phosphorylation of the heavy chain in order to localize to the cleavage furrow of *Dictyostelium* during cytokinesis. This may reflect a need for the myosin to form higher order structures in the form of thick filaments before it can be properly localized to the cleavage furrow.[44] Studies in *Drosophila* S2 cells indicate the initial stage of myosin localization to the cleavage furrow requires Rho1 signalling and Rho kinase phosphorylation of the light chain of myosin II. This is thought to increase thick filament formation.[45] The same study indicates that filamentous actin is not required for the initial localization of myosin II to the cleavage furrow, but is involved in stabilising it once it gets there.

Myosin light chain isoforms show ability to compete for inclusion into structures in muscle cells, with a hierarchical order of binding specificity that mimics the developmental expression of these isoforms. This allows each new isoform expressed to have a higher binding affinity and therefore efficiently replace the previous proteins, while maintaining the stability of the structures. When multiple isoforms are expressed at once, some isoforms are preferentially sorted to the myofibrils, while those with lower affinities are distributed throughout the cytoplasm.[46]

Implications of Tm Sorting

Tm sorting is widespread in a number of cell types, including neurons, epithelial cells and fibroblasts. Although the mechanisms underlying the sorting of Tm isoforms is yet to be fully understood, it is clear that this is a very dynamic and tightly-regulated process. As more examples of Tm sorting are identified it is becoming increasingly clear that specific isoforms are associated with functionally distinct populations of actin filaments.[47] Differential sorting of isoforms is a way to regulate the amount of different Tm isoforms available at specific intracellular sites and therefore control the incorporation of Tms into specific microfilament populations. Because different Tm isoforms have diverse properties and functions with respect to actin and actin-binding proteins (see Chapters 17-21) this sorting can confer specific functional properties to the actin microfilaments and therefore the regulation of Tm sorting can directly contribute to the regulation of actin-filament function.[48]

In the yeast *Saccharomyces cerevisiae*, loss of both Tm genes, TPM1 and TPM2, is lethal and TPM2 cannot compensate for the loss of TPM1 indicating that these two genes have distinct functions.[49] Knockout of the entire αTm or γTm genes in mice is embryonically lethal,[50-52] indicating products of each of these genes are required for cell survival. Knockout of individual isoforms within one gene has much more subtle effects however,[33] indicating that different isoforms from the same gene may be able to compensate for each other. Despite some functional redundancy within genes, it is clear that different Tm isoforms can confer different properties on the actin filament. Tm isoforms show differential abilities to bind actin[31,32] and isoform-specific regulation of the activity of actin-binding proteins myosin,[48,53] ADF/cofilin,[48] gelsolin[54] and formin.[55] These varying properties allow different Tm isoforms to differentially regulate actin filament function.

The large number of Tm isoforms may allow finer regulation of Tm function and activity, as each isoform may be regulated independently. Even isoforms with very similar properties may be regulated differently in time and space, whereas sorting of isoforms with different properties and functions may be a mechanism by which these specific functions can be restricted to the region of the cell where they are required and prevented from being expressed where they are not required. Sorting of Tm isoforms may also help direct the sorting of other cytoskeletal proteins. For example, overexpression of Tm5NM1 is able to recruit myosin II into stress fibres and displace ADF.[48]

Models of Sorting

The central question regarding the mechanism of sorting of Tm isoforms concerns the relative roles of active transport vs. passive diffusion of the molecules. Because Tm isoforms do not appear to contain an intrinsic geographical targeting signal that directs them to a particular region in all cells it is considered unlikely that an active transport system can account for the observed sorting of Tms.[47,56] Instead it appears that multiple regions of the protein and perhaps the protein as a whole are responsible for directing sorting.[56]

The simplest explanation for the accumulation of isoforms in specific structures is the 'molecular sink' model in which isoforms accumulate in structures where they have the highest affinity and are most stable.[47,56] This hypothesis is supported by drug studies, which indicate that fragmentation of actin structures can abolish Tm sorting[6,14] and also correlates with the observations that Tm sorting is flexible throughout development and alters as new structures are formed. Tm isoforms can compete for inclusion into specific actin structures, as demonstrated by the exclusion of HMW Tms from stress fibres in cells overexpressing Tm5NM1.[48]

Tm sorting can be influenced by other actin binding proteins and changes in actin organisation and dynamics. Changes in actin structure and associated proteins will influence the affinity of a particular Tm isoform in any actin-based structure and therefore alter the accumulation of specific Tms at that site. In turn, accumulation of a specific Tm isoform at a particular site in the cell will influence the properties of actin filaments by regulating the association with local actin binding proteins. Thus, collaboration between available Tms and the activity of local actin binding proteins will lead to the local assembly of functionally distinct actin filaments.

An example of this collaborative model is shown in Figure 4. Consider a situation where LIM kinase (LIMK) is active and ADF/cofilin is phosphorylated and inactivated and therefore will not compete with Tms for binding to actin. If myosin light chain kinase (MLCK) is also active, myosin will be phosphorylated and activated, promoting formation of stress fibres which preferentially accumulate the Tm5NM1 isoform. In contrast, if LIMK and MLCK are inactivated, then the equilibrium shifts towards active ADF which competes with some Tms (e.g., Tm5NM1) for actin filament binding, but collaborates with TmBr3 promoting the formation of shorter filaments that incorporate TmBr3 (Fig. 4).[56] In this way, the local active actin binding proteins and a specific Tm(s) act to promote the formation of a functionally specific actin filament at a particular site in the cell. As long as the local signalling and the availability of the specific Tm remain unchanged,

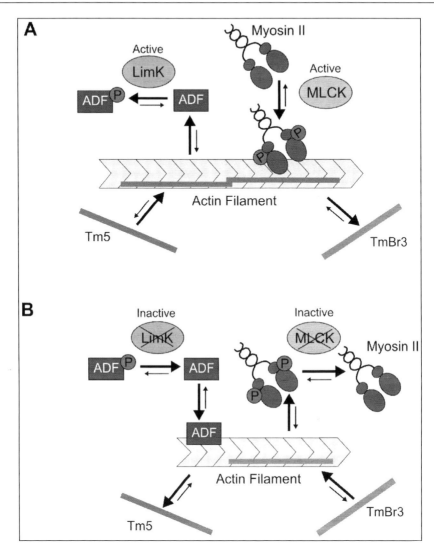

Figure 4. A collaborative model of Tm sorting. Local active actin binding proteins and specific Tms act to promote the formation of functionally specific actin filaments at a particular site in the cell. Local concentrations of all the components will drive competitive/collaborative interactions which will result in assembly of the most thermodynamically stable filaments. A) If LIM kinase and MLCK are active then ADF/cofilin will be inactivated and therefore will not compete with Tms for binding to actin and activated myosin II will promote formation of stress fibres which preferentially accumulate the Tm5NM1 isoform. B) In contrast, if LIMK and MLCK are inactivated then myosin II disengages and the equilibrium shifts towards active ADF which competes with some Tms for actin filament binding, but collaborates with TmBr3, promoting the formation of shorter filaments that favour binding of TmBr3.[56]

the type of actin filament should remain the same. The use of a single type of Tm along the length of the actin filament will also promote fidelity of function along the length of that filament.

Conversely, overexpression of Tm5NM1 will outcompete ADF/cofilin leading to elevated ADF and its subsequent phosphorylation whereas TmBr3 will promote binding of ADF/cofilin to actin filaments.[48] Thus, local concentrations of all the components will drive competitive/collaborative interactions which will result in assembly of the most thermodynamically stable filaments. The spatial segregation of Tm isoforms may therefore be seen as the differential outcomes of these reactions at different sites in the cell.

It appears that cytoskeletal pools of Tm-containing filaments are not fixed in size.[57] Overexpression of exogenous cytoskeletal Tm leads to no decrease in expression of endogenous Tm, indicating the absence of a feedback mechanism to control cytoskeletal Tm expression. This is in contrast to sarcomeric Tms, where overexpression leads to a decrease in endogenous Tm in order to maintain the strict stoichiometry of actin and actin-binding proteins within the sarcomere.[58] Overexpressed cytoskeletal Tms accumulate in the same intracellular locations as endogenous Tm, indicating that these cytoskeletal pools are not saturated with Tm. Increased levels of Tm5NM1 lead to an increase in filamentous actin, indicating a shift in equilibrium towards increased F-actin and filament formation.[57] This suggests that the supply of individual cytoskeletal Tms is limiting for the assembly of actin filaments containing that isoform. This is most consistent with a 'molecular sink' model where Tms define both the pool size and the functional characteristics of specific actin filament populations.

Future Directions

Despite the progress that has been made in understanding how differential sorting of Tm isoforms occurs, there are a number of questions that remain unanswered. It remains to be seen if there is any kind of signal at the destination that is specific for any particular isoform, or if it is indeed simply a matter of actin affinities. It has also not yet been conclusively disproven that there is active transport involved, or what might direct this active transport if it occurred. The role of Tm in structure formation is also yet to be understood. It has been shown that some structures can be perturbed by removal of specific isoforms[6] and knockout studies have indicated that while some compensation by other isoforms can occur within genes, products from both the mammalian α and γ genes are absolutely required for life. It is not clear if an isoform is removed from a structure whether another will step in to take its place, or whether there are some types of actin-filaments that absolutely depend on specific Tm isoforms for their formation and maintenance. Study of knockout mice will be required to unambiguously answer this question.

In conclusion, Tm isoforms show extensive intracellular sorting which results in spatially distinct actin filament populations. Tm isoforms have different properties with respect to actin and actin-binding proteins and can therefore differentially regulate and confer functional differences on these actin filament populations. Although the mechanisms that control the intracellular sorting of Tm isoforms are not well understood, it appears as though many factors may contribute, including actin-filament dynamics, actin-affinity of Tm isoforms and other actin-binding proteins, all of which may favour the accumulation of particular isoforms at cellular sites. In the future, manipulation of the activity of specific actin binding proteins should reveal their role in the restriction of Tms to specific intracellular sites.

Acknowledgements

This work is supported by the Australian National Health and Medical Research Council (NHMRC) (PG, #117409) and funding from the Oncology Children's Foundation. PG is a Principal Research Fellow of the NHMRC (#163626).

References

1. Lin JJ, Hegmann TE, Lin JL. Differential localization of tropomyosin isoforms in cultured nonmuscle cells. J Cell Biol 1988; 107(2):563-572.
2. Schevzov G, Vrhovski B, Bryce NS et al. Tissue-specific tropomyosin isoform composition. J Histochem Cytochem 2005; 53(5):557-570.
3. Percival JM, Thomas G, Cock TA et al. Sorting of tropomyosin isoforms in synchronised NIH 3T3 fibroblasts: evidence for distinct microfilament populations. Cell Motil Cytoskeleton 2000; 47(3):189-208.

4. Percival JM, Hughes JA, Brown DL et al. Targeting of a tropomyosin isoform to short microfilaments associated with the Golgi complex. Mol Biol Cell 2004; 15(1):268-280.
5. Pittenger MF, Helfman DM. In vitro and in vivo characterization of four fibroblast tropomyosins produced in bacteria: TM-2, TM-3, TM-5a and TM-5b are colocalized in interphase fibroblasts. J Cell Biol 1992; 118(4):841-858.
6. Dalby-Payne JR, O'Loughlin EV, Gunning P. Polarization of specific tropomyosin isoforms in gastrointestinal epithelial cells and their impact on CFTR at the apical surface. Mol Biol Cell 2003; 14(11):4365-4375.
7. Temm-Grove CJ, Jockusch BM, Weinberger RP et al. Distinct localizations of tropomyosin isoforms in LLC-PK1 epithelial cells suggests specialized function at cell-cell adhesions. Cell Motil Cytoskeleton 1998; 40(4):393-407.
8. O'Hara SP, Lin JJ. Accumulation of tropomyosin isoform 5 at the infection sites of host cells during Cryptosporidium invasion. Parasitol Res 2006; 99(1):45-54.
9. McMichael BK, Kotadiya P, Singh T et al. Tropomyosin isoforms localize to distinct microfilament populations in osteoclasts. Bone 2006; 39(4):694-705.
10. Burgoyne RD, Norman KM. Immunocytochemical localization of tropomyosin in rat cerebellum. Brain Res 1985; 361(1-2):178-184.
11. Burgoyne RD, Norman KM. Presence of tropomyosin in adrenal chromaffin cells and its association with chromaffin granule membranes. FEBS Lett 1985; 179(1):25-28.
12. Had L, Faivre-Sarrailh C, Legrand C et al. Tropomyosin isoforms in rat neurons: the different developmental profiles and distributions of TM-4 and TMBr-3 are consistent with different functions. J Cell Sci 1994; 107(Pt 10):2961-2973.
13. Weinberger R, Schevzov G, Jeffrey P et al. The molecular composition of neuronal microfilaments is spatially and temporally regulated. J Neurosci 1996; 16(1):238-252.
14. Schevzov G, Gunning P, Jeffrey PL et al. Tropomyosin localization reveals distinct populations of microfilaments in neurites and growth cones. Mol Cell Neurosci 1997; 8(6):439-454.
15. Schevzov G, Bryce NS, Almonte-Baldonado R et al. Specific features of neuronal size and shape are regulated by tropomyosin isoforms. Mol Biol Cell 2005; 16(7):3425-3437.
16. Vrhovski B, Schevzov G, Dingle S et al. Tropomyosin isoforms from the gamma gene differing at the C-terminus are spatially and developmentally regulated in the brain. J Neurosci Res 2003; 72(3):373-383.
17. Perry SV. Vertebrate tropomyosin: distribution, properties and function. J Muscle Res Cell Motil 2001; 22(1):5-49.
18. Kee AJ, Schevzov G, Nair-Shalliker V et al. Sorting of a nonmuscle tropomyosin to a novel cytoskeletal compartment in skeletal muscle results in muscular dystrophy. J Cell Biol 2004; 166(5):685-696.
19. Vlahovich N, Schevzov G, Nair-Shalliker V et al. Tropomyosin 4 defines novel filaments in skeletal muscle associated with muscle remodelling/regeneration in normal and diseased muscle. Cell Motil Cytoskeleton 2008; 65(1):73-85.
20. Heimann K, Percival JM, Weinberger R et al. Specific isoforms of actin-binding proteins on distinct populations of Golgi-derived vesicles. J Biol Chem 1999; 274(16):10743-10750.
21. Rios RM, Bornens M. The Golgi apparatus at the cell centre. Curr Opin Cell Biol 2003; 15(1):60-66.
22. Gao Y, Sztul E. A novel interaction of the Golgi complex with the vimentin intermediate filament cytoskeleton. J Cell Biol 2001; 152(5):877-894.
23. Egea G, Lazaro-Dieguez F, Vilella M. Actin dynamics at the Golgi complex in mammalian cells. Curr Opin Cell Biol 2006; 18(2):168-178.
24. DesMarais V, Ichetovkin I, Condeelis J et al. Spatial regulation of actin dynamics: a tropomyosin-free, actin-rich compartment at the leading edge. J Cell Sci 2002; 115(Pt 23):4649-4660.
25. Hillberg L, Zhao Rathje LS, Nyakern-Meazza M et al. Tropomyosins are present in lamellipodia of motile cells. Eur J Cell Biol 2006; 85(5):399-409.
26. Hannan AJ, Schevzov G, Gunning P et al. Intracellular localization of tropomyosin mRNA and protein is associated with development of neuronal polarity. Mol Cell Neurosci 1995; 6(5):397-412.
27. Du TG, Schmid M, Jansen RP. Why cells move messages: the biological functions of mRNA localization. Semin Cell Dev Biol 2007; 18(2):171-177.
28. Hannan AJ, Gunning P, Jeffrey PL et al. Structural compartments within neurons: developmentally regulated organization of microfilament isoform mRNA and protein. Molecular & Cellular Neurosciences 1998; 11(5-6):289-304.
29. Percival JM. Cell cycle regulation of actin and tropomyosin isoforms [PhD thesis]. Sydney (NSW): University of Sydney 2002.
30. Schevzov G, Lloyd C, Hailstones D et al. Differential regulation of tropomyosin isoform organization and gene expression in response to altered actin gene expression. J Cell Biol 1993; 121(4):811-821.

31. Hammell RL, Hitchcock-DeGregori SE. The sequence of the alternatively spliced sixth exon of alpha-tropomyosin is critical for cooperative actin binding but not for interaction with troponin. J Biol Chem 1997; 272(36):22409-22416.

32. Pittenger MF, Kistler A, Helfman DM. Alternatively spliced exons of the beta tropomyosin gene exhibit different affinities for F-actin and effects with nonmuscle caldesmon. J Cell Sci 1995; 108(Pt 10):3253-3265.

33. Vrhovski B, Lemckert F, Gunning P. Modification of the tropomyosin isoform composition of actin filaments in the brain by deletion of an alternatively spliced exon. Neuropharmacology 2004; 47(5):684-693.

34. Gimona M, Watakabe A, Helfman DM. Specificity of dimer formation in tropomyosins: influence of alternatively spliced exons on homodimer and heterodimer assembly. Proc Natl Acad Sci USA 1995; 92(21):9776-9780.

35. Ridley AJ, Hall A. The small GTP-binding protein rho regulates the assembly of focal adhesions and actin stress fibers in response to growth factors. Cell 1992; 70(3):389-399.

36. Kozma R, Ahmed S, Best A et al. The Ras-related protein Cdc42Hs and bradykinin promote formation of peripheral actin microspikes and filopodia in Swiss 3T3 fibroblasts. Mol Cell Biol 1995; 15(4):1942-1952.

37. Jaffe AB, Hall A. Rho GTPases: biochemistry and biology. Annu Rev Cell Dev Biol 2005; 21:247-269.

38. Bernard O. Lim kinases, regulators of actin dynamics. Int J Biochem Cell Biol 2006; b39(6):1071-1076.

39. Houle F, Rousseau S, Morrice N et al. Extracellular signal-regulated kinase mediates phosphorylation of tropomyosin-1 to promote cytoskeleton remodeling in response to oxidative stress: impact on membrane blebbing. Mol Biol Cell 2003; 14(4):1418-1432.

40. Houle F, Huot J. Dysregulation of the endothelial cellular response to oxidative stress in cancer. Mol Carcinog 2006; 45(6):362-367.

41. Lubit BW, Schwartz JH. An antiactin antibody that distinguishes between cytoplasmic and skeletal muscle actins. J Cell Biol 1980; 86(3):891-897.

42. Herman IM. Actin isoforms. Curr Opin Cell Biol 1993; 5(1):48-55.

43. Kolega J. Cytoplasmic dynamics of myosin IIA and IIB: spatial 'sorting' of isoforms in locomoting cells. J Cell Sci 1998; 111(15):2085-2095.

44. Sabry JH, Moores SL, Ryan S et al. Myosin heavy chain phosphorylation sites regulate myosin localization during cytokinesis in live cells. Mol Biol Cell 1997; 8(12):2605-2615.

45. Dean SO, Rogers SL, Stuurman N et al. Distinct pathways control recruitment and maintenance of myosin II at the cleavage furrow during cytokinesis. Proc Natl Acad Sci USA 2005; 102(38):13473-13478.

46. Komiyama M, Soldati T, von Arx P et al. The intracompartmental sorting of myosin alkali light chain isoproteins reflects the sequence of developmental expression as determined by double epitope-tagging competition. J Cell Sci 1996; 109(8):2089-2099.

47. Gunning PW, Schevzov G, Kee AJ et al. Tropomyosin isoforms: divining rods for actin cytoskeleton function. Trends Cell Biol 2005; 15(6):333-341.

48. Bryce NS, Schevzov G, Ferguson V et al. Specification of actin filament function and molecular composition by tropomyosin isoforms. Mol Biol Cell 2003; 14(3):1002-1016.

49. Drees B, Brown C, Barrell BG et al. Tropomyosin is essential in yeast, yet the TPM1 and TPM2 products perform distinct functions. J Cell Biol 1995; 128(3):383-392.

50. Blanchard EM, Iizuka K, Christe M et al. Targeted ablation of the murine alpha-tropomyosin gene. Circ Res 1997; 81(6):1005-1010.

51. Rethinasamy P, Muthuchamy M, Hewett T et al. Molecular and physiological effects of alpha-tropomyosin ablation in the mouse. Circ Res 1998; 82(1):116-123.

52. Hook J, Lemckert F, Qin H et al. Gamma tropomyosin gene products are required for embryonic development. Mol Cell Biol 2004; 24(6):2318-2323.

53. Fanning AS, Wolenski JS, Mooseker MS et al. Differential regulation of skeletal muscle myosin-II and brush border myosin-I enzymology and mechanochemistry by bacterially produced tropomyosin isoforms. Cell Motil Cytoskeleton 1994; 29(1):29-45.

54. Ishikawa R, Yamashiro S, Matsumura F. Differential modulation of actin-severing activity of gelsolin by multiple isoforms of cultured rat cell tropomyosin. Potentiation of protective ability of tropomyosins by 83-kDa nonmuscle caldesmon. J Biol Chem 1989; 264(13):7490-7497.

55. Wawro B, Greenfield NJ, Wear MA et al. Tropomyosin Regulates Elongation by Formin at the Fast-Growing End of the Actin Filament. Biochemistry 2007; 46(27):8146-8155.

56. Gunning P, O'Neill G, Hardeman E. Tropomyosin-based regulation of the actin cytoskeleton in time and space. Physiological Reviews. 2008;88(1):1-35.

57. Schevzov G, Fath T, Vrhovski B et al. Divergent regulation of the sarcomere and the cytoskeleton. J Biol Chem 2008; 283(1):275-283.

58. Muthuchamy M, Grupp IL, Grupp G et al., Molecular and physiological effects of overexpressing striated muscle beta-tropomyosin in the adult murine heart. J Biol Chem 1995; 270(51):30593-30603.

Human Tropomyosin Isoforms in the Regulation of Cytoskeleton Functions

Jim Jung-Ching Lin*, Robbin D. Eppinga, Kerri S. Warren
and Keith R. McCrae

Abstract

Over the past two decades, extensive molecular studies have identified multiple tropomyosin isoforms existing in all mammalian cells and tissues. In humans, tropomyosins are encoded by *TPM1* (α-*Tm*, 15q22.1), *TPM2* (β-*Tm*, 9p13.2-p13.1), *TPM3* (γ-*Tm*, 1q21.2) and *TPM4* (δ-*Tm*, 19p13.1) genes. Through the use of different promoters, alternatively spliced exons and different sites of poly(A) addition signals, at least 22 different tropomyosin cDNAs with full-length open reading frame have been cloned. Compelling evidence suggests that these isoforms play important determinants for actin cytoskeleton functions, such as intracellular vesicle movement, cell migration, cytokinesis, cell proliferation and apoptosis. In vitro biochemical studies and in vivo localization studies suggest that different tropomyosin isoforms have differences in their actin-binding properties and their effects on other actin-binding protein functions and thus, in their specification of actin microfilaments. In this chapter, we will review what has been learned from experimental studies on human tropomyosin isoforms about the mechanisms for differential localization and functions of tropomyosin. First, we summarize current information concerning human tropomyosin isoforms and relate this to the functions of structural homologues in rodents. We will discuss general strategies for differential localization of tropomyosin isoforms, particularly focusing on differential protein turnover and differential isoform effects on other actin binding protein functions. We will then review tropomyosin functions in regulating cell motility and in modulating the anti-angiogenic activity of cleaved high molecular weight kininogen (HKa) and discuss future directions in this area.

Introduction

Tropomyosin (Tm) is a coiled-coil dimer protein that lies end-to-end in the actin groove and plays important roles in regulating muscle contraction. In addition, tropomyosin provides structural stability of actin filaments and modulates cytoskeleton function.[1-6] In mammals, there are four tropomyosin genes that potentially produce, through alternative splicing, a large number of protein isoforms.[1,2,4-9] Molecular cloning, RT-PCR and Northern blot analyses have identified at least 24 full-length tropomyosin isoforms in rodents. The existence of these isoforms in mouse cells/tissues has been further verified by protein and Western blot analyses.[3,5,9-13] Accumulated lines of evidence support the hypothesis that different tropomyosin isoforms within the cells bind to different populations of actin filaments to create specific structural domains for the actin cytoskeleton that perform their discrete functions. Specific examples of such isoforms that determine or create distinct populations of actin filaments in neuron, epithelial cells and skeletal

*Corresponding Author: Jim Jung-Ching Lin—Department of Biology, University of Iowa, 340BBE, Iowa City, IA 52242-1324, U.S.A. Email: jim-lin@uiowa.edu

Tropomyosin, edited by Peter Gunning. ©2008 Landes Bioscience
and Springer Science+Business Media.

muscle, have been extensively reviewed in three excellent articles.[2,4,5] In addition, a recent article has comprehensively reviewed the historical aspects of tropomyosin structure and function, the molecular basis of tropomyosin diversity, tropomyosin isoform-based regulation of actin dynamics and tropomyosin in human disease.[3] In this chapter, we focus our discussion on the existence, the differential localization and the differential functions of human tropomyosin isoforms. Where possible, the results from studies with rodent tropomyosin isoforms will be related to the discussion of human tropomyosin isoforms.

Human Tropomyosin Gene Organization and Isoforms

To understand how human tropomyosin isoforms can specify functional diversity of actin filaments, we first need to categorize how many tropomyosin genes and isoforms exist in humans. Recent advances in the human genome project, functional genomics, gene cloning and expression profiling lead to a summary that in humans, 4 tropomyosin genes, *TPM1* (previously named α-*Tm*), *TPM2* (β-*Tm*), *TPM3* (γ-*Tm*, *hTm30nm* or *hTmnm*) and *TPM4* (δ-*Tm*, *hTm30pl* or *hTmpl*) are localized to chromosomes, 15q22.1 (Hs.133892), 9p13.2-p13.1 (Hs.300772), 1q21.2 (Hs.644306) and 19p13.1 (Hs. 631618, http://www.ncbi.nlm.nih.gov/UniGene/clust.cgi), respectively. As shown in Figure 1, human tropomyosin genes generate, through the use of alternatively spliced exons, different promoters and different poly(A) additional signals, at least 22 different mRNAs with full-length open reading frames, which have been cloned from various human tissues and cells. The exon and intron organization of these genes are very similar to that of rodent tropomyosin genes,[3] except that in the rodent δ-*Tm* gene, there are no equivalent exons 1a and 2 found so far. Based on the current cDNA data, only *TPM1* gene utilized alternative exon 2a or 2b. The *TPM2* and *TPM4* genes did not use alternative exons for exon 1 and 6, respectively. For a convenient comparison in the literature, the names of related isoforms in rodents (Tm) are given in parentheses after each of the human tropomyosin (hTm) (Fig. 1). These tropomyosin isoforms are traditionally classified into two major groups, high molecular weight (HMW) isoforms containing 284-285 amino acids (aa) except hTm1-1 and low molecular weight (LMW) isoforms containing 245-248 aa and they are expressed differentially in various tissues and cell types.

Muscle Tropomyosin Isoforms

The principal tropomyosin isoforms found in human striated muscles are α-fast tropomyosin (αf-Tm)/hTmskα1 from the *TPM1* gene, β-tropomyosin (β-Tm)/hTmskβ from the *TPM2* gene and α-slow tropomyosin (αs-Tm)/hTmskα2 from the *TPM3* gene. In adult human hearts, β to α tropomyosin ratio is about 1:4.8, whereas adult mouse hearts contain almost exclusively the α isoform.[14] The slow-twitch muscle isoform, hTmskα2, was cloned from human skeletal muscle[15] but has not been detected in human heart.[14,16] Adult mouse hearts also express very little α-slow muscle (αs-Tm) isoform.[17] In addition to hTmskα1, the human heart expresses hTmskα1-1 isoform utilizing exon 2a of the *TPM1* gene.

In smooth muscle-enriched tissues such as placenta and uterus, hTmsmα and hTmsmα-1 from the *TPM1* gene, hTm1 from the *TPM2* gene and hTm5 from the *TPM3* gene have been cloned. In addition, both *hTmsmα* and *hTm1* messages are detected in human stomach, another smooth muscle-enriched tissue, by Northern blot analysis.[16] Therefore, human muscle tropomyosin isoforms include hTmskα1, hTmskβ, hTmskα2 and hTmskα1-1 in striated muscle, hTmsmα, hTm1 and hTmsmα-1 in smooth muscle.

Nonmuscle/Cytoskeletal Tropomyosin Isoforms

Protein and cloning studies from human nonmuscle cell lines such as MRC-5, HuT-11, HuT-14 and WI-38 have previously identified at least eight tropomyosin isoforms. These are hTm2, hTm3, hTmsmα, hTm5a and hTm5b from the *TPM1* gene, hTm1 from the *TPM2* gene, hTm5 from the *TPM3* gene and hTm4 from the *TPM4* gene.[16,18-22] Further cloning from placenta and placenta choriocarcinoma libraries identifies hTm2, hTm3, hTm3-1, hTmsmα-1 and hTm5b from the *TPM1* gene, hTm1 from the *TPM2* gene, mutant hTm5 from the *TPM3* gene and hTm4 from the *TPM4* gene. Therefore, two more isoforms, hTmsmα-1 and hTm3-1, are included in the

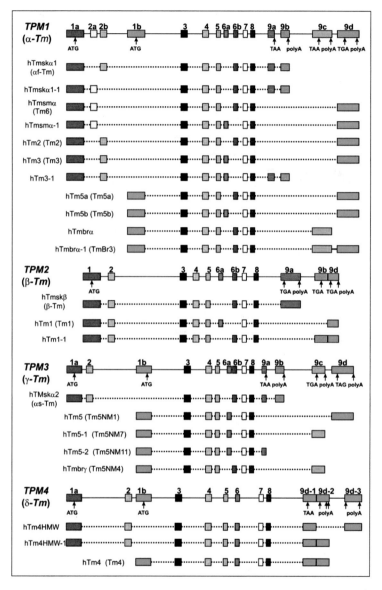

Figure 1. Schematic diagram of human tropomyosin gene organization and isoform diversity. In humans, there are 4 tropomyosin genes, *TPM1* (α-*Tm*), *TPM2* (β-*Tm*), *TPM3* (γ-*Tm*) and *TPM4* (δ-*Tm*), located in different chromosomes. The exon (indicated by the colored box) and intron (indicated by the solid line) organization of these genes is very similar. After splicing out the intron (indicated by the dashed line), each gene is capable of generating multiple mRNAs that encode different proteins. The isoforms that are listed under each gene have been detected in human tissues and/or cell lines and their cDNAs with full-length open reading frame have been cloned. Isoform variation occurs at both N- and C-termini, as well as an internal exon 6. However, alternative usages of the exon 1 for the *TPM2* gene and the exon 6 for the *TPM4* gene have not been detected. The corresponding isoforms found in rodents and named by Gunning's group[3] are included in parentheses. The isoforms hTm4 and hTm5 are synonymous with hTmpl and hTmnm, respectively.[21,22]

nonmuscle tropomyosin list. As previously reported for rat brain,[10] human brain also expresses its own specific isoforms, hTmbrα and hTmbrα-1 from the *TPM1* gene and hTmbrγ from the *TPM3* gene. However, differing from rat brain, human brain expresses muscle isoform hTmskβ from the *TPM2* gene. Full-length cDNA clones encoding hTmbrα, hTmskβ and hTMbrγ have been obtained from a human fetal brain library, whereas hTmbrα, hTmbrα-1 and hTmskβ were cloned from adult human brain and hippocampus libraries (Table 1). Both hTmbrα and hTmbrα-1 have the same protein sequence with 245 residues, whereas hTmbrγ contains 247 residues. Other brain-specific tropomyosin isoforms (TmBr1 and TmBr2) derived from the rodent α-*Tm* gene have not been found in human brain. Interestingly, both human fetal and adult brains express the HMW muscle tropomyosin (hTmskβ). The localization and function of hTmskβ and brain-specific isoforms (hTmbrα, hTmbrα-1 and hTmbrγ) in the brain remain to be determined. Early studies on cardiomyocytes and skeletal muscles unambiguously showed the presence of nonmuscle tropomyosin isoforms in adult muscles,[3,6,14,23-27] which performed important roles in regulating actin dynamics and functions. Therefore, the division between muscle and nonmuscle tropomyosin isoforms based on tissue types may not be suitable and we will refer these nonmuscle forms as cytoskeletal isoforms.

Similar to erythrocytes,[28,29] Jurkat T-cells express hTm5b and hTm5. It has been shown that both hTm5 and hTm5b bind more strongly to tropomodulin, a tropomyosin-binding and actin filament capping protein, than other tropomyosin isoforms.[28-30] In erythrocytes, the hTm5-tropomodulin or hTm5b-tropomodulin complexes together with spectrin, adducin, capZ, protein 4.1 and 4.9 provide a membrane skeletal network for membrane stability under mechanical stress.[31] Tropomyosin-tropomdulin complexes appear to stabilize and limit actin into a short filament

Table 1. *Summary of human tropomyosin isoforms, GenBank accession numbers for full-length cDNA clones and expressed tissues/cells*

Tropomyosin Isoforms and Predicted aa Residues	Accession Number	Expressed Tissues/Cells
hTmskα1 (αf-Tm), 284aa	M19713, AY640415, NM_001018005	Skeletal muscle, cardiac muscle
hTmskβ (β-Tm), 284aa	X06825, CR614416, CR615839, NM_003289	Skeletal muscle, cardiac muscle, fetal brain, adult brain
hTmskα2 (αs-Tm), 285aa	X04201, BC008407, BC008425, NM_152263	Skeletal muscle
hTmskα1-1, 284aa	AY640414	Cardiac muscle
hTmsmα (Tm6), 284aa	AL050179, NM_001018007	Adult uterus, cell lines: MRC-5, WI-38
hTmsmα-1, 284aa	CR594134, CR622076, NM_001018020	Placenta
hTm1 (Tm1), 284aa	CR626020, AK223258, BC011776, M75165, M74817, NM_213674	Placenta, stomach mucosa, cell lines: MRC-5, WI-38, and T84, pancreatic adenocarcinoma, colon, colon carcinoma
hTm1-1, 322aa	CR590682	HeLa
hTm2 (Tm2), 284aa	CR598963, CR626242, NM_001018004	Fetal liver, placenta, cell lines: MRC-5, HuT-14 and T84

continued on next page

Table 1. Continued

Tropomyosin Isoforms and Predicted aa Residues	Accession Number	Expressed Tissues/Cells
hTm3 (Tm3), 284aa	CR623950, CR610885, NM_001018006	Placenta, neuroblastoma, cell lines: MRC-5, HuT-14, WI-38 and T84
hTm3-1, 284aa	BC007433, NM_000366	placenta choriocarcinoma
hTm4 (Tm4), 248aa	X05276, M12127, CR599958, BC002827, BC037576, BC067225, NM_003290	Cell lines: MRC-5, HuT-14, WI-38, HeLa and T84, placenta choriocarcinoma, eye retinoblastoma, testis embryonal carcinoma
hTm4HMW, 284aa	AK023385	Ovary tumor tissue
hTm4HMW-1, 284aa	CR599958	HeLa
hTm5 (Tm5NM1), 248aa	X04588, CR618509, AK026559, CR617822, BC072428, CR597930, BC015403, BC000771, BC017195, NM_153649	Cell lines: MRC-5, HuT-14, WI-38, T84, and KATO III, Jurkat T-cell, uterus leiomyosarcoma, leukocytes, fetal liver, bone osteosarcoma, kidney renal cell adenocarcinoma, placenta choriocarcinoma
hTm5-1/TC22 (Tm5NM7), 247aa	AY004867, NM_001043352	Colon carcinoma T84
hTm5-2 (Tm5NM11), 247aa	AF474157	Leukocytes from skeletal muscle
hTm5a (Tm5a), 248aa	L02922* (clone pSNL30-5)	Cell lines: WI-38
hTm5b (Tm5b), 248aa	CR501288, CR604708, CR590047, X12369, CR604315, CR602634	Placenta, cell lines: WI-38, Jurkat T-cell, fetal and adult liver, neuroblastoma
hTmbrα, 245aa	CR603337, CR623323 BC050473, NM_001018008	Fetal and adult brain, hippocampus
hTmbrα-1 (TmBr3), 245aa	AB209041	Brain
hTmbrγ (hTm5NM4), 247aa	CR589996, NM_001043353	Fetal brain

The tropomyosin isoform listed in the parenthesis represents the known rodent homolog of human isoform.
*L02922 represents exon 1b sequence derived from clone pSNL30-5, which contains a 1.5 kb cDNA insert encoding aa #3-248 of hTm5a.16

(protofilament) with a length of only one tropomyosin molecule. Selective removal of these tropomyosins from erythrocyte membrane impairs the membrane mechanical stability, as assayed by the resistance to shear in the ektacytometer. The addition of these erythrocyte tropomyosins back to tropomyosin-depleted membranes reverses the loss of stability. This stabilizing effect appears to be highly isoform-specific, because the HMW tropomyosin isoforms cannot restore the mechanical stability.[32] These results clearly demonstrate the differential functions among tropomyosin isoforms.

Liver expresses hTm2, hTm5b and hTm5. Tropomyosin isoforms, hTm3, hTm5b and hTm5 mutant were found in a neuroblastoma library. From the *TPM2* gene, hTm1 has been found in pancreatic adenocarcinoma and colon epithelia. In addition, hTm5 has been cloned from bone osteosarcoma and kidney renal cell adenocarcinoma. From the *TPM4* gene, hTm4 has been found in eye retinoblastoma and embryonic carcinoma testis. Colon cancer cell line T84 expresses a new isoform related to hTm5, hTm5-1 (also named TC22), in addition to hTm1, hTm4 and hTm5.[33] Characterization of TC22 reveals that it is preferentially associated with colonic neoplasia and carcinoma. This TC22 may provide a useful biomarker for surveillance of colon cancer. Leukocytes from skeletal muscle appear to express another isoform related to hTm5, hTm5-2 (Tm5NM11 rodent homologue), from the *TPM3* gene.

HeLa cells express an unusual large tropomyosin (322 amino acid residues) hTm1-1 from the *TPM2* gene and hTm4HMW-1 from the *TPM4* gene. Tumor tissue of ovary expresses another HMW isoform of hTm4, hTm4HMW. Thus, at least 22 different tropomyosin isoforms are found in various human muscle and nonmuscle tissues and cells. Table 1 summarizes these isoforms with GenBank accession numbers for their full-length cDNA clones, which were obtained from the listed tissue/cell libraries.

Strategies and Evidence for Differential Localization of Tropomyosins within the Cells

Actin filaments are believed to provide protrusive and contractile properties to the cell during movement and cytokinesis, to contribute to vesicle movement and to change and maintain cell shape,[1,34-38] but the mechanisms controlling their dynamics are not completely understood. A number of regulatory mechanisms, employing many actin binding proteins, have evolved to control the dynamics of actin filaments.[34,38] These regulatory activities (and an example of their corresponding actin-binding proteins) include: G-actin monomer sequestering (thymosin β4), ADP-actin to ATP-actin nucleotide exchange (profilin), actin nucleation (formins), branching actin polymerization (Arp2/3), linear actin polymerization (formins), actin filament capping (capping protein), actin filament severing (cofilin), actin filament stabilization (tropomyosin), actin filament cross-linking and/or bundling (fascin) and actin filament contraction (myosin II).

Tropomyosin, when bound to actin filaments, influences the actin-activated myosin activity, increases actin filament stability and modulates the activities of other actin binding proteins.[3,6-8] Early studies have shown that muscle tropomyosin isoforms after phosphorylation increase their head-to-tail polymerization and promote actin activated myosin activity.[3] A few cytoskeletal tropomyosin isoforms, such as Tm1 in the oxidative stressed cells or Tm2 during agonist-dependent receptor internalization, can undergo phosphorylation and possibly change their ability to modulate actin dynamics.[39,40] However, most of the cytoskeletal tropomyosin isoforms purified from chick, rat and human nonmuscle cells do not have detectable posttranslational modifications such as phosphorylation or methylation.[41-43] In order for actin filaments to effectively perform the above listed functions, nonmuscle cells express multiple isoforms of tropomyosin and differentially localize them in a temporospatially regulated manner where they collaborate with other actin binding proteins to influence actin dynamics.

Different Tropomyosin Isoforms Occupy Slightly Different Positions along Actin Filaments

In striated muscle, actomyosin contraction is switched on by calcium binding to troponin complex, resulting in the movement of tropomyosin, presumably from a position which sterically and allosterically hinders actin-myosin interaction.[44,45] Different tropomyosin isoforms (αf-Tm, β-Tm and αs-Tm) may occupy different positions on the thin filaments,[46,47] thus regulating different types of contractile forces.[17,48] Several lines of evidence supporting this claim include tropomyosin isoform switching from 80% αf-Tm and 20% β-Tm in fetal heart to almost exclusively αf-Tm in adult mouse heart,[25,49] the re-expression of β-Tm in adult heart during pressure overload-induced hypertrophy,[24] various myopathies caused by muscle tropomyosin missense mutations[50-56] and altered systolic function in the transgenic mouse heart overexpressing β-Tm[49,57] or αs-Tm.[48]

Smooth muscle and nonmuscle cells do not express troponin complex and the mechanism of tropomyosin-mediated stimulation of myosin is not clear. In these cells, phosphorylated myosin might move tropomyosin into a position that favors myosin activation[58,59] and this movement might be regulated by caldesmon,[60] a multiple interacting protein that binds Ca^{2+}-calmodulin, tropomyosin, myosin and actin.[61] Caldesmon inhibits actin-activated myosin ATPase in vitro, but full inhibition requires the presence of tropomyosin.[62,63] Caldesmon-tropomyosin regulation affects phosphate release of myosin[64,65] and may block myosin-actin interaction. Fluorescence resonance energy transfer studies using tagged tropomyosin in reconstituted thin filaments show that caldesmon interacts with and alters the position of tropomyosin and thereby potentially limits the ability of myosin heads to move tropomyosin to a position favoring ATPase activation.[60] Different tropomyosin isoforms in the presence of caldesmon may occupy different position along actin filaments and subsequently affect the actin dynamics. The evidences consistent with this claim include that fibroblast caldesmon enhances the binding of LMW tropomyosin isoforms to actin filaments greater than HMW isoforms;[66-68] and that overexpression of caldesmon fragment containing actin-, tropomyosin- and Ca^{2+}/calmodulin-binding sites in cells prevents LMW isoforms from turnover, thus stabilizing actin bundles.[69]

In Vitro Biochemical Properties Differ among Tropomyosin Isoforms

Biochemical studies show that cytoskeletal[67,70,71] and smooth muscle tropomyosins,[71-73] when bound to actin, enhance the myosin ATPase activity in a calcium independent manner. The degree of effect varies between isoforms. For instance, under the same conditions, the HMW hTm3 increases the myosin ATPase activity 1.5 fold over actin alone, whereas the LMW hTm5 increases myosin activity 4.7 fold.[67] Enhanced actin-myosin stimulation by cytoskeletal tropomyosin contrasts with the effect of skeletal muscle tropomyosin, which has been reported to inhibit the myosin ATPase activity.[6,74,75] Studies with chicken homologues of αf-Tm and Tm3 and with *Xenopus* homolog of Tm5b also reveal that different tropomyosin isoforms when bound to actin filaments differ in their ability to regulate myosin II and brush border myosin I ATPase activity, as well as the activity assayed by in vitro motility.[76]

Tropomyosin can influence actin dynamics independent of myosin II by binding and stabilizing actin filaments. Different tropomyosin isoforms exhibit different actin binding kinetics. Evidence to support this has been reviewed several times.[3,7,8] For example, the LMW hTm5 binds more stronger than HMW hTm3 to actin filaments, however, the binding of hTm3 exhibits higher cooperativity than hTm5.[67] When the affinity for actin filaments was compared between recombinant rat tropomyosin isoforms with the same C-terminal sequence, LMW Tm5b > HMW Tm2 > HMW Tm3 > LMW Tm5a[77] and when all isoforms with the same internal exon sequence were compared, LMW Tm5a > HMW Tm2 > HMW αf-Tm > HMW TmBr1 = LMW TmBr3.[78] There appears to be no correlation between the size of isoforms and actin binding affinity; rather the spliced exons at the internal and at both N- and C-termini of tropomyosin are the determinants of actin affinity. It has been shown that native muscle tropomyosins exist in heterodimers, which have different properties from homodimers.[79,80] Although most of the cytoskeletal tropomyosin isoforms purified from fibroblasts have been shown to exist in homodimers,[41,42] it is possible that the ability of tropomyosin isoforms to form heterodimer inside the cell may also affect their actin binding affinity.[79-82]

Tropomyosin promotes the stress fiber formation by repressing the branching activities of Arp2/3[83,84] and encouraging the actin bundling abilities of formins.[85] Tropomyosin can stabilize these bundles by protecting actin filaments from the depolymerizing or severing actions of cofilin,[86-88] DNase I,[89] gelsolin[90-92] and villin.[93,94] Tropomyosin can also limit actin depolymerization by working with tropomodulin to cap the pointed ends of actin filaments[95] and by repressing depolymerization from the pointed end of actin filaments independent of[96] or in spite of[92] capping proteins. Tropomyosin also antagonizes the bundling ability of villin[93] and fascin.[97,98] Thus, tropomyosin is a universal regulator for actin filament dynamics. The question is whether different tropomyosin isoforms regulate these activities differentially. There are very few report in which human tropomyosin has been used to address this question. However, it has been shown that rat recombinant Tm5a is the strongest inhibitor of Arp2/3 branching activity, followed by Tm2 and then αf-Tm isoform.[84] This differential effect is consistent with the differential localization of tropomyosin isoforms. The LMW Tm5a can be found in lamella and near lamellipodia,[43,99-103] regions of highly dynamic actin. The HMW Tm2 is mainly localized to the stress fibers, whereas the αs-Tm is found in the relatively stable thin filaments of muscle cells. Emerging conclusion from these studies and others is that collaborative activities among Arp2/3, profilin, capping protein and cofilin at the leading edges of migrating cells regulate actin assembly and disassembly, which can drive lamellipodial motility.[1,38] Although tropomyosin plays no direct role in lamellipodial assembly, LMW tropomyosin isoform localized to this region can limit the size of lamellipodium.[104]

Tropomyosins Have Isoform-Specific Turnover Rates in Human Cell Lines

One consistent hallmark of transformation is the suppressed expression of one or more of the HMW tropomyosin isoforms.[3,8,105] This isoform-specific down-regulation correlates to a deranged actin cytoskeleton, few actin stress fibers and a more rounded morphology, suggesting a role of HMW tropomyosin isoforms for protecting and organizing actin filaments. Restoration of Tm1 expression reorganizes stress fibers and suppresses the malignant growth of ras- and src-transformed cells.[106,107] TGF-β treatment of epithelial cells and several transformed cells but not high-grade, metastatic carcinoma MDA-MB-231 cells induces the expression of HMW tropomyosin isoforms from *TPM1* and *TPM2* genes and subsequently restores actin stress fibers and inhibits cell migration.[108] The mechanism for the failure of TGF-β to induce stress fiber and inhibit cell motility in MDA-MB-321 cells is that the methylation of *TPM1* proximal promoter in these tumor cells silences the expression of *TPM1* but not *TPM2* and then alters TGF-β tumor suppressor function.[109]

Besides the suppression of isoform-specific synthesis, protein turnover may also contribute to the disappearance of HMW isoforms from actin stress fibers. We have performed metabolic pulse-chase labeling studies using human fibroblast KD, chemically transformed HuT-11 and bladder carcinoma EJ cells to determine the turnover rates of individual tropomyosin isoforms and to address whether turnover rates change in transformed cells. The tropomyosin profiles for the 3 human cell lines are shown in Figure 2, a 2D gel analysis of extracts from cells that were pulse-labeled with [^{35}S]-methionine. KD (A) and HuT-11 (B) both express detectable amounts of the tropomyosin isoforms, hTm1, hTm2, hTm3, hTm4 and hTm5, as previously demonstrated.[110] The criteria used to identify the 2D gel spots as tropomyosin species included immunoprecipitation, microfilament association and heat stability.[110] EJ (C) extracts do not express enough hTm1 and hTm4 to analyze. The intensity of the autoradiograph spots of individual tropomyosin isoform at each chase point were compared (Fig. 2 graphs). It is clear that the HMW tropomyosins have, as a group, much faster turnover than the LMW isoforms. In all lines, the hTm1, hTm2 and hTm3, have short half-lives between 1.5 and 8.25 hours, whereas the hTm4 and hTm5 have half-lives greater than 20 hours. Interestingly, the stability of individual tropomyosin isoforms expressed in transformed cell lines is not different from the relative stability of the corresponding isoforms in normal KD cells. Similar results have also obtained from rat NRK cells; the HMW isoforms, Tm1, Tm2 and Tm3, turn over more rapidly than the LMW, Tm4 and Tm5.[111] Although the turnover rates of tropomyosins do not change significantly in human transformed cells tested so far, the HMW tropomyosin from TGF-α treated NRK cells are even more rapidly degraded in a proteosome-dependent manner,[111] suggesting that the level of HMW tropomyosin isoforms and their cytoskeletal association can be rapidly inhibited and precede the appearance of phenotypic transformation.

Tropomyosin Isoforms Localize Differentially Within the Cell

In nonmuscle cells, tropomyosin isoforms differentially localizes to stress fibers, lamella and the contractile ring.[8,101,112] When tropomyosin isoforms are overexpressed, they localize to the

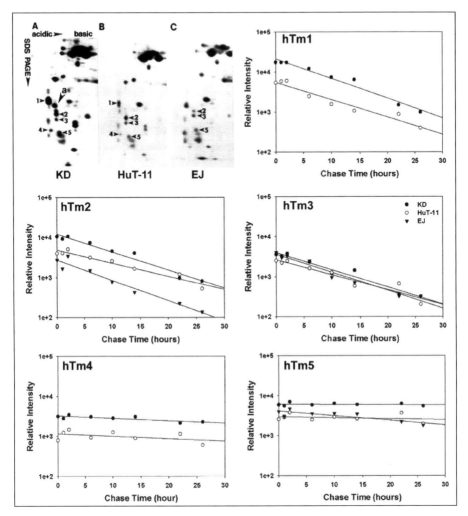

Figure 2. Two-dimensional gel analyses of human tropomyosin isoforms and their turnover rates in cultured cell lines. Cells from a human lip fibroblast line (KD), a chemically transformed derivative of KD (HuT-11) and a human bladder carcinoma line (EJ) were pulse-labeled with [^{35}S]-methionine. Total protein extracts were resolved by 2D gel electrophoresis and portions of the autoradiograms are shown in A-C. The multiple isoforms of tropomyosin are indicated with arrowheads, labeled 1 for hTm1, 2 for hTm2, 3 for hTm3, a for hTm3-1, 4 for hTm4 and 5 for hTm5. The hTm isoform identity was assigned based on relative 2D gel positions as compared with previously reported 2D profiles in Lin et al.[110] Pulse-chase experiments were performed to examine hTm isoform turnover. Labeled cell extracts were collected throughout the chase, separated by 2D gel electrophoresis and exposed to film. Autoradiograph images were acquired and analyzed by Image-1/AT image processing system (Universal Imaging Corp, West Chester, PA). The relative intensity values for the tropomyosin isoform autoradiograph spots at each time point were plotted against the chase time. The high molecular weight isoforms (hTm1, hTm2 and hTm3) had, as a group, much faster turnover than the low molecular weight isoforms (hTm4 and hTm5). Interestingly, these isoforms with more rapid turnover rate are normally reduced in many phenotypically transformed cells, suggesting a plausible mechanism for tropomyosin regulation of cytoskeletal reorganization.

same locations as their endogenous counterparts.[101,102,113] LMW tropomyosins and few HMW tropomyosins have been observed in the lamella and in ruffling regions of normal and transformed cells of human, chick and rodent.[4,43,83,99,101,114] The evidences for the differential localizations of tropomyosin isoforms within neurons, epithelial cells, fibroblasts, osteoclasts and skeletal muscle have been comprehensively reviewed.[3] The compelling evidence has also suggested that the sorting mechanisms for tropomyosin localization involve the differences in the intrinsic properties of tropomyosins, in the actin isoforms and in the ability of tropomyosin isoforms to collaboratively interact with other actin-binding proteins.[3] As a result, the differential localization of tropomyosin isoforms may determine and specify functionally distinct actin compartments. Conversely, the precise type of actin filament and its function may determine the tropomyosin isoform present.[2-5,8,99,115-117] For examples, human erythrocytes express hTm5 and h1m5b but not HMW tropomyosin isoforms, which assemble into membrane skeletal network for membrane stability.[28,32] Surface expression of hTm5 but not hTm1 or hTm4 has been detected in colonic epithelial cells but not in ileal epithelial cells,[118] suggesting that this subset of hTm5 can act as an autoantigen in the pathogenesis of ulcerative colitis.

Tropomyosin Isoforms Regulate Actin Cytoskeleton Functions

A general way that cells regulate actin filament function is by changing the compliment of tropomyosin isoforms through the control of gene expression. Changes from nonmuscle to muscle and embryonic to adult tropomyosin isoforms are associated with embryogenesis and differentiation.[24,25,27,119,120] A reverse scenario, down regulation of HMW tropomyosin isoforms, is observed during transformation.[3,8,105] The control of tropomyosin isoform expression in response to signals likely includes transcriptional control such as use of different promoters and poly(A) additional signals and posttranscriptional control such as use of alternatively spliced exons. The recent discovery that *TPM1* is one of target genes for a naturally occurring small noncoding RNA, microRNA-21 (*mir-21*)[121] has added another level of posttranscriptional control of tropomyosin isoform expression. The *mir-21* binding site is located within the 3'-untranslated region of *hTmskα1*, *hTmskα1-1* and *hTm3-1* messages. The isoform hTm3-1, which differs from hTm3 only at the C-terminus, may represent a protein labeled "a" in Fig. 2A and in our previously published 2D gel analysis, that is significantly down-regulated in many human tumor cell lines, including breast adenocarcinoma MCF-7.[110]

Roles of Tropomyosin Isoforms in Vesicle Transport

A role for tropomyosin isoforms in vesicle movement was first indicated by microinjection of an antibody that recognizes an epitope on tropomyosins 1, 3a and 3b (chicken homologues of hTm2, hTm5 and hTm4, respectively) from motile chicken embryo fibroblasts.[122,123] Injection of the antibody slowed the saltatory movement of vesicles/granules, suggesting that when cells are moving, the tropomyosins that lie on microfilaments change conformation to display the epitope and to allow efficient vesicle/granule transport.[124] Further evidence for differential function of tropomyosin isoforms in intracellular transport was obtained from microinjection of hTm3 and hTm5 into NRK cells.[113] Injection of hTm3, but not hTm5, induced the retrograde transport of organelles to the cell center. Both myosin I and cytoplasmic dynein were found to redistribute together with the translocated organelles.[113] Furthermore, Golgi-derived vesicles prepared from rat liver contained actin and Tm5NM2 isoform, but not other tropomyosin isoforms.[115] The isoform-specific association identified by the isoform-specific antibody and by transient expression of YFP-tagged tropomyosin isoforms into NIH3T3 cells may specify this population of actin filaments for transporting Golgi vesicles.[115,125] Unfortunately, the human homologue of Tm5NM2 has not been identified yet. The CG3 antibody recognizes hTm5, a homologue of Tm5NM1 and also stains the perinuclear (Golgi) region of human culture cells, in addition to ruffles and stress fibers.[43] Perhaps a subset of the hTm5 associates with Golgi-derived vesicles in human cells.

Roles of Tropomyosin Isoforms in Cell Migration

Tropomyosins have also been implicated in cell migration. LMW hTm5 localizes to the lamella, whereas both LMW (hTm5) and HMW (hTm2 and hTm3) isoforms localize to stress fibers.[43] Based on this localization and the ability of tropomyosin to antagonize Arp2/3 and cofilin, tropomyosin may confine Arp2/3 and cofilin activity to the leading edge and thereby define the lamellipodia.[83] Consistent with this, microinjection of rabbit skeletal muscle tropomyosin into PtK cells resulted in the loss of lamellipodia and also caused a 3.5-fold increase in myosin-dependent retrograde actin flow.[102] These data parallel the observation that hTm3 injection causes retrograde organelle movement and increased actin-arc structures in lamellipodia-like structures.[113] Interestingly, the tropomyosin-mediated loss of lamellipodia did not slow cell migration. Rather cells migrated more rapidly but lost directional control.[102] Therefore, it seems that tropomyosins play a decisive role at the base of the lamellipodia to drive cell migration, perhaps by stabilizing rearward flow of actin bundles in the lamella. Alternatively, tropomyosin might activate lamellar myosin which is known to be important for generating retrograde flow forces.[102,126,127] Additional support for this latter hypothesis comes from in vitro motility assays in which tropomyosin can enhance myosin function.[67,128]

Several studies have also suggested the importance of tropomyosin in tumorigenesis and metastasis.[105] Although it is clear that tropomyosin can stabilize stress fibers, the mechanisms for tropomyosin expression in response to tumorigenesis is complex and remain unclear. TGF-β stimulates up-regulation of tropomyosins and stress fibers in human cervical carcinoma SiHa and lung epithelial A549 cells.[108] This up-regulation is clearly mediated by *Smad* and p38Mapk signaling pathways. However, in metastatic breast cancer MDA-MB-231 cells, TGF-β fails to induce the up-regulation of tropomyosin and stress fibers.[108] Instead, TGF-β greatly stimulates the migration of MDA-MB-231 cells in a wound-healing assay.[129] Interestingly, MDA-MB-231 cells have been shown to express constitutively active Ras-ERK signaling,[130,131] which can be responsible for down-regulation of tropomyosin and disruption of actin stress fibers.[132,133] To support this possibility, pharmacological inhibitors have been used to block the Raf-ERK pathway in this cell line. The treated cells showed a significantly increase in TGF-β-induction of Tm1 expression and stress fiber formation, leading to inhibit cell migration.[108] Therefore, a thorough dissection of signaling pathways that control tropomyosin isoform expression will certainly advance our understanding of the mechanisms underlying cancer cell metastasis.

Recently, tropomyosins have been shown to function at the host-parasite interface. Cryptosporidiosis is an opportunistic disease that can be fatal to immunocompromised patients, such as AIDS patients and immunosupressed, organ-transplant patients.[134] The infection is transmitted by *Cryptosporidium* oocysts in a fecal-to-oral route to the epithelial cells of the gastrointestinal tract. During *C. parvum* infection, the anterior end of the oocyst comes into the proximity of the host cell apical membrane, triggering the host cell membrane to extend and enclose the parasite to form a parasitophorous vacuole.[135,136] The developing parasite becomes intracellular but still remains extracytoplasmic. In addition to host cell membrane extension, at the host-parasite interface within the host cell cytoplasm, an electron-dense band containing actin but devoid of membrane is quickly formed, implying host actin cytoskeleton remodeling. During *C. parvum* infection, the hTm5 isoform, but not hTm1 and hTm4, colocalizes to the infection sites with a novel parasite antigen, CP2.[137] Cells overexpressing hTm5 but not mutant chimeric isoform hTm5/3 or hTm3 exhibit a significant enhancement in the infection rate of the parasites.[137] This together with the findings that actin and actin associated proteins such as villin, α-actinin, ezrin, Arp2/3 complex, VASP, N-WASP are present at these infection sites, suggests that a localized induction of actin associated and membrane protrusive machinery, including specific tropomyosin isoform, facilitates parasite invasion. Similarly, upon entry into cultured nonmuscle cells, *Salmonella* and *Shigella* species are surrounded by a transient, tropomyosin-rich cytoskeleton compartment that is thought to be important for generating the forces required for internalization.[138,139]

Roles of Tropomyosin Isoforms in Cytokinesis

Tropomyosin is thought to regulate furrow progression and the maintenance of cell shape during cytokinesis in mammals. In addition to that many of tropomyosin isoforms are observed within the cleavage furrow of cells in tissue and in cell culture (Fig. 3),[8,112,140] evidence for a functional role has come from over-expression studies using normal and mutant forms of tropomyosin. CHO cell

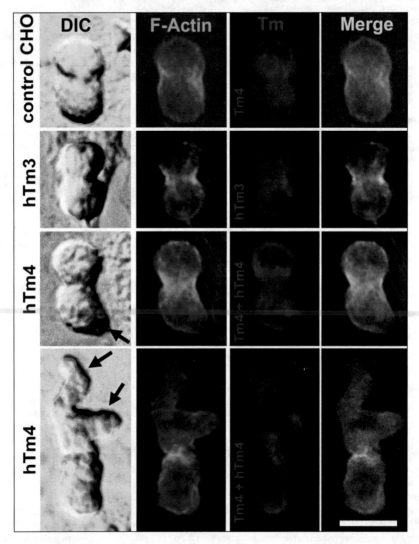

Figure 3. Overexpression of hTm3 or hTm4 isoforms generates different phenotypes during cytokinesis. Confocal stacks of non-expressing CHO cells or cells that express hTm3 or hTm4 that were double-labeled with FITC phalloidin (green) for actin filaments and with either LC24 antibody for hTm4 or CGβ6 antibody for hTm3 (red). LC24 also recognizes endogenous CHO Tm4 that like hTm5 and hTm3,[140] is located along the cell equator and is somewhat enriched in the cell periphery. Overexpressed hTm4 displays a similar pattern with more enrichment in the periphery. These cells, like those that express hTm5/3[141] or hTm5 but unlike those that express hTm3,[140] produce bulges (arrows) that disrupt cell symmetry during cytokinesis.

lines that over-express the chimeric proteins hTm5/3 or hTm5/2 lead to polyploidy and produce large membrane protrusions during cytokinesis.[114,141] Since hTm5/3 binds tightly to actin and increases readily the myosin ATPase activity,[67] it is possible that this fusion protein produces too much force on cell cortex to form large membrane protrusions. Similarly, overexpression of Tm1 in a *v-Ki-ras*-transformed, serum-starved, NIH3T3 cell leads to a greater percent of cells in G2-M phase and a 10-fold increase in binucleated cells compared to controls, suggesting that cytokinesis had been delayed.[142] Overexpression of a chimeric fusion of HMW tropomyosins, Tm1-Tm2, also increases polyploidy in the *v-Ki-ras*-transformed NIH-3T3 cells compared to control cells and cells that express the reciprocal chimeric protein Tm2-Tm1.[143]

Overexpressed hTm5/3 localizes preferentially to the peripheral cortex of dividing cells, in addition to the contractile ring.[140] This localization of hTm5/3 did not significantly alter the endogenous actin or myosin distribution. However, cells expressing hTm5/3 were faster to complete the first phase of cytokinesis (anaphase to 50% cytokinesis).[140] As reported previously,[141] hTm5/3-expressing cells showed a number of membrane alterations that, in some ways resembled blebs. However, these membrane protrusions were larger and less dynamic than blebs and represented the bulging of the entire submembranous actin cortex, rather than a dissociation of the membrane from the actin cortex.[144] Together, these data suggest that the tropomyosin chimera could alter cleavage furrow dynamics by changing the actomyosin properties in the peripheral cortex. To our surprise, cells that overexpress hTm5 also exhibited the large bulges to a lesser extent and were faster to progress from anaphase to 50% cytokinesis, even though hTm5 localized preferentially to the furrow region.[140] Similar phenotypes, faster to progress from anaphase start to 50% cytokinesis and large bulges formed, were observed for dividing cells expressing hTm4 (Fig. 3 and Table 2). Interestingly, cells expressing the HMW hTm3 were neither faster through cytokinesis nor did they produce bulges (Fig. 3 and Table 2).[140] We conclude that LMW tropomyosins but not HMW tropomyosins are important regulators of cell symmetry and furrow progression in CHO cells and that these LMW tropomyosins perform their roles by regulating actin and myosin in both the cleavage furrow and the cortical actin network.

Table 2. The incidence of abnormal morphology (bulges) in non-expressing cells and cells expressing hTm3, hTm4, hTm5 or hTm5/3 during cytokinesis

Force-Expressed Proteins	Stable Cell Line	Number of Cells Analyzed	Number of Bulged Cells (% of Total)	p Value
none	Di61	19	0 (0%)	NS
hTm3	C73	21	0 (0%)	–
hTm4	C14	15	10 (66.7%)	<0.0001
hTm4	C11	13	9 (69.2%)	<0.0001
hTm5	C14	26	6 (23.1%)	0.0265
hTm5/3	C70	28	18 (64.3%)	<0.0001

As shown previously[140], cells expressing hTm5 (C14) and hTm5/3 (C70, a chimeric tropomyosin mutant) but not hTm3 (C73) produce large protracted membrane bulges during cytokinesis, suggesting a compromised regulation of the cortical actin cytoskeleton. Similarly, two cell lines stably expressing hTm4 (C14 and C11) exhibit bulge morphology during cytokinesis (Fig. 3), whereas the non-expressing, but G418-resistant line (Di61) did not produce any membrane bulges. Thus, bulge formation during cytokinesis seems to be a feature associated with over-expression of LMW tropomyosins, hTm4 and hTm5, suggesting that cortical dynamics of actin filaments are regulated differently by different tropomyosin isoforms. Data are from cells imaged live from metaphase to 50% cytokines. Statistics were performed with SigmaStat 3.1 using Fisher's exact test. NS, not significant ($p > 0.05$).

A Potential Role for Tropomyosin in Angiogenesis

Angiogenesis may be regulated through the actions of naturally-acting inhibitors.[145] Many of these are proteolyzed or otherwise conformationally-altered polypeptides whose parental proteins are extracellular matrix proteins[146] or members of coagulation pathways.[147] One such inhibitor, cleaved HMW kininogen (HKa), is derived from single chain HMW kininogen (HK), a member of the intrinsic coagulation pathway, following cleavage by kallikrein. HKa induces apoptosis of proliferating endothelial cells and inhibits angiogenesis in vivo.[148,149]

HK binds to several sites on endothelial cells, including the receptor for the globular head of C1q (gC1qR),[150,151] cytokeratin 1,[152] urokinase receptor[153] and proteoglycans.[154] However, functional studies using proliferating endothelial cells did not support a role for any of these receptors in mediating the antiangiogenic activity of HKa.[148,155] These observations suggested that another binding site might mediate the antiangiogenic activity of HKa. Based on a report that demonstrated cross-reactivity between an antibody reactive with an endostatin-binding cyclic peptide and hTm3,[156] as well as molecular modeling (threading) studies performed in collaboration with Dr Yuan Ping-Pang (Mayo Clinic) that suggested structural homology between HKa and endostatin, it was hypothesized that tropomyosin might mediate the antiangiogenic activity of HKa. Subsequent studies demonstrated a central role for tropomyosin in mediating HKa-induced apoptosis of proliferating endothelial cells.[155] First, the anti-tropomyosin monoclonal antibody (mAb) TM-311 blocked the HKa-mediated endothelial apoptosis and the anti-angiogenesis activity of HKa in the chick chorioallantoic membrane assay.[155] Moreover, the binding of HKa to proliferating endothelial cells or purified chicken gizzard tropomyosin was potently inhibited by mAb TM-311. These findings confirmed the role of tropomyosin in mediating the anti-angiogenic activity of HKa and implied that tropomyosin must be expressed on the endothelial cell surface.[155] However, cell surface localization of tropomyosin is in marked contradistinction to conventional thought and thus, these observations prompted additional studies to characterize the expression of tropomyosin by human endothelial cells.

First, staining of unpermeabilized confluent cells with mAb TM-311 revealed a faint, diffuse background stain, while staining of subconfluent proliferating cells revealed a pattern strongly suggestive of cell surface tropomyosin expression.[155] Second, immunoprecipitation of surface-labeled extracts of proliferating endothelial cells with mAb TM-311 revealed a labeled protein of ~36 kDa, consistent with the size of tropomyosin.[155] Third, chemical cross-linking of biotinylated HKa with proliferating endothelial cells led to its incorporation into a 150 kDa HKa-tropomyosin complex, recognized by both mAb TM-311 and anti-HKa antibodies.[155] Hence, these results support that cell surface tropomyosin functions as a binding site for HKa on proliferating endothelial cells.

Though intriguing, these results raise many questions. First, it is unclear which of tropomyosin isoforms are expressed by endothelial cells. Our studies suggest that at the least, human umbilical vein endothelial cells (HUVEC) express hTm2, hTm3, hTm4 and hTm5, as well as hTm5-1 (TC22) (unpublished data). Deletion of a specific isoform would be the most straightforward approach to this dilemma, however the complex splice patterns of tropomyosin make selective deletion of an isoform difficult.[3,5,8] Moreover, whether endothelial cells from different vascular beds (i.e., microvascular, renal, etc) express the same repertoire of tropomyosins as HUVEC is uncertain.[100] Indeed, several monoclonal anti-tropomyosin antibodies of varying specificity inhibit HKa-induced endothelial cell apoptosis and may also directly affect endothelial proliferation. Some of these directly block proliferation, much like HKa, while others, such as CGβ6, against hTm2 and hTm3, appear to stimulate endothelial cell proliferation (unpublished data).

Externalization of tropomyosin by endothelial cells may be representative of a cellular stress response, which has been associated with externalization of several proteins in endothelial and other cell types. In some cases, the externalized proteins have served as receptors for plasma proteins and mediated cellular events occurring as a consequence of ligand binding. For example, actin may be externalized to the endothelial cell surface,[157,158] where it may function as a receptor for the proangiogenic molecule angiogenin[157] and for plasminogen.[158] The gC1qR, a kininogen binding and complement activating protein, is another protein once thought to be exclusively intracellular that is externalized by endothelial cells.[159,160] Other proteins once considered purely intracellular that have been localized to the cell surface include annexin A2[161] and several heat shock proteins involved in signaling and modulation of the immune response.[162]

Another question that remains unanswered is the mechanism by which ligand binding to cell surface tropomyosin affects cell proliferation responses. As a cytoskeletal protein, tropomyosin is not thought to contribute to activation of transmembrane signaling pathways. Moreover, our studies suggest that cell surface tropomyosin is reversibly bound to the endothelial cell surface, implying that it might be associated with another protein(s) capable of mediating transmembrane signal transduction. Thus, future studies designed to define the binding sites for tropomyosin on the cell surface may provide new insight into potential biologic roles of cell surface tropomyosin on endothelial cells.

Finally, all the work addressing cell surface expression of tropomyosin by endothelial cells has been performed in vitro and expression of tropomyosin on the surface of endothelial cells in vivo has yet to be conclusively demonstrated. However, precedent does exist for externalization of tropomyosin in vivo. Specifically, the observation that patients with ulcerative colitis develop an autoimmune response to hTm5 involving complement fixing IgG1 antibodies,[163,164] coupled with immunohistochemical staining patterns demonstrating a cell surface expression pattern of hTm5 in colonic epithelium,[165] strongly suggest externalization of tropomyosin in vivo. Moreover, cell culture experiments have demonstrated a specific pathway of hTm5 externalization by primary colon epithelial and LS180 colon cancer cells, in which tropomyosin is externalized as a complex with membrane-associated colon epithelial protein.[118]

Future Directions

It is clear that different tropomyosin isoforms play distinct roles in regulating cell motility including vesicle transport, cell migration and cytokinesis. The in vitro characterizations such as actin binding properties and effects of tropomyosin isoform on other actin-binding protein functions have begun to provide an understanding of how tropomyosin isoforms differentially regulate actin dynamics for controlling cell motility. However, the in vitro studies with purified native or recombinant cytoskeletal tropomyosins have, thus far been performed almost exclusively with muscle α-actin. It is now known that actin isoforms also play important roles in tropomyosin isoform sorting and function; thus, these in vitro experiments should be performed on nonmuscle actin isoforms. Wild type and mutant nonmuscle actin have been successfully purified from yeast in a large enough quantity for biochemical characterizations.[166] These investigators are currently using the baculovirus expression system to express and purify human γ-nonmuscle actin. Thus, it will be feasible to use nonmuscle β- and γ-actin in future in vitro studies on tropomyosin isoform effects on actin dynamics.

The in vivo studies with many transformed cells and TGF-β-treated cells have revealed a critical role for tropomyosins in regulating the actin cytoskeleton during cell motility.[105,108] The TGF-β signaling pathway is a major cellular growth inhibitory and proapoptotic pathway in many cell types and is also required for metastasis of many different types of tumor cells.[167] A mechanistic understanding of tropomyosin involvement in these superficially opposite effects of TGF-β on proliferation, apoptosis and cell motility remain unclear. The dissection of the TGF-β signal pathway and the study of its cross-talk with other signaling pathways such as Ras, integrin, etc. will advance our understanding of cancer cell biology, metastasis and actin cytoskeleton remodeling. Molecular studies using transgenic mouse models overexpressing and knockout animals with deletions of specific tropomyosin isoforms will be a fruitful approach to study isoform-specific function in vivo. The investigation of tropomyosin isoform alterations in human diseases such as cancer and angiogenesis, myopathy, inflammatory ulcerative colitis, Behcet's disease with posterior uveitis,[168] essential hypertension[169] and polycystic kidney disease[170] will greatly facilitate the development of complementary animal models displaying similar pathophysiology.

Acknowledgements

We would like to thank Jenny L-C. Lin and Alisa Van Winkle for excellent technical supports. This work was supported in part by grants HD18577 and HL76810 from the National Institutes of Health, USA.

References

1. Cooper JA. Actin dynamics: tropomyosin provides stability. Curr Biol 2002; 12:R523-R525.
2. Gunning P, Hardeman E, Jeffrey P et al. Creating intracellular structural domains: spatial segregation of actin and tropomyosin isoforms in neurons. Bioessays 1998; 20:892-900.
3. Gunning P, O'Neill G, Hardeman E. Tropomyosin-based regulation of the actin cytoskeleton in time and space. Physiol Rev 2008; 88(1):1-35.
4. Gunning P, Weinberger R, Jeffrey P et al. Isoform sorting and the creation of intracellular compartments. Annu Rev Cell Dev Biol 1998; 14:339-372.
5. Gunning PW, Schevzov G, Kee AJ et al. Tropomyosin isoforms: divining rods for actin cytoskeleton function. Trends Cell Biol 2005; 15:333-341.
6. Perry SV. Vertebrate tropomyosin: distribution, properties and function. J Muscle Res Cell Motil 2001; 22:5-49.
7. Pittenger MF, Kazzaz JA, Helfman DM. Functional properties of nonmuscle tropomyosin isoforms. Curr Opin Cell Biol 1994; 6:96-104.
8. Lin JJ, Warren KS, Wamboldt DD et al. Tropomyosin isoforms in nonmuscle cells. Int Rev Cytol 1997; 170:1-38.
9. Lees-Miller JP, Helfman DM. The molecular basis for tropomyosin isoform diversity. BioEssays 1991; 13:429-437.
10. Lees-Miller JP, Goodwin LO, Helfman DM. Three novel brain tropomyosin isoforms are expressed from the rat α-tropomyosin gene through the use of alternative promoters and alternative RNA processing. Mol Cell Biol 1990; 10:1729-1742.
11. Dufour C, Weinberger RP, Schevzov G et al. Splicing of two internal and four carboxyl-terminal alternative exons in nonmuscle tropomyosin 5 premRNA is independently regulated during development. J Biol Chem 1998; 273:18547-18555.
12. Goodwin LO, Lees-Miller JP, Leonard MA et al. Four fibroblast tropomyosin isoforms are expressed from the rat a-tropomyosin gene via alternative RNA splicing and the use of two promoters. J Biol Chem 1991; 266:8408-8415.
13. Wieczorek DF, W.SC, Nadal-Ginard B. The rat alpha-tropomyosin gene generates a minimum of six different mRNAs coding for striated, smooth and nonmuscle isoforms by alternative splicing. Mol Cell Biol 1988; 8:679-694.
14. Marston SB, Redwood CS. Modulation of thin filament activation by breakdown or isoform switching of thin filament proteins. Circ Res 2003; 93:1170-1178.
15. Reinach FC, Macleod AR. Tissue-specific expression of the human tropomyosin gene involved in the generation of the trk oncogene. Nature 1986; 322:648-650.
16. Novy RE, Lin JL-C, Lin CS et al. Human fibroblast tropomyosin isoforms: characterization of cDNA clones and analysis of tropomyosin isoform expression in human tissues and in normal and transformed cells. Cell Motil Cytoskeleton 1993; 25:267-281.
17. Pieples K, Wieczorek DF. Tropomyosin 3 increases striated muscle isoform diversity. Biochemistry 2000; 39:8291-8297.
18. Lin CS, Leavitt J. Cloning and characterization of a cDNA encoding transforming-senstive tropomyosin isoform 3 from tumorigenic human fibroblasts. Mol Cell Biol 1988; 8:160-168.
19. MacLeod AR, Gooding C. Human hTMα gene: Expression in muscle and nonmuscle tissue. Mol Cell Biol 1988; 8:433-440.
20. MacLeod AR, Houlker C, Reinach FC et al. A muscle-type tropomyosin in human fibroblasts: Evidence for expression by an alternative RNA splicing mechanism. Proc Natl Acad Sci USA 1985; 82:7835-7839.
21. MacLeod AR, Houlker C, Reinach FC et al. The mRNA and RNA copy pseudogenes encoding TM30$_{nm}$, a human cytoskeletal tropomyosin. Nucleic Acids Res 1986; 14:8413-8426.
22. MacLeod AR, Talbot K, Smillie LB et al. Characterization of a cDNA defining a gene family encoding TM30$_{pl}$, a human fibroblast tropomyosin. J Mol Biol 1987; 194:1-10.
23. Kee AJ, Schevzov G, Nair-Shalliker V et al. Sorting of a nonmuscle tropomyosin to a novel cytoskeletal compartment in skeletal muscle results in muscular dystrophy. J Cell Biol 2004; 166:685-696.
24. Izumo S, Nadal-Ginard B, Mahdavi V. Protooncogene induction and reprogramming of cardiac gene expression produced by pressure overload. Proc Natl Acad Sci USA 1988; 85:339-343.

25. Muthuchamy M, Pajak L, Howles P et al. Developmental analysis of tropomyosin gene expression in embryonic stem cells and mouse embryos. Mol Cell Biol 1993; 13:3311-3323.
26. L'Ecuyer TJ, Schulte D, Lin JJ-C. Thin filament changes during in vivo rat heart development. Pediatr Res 1991; 30:232-238.
27. Wang S-M, Wang S-H, Lin JL-C et al. Striated muscle tropomyosin-enriched microfilaments of developing muscles of chicken embryos. J Muscle Res Cell Motil 1990; 11:191-202.
28. Sung LA, Gao K-M, Yee LJ et al. Tropomyosin isoform 5b is expressed in human erythrocytes: implications of tropomodulin-TM5 or tropomodulin-TM5b complexes in the protofilament and hexagonal organization of membrane skeletons. Blood 2000; 95:1473-1480.
29. Sung LA, Lin JJ-C. Erythrocyte tropomodulin binds to the N-terminaus of hTM5, a tropomyosin isoform encoded by the γ-tropomyosin gene. Biochem Biophys Res Commun 1994; 201:627-634.
30. Vera C, Sood A, Gao KM et al. Tropomodulin-binding site mapped to residues 7-14 at the N-terminal heptad repeats of tropomyosin isoform 5. Arch Biochem Biophys 2000; 378:16-24.
31. Mohandas N, Evans E. Mechanical properties of the red cell membrane in relation to molecular structure and genetic defects. Annu Rev Biophys Biomol Struct 1994; 23:787-818.
32. An X, Salomao M, Guo X et al. Tropomyosin modulates erythrocyte membrane stability. Blood 2007; 109:1284-1288.
33. Lin JL, Geng X, Bhattacharya SD et al. Isolation and sequencing of a novel tropomyosin isoform preferentially associated with colon cancer. Gastroenterology 2002; 123:152-162.
34. Pollard TD, Blanchoin L, Mullins RD. Molecular mechanisms controlling actin filament dynamics in nonmuscle cells. Annu Rev Biophys Biomol Struct 2000; 29:545-576.
35. Theriot JA, Mitchison TJ. Actin microfilament dynamics in locomoting cells. Nature 1991; 352:126-131.
36. Carthew RW. Adhesion proteins and the control of cell shape. Curr Opin Genet Dev 2005; 15:358-363.
37. Smythe E, Ayscough KR. Actin regulation in endocytosis. J Cell Sci 2006; 119:4589-4598.
38. Pollard TD, Borisy GG. Cellular motility driven by assembly and disassembly of actin filaments. Cell 2003; 112:453-465.
39. Houle F, Rousseau S, Morrice N et al. Extracellular signal-regulated kinase mediates phosphorylation of tropomyosin-1 to promote cytoskeleton remodeling in response to oxidative stress: Impact on membrane blebbing. Mol Biol Cell 2003; 14:1418-1432.
40. Prasad SVN, Jayatilleke A, Madamanchi A et al. Protein kinase activity of phosphoinositide 3-kinase regulates β-adrenergic receptor endocytosis. Nat Cell Biol 2005; 7:785-796.
41. Matsumura F, Yamashiro-Matsumura S. Purification and characterization of multiple isoforms of tropomyosin from rat cultured cells. J Biol Chem 1985; 260:13851-13859.
42. Lin JJ, Helfman DM, Hughes SH et al. Tropomyosin isoforms in chicken embryo fibroblasts: purification, characterization and changes in Rous sarcoma virus-transformed cells. J Cell Biol 1985; 100:692-703.
43. Lin JJ-C, Hegmann TE, Lin JL. Differential localization of tropomyosin isoforms in cultured nonmuscle cells. J Cell Biol 1988; 107:563-572.
44. Vibert P, Craig R, Lehman W. Steric-model for activation of muscle thin filaments. J Mol Biol 1997; 266:8-14.
45. Kress M, Huxley HE, Faruqi AR et al. Structural changes during activation of frog muscle studied by time-resolved X-ray diffraction. J Mol Biol 1986; 188:325-342.
46. McKillop DF, Geeves MA. Regulation of the interaction between actin and myosin subfragment 1: evidence for three states of the filament. Biophys J 1993; 65:693-701.
47. Lehman W, Hatch V, Korman V et al. Tropomyosin and actin isoforms modulate the localization of tropomyosin strands on actin filaments. J Mol Biol 2000; 302:593-606.
48. Pieples K, Arteaga G, Solaro RJ et al. Tropomyosin 3 expression leads to hypercontractility and attenuates myofilament length-dependent Ca²⁺ activation. Am J Physiol Heart Circ Physiol 2002; 283: H1344-H1353.
49. Muthuchamy M, Grupp I, Grupp G et al. Molecular and physiological effects of overexpressing striated muscle β-tropomyosin in the adult murine heart. J Biol Chem 1995; 270:30593-30603.
50. Ochala J, Li M, Tajsharghi H et al. Effects of a R133W β-tropomyosin mutation on regulation of muscle contraction in single human muscle fibers. J Physiol 2007; 581:1283-1292.
51. Bos JM, Ommen SR, Ackerman MJ. Genetics of hypertrophic cardiomyopathy: one, two, or more diseases? Curr Opin Cardiol 2007; 22:193-199.
52. Golitsina N, An Y, Greenfield NJ et al. Effects of two familial hypertrophic cardiomyopathy-causing mutations on α-tropomyosin structure and function. Biochemistry 1997; 36:4637-4642.
53. Moraczewska J, Greenfield NJ, Liu Y et al. Alteration of tropomyosin function and folding by a nemaline myopathy-causing mutation. Biophys J 2000; 79:3217-3225.

54. Boussouf SE, Maytum R, Jaquet K et al. Role of tropomyosin isoforms in the calcium senstivity of stri-ated muscle thin filaments. J Muscle Res Cell Motil 2007; 28:49-58.
55. Laing NG, Wilton SD, Akkari PA et al. A mutation in the α tropomyosin gene TPM3 associated with autosomal dominant nemaline myopathy. Nat Gent 1995; 9:75-79.
56. Tajsharghi H, Kimber E, Holmgren D et al. Distal arthrogryposis and muscle weakness associated with a β-tropomyosin mutation. Neurology 2007; 68:772-775.
57. Palmiter KA, kitada Y, Muthuchamy M et al. Exchange of β- for α-tropomyosin in hearts of transgenic mice induces change in thin filament response to Ca^{2+} strong cross-bridge binding and protein phos-phorylation. J Biol Chem 1996; 271:11611-11614.
58. Graceffa P. Phosphorylation of smooth muscle myosin heads regulates the head-induced movement of tropomyosin. J Biol Chem 2000; 275:17143-17148.
59. Graceffa P. Movement of smooth muscle tropomyosin by myosin heads. Biochemistry 1999; 38:11984-11992.
60. Graceffa P, Mazurkie A. Effect of caldesmon on the position and myosin-induced movement of smooth muscle tropomyosin bound to actin. J Biol Chem 2005; 280:4135-4143.
61. Sobue K, Sellers JR. Caldesmon, a novel regulatory protein in smooth muscle and nonmuscle actomyosin systems. J Biol Chem 1991; 266:12115-12118.
62. Smith CW, Pritchard K, Marston SB. The mechanism of Ca^{2+} regulation of vascular smooth muscle thin filaments by caldesmon and calmodulin. J Biol Chem 1987; 262:116-122.
63. Chalovich JM, Cornelius P, Benson CE. Caldesmon inhibits skeletal actomyosin subfragment-1 ATPase activity and the binding of myosin subfragment-1 to actin. J Biol Chem 1987; 262:5711-5716.
64. Marston S. Aorta caldesmon inhibits actin activation of thiophosphorylated heavy meromyosin Mg2+-ATPase activity by slowing the rate of product release. FEBS Lett 1988; 238:147-150.
65. Horiuchi KY, Samuel M, Chacko S. Mechanism for the inhibition of acto-heavy meromyosin ATPase by the actin/calmodulin binding domain of caldesmon. Biochemistry 1991; 30:712-717.
66. Yamashiro-Matsumura S, Matsumura F. Characterization of 83-kilodalton nonmuscle caldesmon from cultured rat cells: stimulation of actin binding of nonmuscle tropomyosin and periodic localization along microfilaments like tropomyosin. J Cell Biol 1988; 106:1973-1983.
67. Novy RE, Sellers JR, Liu LF et al. In vitro functional characterization of bacterially expressed human fibro-blast tropomyosin isoforms and their chimeric mutants. Cell Motil Cytoskeleton 1993; 26:248-261.
68. Pittenger MF, Kistler A, Helfman DM. Alternatively spliced exons of the βTM gene exhibit different affinities for F-actin and effects with nonmuscle caldesmon. J Cell Sci 1995; 108:3253-3265.
69. Warren KS, Lin JL, Wamboldt DD et al. Overexpression of human fibroblast caldesmon fragment con-taining actin-, Ca++/calmodulin- and tropomyosin-binding domains stabilizes endogenous tropomyosin and microfilaments. J Cell Biol 1994; 125:359-368.
70. Nosaka S, Onji T, Shibata N. Enhancement of actomyosin ATPase activity by tropomyosin. Recom-bination of myosin and tropomyosin between muscles and platelet. Biochim Biophys Acta 1984; 788:290-297.
71. Sobieszek A, Small JV. Regulation of the actin-myosin interaction in vertebrate smooth muscle: activa-tion via a myosin light-chain kinase and the effect of tropomyosin. J Mol Biol 1977; 112:559-576.
72. Sobieszek A, Small JV. Effect of muscle and nonmuscle tropomyosins in reconstituted skeletal muscle actomyosin. Eur J Biochem 1981; 118:533-539.
73. Sobieszek A. Steady-state kinetic studies on the actin activation of skeletal muscle heavy meromyosin sub-fragments. Effects of skeletal, smooth and nonmuscle tropomyosins. J Mol Biol 1982; 157:275-286.
74. Lehrer SS, Morris EP. Dual effects of tropomyosin and troponin-tropomyosin on actomyosin subfrag-ment 1 ATPase. J Biol Chem 1982; 257:8073-8080.
75. Eaton BL, Kominz DR, Eisenberg E. Correlation between the inhibition of the acto-heavy meromyosin ATPase and the binding of tropomyosin to F-actin: Effects of Mg++, KCl, troponin I and Troponin C. Biochemistry 1975; 14:2718-2724.
76. Fanning AS, Wolenski JS, Mooseker MS et al. Differential regulation of skeletal muscle myosin-II and brush border myosin-I enzymology and mechanochemistry by bacterially produced tropomyosin isoforms. Cell Motil Cytoskeleton 1994; 29:29-45.
77. Pittenger MF, Helfman DM. In vitro and in vivo characterization of four fibroblast tropomyosins produced in bacteria:TM-2, TM-3, TM-5a and TM-5b are colocalized in interphase fibroblasts. J Cell Biol 1992; 118:841-858.
78. Moraczewska J, Nickolson-Flynn K, Hitchcock-DeGregori SE. The ends of tropomyosin are major determinants of actin affinity and myosin subfragment 1-induced binding to F-actin in the open state. Biochemistry 1999; 38:15885-15892.
79. Jancso A, Graceffa P. Smooth muscle tropomyosin coiled-coil dimers: subunit composition, assembly and end-to-end interaction. J Biol Chem 1991; 266:5891-5897.

80. Sanders C, Burtnick LD, Smillie LB. Native chicken gizzard tropomyosin is predominantly a beta gamma-heterodimer. J Biol Chem 1986; 261:12774-12778.
81. Gimona M, Watakabe A, Helfman DM. Specificity of dimer formation in tropomyosins: influence of alternatively spliced exons on homodimer and heterodimer assembly. Proc Natl Acad Sci USA 1995; 92:9776-9780.
82. Prasad GL, Fuldner RA, Braverman R et al. Expression, cytoskeletal utilization and dimer formation of tropomyosin derived from retroviral-mediated cDNA transfer. Metabolism of tropomyosin from transduced cDNA. Eur J Biochem 1994; 224:1-10.
83. DesMarais V, Ichetovkin I, Condeelis J et al. Spatial regulation of actin dynamics: a tropomyosin-free, actin-rich compartment at the leading edge. J Cell Sci 2002; 115:4649-4660.
84. Blanchoin L, Pollard TD, Hitchcock-DeGregori SE. Inhibition of the Arp2/3 complex-nucleated actin polymerization and branch formation by tropomyosin. Curr Biol 2001; 11:1300-1304.
85. Wawro B, Greenfield NJ, Wear MA et al. Tropomyosin regulates elongation by formin at the fast-growing end of the actin filament. Biochemistry 2007; 46:8146-8155.
86. Bernstein BW, Bamburg JR. Tropomyosin binding to F-actin protects the F-actin from disassembly by brain actin-depolymerizing factor (ADF). Cell Motil 1982; 2:1-8.
87. Ono S, Ono K. Tropomyosin inhibits ADF/cofilin-dependent actin filament dynamics. J Cell Biol 2002; 156:1065-1076.
88. Nishida E, Muneyuki E, Maekawa S et al. An actin-depolymerizing protein (destrin) from porcine kidney. Its action on F-actin containing or lacking tropomyosin. Biochemistry 1985; 24:6624-6630.
89. Hitchcock SE, Carisson L, Lindberg U. Depolymerization of F-actin by deoxyribonuclease I. Cell 1976; 7:531-542.
90. Ishikawa R, Yamashiro S, Matsumura F. Annealing of gelsolin-severed actin fragments by tropomyosin in the presence of Ca²⁺. Potentiation of the annealing process by caldesmon. J Biol Chem 1989; 264:16764-16770.
91. Fattoum A, Hartwig JH, Stossel TP. Isolation and some structural and functional properties of macrophage tropomyosin. Biochemistry 1983; 22:1187-1193.
92. Nyakern-Meazza M, Narayan K, Schutt CE et al. Tropomyosin and gelsolin cooperate in controlling the microfilament system. J Biol Chem 2002; 277:28774-28779.
93. Burgess DR, Broschat KO, Hayden JM. Tropomyosin distinguishes between the two actin-binding sites of villin and affects actin-binding properties of other brush border proteins. J Cell Biol 1987; 104:29-40.
94. Kobayashi R, Nonomura Y, Okano A et al. Purification and some of the properties of porcine kidney tropomyosin. J Biochem (Tokyo) 1983; 94:171-179.
95. Fischer RS, Fowler VM. Tropomodulins: life at the slow end. Trends Cell Biol 2003; 13:593-601.
96. Broschat KO, Weber A, Burgess DR. Tropomyosin stabilizes the pointed end of actin filaments by slowing depolymerization. Biochemistry 1989; 28:8501-8506.
97. Matsumura F, Yamashiro-Matsumura S. Modulation of actin-bundling activity of 55-kDa protein by multiple isoforms of tropomyosin. J Biol Chem 1986; 261:4655-4659.
98. Bryan J, Edwards R, Matsudaira P et al. Fascin, an echinoid actin-bundling protein, is a homolog of the Drosophila singed gene product. Proc Natl Acad Sci USA 1993; 90:9115-9119.
99. Bryce NS, Schevzov G, Ferguson V et al. Specification of actin filament function and molecular composition by tropomyosin isoforms. Mol Biol Cell 2003; 14:1002-1016.
100. Schevzov G, Vrhovski B, Bryce NS et al. Tissue-specific tropomyosin isoform composition. J Histochem Cytochem 2005; 53:557-570.
101. Hillberg L, Zhao Rathje LS, Nyakern-Meazza M et al. Tropomyosins are present in lamellipodia of motile cells. Eur J Cell Biol 2006; 85:399-409.
102. Gupton SL, Anderson KL, Kole TP et al. Cell migration without a lamellipodium: translation of actin dynamics into cell movement mediated by tropomyosin. J Cell Biol 2005; 168:619-631.
103. Temm-Grove CJ, Guo W, Helfman DM. Low molecular weight rat fibroblast tropomyosin 5 (TM5): cDNA cloning, actin-binding, localization and coiled-coil interactions. Cell Motil Cytoskel 1996; 33:223-240.
104. Iwasa JH, Mullins RD. Spatial and temporal relationships between actin-filament nucleation, capping and disassembly. Curr Biol 2007; 17:395-406.
105. Prasad GL. Regulation of the expression of tropomyosins and actin cytoskeleton by ras transformation. Meth Enzymol 2005; 407:410-422.
106. Prasad GL, Fuldner RA, Cooper HL. Expression of transduced tropomyosin 1 cDNA suppresses neoplastic growth of cells transformed by the ras oncogene. Proc Natl Acad Sci USA 1993; 90:7039-7043.
107. Prasad GL, Masuelli L, Raj MH et al. Suppression of src-induced transformed phenotype by expression of tropomyosin -1. Oncogene 1999; 18:2027-2031.

108. Bakin AV, Safina A, Rinehart C et al. A critical role of tropomyosins in TGF-β regulation of the actin cytoskeleton and cell motility in epithelial cells. Mol Biol Cell 2004; 15:4682-4694.
109. Varga AE, Storman NV, Zheng Q et al. Silencing of the tropomyosin-1 gene by DNA methylation alters tumor suppressor function of TGF-β. Oncogene 2005; 24:5043-5052.
110. Lin JJ-C, Yamashiro-Matsumura S, Matsumura F. Microfilaments in normal and transformed cells: Changes in the multiple forms of tropomyosin. Cancer Cells 1984; 1:57-65.
111. Warren RH. TGF-α-induced breakdown of stress fibers and degradation of tropomyosin in NRK cells is blocked by a proteosome inhibitor. Exp Cell Res 1997; 236:294-303.
112. Hughes JA, Cooke-Yarborough CM, Chadwick NC et al. High-molecular-weight tropomyosins localize to the contractile rings of dividing CNS cells but are absent from malignant pediatric and adult CNS tumors. Glia 2003; 42:25-35.
113. Pelham RJJ, Lin JJ-C, Wang Y-L. A high molecular mass nonmuscle tropomyosin isoform stimulates retrograde organelle transport. J Cell Sci 1996; 109:981-989.
114. Warren KS, Lin JL, McDermott JP et al. Forced expression of chimeric human fibroblast tropomyosin mutants affects cytokinesis. J Cell Biol 1995; 129:697-708.
115. Heimann K, Percival JM, Weiberger R et al. Specific isoforms of actin-binding proteins on distinct populations of Golgi-derived vesicles. J Biol chem 1999; 274:10743-10750.
116. Schevzov G, Gunning P, Jeffrey PL et al. Tropomyosin localization reveals distinct populations of microfilaments in neurites and growth cones. Mol Cellul Neurosci 1997; 8:439-454.
117. Stehn JR, Schevzov G, O'Neill GM et al. Specialisation of the tropomyosin composition of actin filaments provides new potential targets for chemotherapy. Curr Cancer Drug Targets 2006; 6:245-256.
118. Kesari KV, Yoshizaki N, Geng X et al. Externalization of tropomyosin isoform 5 in colon epithelial cells. Clin Exp Immunol 1999; 118:219-227.
119. Lin JJ, Lin JL. Assembly of different isoforms of actin and tropomyosin into the skeletal tropomyosin-enriched microfilaments during differentiation of muscle cells in vitro. J Cell Biol 1986; 103:2173-2183.
120. L'Ecuyer TJ, Schulte D, Lin JJ. Thin filament changes during in vivo rat heart development. Pediatr Res 1991; 30:232-238.
121. Zhu S, Si M-L, Wu H et al. MicrRNA-21 targets the tumor suppressor gene tropomyosin 1 (TPM1). J Biol Chem 2007; 282:14328-14336.
122. Lin JJ-C, Chou CS, Lin JL-C. Monoclonal antibodies against chicken tropomyosin isoforms: production, characterization and application. Hybridoma 1985; 4:223-242.
123. Hegmann TE, Lin JL-C, Lin JJ-C. Motility-dependence of the heterogenous staining of culture cells by a monoclonal anti-tropomyosin antibody. J Cell Biol 1988; 106:385-393.
124. Hegmann TE, Lin JL-C, Lin JJ-C. Probing the role of nonmuscle tropomyosin isoforms in intracellular granule movement by microinjection of monoclonal antibodies. J Cell Biol 1989; 109:1141-1152.
125. Percival JM, Hughes JAI, Brown DL et al. Targeting of a tropomyosin isoform to short microfilaments associated with the Golgi complex. Mol Biol Cell 2004; 15:268-280.
126. Cai Y, Biais N, Giannone G et al. Nonmuscle myosin IIA-dependent force inhibits cell spreading and drives F-actin flow. Biophys J 2006; 91:3907-3920.
127. Kovar DR. Intracellular motility: myosin and tropomyosin in actin cable flow. Curr Biol 2007; 17: R244-247.
128. Collins K, Matsudaira P. Differential regulation of vertebrate myosins I and II. J Cell Sci Suppl 1991; 14:11-16.
129. Bakin AV, Rinehart C, Tomlinson AK et al. p38 mitogen-activated protein kinase is required for TGFβ-mediated fibroblastic transdifferentiation and cell migration. J Cell Sci 2002; 115:3193-3206.
130. Kozma SC, Bogaard MC, Buser K et al. The human c-Kirstein ras gene is activated by a novelmutation in codon 13 in the breastcarcinomacell line MDA-MB321. Nucleic Acids Res 1987; 15:5963-5971.
131. Ogata H, Sato H, Takatsuka J et al. Human breast cancer MDA-MB-321 cells fail to express the neurofibromin protein, lack its type 1 mRNA isoform and slow accumulation of P-MAPK and activated Ras. Cancer Lett 2001; 172:159-164.
132. Ljungdahl S, Linder S, Franzen B et al. Down-regulation of tropomyosin-2 expression in c-jun-transformed rat fibroblasts involves induction of a MEK1-dependent autocrine loop. Cell Growth Differ 1998; 9:565-573.
133. Shields JM, Mehta H, Pruitt K et al. Opposing roles of the extracellular signal-regulated kinase and p38 mitogen-activated protein kinase cascades in Ras-mediated downregulation of tropomyosin. Mol Cell Biol 2002; 22:2304-2317.
134. O'Donoghue PJ. Cryptosporidium and cryptosporidiosis in man and animals. Int J Parasitol 1995; 25:139-195.
135. Forney JR, DeWald DB, Yang SG et al. A role for host phosphoinositide 3-kinase and cytoskeletal remodeling during Cryptosporidium parvum infection. Infect Immun 1999; 67:844-852.

136. Marcial MA, Madara JL. Cryptosporidium: cellular localization, structural analysis of absorptive cell-parasite membrane-membrane interactions in guinea pigs and suggestion of protozoan transport by M cells. Gastroenterology 1986; 90:583-594.

137. O'Hara SP, Lin JJ. Accumulation of tropomyosin isoform 5 at the infection sites of host cells during Cryptosporidium invasion. Parasitol Res 2006; 99:45-54.

138. Finlay BB, Ruschkowski S, Dedhar S. Cytoskeletal rearrangements accompanying salmonella entry into epithelial cells. J Cell Sci 1991; 99(Pt 2):283-296.

139. Gruenheid S, Finlay BB. Microbial pathogenesis and cytoskeletal function. Nature 2003; 422:775-781.

140. Eppinga RD, Li Y, Lin JL-C et al. Tropomyosin and caldesmon regulate cytokinesis speed and membrane stability during cell division. Arch Biochem Biophys 2006; 456:161-174.

141. Wong K, Wessels D, Krob SL et al. Forced expression of a dominant-negative chimeric tropomyosin causes abnormal motile behavior during cell division. Cell Motil Cytoskel 2000; 45:121-132.

142. Bharadwaj S, Hitchcock-DeGregori S, Thorburn A et al. N terminus is essential for tropomyosin functions: N-terminal modification disrupts stress fiber organization and abolishes anti-oncogenic effects of tropomyosin-1. J Biol Chem 2004; 279:14039-14048.

143. Bharadwaj S, Shah V, Tariq F et al. Amino terminal, but not the carboxy terminal, sequences of tropomyosin-1 are essential for the induction of stress fiber assembly in neoplastic cells. Cancer Lett 2005; 229:253-260.

144. Charras GT, Hu CK, Coughlin M et al. Reassembly of contractile actin cortex in cell blebs. J Cell Biol 2006; 175:477-490.

145. Nyberg P, Xie L, RK. Endogenous inhibitors of angiogenesis. Cancer Res 2005; 65:3967-3979.

146. Sund M, Xie L, Kalluri R. The contribution of vascular basement membranes and extracellular matrix to the mechanics of tumor angiogenesis. APMIS 2004; 112:450-462.

147. Browder T, Folkman J, Pirie-Shepard S. The hemostatic system as a regulator of angiogenesis. J Biol Chem 2000; 275:1521-1524.

148. Zhang J-C, Claffey K, Sakthivel R et al. Cleaved high molecular weight kininogen promotes endothelial cell apoptosis and inhibits angiogenesis in vivo. FASEB J 2000; 14:2589-2600.

149. Zhang J-C, Qi X, Juarez J et al. Inhibition of angiogenesis by two-chain high molecular weight kininogen (HKa) and kininogen-derived polypeptides. Can J Physiol Pharmacol 2002; 80:85-90.

150. Joseph K, Ghebrehiwet B, Peerschke EIB et al. Identification of the zinc-dependent endothelial cell binding protein for high molecular weight kininogen and factor XII: Identify with the receptor that binds to the globular "heads" of C1q (gC1q-R). Proc Natl Acad Sci USA 1996; 93:8552-8557.

151. Herwald H, Dedio J, Kellner R et al. Isolation and characterization of the kininogen binding protein p33 from endothelial cells. J Biol Chem 1996; 271:13040-13047.

152. Hasan AAK, Zisman T, Schmaier AH. Identification of cytokeratin as a binding protein and presentation receptor for kininogens on endothelial cells. Proc Natl Acad Sci USA 1998; 95:3615-3620.

153. Colman RW, Pixey RA, Najamunnisa S et al. Binding of high molecular weight kininogen to human endothelial cells is mediated via a site within domains 2+3 of the urokinase receptor. J Clin Invest 1997; 100:1481-1487.

154. Renne T, Dedio J, David G et al. High molecular weight kininogen utilizes heparan sulfate proteoglycans for accumulation on endothelial cells. J Biol Chem 2000; 275:33688-33696.

155. Zhang J-C, Donate F, Qi X et al. The antiangiogenic activity of cleaved high molecular weight kininogen is mediated through binding to endothelial cell tropomyosin. Proc Natl Acad Sci USA 2002; 99:12224-12229.

156. MacDonald NJ, Shivers WY, Narum DL et al. Endostatin binds tropomyosin: A potential modulator of the anti-tumor activity of endostatin. J Biol Chem 2001; 276(27):25190-25196.

157. Moroianu J, Fett JW, Riordan JF et al. Actin is a surface component of calf pulmonary artery endothelial cells in culture. Proc Natl Acad Sci USA 1990; 90:3815-3819.

158. Dudani AK, Ganz PR. Endothelial cell surface actin serves as a binding site for plasminogen, tissue plasminogen activator and lipoprotein(a). Br J Haematol 1996; 95:168-178.

159. Dedio J, Muller-Esterl W. Kininogen binding protein p33/gC1qR is localized in the vesicular fraction of endothelial cells. FEBS Lett 1996; 399:255-258.

160. Dedio J, Jahnen-Dechent W, Bachmann M et al. The multiligand-binding protein gC1qR, putative C1q receptor, is a mitochondrial protein. J Immunol 1998; 160:3534-3542.

161. Ling Q, Jacovina AT, Deora A et al. Annexin II regulates fibrin homeostasis and neoangiogenesis in vivo. J Clin Invest 2004; 113:38-48.

162. Joseph K, Tholanikunnel BG, Kaplan AP. Heat shock protein 90 catalyzes activation of the prekallikrein-kininogen complex in the absence of factor XII. Proc Natl Acad Sci USA 2002; 99:896-900.

163. Taniguchi M, Geng X, Glazier KD et al. Cellular immune response against tropomyosin isoform 5 in ulcerative colitis. Clin Immunol 2001; 101:289-295.

164. Ebert EC, Geng X, Glazier KD et al. Autoantibodies against human tropomyosin isoform 5 in ulcerative colitis destroys colonic epithelial cells through antibody and complement-mediated lysis. Cell Immunol 2006; 244:43-49.
165. Mirza ZK, Sastri B, Lin JJ-C et al. Autoimmunity against human tropomyosin isoforms in ulcerative colitis. localization of specific human tropomyosin isoforms in the intestine and extraintestinal organs. Inflamm Bowel Dis 2006; 12:1036-1043.
166. Cook RK, Blake WT, Rubenstein PA. Removal of the amino-terminal acidic residues of yeast actin: studies in vitro and in vivo. J Biol Chem 1992; 267:9430-9436.
167. Roberts AB, Wakefield LM. The two faces of transforming growth factor β in carcinogenesis. Proc Natl Acad Sci USA 2003; 100:8621-8623.
168. Mahesh SP, Li Z, Buggage R et al. Alpha tropomyosin as a self-antigen in patients with Behcet's disease. Clin Exp Immunol 2005; 140:368-375.
169. Dunn SA, Mohteshamzadeh M, Daly AK et al. Altered tropomyosin expression in essential hypertension. Hypertension 2003; 41:347-354.
170. Li Q, Dai Y, Guo L et al. Polycystin-2 associates with tropomyosin-1, an actin microfilament component. J Mol Biol 2003; 325:949-962.

CHAPTER 17

Tropomyosins Regulate the Impact of Actin Binding Proteins on Actin Filaments

Uno Lindberg,* Clarence E. Schutt, Robert D. Goldman,
Maria Nyåkern-Meazza, Louise Hillberg, Li-Sophie Zhao Rathje
and Staffan Grenklo

Abstract

The state of actin depends intimately on its interaction partners in eukaryotic cells. Classically, the cooperative force-generating acto-myosin couple is turned off and on by the calcium-dependent binding and release of tropomyosin molecules. The situation with nonmuscle cells appears to be much more complicated, with tropomyosin isoforms regulating the kinds of tension-producing and stress-bearing structures formed of actin filaments. The polymerization of even the shortest gelsolin-capped filaments is efficiently promoted by the binding of tropomyosin, for example, a process that might occur all the way out to the leading edges of advancing cells. Recently, multimers of tropomyosin have been discovered that appear to be assembly intermediates, formed from identical tropomyosin molecules, which act as ready pools of tropomyosin during the catalytic formation of lamellipodia and filopodia. Remarkably, these multimers apparently reform during the disassembly of cellular actin-containing structures. The existence of these recyclable, tropomyosin isoform-specific structures suggests how cells prevent nonproductive association of non-identical, but closely similar, tropomyosin isoforms.

The Actin Microfilament System

As expressed earlier in this book, tropomyosins (Tm) are perhaps the most important elements in the regulation of the microfilament (MF)-system, driving such diverse cellular processes as cell motility and migration, phagocytosis, vesicle movement and cytokinesis. A highly dynamic, concentrated and well organized weave of actin microfilaments, juxtaposed to the inside of the plasma membrane, shapes cells and governs their integrity (Fig. 1).[1,2] Transmembrane proteins, directly linked to the sub-membranous actin force generating system control the MF-system via the basic processes of polymerization, cross-linking and depolymerization, as seen in response to growth factors, cytokines and other manifestations of the exterior world experienced by cells (reviewed by[3-5]). Likely, tropomyosins influence all these steps of the cell motility (CM) cycle.

Cell surface protrusions like lamellipodia and filopodia are structured out of actin microfilaments, the assembly of which takes place at the advancing edge.[6-8] Polymerization of actin most likely provides the force for growth of these protrusions[4] and myosin-dependent processes translocate molecules and particles along formed MF-arrangements. For instance, adhesion proteins

*Corresponding Author: Uno Lindberg—Karolinska Institutet, Department of Microbiology, Tumor Biology and Cell Biology, Nobels väg 16, SE 171 77 Stockholm, Sweden. Email: uno.lindberg@ki.s

Tropomyosin, edited by Peter Gunning. ©2008 Landes Bioscience and Springer Science+Business Media.

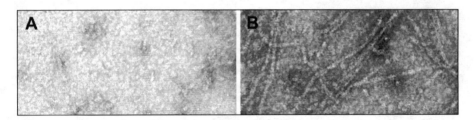

Figure 1. Annealing of gelsolin-capped actin filaments analyzed by electron microscopy. Panel (A) shows gelsolin and actin mixed in a 1:3 molar ratio and Panel (B) a mixture as in (A) after the addition of 10 μM α-tropomyosin.

(like integrins) are transported by a myosin X-dependent process to the tip of filopodia,[9] where they become involved in the establishment of adhesion sites, specialized, multiprotein structures connecting actin filament arrangements to extracellular structures.[10,11] Microfilament ensembles combine with myosin to translocate cells.[12] In tissues, cell:cell adhesions variously engage different kinds of transmembrane proteins[13] linked to actin microfilament arrangements inside partner cells. All these processes appear to be controlled by Tm isoforms specialized for the tasks at hand.[14,15]

There is evidence that the capacity of tropomyosins to supervene in the control of the MF-system depends both on direct blocking of the binding site and on the induction of conformational changes along the filament, thus competing with or counteracting the binding effects of other actin-filament binding proteins. This is exemplified by the effects of tropomyosin on a number of actin-binding proteins; ADF/cofilin family of proteins (here referred to as cofilin), gelsolin, the Arp2/3 complex, as well as myosin, all of which are influenced in their binding to actin filaments.

Cofilin and Arp2/3

Cofilin is an actin filament-depolymerizing factor, with the additional capacity to sever actin filaments. A number of different factors influence the activity of cofilin; changes in pH, phosphorylation, binding to polyphosphoinositides[16-18] (see also Chapter 18). Cofilin has been proposed to be of decisive importance in the earliest phase of growth factor-induced cell motility. There is experimental evidence that stimulation of motile cells induces the release of plasma membrane-bound cofilin and that the released cofilin is active and severs newly formed actin filaments and furthermore that the resulting increase in the number of actin filament growth points is further augmented by branch formation during Arp2/3, WASP (WAVE)-dependent polymerization of actin.[19,20] However in vitro, both cofilin severing and branch formation by the Arp2/3 WASP (WAVE) system are inhibited by tropomyosin[21,22] although this is isoform dependent because some Tms collaborate with cofilin binding (Chapter 18). It is notable that tropomyosin, is needed in budding yeast (*Sacharomyces cereviciae*) for the formation of the actin cable that connects the mother cell with the bud[23] and that tropomyosin in vitro regulates elongation by formin at the fast-growing end of the actin filament.[24] Thus, the fact that Tm isoforms have access to the space closest to the advancing edges of lamellipodia implies that the distinct roles of cofilin as well as Arp2/3 in polymerization of actin in vivo have to be further clarified. Detailed studies of the Arp2/3-dependent branch formation in vitro has revealed that there is a slow debranching linked to hydrolysis of ATP on one of the actin-related proteins (arp2) of the Arp2/3 complex.[25] The effect of tropomyosin on this process remains to be studied.

Gelsolin

Gelsolin is an abundant protein present all over the cell, including lamellipodia.[26,27] It severs actin filaments in the presence of Ca^{2+} ions, after which gelsolin remains as a cap bound to the (+)-end (fast growing end or barbed end) of one of the fragments produced.[28] In this position it inhibits monomer addition. Villin has similar activities and both villin and gelsolin can nucleate actin polymerization in the presence of Ca^{2+} ions, with a resulting polymerization, which proceedes by addition of actin monomers onto the (−)-end of the actin oligomers/filaments.[29] The structure of gelsolin in different states has been solved and models of how gelsolin might sever actin filaments have been presented.[30-32]

Two Distinct Actin Filament Conformations

Several lines of evidence indicate that actin filaments can exist in at least two distinct conformational states depending on the type of ligand bound to the polymer. Firstly, the binding of gelsolin to the (+)-end of an actin filament affects the polymer conformation, stabilizing the filament in a state, which binds cofilin with increased affinity.[33] Biochemical data suggest that this effect of gelsolin on the cofilin-binding to actin propagates 10-20 monomers from the gelsolin-capped (+)-end of the filament.[34] Evidence obtained by electron microscopy and time-resolved phosphorescence and absorption anisotropy suggest that the effect of gelsolin may extend over longer distances, involving changes in the helicity and torsional flexibility of the actin filament.[35-37]

Secondly, cofilin and some tropomyosin isoforms exhibit mutually exclusive binding to actin filaments. This appears not to be due to steric hindrance, since the two proteins do not have overlapping binding sites on actin filaments.[16,22,38,39] Phalloidin can bind tropomyosin-decorated actin filaments,[40] whereas it cannot bind to cofilin-decorated filaments,[34] suggesting that cofilin and some tropomyosins stabilize different conformers of the actin filament. It may be, however, that some Tms like TmBr3 actually cooperate with cofilin binding (Chapter 18). As mentioned above, the relative affinity of cofilin for actin filaments is increased by gelsolin,[33] whereas phalloidin is displaced by binding of gelsolin.[41] Thus, some tropomyosins and phalloidin appear to stabilize one state of the actin filament and gelsolin and cofilin another. Binding of cofilin to filamentous actin changes the helical twist and the torsional flexibility of the actin filament,[42] but whether this state is related to the gelsolin-induced state is unclear. The observations described below further support the existence of multiple conformations of the actin filament accessible via cooperative transitions along the length of the filaments induced (or stabilized) by binding of different actin-binding proteins (see Chapters 7 and 15).

It was discovered a long time ago that tropomyosin can anneal actin fragments and also gelsolin capped oligomers, into long filaments.[43] In the latter case this illustrates that tropomyosin must have a strong effect on the conformation of the oligomers, so much so that the capping effect of gelsolin is eliminated.[44] Tropomyosin-decorated actin filaments are protected from severing by gelsolin, a protection strengthened by the binding of caldesmon to the tropomyosin-decorated filaments.[43,45] These results demonstrate that tropomyosin stabilizes a state incompatible with gelsolin-binding to the (+)-end. It is still far from clear how the deployment of these actin-binding proteins is dictated by signal transduction during the motile activity of cells and it is possible that signal transduction pathways converging on cofilin,[45,46] also influence the activity of tropomyosin.

Observations that skeletal α-tropomyosin efficiently anneals even the smallest gelsolin:actin complexes (G1:A3)[44] is interesting from many points of view (Figs. 1, 2). This effect on the (+)-end of the actin filament, if shared with nonmuscle tropomyosins, suggests a role for tropomyosin at the very onset of actin polymerization in stimulated cells, even before significant elongation of filaments has taken place. This also suggests the possibility that gelsolin:actin complexes appearing in the cytoplasm of cells are converted into long filaments by tropomyosin, a process which could contribute to the formation of cortical weaves of actin microfilaments. Clearly, tropomyosin is essential in protecting filaments from severing by either gelsolin or cofilin in connection to growth of the filaments. Furthermore, nonmuscle tropomyosin likely influences force generation in the MF-system, in analogy with the role of tropomyosin in Ca^{2+}-regulation of muscle contraction (see Chapters 8, 9). Finally, there is reason to believe that tropomyosin plays essential roles in directing the formation of actin filaments in locations requiring functionally specific filament populations. For example, LMW but not HMW Tms are located in the motile areas of cells.[47]

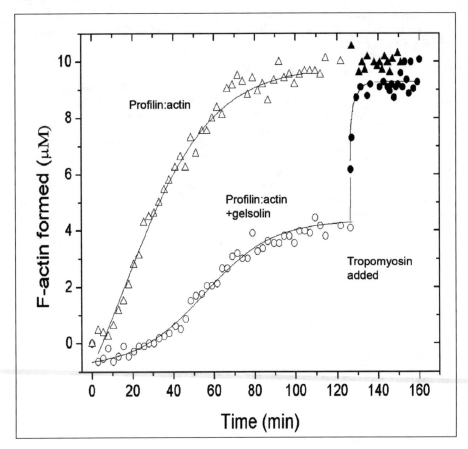

Figure 2. Effect of adding α-tropomyosin to gelsolin-capped actin filaments formed in the presence of gelsolin (and profilin). During incubation of profilin:actin under polymerizing conditions actin filament form and the concentration of free profilin increases till a steady state situation is reached. In the presence of gelsolin the (+)-end of formed filaments will be capped by the gelsolin, which in the presence of released profilin results in a lower plateau. Subsequent addition of tropomyosin results in rapid dissociation of the gelsolin and polymerization to a higher level coinciding with that reached in the absence of gelsolin.

Tropomyosin in Lamellipodia

Applying antibodies to HMW tropomyosin isoforms Tm1, 2 and 3; (abTM311, Sigma) and to low molecular weight Tm isoforms 4 and 5 in indirect immunofluorescence, has revealed a diffuse tropomyosin-specific staining all over the cell (crucially also close to advancing edges of lamellipodia harboring actin polymerization machineries), intense periodic staining over stress fibers and finally a granulated tropomyosin-specific staining, which reaches the outer parts of lamellipodia.[47] Imaging of live cells expressing GFP-tagged tropomyosin demonstrates the presence of tropomyosin at the very edge of advancing lamellipodia involved in forming filamentous structures, moving away from the edge towards the center of the cell, where they join larger conglomerates of GFP-tropomyosin containing structures in the convergence zone between lamellipodia and the rest of the leading lamellum.[47] Analyzing cells with indirect immunofluorescence shows a variation in the number density of dot-like Tm-positive structures, depending on the procedure used for fixation of the cells, suggesting the loss of soluble Tm-containing structures (Grenklo et al, unpublished).

Cytosolic Tm

Lin and coworkers long ago reported results indicating small amounts of soluble tropomyosin.[48] We have found that gentle extraction of cultured cells or tissues, with detergent (NP40 or Triton X100) leaves the cytomatrix (microfilaments, microtubules and cytokeratins) and nuclei seemingly undisturbed on the solid substratum, on which the cells are grown. Staining of cells for tropomyosin, before and after such extraction, clearly demonstrates removal of Tm positive material with the cytosol (Fig. 3). Figure 4 illustrates the fractionation of the cytosol from rat fibroblasts by gel filtration on Superose 6. Analysis of the fractions by polyacrylamide gelelectrophoresis followed by Western blotting shows the presence of tropomyosin isoforms as structures apparently larger than Tm dimers. Notably, more than 90% of the soluble tropomyosins (HMW Tm 1, 2 and 3 and LMW Tm 4) appear in such protein structures. Thus, the Tm positive material, which disappeared by extracting the cells, as seen by immunofluorescence (compare Fig. 3A and B), is recovered mostly as discrete Tm isoform-specific structures on gel filtration. The size of these tropomyosin structures was estimated to 180,000 and 250,000 for the LMW and HMW Tms, respectively, suggesting that they consist of multimers of Tm dimers. The relative amount of soluble tropomyosin in cells compared with the amount present in the cytomatrix varies between 10-30% of the total Tm, depending on cell type and state of activity. Co-staining of cells with antibodies to different Tm isoforms and fractionation of tagged tropomyosin isoforms confirm that the tropomyosin multimers are isoform specific and that their apparent molecular weights is mostly determined by the tropomyosins in question. Analysis of the fractions also revealed variable amounts of β-actin co-eluting with LMW Tm isoforms. Non-muscle γ-actin on the other hand has not been detected in the tropomyosin containing fractions of cells studied so far.

Significance of Cytosolic Tm Multimers

Rapid changes in the levels of Tm1 and Tm4 isoform multimers subsequent to stimulation of starved cells with growth factors indicates that the Tm multimers are assembly intermediates in the control of the MF-system turnover (Grenklo et al unpublished). The levels of both forms decreased during the first minute of stimulation and then increased again during the subsequent 2 minutes, reflecting major reorganizations in the MF-system. There was no detectable change in the size distribution of Tm1 for various times of stimulation. However, in the case of Tm4, there was a broadening of the Tm peak with longer stimulation times, with significant amounts of Tm appearing in complexes of size intermediate between the multimers and Tm dimers. During the same time period, there was no significant change in either Tm2 or Tm3.

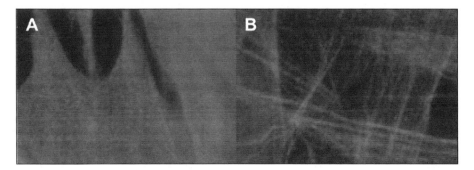

Figure 3. Effect of extraction of fibroblasts with detergents in a buffer stabilizing microfilaments and microtubules and intermediate filaments. Panel (A) and (B) show cells stained for HMW TM1, 2 and 3; panel A before and panel B after extraction with a detergent-containing buffer. Note that extraction had caused a significant decrease in Tm positive staining.

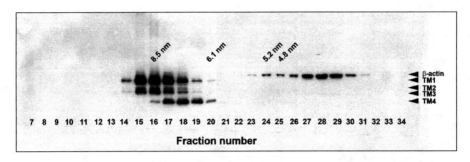

Figure 4. Fractionation of gel exclusion chromatography of a cytosolic extract of rat embryo fibroblasts. The extract made under conditions stabilizing actin microfilaments,[57] was fractionated on Superose 6 under the same conditions. TM isoforms were detected using PAGE followed by Western blotting. Ninety percent of the cytosolic TM appears as multimers in the chromatogram; apparent molecular weights of 180,000 and 250,000 for the LMW and HMW Tm, respectively. The analysis for β-actin shown was performed with the β-actin specific monoclonal antibody AC14 (Sigma).

High Resolution Crystal Structures of Actin Filaments

Considering the multitude of roles the actin MF-system plays in eukaryotic cells, the determination of the high resolution structure of the actin filament would seem to be one of the most important tasks in structural biology. A model of the actin filament was proposed in 1990 in conjunction with the solving of the crystal structure of the DNase I:actin (monomer) complex,[49] a model which, despite a number of shortcomings, has become accepted as a good working model of the actin filament.[50] Crystals of the profilin:actin (monomer) complex contain an actin structure referred to as the actin ribbon, which in many respects resembles an actin filament as seen by electron microscopy (notably, the actin filament seen by EM is a twisted ribbon,[51,52]) but which also differs from that and from the filament model, in several important respects.[53] The actin ribbon seen in the profilin:actin crystals is proposed to be an untwisted and slightly elongated form of the classical helical filament. Since the ribbon contains ATP, it is a metastable state of the actin filament and it is proposed that a ribbon → helix transition, accompanied by the hydrolysis of ATP, generates forces in the 100 pN range. In the context of muscle contraction, this model requires that tropomyosin responds to successive waves of ribbon to helix transitions along actin by integrating and transmitting the resulting forces to the Z-disc.[54] This model operates at high thermodynamic efficiencies and resolves a number of paradoxes that arise when in vitro motility data are interpreted in terms of the standard myosin cross-bridge theory.[55]

Concluding Remarks

The presence of tropomyosins close to the advancing edge of lamellipodia and in filopodia, where actin polymerization takes place and in the pools of Tm in response to stimulation of cells with growth factors, strongly suggests that the role of Tm has to be taken into account in modeling mechanisms of actin filament formation in cells. This conclusion is strengthened by observations on the effects of over-expressing various Tm isoforms on specific processes linked to the MF-system.[15] It is still not clear what Tm is doing, apart from stabilizing newly formed actin filaments, but in view of their effects on the actin filament (+)-end and on formin activity in vitro, it seems plausible that Tms must be involved in the early phases of filament formation. The discovery of Tm isoform-specific multimers in the cytosol uncovers a new level of control in the MF-system, namely the requirement for a stable, diffusible, storage form. It is important to find the factors controlling the release of Tm in functional form (likely Tm dimers) from these particles at sites of actin filament elongation and the mechanisms involved in reforming Tm particles during global reorganization of the MF-system. Whether the release switch involves H_2O_2 or some other oxidative agent remains to be seen. Recent reports describing the involvement of phosphorylation by kinase specific for the activation of tropomyosin[56] and with undisputable effects on the recruitment of certain Tms in processes requiring actin filament formation must also be taken into account. The demonstration that the cytoplasm is populated by distinct isoform-specific multimers of tropomyosin emphasizes the concept of "Tm-sorting", namely, how are these subtly-different assembly units cycled and redeployed as cells shift form in response to stimulation?

Acknowledgements

Gratefully acknowledge the generosity of Ingemar Ernberg for space and inspiring discussions. This work was supported by grants from the Swedish Cancer Society, Swedish research council and from the Nancy Lurie Marks Family Foundation.

References

1. Hoglund AS, Karlsson R, Arro E et al. Visualization of the peripheral weave of microfilaments in glia cells. J Muscle Res Cell Motil 1980; 1:127-46.
2. Small JV, Rinnerthaler G, Hinssen H. Organization of actin meshworks in cultured cells: the leading edge. Cold Spring Harb Symp Quant Biol 1982; 46(Pt 2):599-611.
3. Lindberg U, Karlsson R, Lassing I et al. The microfilament system and malignancy. Semin Cancer Biol 2007; 18:2-11
4. Pollard TD, Borisy GG. Cellular motility driven by assembly and disassembly of actin filaments. Cell 2003; 112:453-65.
5. Small JV, Stradal T, Vignal E et al. The lamellipodium: where motility begins. Trends Cell Biol 2002; 12:112-20.
6. Danuser G, Oldenbourg, R. Probing f-actin flow by tracking shape fluctuations of radial bundles in lamellipodia of motile cells. Biophys J 2000; 79:191-201.
7. Theriot JA, Mitchison TJ. Comparison of actin and cell surface dynamics in motile fibroblasts. J Cell Biol 1992; 119:367-77.
8. Watanabe N, Mitchison TJ. Single-molecule speckle analysis of actin filament turnover in lamellipodia. Science 2002; 295:1083-6.
9. Zhang H, Berg JS, Li Z et al. Myosin-X provides a motor-based link between integrins and the cytoskeleton. Nat Cell Biol 2004; 6:523-31.
10. Geiger B, Bershadsky A. Exploring the neighborhood: adhesion-coupled cell mechanosensors. Cell 2002; 110:139-42.
11. Geiger B, Bershadsky A, Pankov R et al. Transmembrane crosstalk between the extracellular matrix—cytoskeleton crosstalk. Nat Rev Mol Cell Biol 2001; 2:793-805.
12. Schwartz MA, Horwitz AR. Integrating adhesion, protrusion and contraction during cell migration. Cell 2006; 125:1223-5.
13. Nelson WJ, Drees F, Yamada S. Interaction of cadherin with the actin cytoskeleton. Novartis Found Symp 2005; 269:159-68; discussion 168-77:223-30.
14. Gunning P, O'Neill G, Hardeman E. Tropomyosin-based regulation of the actin cytoskeleton in time and space. Physiol Rev 2008; 88:1-35.
15. Gunning PW, Schevzov G, Kee AJ et al. Tropomyosin isoforms: divining rods for actin cytoskeleton function. Trends Cell Biol 2005; 15:333-41.
16. Bamburg JR. Proteins of the ADF/cofilin family: essential regulators of actin dynamics. Annu Rev Cell Dev Biol 1999; 15:185-230.
17. Bamburg JR, Wiggan OP. ADF/cofilin and actin dynamics in disease. Trends Cell Biol 2002; 12:598-605.
18. McGough A. F-actin-binding proteins. Curr Opin Struct Biol 1998; 8:166-76.
19. DesMarais V, Macaluso F, Condeelis J et al. Synergistic interaction between the Arp2/3 complex and cofilin drives stimulated lamellipod extension. J Cell Sci 2004; 117:3499-510.
20. van Rheenen J, Song X, van Roosmalen W et al. EGF-induced PIP2 hydrolysis releases and activates cofilin locally in carcinoma cells. J Cell Biol 2007; 179:1247-59.
21. Blanchoin L, Pollard TD, Hitchcock-DeGregori SE. Inhibition of the Arp2/3 complex-nucleated actin polymerization and branch formation by tropomyosin. Curr Biol 2001; 11:1300-4.
22. Ono S, Ono K. Tropomyosin inhibits ADF/cofilin-dependent actin filament dynamics. J Cell Biol 2002; 156:1065-76.
23. Evangelista M, Zigmond S, Boone C. Formins: signaling effectors for assembly and polarization of actin filaments. J Cell Sci 2003; 116:2603-11.

24. Wawro B, Greenfield NJ, Wear MA et al. Tropomyosin regulates elongation by formin at the fast-growing end of the actin filament. Biochemistry 2007; 46:8146-55.
25. Le Clainche C, Pantaloni D, Carlier MF. ATP hydrolysis on actin-related protein 2/3 complex causes debranching of dendritic actin arrays. Proc Natl Acad Sci USA 2003; 100:6337-42.
26. Cooper JA, Bryan J, Schwab B 3rd et al. Microinjection of gelsolin into living cells. J Cell Biol 1987; 104:491-501.
27. Cooper JA, Loftus DJ, Frieden C et al. Localization and mobility of gelsolin in cells. J Cell Biol 1988; 106:1229-40.
28. Janmey PA, Chaponnier C, Lind SE et al. Interactions of gelsolin and gelsolin-actin complexes with actin. Effects of calcium on actin nucleation, filament severing and end blocking. Biochemistry1985; 24:3714-23.
29. Glenney JR Jr, Kaulfus P, Weber K. F actin assembly modulated by villin: Ca++-dependent nucleation and capping of the barbed end. Cell 1981; 24:471-80.
30. Burtnick LD, Koepf EK, Grimes J et al. The crystal structure of plasma gelsolin: implications for actin severing, capping and nucleation. Cell 1997; 90:661-70.
31. Burtnick LD, Robinson RC, Choe S. Structure and function of gelsolin. Results Probl Cell Differ 2001; 32:201-11.
32. McGough AM, Staiger CJ, Min JK et al. The gelsolin family of actin regulatory proteins: modular structures, versatile functions. FEBS Lett 2003; 552:75-81.
33. Ressad F, Didry D, Xia GX et al. Kinetic analysis of the interaction of actin-depolymerizing factor (ADF)/cofilin with G- and F-actins. Comparison of plant and human ADFs and effect of phosphorylation. J Biol Chem 1998; 273:20894-902.
34. Ressad F, Didry D, Egile C et al. Control of actin filament length and turnover by actin depolymerizing factor (ADF/cofilin) in the presence of capping proteins and ARP2/3 complex. J Biol Chem 1999; 274:20970-6.
35. Orlova A, Egelman EH. Structural dynamics of F-actin: I. Changes in the C terminus. J Mol Biol 1995; 245:582-97.
36. Orlova A, Prochniewicz E, Egelman EH. Structural dynamics of F-actin: II. Cooperativity in structural transitions. J Mol Biol 1995; 245:598-607.
37. Prochniewicz E, Zhang Q, Janmey PA et al. Cooperativity in F-actin: binding of gelsolin at the barbed end affects structure and dynamics of the whole filament. J Mol Biol 1996; 260:756-66.
38. Bernstein BW, Painter WB, Chen H et al. Intracellular pH modulation of ADF/cofilin proteins. Cell Motil Cytoskeleton 2000; 47:319-36.
39. Nishida E, Maekawa S, Sakai H. Cofilin, a protein in porcine brain that binds to actin filaments and inhibits their interactions with myosin and tropomyosin. Biochemistry 1984; 23:5307-13.
40. De La Cruz E, Pollard TD. Transient kinetic analysis of rhodamine phalloidin binding to actin filaments. Biochemistry 1994; 33:14387-92.
41. Allen PG, Janmey PA. Gelsolin displaces phalloidin from actin filaments. A new fluorescence method shows that both Ca^{2+} and Mg^{2+} affect the rate at which gelsolin severs F-actin. J Biol Chem 1994; 269:32916-23.
42. McGough A, Pope B, Chiu W et al. Cofilin changes the twist of F-actin: implications for actin filament dynamics and cellular function. J Cell Biol 1997; 138:771-81.
43. Ishikawa R, Yamashiro S, Matsumura F. Annealing of gelsolin-severed actin fragments by tropomyosin in the presence of Ca^{2+}. Potentiation of the annealing process by caldesmon. J Biol Chem 1989; 264:16764-70.
44. Nyakern-Meazza M, Narayan K, Schutt CE et al. Tropomyosin and gelsolin cooperate in controlling the microfilament system. J Biol Chem 2002; 277:28774-9.
45. Amano T, Tanabe K, Eto T et al. LIM-kinase 2 induces formation of stress fibres, focal adhesions and membrane blebs, dependent on its activation by Rho-associated kinase-catalysed phosphorylation at threonine-505. Biochem J 2001; 354:149-59.
46. Dan C, Kelly A, Bernard O et al. Cytoskeletal changes regulated by the PAK4 serine/threonine kinase are mediated by LIM kinase 1 and cofilin. J Biol Chem 2001; 276:32115-21.
47. Hillberg L, Zhao Rathje LS, Nyakern-Meazza M et al. Tropomyosins are present in lamellipodia of motile cells. Eur J Cell Biol 2006; 85:399-409.
48. Lin JJ, Matsumura F, Yamashiro-Matsumura S. Tropomyosin-enriched and alpha-actinin-enriched microfilaments isolated from chicken embryo fibroblasts by monoclonal antibodies. J Cell Biol 1984; 98:116-27.
49. Holmes KC, Popp D, Gebhard W et al. Atomic model of the actin filament. Nature 1990; 347:44-9.

50. Poole KJ, Lorenz M, Evans G et al. A comparison of muscle thin filament models obtained from electron microscopy reconstructions and low-angle X-ray fibre diagrams from non-overlap muscle. J Struct Biol 2006; 155:273-84.
51. Lepault J, Erk I, Nicolas G et al. Time-resolved cryo-electron microscopy of vitrified muscular components. J Microsc 1991; 161:47-57.
52. Narita A, Maeda Y. Molecular determination by electron microscopy of the actin filament end structure. J Mol Biol 2007; 365:480-501.
53. Schutt CE, Rozycki MD, Myslik JC et al. A discourse on modeling F-actin. J Struct Biol 1995; 115:186-98.
54. Schutt CE, Lindberg U. Actin as the generator of tension during muscle contraction. Proc Natl Acad Sci USA 1992; 89:319-23.
55. Schutt CE, Lindberg U. Muscle contraction as a Markov process. I: Energetics of the process. Acta Physiol Scand 1998; 163:307-23.
56. Houle F, Poirier A, Dumaresq J et al. DAP kinase mediates the phosphorylation of tropomyosin-1 downstream of the ERK pathway, which regulates the formation of stress fibers in response to oxidative stress. J Cell Sci 2007;120: 3666-77.
57. Blikstad I, Carlsson L. On the dynamics of the microfilament system in HeLa cells. J Cell Biol 1982; 93:122-8.

CHAPTER 18

Tropomyosin and ADF/Cofilin as Collaborators and Competitors

Thomas B. Kuhn and James R. Bamburg*

Abstract

Dynamics of actin filaments is pivotal to many fundamental cellular processes such as cytokinesis, motility, morphology, vesicle and organelle transport, gene transcription and senescence. In vivo kinetics of actin filament dynamics is far from the equilibrium in vitro and these profound differences are attributed to large number of regulatory proteins. In particular, proteins of the ADF/cofilin family greatly increase actin filament dynamics by severing filaments and enhancing depolymerization of ADP-actin monomers from their pointed ends. Cofilin binds cooperatively to a minor conformer of F-actin in which the subunits are slightly under rotated along the filament helical axis. At high stoichiometry of cofilin to actin subunits, cofilin actually stabilizes actin filaments. Many isoforms of tropomyosin appear to compete with ADF/cofilin proteins for binding to actin filaments. Tropomyosin isoforms studied to date prefer binding to the "untwisted" conformer of F-actin and through their protection and stabilization of F-actin, recruit myosin II and assemble different actin superstructures from the cofilin-actin filaments. However, some tropomyosin isoforms may synergize with ADF/cofilin to enhance filament dynamics, suggesting that the different isoforms of tropomyosins, many of which show developmental or tissue specific expression profiles, play major roles in the assembly and turnover of actin superstructures. Different actin superstructures can overlap both spatially and temporally within a cell, but can be differentiated from each other based upon their kinetic and kinematic properties. Furthermore, local regulation of ADF/cofilin activity through signal transduction pathways could be one mechanism to alter the dynamic balance in F-actin-binding of certain tropomyosin isoforms in subcellular domains.

Introduction

In the contractile units of muscle cells, actin filaments are stable and highly organized in sarcomeres for optimal interactions with the bipolar myosin II motor protein to achieve optimal sliding of the actin during muscle contraction. However, in the muscle cell cortex and in nonmuscle cells, actin undergoes rapid assembly and disassembly and often carries out motile functions in the absence of motor protein binding. To understand this dynamic behavior of actin and the role of other actin binding proteins in regulating it, it is necessary to first provide a short overview of actin dynamics.

Actin is ubiquitously expressed in all eukaryotic cells and is one of the most abundant cellular proteins with an estimated concentration of 50-200 μM (2-8 mg/ml). Of the six isoforms expressed in mammals, four are expressed in a muscle specific fashion whereas the cytoplasmic

*Corresponding Author: James R. Bamburg—Department of Biochemistry and Molecular Biology Colorado State University Fort Collins, CO 80523-1870.
Email: jbamburg@lamar.colostate.edu

Tropomyosin, edited by Peter Gunning. ©2008 Landes Bioscience and Springer Science+Business Media.

β-actin and γ-actin isoforms are found in all nonmuscle cell types. The 375 amino acid highly conserved monomeric actin (MW 42.5 kD) folds into a compact globular structure composed of four lobes, two of which are separated by a characteristic cleft, the site of adenine nucleotide binding, with a flexible hinge region in the cleft floor.[1,2] Under physiological salt concentrations in vitro, monomeric globular actins (G-actin) slowly organize end-to-end and side-to-side through noncovalent forces to create trimeric nuclei to which actin subunits rapidly assemble into a twisted polar two-stranded helical filament (F-actin) with an axial rise of 2.75 nm and a rotation of $-167°$ per actin subunit.[3,4] Hydrolysis of ATP to ADP-Pi occurs within 1-2 s after assembly, followed by the much slower ($t_{1/2}$ = 600 s) loss of Pi, which elicits a structural change that has profound effects on the kinetic and thermodynamic characteristics of actin.[5] Each end of the polar filament maintains a different equilibrium monomer concentration (critical concentration). The polar nature of the F-actin is readily observed by decoration with proteolytic fragments of myosin II, which form a characteristic arrowhead structure giving rise to the nomenclature in which the fast growing end is referred to as the barbed end and the slow growing end as the pointed end.[5] At steady state, ATP-bound G-actin monomers rapidly polymerize onto the barbed end of filaments, undergo rapid ATP hydrolysis and slow Pi loss and subunits depolymerize off the pointed end of filaments as ADP-bound G-actin monomers, a process known as treadmilling (Fig. 1). In vitro the actin filament growth rate is 0.03 μm/sec with a treadmilling rate of 0.3/sec and a free G-actin concentration of 0.1 μM.[5] Significantly, filament growth rates in vivo range from 2 to 20 μm/sec with a treadmilling rate of 20-200/sec and a G-actin concentration of 2 to 20 μM. This considerable discrepancy in the filament dynamics in vitro compared to in cells underscores the critical function of regulatory proteins implicated in nucleating filament growth, capping filament ends, severing filaments, or sequestering G-actin monomers.[5-8]

Actin filament dynamics plays a pivotal role in many fundamental cellular processes including cytokinesis, motility, contractility, cell morphology, organelle transport, organelle localization and

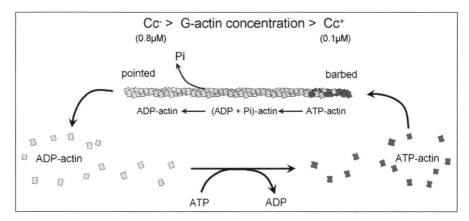

Figure 1. Steady-state behavior of actin under physiological ionic conditions. ATP-actin subunits (red/black) add onto the barbed end of F-actin, undergo hydrolysis of the ATP within 1-2 s (orange/gray) and eventually the inorganic phosphate dissociates leaving ADP-actin (green/light gray) as the major form at the pointed end. ADP-actin dissociates from the pointed end and nucleotide exchange occurs on the free actin subunits. In vivo, ADF/cofilin proteins enhance turnover by severing filaments and increasing the depolymerization rate, whereas profilin supports nucleotide exchange and polymerization of ATP-actin monomers. The treadmilling, which occurs at actin monomer concentrations between the critical concentrations for the two ends, depends on the maintenance of ATP, since the bound nucleotide on actin will equilibrate with the adenine nucleotide pool. At actin monomer subunit concentrations above 0.8 μM, actin will assemble onto both ends and below 0.1 μM, actin will dissociate from both ends. A color version of this figure is available at www.Eurekah.com.

function and compartmentalization of the cytosol.[9-12] For instance a cell of 20 μm in diameter has the capacity to compartmentalize metabolic and signal transduction pathways utilizing the plasma membrane surface area of roughly 700 μm². In contrast, its actin filament network provides over 45,000 μm² of scaffolding area. It is not surprising therefore that glycolytic enzymes, nonreceptor tyrosine kinases, lipid kinase, phospholipases, elongation factors of protein synthesis, ion channels and transporters and even nuclear events are all intimately linked to the dynamics of actin filaments.

Recently, it has been recognized that all eukaryotic cells exhibit many distinct actin filament superstructures based on the ability of other proteins to organize filaments into bundles or gels (reviewed in ref. 13). Bundles have adjacent filaments with either parallel or antiparallel orientation, depending on the nature of the cross-linking protein. Gels can form from filaments that are branched or cross-linked by other proteins or protein complexes. While each of these superstructures may have its separate spatial and temporal regulation, recent findings show that different superstructures can overlap each other in space and time and their dynamic regulation, although independent, must be highly coordinated.[13] The turnover of actin filaments within these actin superstructures may be quite different with some, such as those in the leading edge of migrating cells, having a high turnover of recycling subunits and others, such as anchoring cables or stress fibers, forming longer lived structures. One key to understanding the in vivo dynamics of actin filaments is an understanding of the role of members of the ADF(actin depolymerizing factor)/cofilin family and its enhancers, Srv2/Cap and profilin, which collaborate in the rapid turnover of F-actin and tropomyosins (Tms), most isoforms of which stabilize actin filaments.[8,14] In this chapter we will elaborate on findings illuminating the interplay between ADF/cofilin and Tms in cytokinesis, cell motility, membrane trafficking and cell survival/senescence.

Mechanisms of ADF/Cofilin Mediated Actin Turnover

In vitro Studies of ADF/Cofilin on Actin Dynamics: Actin filament dynamics is the cumulative expression of several reactions each with its own kinetics and affinity of reaction partners: polymerization of ATP-G-actin or profilin-ATP-actin onto filament barbed ends, depolymerization of ADP-G-actin monomers off filament pointed ends, ATP hydrolysis in actin subunits in filaments, dissociation of Pi from the filament and nucleotide exchange of G-actin monomers. ADF/cofilin proteins can affect most of these processes.

An ADF/cofilin (AC) has been identified in higher plants, yeasts and fungi, protists and every phyla in the animal kingdom in which they have been sought suggesting they are ubiquitous in all eukaryotes that express actin.[8] AC proteins from different organisms vary in MW (15 to 21 kDa) and exhibit up to 70% amino acid identity within one organism but less than 40% when compared across organisms. For example, mouse ADF and mouse cofilin are 70% identical but yeast cofilin is only 41% identical to mouse cofilin. Single cell organisms express a single member of this family whereas metazoans usually express two or three members, suggesting these isoforms have evolved to fulfill specific functions or for tissue specific regulation of their expression.[15]

All members share the ADF-homology (ADF-H) domain as a structural motif. The minimal ADF-H, found in the 118 amino acid *Toxoplasma gondii* ADF, is a hydrophobic core of 4 β-sheets enclosed by 4 α-helices. Interestingly, this structural motif is utilized in other families of actin binding proteins with different activities. The ADF-H is repeated twice in twinfilins, which serve mainly as actin monomer sequestering proteins with some severing activity, three times in the severing proteins fragmin and severin and in the barbed end capping protein and six times in the gelsolin family proteins, which have calcium-dependent actin filament severing and barbed end capping activities.[16]

There are three isoforms of AC proteins expressed in mammals: ADF, cofilin-1 and cofilin-2.[17] Cofilin-1 is expressed in the oocyte and is ubiquitously expressed during development, disappearing from skeletal muscle shortly after myoblast fusion when it is replaced with the muscle isoform, cofilin-2. Cofilin-2, however, is not muscle specific in that an alternatively spliced version of the mRNA with the identical coding sequence for cofilin-2 is expressed at lower levels in many different tissues and in tissue culture cell lines.[18] All three isoforms from higher vertebrates contain two sequence insertions (loops in the ADF-H structure) both serving as nuclear translocation sequences, one of which is critical for nuclear translocation.[19,20] Binding to actin monomer and to one subunit in a filament is attributed to a set of charged residues along a major α-helix and a second set of charged residues is critical for interacting with a second subunit along the long axis of the actin filament (F-actin binding).[21,22] AC proteins bind cooperatively to actin filaments resulting in localized regions of an actin filament saturated with AC proteins.[23,24] This cooperative interaction occurs on actin filaments in a minor "twisted" state and stabilizes the filaments in the twisted form in which each subunit has about a 5° rotation (162° vs 167°) and the helical crossover shifts from about 35 nm to 25 nm along the filament without affecting the overall 2.75 nm rise/subunit (Fig. 2).[25] Moreover, this change in filament structure masks the binding site for phalloidin, fluorescent derivatives of which are commonly used to stain for F-actin. Although cofilin saturation of actin filaments confers a stability upon the filament, low amounts of partial decoration seems to confer an instability, which leads to severing, one of the primary activities of AC proteins.[26] This severing is greatly enhanced on filaments that are attached to other structures suggesting a mechanism of allosteric and cooperative destabilization.[27] Binding of AC proteins along an actin filament enhances the loss of Pi and thus aids in the rapid conversion of an ADP-Pi region of a filament to an ADP-actin region.[28] AC proteins also enhance the rate of depolymerization at pointed ends of filaments, over 20 times at an actin/AC ratio of 1:8, although this rate does not exceed that of naked F-actin alone when diluted below critical concentration of the pointed end.[6,26] The severing and depolymerizing activities of AC proteins can be uncoupled by point mutations in AC.[29] Taken together these activities greatly increase the concentration of free actin filament ends, which explains their positive contribution to actin filament dynamics. AC proteins exhibit a higher affinity for Mg-ADP-G-actin compared to Mg-ATP-G-actin, although

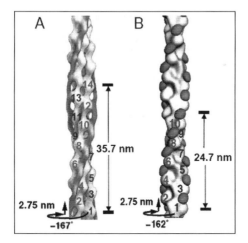

Figure 2. The relative rotations of actin subunits within a filament favor either tropomyosin or cofilin binding. The actin filament can be described as a single left handed helix in which every subunit is included. Subunits in F-actin alone tends to occupy two favored rotation states, the major state (A) with rotations of about –165-167°/per subunit and a minor state (B) with rotations between –158 and 162°/subunit.[22,25] Only a few tropomyosin isoforms (mostly muscle specific ones) bound to F-actin (skeletal muscle alpha isoform) have been examined structurally and these prefer to bind to the major rotation state (A), whereas cofilin prefers to bind to actin in the minor rotation state (B). Each form of actin has the same rise per subunit of 2.75 nm. The actin filament also can be described as two slowly twisting helices of alternating subunits (red and blue numbers in figure). Each half turn of the twist gives rise to the "crossover", which for F-actin alone is about 13-14 subunits and for cofilin-saturated F-actin is about 10 subunits. For this reason, cofilin is often said to bind to a "twisted" form of F-actin.

this difference is much greater for cofilin than for ADF.[30] Significantly, cofilin at near equal molar ratios to Mg-ATP-G-actin induces nucleation of assembly whereas ADF does not.[26,30,31] Spontaneous nucleotide exchange is very slow on the AC-actin complex.[23,24,32] However, Srv2/Cap can bind directly to the cofilin-actin complex and enhance nucleotide exchange by stabilizing the nucleotide-free actin and displacing cofilin.[33-35] Profilin, binding to ADP-actin, also greatly enhances nucleotide exchange thereby creating a profilin-ATP-G-actin pool ready for a new polymerization cycle.[35,36] Together AC proteins and profilin speed up actin filament turnover in vitro more than 100 fold.

The activity of AC proteins is regulated by many factors.[8] Phosphorylation of Ser3 inactivates AC proteins and can be mimicked by the S3E mutation, which is minimally active.[37] In contrast, the S3A mutation is not phosphorylatable and thus serves as a potentially active nonphospho-regulated AC mutant. In vivo, AC phosphorylation is catalyzed by LIM kinases 1 and 2, which are regulated by RhoGTPases, or by TES kinases, which are regulated by binding to actopaxin at focal adhesions.[38-40] The slingshot phosphatases and chronophin are implicated in the dephosphoryla-tion of AC proteins.[41-43] Phosphoinositol 4-phosphate (PIP) and 4,5 phosphate (PIP$_2$) inhibit AC activity by binding to the actin binding site and both phosphoinositides are important for the regulation of cell morphology and motility.[44,45] Finally, cofilin activity is modulated by the actin interacting protein 1 (Aip1), which enhances cofilin binding to F-actin and promotes filament severing and turnover.[46-49]

In Vivo Studies on AC Activity

In three different cell lines, siRNA silencing of either ADF, cofilin-1 or cofilin-2 resulted in more actin filaments, larger cell size, reduced cell motility and decreased cytokinesis.[50] Cellular deficiencies by knock down of cofilin could be rescued by ADF overexpression and vice versa. Nevertheless, results from many studies suggest that ADF and the cofilins likely have distinct roles not only within an organism but also within a single cell. The expression of ADF but not cofilin is regulated by the actin monomer pool.[51] The cellular distribution of cofilin remained with the F-actin pool whereas ADF distributed more with the actin monomer pool in cultured Swiss 3T3 mouse fibroblasts in which pH was jump-shifted.[52] ADF is the predominant AC protein in epithelial cells, which efficiently supports actin filament turnover with a strong pH dependence.[17] Cofilin 2, the prominent isoform expressed in muscle, had a weak effect on actin filament turn-over and also a lesser pH dependence. Finally, a comparative study in which siRNA was used to downregulate the expression of ADF (destrin) or cofilin in a colorectal cancer cell line expressing 17% ADF and 83% cofilin showed silencing of either ADF or cofilin increased the number of multinucleated cells, altered polarized lamellipodium protrusions, caused a redistribution of paxil-lin and enhanced adhesion.[53] However, silencing expression of ADF but **not** cofilin decreased cell migration on collagen I and invasion through matrigel that was stimulated by bombesin. Moreover, silencing of ADF but not cofilin caused phosphorylation of p130^{CAS} suggesting that ADF but not cofilin is a significant regulator of various processes important for the invasive phenotype of human colorectal cancer cells.[53]

In Vitro Effects of Tm on AC-Induced Actin Dynamics

Actin filaments saturated with skeletal muscle tropomyosin (Tm) are relatively resistant to the depolymerizing effects of chick ADF.[54] Surprisingly, actin filaments saturated with a mixture of Tm isoforms isolated from brain are even more resistant to ADF-induced depolymerization.[55] When both brain Tm and ADF were added simultaneously to F-actin there was virtually no protection, demonstrating the need for Tm to have bound to the F-actin to block the ADF effects. Addition of excess cofilin to actin-Tm complexes caused the dissociation of Tm,[56] the first studies to directly demonstrate the competitive nature of the binding between cofilin and Tm although the binding sites between cofilin and Tm are not overlapping.[57] However, the preference of cofilin for binding the "twisted" form of the actin filament and the preference of Tm for the nontwisted form, coupled with the ability of both cofilin and Tm to bind F-actin cooperatively, explains their competitive interactions with F-actin. Actin filaments containing Tm interact very well with myosin II but displacing the Tm with cofilin disrupts myosin II binding.[56] Tm also inhibits spontaneous actin filament depolymerization and Arp2/3 complex supported nucleation.[58,59] The above studies were the first to suggest that cofilin and Tm could specify unique populations of actin filaments that had different interactions with motor proteins and/or branching/nucleators and thus could have different cellular functions. It is interesting to note that many of these studies were completed prior to the recognition of the complexity of the Tm isoforms and even before the relationship between ADF and cofilin was established.

The multiple genes for Tm and the ability of many transcripts to undergo alternative splicing generate over 40 isoforms, mostly nonmuscle type.[14] These generally fall into two categories, the low molecular weight (248 amino acids) and the high molecular weight (284 amino acids). Tm isoforms exert distinct functions on actin filament dynamics in different cell types and splice forms are not only developmentally regulated but even in a single cell they are differentially compartmentalized.[60-62] Several of these Tm isoforms increase the stiffness of actin filaments and stabilize the "untwisted" form, which could diminish the ability of AC to bind by greatly reducing the population of subunits in the more "twisted" conformation. However, it seems likely that even Tm-saturated filaments can undergo some natural "twisiting" to explain why high cofilin concentrations can drive off the bound Tm.[56] The affinity of different Tm isoforms for actin filaments is variable (see Chapters 6 and 15 this volume) and the complexity is increased by the fact that multiple Tm isoforms may be able to bind cooperatively to single actin filaments (see chapters 7 and 15).[63] Furthermore, it is not clear if all Tm isoforms occupy the same binding sites along an actin filament or if some isoforms may have higher affinities for minor "twisted" forms of F-actin as is suggested by in vivo studies discussed below.

The role of Tm in modulating the ability of Aip1 to enhance cofilin-induced actin dynamics has only been examined in one in vitro system. Analysis of the effects of muscle Tm on actin disassembly by the combined activity of *Caenorhabditis elegans* Aip1 (UNC-78) and cofilin (UNC-60B), demonstrated that Tm protected the actin from disassembly.[64]

In Vivo Evidence for Competition and Synergy between AC Proteins and Tms

The dynamics, structural organization and subcellular localization of actin filaments is the result of an intricate interplay among many actin binding proteins, their isoforms and expression patterns. Clearly, the dramatic effects of either AC proteins or Tm isoforms on actin filament turnover poses the question what the parameters are that determine whether activities from these two families act in synergy or in competition.

Genetic evidence from model systems including yeast, *Drosophila melanogaster* and *C. elegans*, all of which have a fewer genes for AC and Tms and less alternatively spliced variants than mammalian systems, supports a competition between AC and Tm for actin turnover and stabilization. Actin filament structures in yeast fall in two classes, specifically those localized in the cortical patches and those cable-like structures spanning the entire cell volume (see Chapter 14 for a discussion of yeast actin and Tm). While actin turnover is high in cortical patches, longitudinal cables are rather stable. Not surprisingly, cofilin is high in cortical patches whereas the two yeast Tm isoforms (Tpm1p and Tpm2p) are abundant in cables.[65,66] A genetic approach in yeast demonstrated that the severing activity and the depolymerizing activities of cofilin could be separated by specific mutations. Expressing the severing-defective yeast cofilin disrupted actin filament turnover and organization as well as cell viability.[21] In contrast, expressing the depolymerization defective cofilin mutation had no phenotype.[29] Both Tpm1p and Tpm2p bind to actin filaments in a saturable manner with Tpm2p having slightly higher affinity. Deletion of Tpm1p disrupted actin cables as the major phenotype while deletion of Tpm2p had no apparent effect.[65] However loss of both Tm isoforms is lethal. In yeast expressing a polymerization defective actin, the V226G and L267G double mutation, the critical actin concentration for filament formation is about 200 fold higher than for WT actin.[67] Interestingly, expressing either Tpm1p or Tpm2p were able to rescue actin filament formation by lowering the critical concentration 20 fold. Studies in yeast also show that Aip1 works in cooperation with cofilin to enhance actin filament dynamics, even on the Tpm1p-containing actin cables.[48] Competition between Tpm1p for stabilizing cable filaments and Aip1/cofilin for their turnover was demonstrated by the ability of an Aip1 deletion mutant to rescue the growth and loss-of cable defect of a temperature-sensitive Tpm1p mutant.[48]

Modification of the N terminus of Tm greatly alters its function.[68] Expressing Tm containing an N terminal HA epitope no longer stabilizes actin filaments and delays cytokinesis because of its diminished F-actin-binding capability. Notably, expression of HA-tagged Tm caused a decline in cofilin phosphorylation, whereas overexpression of normal Tm increased the inactive, phospho-form of cofilin consistent with its effects on actin filament stabilization.

Several studies in *C. elegans* shed more light on the antagonism between Tm and AC proteins. The unc60 gene encodes two AC isoforms, UNC60A and B, both products of alternative splicing.[69] UNC60B is expressed in body wall muscle cells and mutations within UNC60B cause major disruption of actin filaments. Although UNC60B binds to actin filaments, neither severing nor depoymerization activity is observed in vivo. On the other hand, UNC60B does exhibit typical AC activities in vitro suggesting that in vivo other factors function to stabilize actin filaments.[70] The four *C. elegans* Tm isoforms (CeTm) are derived from a single gene through alternative splicing; mutations of this gene result in sever phenotype changes.[71] Purified CeTm and UNC60B both bound actin filaments in a mutually exclusive manner in accordance with previous findings. Also, CeTm negated actin filament depolymerization in the presence of UNC60B. CeTm is a major component of isolated CE actin filaments and, in a reconstitution experiment, revealed a dose dependent exclusion of UNC60B. During muscle development, CeTm and UNC60B displayed differential localization patterns with CeTm present in myofibrils and UNC60B diffusely in the cytoplasm. Silencing CeTm by siRNA caused substantial disorganization of actin filaments and a motility defective phenotype. In sharp contrast, silencing CeTm had minimal effects in a strain of *C. elegans* expressing a loss of fuction mutant AC, which maintains interaction with G-actin but is unable to bind or to sever F-actin. The simplest interpretation for this finding is that in a cell with reduced cofilin activity, actin filament turnover is inherently reduced and could adsorb a loss of Tm without a significant impact on actin filament dynamics. This elegant study provided both in vitro and in vivo evidence for the competition between AC and Tm in actin filament dynamics. Furthermore, Aip1 in the presence of AC contributes to actin filament depolymerization in vivo in *C elegans*. The CE Aip1 (UNC78) enhances dynamics of cofilin (UNC60B)-bound actin filaments and CeTm was antagonistic to Aip1 and cofilin in body wall muscle actin filament disassembly.[64,72]

Thus far, a large body of evidence from model systems described above supports the notion that Tm isoforms antagonize AC proteins in vivo and in vitro. However, similar investigations in higher vertebrates suggest some of the more than 40 Tm isoforms are antagonistic to AC whereas others may work cooperatively with AC to enhance actin filament dynamics. The picture of how Tms affect actin dynamics through the recruitment and regulation of other actin binding proteins is complex. First, different Tm isoforms have different affinities for actin filaments and bind at different sites along actin filaments.[63] Manipulation in the cellular expression of Tm5NM1 and TmBr3 resulted in isoform-specific changes in cell morphology and migration as well as in actin filament organization.[61] Whereas overexpression of TmBr3 caused a loss of stress fibers and increased the formation of lamellipodia, overexpression of Tm5NM1 has the opposite effect. These Tms clearly interact with actin filaments, which exhibit most likely a distinct molecular composition due to their spatially distinct cellular localization. In developing neurons, initially the Tm isoform Tm5NM1/2 is localized in axons but is later replaced by TmBr3, an adult neuron-specific Tm.[60] Such subtle differences in the composition of Tm was demonstrated even in neuronal growth cones and correlated with specific actin filament structures.[73,74]

Expression of Tm isoforms also correlates with major changes in the activities of other actin binding proteins. Stable cell lines overexpressing different levels of the Tm5NM1 isoform, showed a direct correlation between the level of Tm5NM1 expressed and myosin II activity (measured as phosphorylated myosin light chain) and an inverse correlation with cofilin activity.[61] Cells

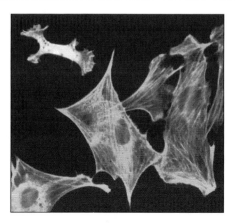

Figure 3. Alteration in tropomyosin isoform expression alters cell morphology and migratory behavior. Clonally selected line of B35 cells expressing high levels of Tm5NM1 were transfected with plasmids for expression of GFP (green cell) and TmBr3.[61] Cells were fixed and stained for F-actin with rhodamine phalloidin (red). Cells expressing high levels of Tm5NM1 are very spread-out and nonmotile with taught membranes and many stress fibers. When TmBr3 is expressed, the stress fibers disappear and ruffling membrane and lamellipodia appear. These cells are much more motile. Cofilin is associated with actin filaments in the TmBr3-expressing cells (not shown) but most cofilin is phosphorylated and diffuse in the Tm5NM1-expressing cells (adapated from ref. 61). A color version of this figure is available at www.eurekah.com.

expressing the highest Tm5NM1 were very broadly spread and had taut membranes indicative of contraction of sub-membrane associated actin filaments. Stable cell lines overexpressing different levels of the TmBr3 isoform showed no changes in either phospho-myosin light chain or phospho-cofilin and remained small and motile with many regions of ruffling membrane indicative of highly dynamic actin. Furthermore, when cells expressing the highest levels of Tm5NM1 were transiently transfected with a plasmid expressing TmBr3, the cells became smaller and stress fibers disappeared being replaced by ruffling membrane (Fig. 3).[61] Thus the Tm isoforms can specify the functional properties of actin and the proteins with which they can interact.

Tms are also critical in cytokinesis and were identified in the contractile ring.[75] In fission yeast, the Tm cdc8 is required for the stabilization of the contractile ring and Tm4 and Tm5 were found in the contractile ring of CHO cells (for more details, see Chapters 14 and 16).[76,77] In dividing astrocytes, Tm1 and/or Tm6 are associated with contractile rings.[78] Altering expression levels of Tms has functional consequences for cytokinesis. Overexpression of Tm1 resulted in a dramatic increase of multinucleated cells, an indication for impaired cytokinesis although cleaveage furrows exhibited a normal morphology (Thoms and Gunning, personal communication). AC proteins are also necessary for cytokinesis and are constituents of the contractile ring, suggesting the competition between Tms and ACs is significant in regulating the underlying actin filament dynamics. Indeed, overexpression of Tm1 virtually eliminated the accumulation of cofilin in contractile rings. Impairment of cytokinesis as a result of Tm1 overexpression was compensated by overexpression of cofilin thus establishing a functional competition supporting physiological actin filament dynamics (Thoms and Gunning, personal communication). Together, it is feasible that Tms impart a broad range of stabilization to actin filaments as a consequence of different affinities, distinct binding sites in actin filaments, differential expression pattern in cell types and ultimately variation in the composition within different compartments of a single cell. Progress in understanding of the functions of Tms is hampered by the large number of Tm splice variants and their spatial and temporal expression patterns in the developing and adult organism, which infers unique functions in different subcellular compartments. All these parameters illuminate how complex the influence of Tms could be regarding the recruitment and regulation of other actin binding proteins.

Regulation of AC and Role of AC Activity in Tm Selection and Actin Binding

Tms significantly contribute to actin filament dynamics with outcomes ranging from stabilization to increased turnover depending on the repertoire of Tms, the cellular localization and the molecular composition of actin filaments, which includes AC proteins. The question arises whether the influence of Tms on actin filament dynamics derives from their interaction (1) solely with actin filaments, (2) with other actin binding proteins such as ACs, or (3) a combination of both. Actin filaments decorated with different Tms exhibited varying sensitivities to cytochalasin D treatment.[79] Actin filaments decorated with low molecular weight Tms were much more resistant compared to actin filaments bound with high molecular weight Tms. In nonmuscle cells, Tm is bound either on the inner or the outer domain of actin, which depends on the specific actin and/or Tm isoform.[63] The differences in binding sites results from minor amino acid sequence differences among Tms, which could influence the effect on other actin binding proteins (see chapters 7 and 17). As mentioned above, overexpression of Tm5NM1 increases myosin interaction with actin filaments.[61] Furthermore, myosin variants were mislocalized in dendrites, neuronal growth cones greatly increased in surface area and myosin heavy chain IIB was localized to actin filaments in filopodia, a rather unusual distribution. These experimental results suggest that Tm isoforms can preferentially accumulate myosin at sites of high affinity Tm-actin filament interactions. Overexpression of the Tm5NM1 isoform increased the amount of phosphorylated, inactive AC, which could arise from Tm5NM1 displacing AC from actin filaments and increasing its accessibility to LIMK. Transient TmBr3 overexpression in these Tm5NM1-expressing cells restored normal cofilin activity and cell morphology, suggesting that Tm isoform affects the activity of AC proteins and thus their interaction with actin filaments. In lieu of the differential affinities of Tms and the variations in their binding sites on actin filaments, it is feasible that individual Tms could generate synergy of interactions with distinct repertoires of actin binding proteins.

Tm Isoforms Are Functionally Distinct

The plethora of Tm isoforms encoded by 4 genes are mostly expressed in nonmuscle cells and all exhibit three fundamental functions albeit to varying degrees: (1) interaction with actin filaments, (2) altering myosin activity and (3) influencing AC activity.[14] Their expression patterns change during development and their composition is distinct in subcellular compartments (see chapters 4 and 15). To further our understanding of the particular function, altering the expression of Tm isoforms represents one approach. The tissue-specific expression and subcellular distribution of Tms, which is highly conserved across species, implies a very specific function of individual Tms.[80] Global elimination of the γTm gene was lethal; products of the γTm gene are implicated in Golgi vesicle transport, neuronal polarity and axon outgrowth.[60,62,73] The *S. cerevisae* TM isoforms Tpm1p and Tpm2p are required for growth and secretion, respectively and the *S. pombe* Tm cdc8 is necessary for cytokinesis. An extensive study using antibodies directed against various Tm isoforms revealed a complex tissue and subcellular distribution.[80] For instance, TmBr1 and 3 were localized to the cell periphery and ruffling membranes whereas Tm1, 2, 3 and 6, were associated with stress fibers.[62] Manipulation of Tm5NM1 and TmBr3 in B35 neuro-epithelial cells clearly showed that each Tm isoform caused opposing effects on actin filament dynamics.[61,74] Although our knowledge is incomplete, Tms from different genes are clearly not redundant in their function but have specific functions that cannot be substituted for by just any Tm gene products.

Competition and Synergy between AC and Tm in Selected Cellular Processes

Tms provide a broad range of influence on actin filament dynamics by altering the molecular composition of actin filaments and their interactions with other actin binding proteins. Distinct

Tm isoforms bind to actin filaments with varying affinities and binding sites and exhibit specific tissue and subcellular localization (see Chapters 4 and 15). As has been documented above, the interplay between Tms and ACs can be competitive or cooperative in the regulation of actin filament dynamics. Here we will discuss how these aspects are reflected in a few essential cellular processes.

Cytokinesis

During mitosis, the plane of division of the future daughter cells is established during anaphase and a constriction of the plasma membrane reveals a distinct morphological structure, the cleavage furrow. The furrow is formed from contraction of an actomyosin ring in the cell cortex and the regulated mechanism of its progressive contraction underlies the phenomenon of cytokinesis.[81] Many studies provide evidence that de novo actin filament formation is required.[82,83]

In the fission yeast *S. pombe*, actin filaments are organized as cortical patches at the growing ends and as thick bundles along the long axis of the cells.[84,85] During cytokinesis, cortical actin patches dissolve and new actin filament structures are established to form a contractile ring.[86] These actin filament rearrangements require the activity of several regulatory proteins such as profilin, formin, IQGAP, Arp2/3 and ADF/cofilin (Adf1) and tropomyosins.[83,87-91] Downregulation of ADF/cofilin activity inhibits cytokinesis but does not prevent its initiation,[50,89,90] even though ADF/cofilin is present in the cleavage furrow early during cytokinesis.[87] In fission yeast, the AC member Adf1 was shown to play a key role in the progression of cytokinesis.[92] Suppression of Adf1 abolished actin filament reorganization in cells entering mitosis whereas overexpression resulted in the depolymerization of cortical patches as well as the contractile ring. One proposed function of Adf1 supports the timely depolymerization of actin filaments in patches in but it also assists in the transport of actin monomers to their new location in support of the formation of the contractile ring. Phosphoregulation of cofilin has not been demonstrated in yeast and this is supported by the finding that the active cofilin S4A mutation, which cannot be phosphorylated, evoked no defects in patch dissolution and contractile ring formation in yeast. Thus the interaction of yeast Adf1 with actin filaments underlies a different regulation. Interestingly, Adf1 is associated with actin filaments in the contractile ring but not in cytosolic cables suggesting an active exclusion of Adf1 from stable actin filaments, although in vitro ADF1 can bind actin filaments. Tm (cdc8 in *S. pombe*) is a prime candidate for excluding Adf1 from the cables and indeed cdc8 does interfere with Adf1 binding to actin filaments in vitro.[92] In the absence of cdc8, Adf1 completely disassembled actin filaments of the contractile ring demonstrating that a balance between Adf1 and cdc8 activities is necessary to maintain a functional contractile ring. Analysis of Adf1 mutants that disrupt either severing (S120A) or depolymerizing (Y82F) activity revealed that CofilinY82F could restore a proper contractile ring in Adf1-depleted cells whereas cofilin S120A was ineffective. This study suggests that the severing activity of cofilin is essential and demonstrates an antagonist role between AC proteins and Tm in modulating actin filament dynamics during cytokinesis.

Cell Motility

Cell migration is essential for proper development of multicellular organisms as well as for the maintenance of tissue integrity. However, as is evident in metastasis and the formation of secondary tumors, aberrant cell migration can be harmful. Polarized migration of cells is highly directed and is morphologically associated with a leading edge lamellipodium at the front of a broad lamella. Cell migration depends on highly regulated and coordinated dynamics of actin filament structures within the leading edge of cells. Our rather simplistic view of the leading edge of advancing cells with an underlying rapid actin filament turnover has seen a rigorous revision over the past few years due to the discovery of new actin binding proteins and a more detailed understanding of their function. Two spatially distinct subdomains within the leading edge of migrating cells have been identified each characterized by a unique regulation of actin filament dynamics and distinct molecular composition.[93] These two distinct subcompartments of actin filaments are defined by four measurable criteria: (1) unique molecular composition, (2) spatial difference in rates of actin filament turnover (kinetics), (3) rate of actin filament translocation (kinematics) and (4) mechanism of actin filament translocation (kinematics).[94] In the 2 to 4 μm wide, Arp2/3 complex containing lamellipodial region under the plasma membrane, intense treadmilling and rapid retrograde flow occur due to assembly of actin at the membrane and severing and depolymerization of actin filaments at the rear of this zone (kinetics). At the interface between the lamellipodium and lamella reside the major sites of adhesive contacts to the extracellular environment. The lamella, a region behind the lamellipodium but within 3 to 15 μm of the leading edge, contains Tm and myosin II. Although spatially random spots of actin filament turnover occur in the lamella, a slower myosin-dependent retrograde flow accumulates these filaments in a zone, often referred to as an actin arc, further back in the cytoplasm.

Maintenance of a polarized migrating phenotype requires active ADF/cofilin; over expression of LIMK1 causes the loss of polarity but polarity can be rescued by expression of a nonphospho-regulatable form of cofilin.[95] Tm plays a critical role in maintaining the spatial separation of two actin filament pools, with a clear difference between normal and malignant cells (see Chapter 10).[96] Acute addition of TGF-β to epithelial cells induces membrane ruffling tied to enhanced motility but over a prolonged period results in the formation of stress fibers and reduced cell motility. The long-term effects required protein synthesis and expression of several actin binding proteins, among them Tm. Stress fiber formation was absent without Tm expression, evidence that supports Tm stabilizing contractile actin filaments. Interestingly, stress fiber formation in response to TGF-β was not observed in metastatic cells and was linked to hyperactivity of the ras-ERK signaling pathway. No change in the degree of cofilin phosphorylation was determined. Presumably, the loss of TGF-β responsiveness could contribute to the metastatic phenotype of tumor cells.

In epithelial cells, endogenous Tm is localized to the lamella with little to none in the lamellipodium. Yet after injection of skeletal Tm (skTm) into these cells, skTm extended out to the leading edge.[94] Concomitant with a depletion of Arp2/3 and ADF, there is a loss of the lamellipodium indicated by changes in both the kinetics and kinematics of actin filament dynamics. Over abundance of skTm also increased myosin II interaction with actin filaments. Importantly, cell motility was not eliminated but protrusion time and retraction times of membrane ruffles was altered. These results demonstrate that lamellipodial activity is not necessary for cell migration; however, directional migration in response to extracellular cues probably does require a lamellipodium in order to modulate localized actin assembly and turnover in response to extracellular signals. One concern of this study is the utilization of a skeletal muscle Tm isoform in an epithelial cell environment, especially given the non redundancy and cell type-specific functions of many Tm isoforms. Furthermore, a clear border between lamella and lamellipodium is not a necessity and these domains could substantially overlap.[97]

A more recent study demonstrated that changes in Tm levels have a direct influence on cofilin and its activity. Downregulation of Tm resulted in a substantial enlargement of the lamellipodium at the expense of the lamella, whereas elimination of cofilin in a *Drosophila* cell line had the opposite effect, an expansion of the lamella at the expense of the lamellipodium and an increase in Tm decoration of actin filaments.[98] In contrast, enhancement of lamellipodial cofilin activity accelerates F-actin turnover and retrograde flow, resulting in widening of the lamellipodium.[99] This is accompanied by increased spatial overlap of the lamellipodium and lamella networks and reduced cell edge protrusion efficiency. Thus, the leading edge of the cell has multiple actin superstructures; the lamellipodium consisting of a submembraneous domain rich in Arp2/3 complex branched filaments and an ADF/cofilin enriched domain and the lamella, enriched in linear actin filament bundles containing Tm and myosin, some of which can overlap the lamellipodial structures (Fig. 4).

Golgi Membrane Sorting and Vesicle Dynamics

The Golgi apparatus is the cellular hub for sorting proteins through numerous vesicle trafficking pathways to and from the plasma membrane, lysosomes, endosomes and endoplasmic reticulum (ER). Many regions of the plasma membrane on most cells are quite dynamic undergoing endocytosis and exocytosis, increasing membrane area during development, especially in highly

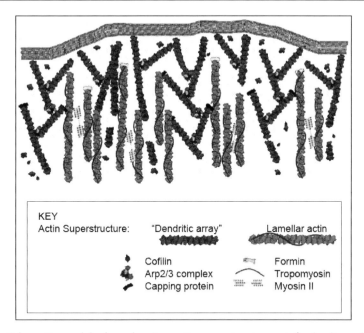

Figure 4. Schematic model of overlapping actin superstructures at the leading edge. The Arp2/3 complex branched actin filaments of the lamellipodial "dendritic array" (red/dark gray) are responsible for much of the membrane protrusive activity driven by actin assembly. Filaments of this superstructure grow for short periods and then are capped by barbed end capping protein (black) as they undergo retrograde flow due to array treadmilling. Cofilin binds to the distal (ADP-actin) subunits and disassembles the filaments for subunit recycling. The tropomyosin-containing filaments of the lamella (green/light gray) can overlap this region. Formins help nucleate linear bundles of actin, which bind tropomyosin and recruit myosin II for contractile events. These filaments also undergo retrograde flow due to myosin-dependent contraction. The two different networks can be distinguished by their kinetic and kinematic properties measured using fluorescence speckle microscopy.[97,99]

asymmetric cells such as neurons. Thus the maturation, modification and delivery of membrane proteins via the Golgi apparatus are essential. Treatment of cells with actin filament disrupting toxins such as latrunculins or cytochalasins resulted in severe alterations to the Golgi morphology and disrupted some aspects of vesicle trafficking, suggesting a vital role for actin at the Golgi.[77] In addition, β and γ-actin have been found in association with Golgi membranes, as well as other actin binding proteins including myosin II, tropomyosin isoform Tm5NM1, profilin, gelsolin and AC.[65,100-102] In yeast and mammals, post Golgi vesicle trafficking requires myosin II and V, profilin and tropomyosin.[65,103] Evidently, actin filament dynamics is necessary for the positioning of the Golgi apparatus, at least some form of vesicle budding and retrograde vesicle traffic from Golgi to ER. Of particular interest is the fact that in neurons trafficking of vesicles from the trans Golgi to axons but not to the somatodendritic domain requires cofilin-driven actin dynamics.[104] Thus, whatever the mechanism for actin involvement in Golgi in vesicle sorting, it applies only to a selected population of vesicles and is not a general mechanism required for all Golgi-derived vesicles. Presumably this will be dictated by either specific cytoplasmic proteins or lipids, which can recruit specific families of proteins to modulate actin-vesicle interactions.

The role of Tms in Golgi function, specifically the Tm isoforms Tm5NM1 and 2, have been studied.[79] Both isoforms are generated from the γTm gene through alternative splicing and differ only in the differential splicing of exon 6. Most interestingly, Tm5NM1 is exclusively localized to stress fibers whereas Tm5NM2 is concentrated at the Golgi and is associated with a subpopulation of vesicles containing short actin filaments. ARF-1 is essential for targeting Tm5NM2 to the Golgi. Presumably, short stable actin filaments are a prerequisite for the tethering vesicles during short range transport and/or budding. Thus, Tm5NM2 could support this network of short actin filaments by protecting against severing and/or depolymerizing activity of AC proteins. Manipulation of cofilin or LIMK 1 substantially affects the dynamics of the Golgi apparatus.[104] LIMK 1 through its LIM domain is localized to the Golgi and one of its primary functions is the regulation of actin dynamics through phosphorylation of cofilin (i.e., inactivation). Overexpression of active LIMK1 dampens Golgi tubule dynamics but these can be restored by expressing a nonphosphorylatable form of active cofilin (S3A). That cofilin is working via enhancing actin dynamics was demonstrated by titrating in the actin filament stabilizing drug jasplakinolide, which in a dose-dependent fashion dampened the enhanced Golgi tubule dynamics induced by cofilin S3A.[104] In support of this model, a kinase dead version of LIMK1 works in a dominant interfering fashion to alter Golgi morphology similarly to the cofilin S3A. The trans-Golgi tubule network undergoes a loss of compaction, elongated cisternae, enhanced tubule formation and over long time periods, the fragmentation of the Golgi. Thus, proper protein membrane protein sorting/delivery through the Golgi may depend extensively on a tight regulation of the organization and dynamics of short actin filament through an interplay between AC proteins and Tm isoforms. This is an area ripe for further investigation.

Cell Survival/Senescence

Because actin filaments are linked to so many vital cellular processes, it is not surprising that cell viability is linked to actin filament dynamics. However, recent findings attribute a vital function of actin filament dynamics to cellular senescence and apoptosis, both stringently regulated processes. Yeast serves as an excellent model because only one single actin isoform is expressed. Cytoplasmic actin cables in yeast have been long known to support distribution of new mitochondria to budding daughter cells. However, new findings reveal that the filament status of actin is directly impacting cell survival.[105] Reduction of actin filament turnover and accumulation of actin filaments increased the formation of reactive oxygen species (ROS) and induced apoptosis and senescence whereas increasing actin filament turnover shows a concomitant decrease in ROS production and increased viability.[106] Interestingly, many known extrinsic stresses induce actin filament formation and clumping in cells preceding apoptosis. Moreover, actin accumulations such as cofilin-actin rods are associated with many neurodegenerative disorders.[107] Actin filaments physically interact with VDAC channels of mitochondria, one component of the permeability transition pore, thus modulating ROS leakage.[106,108] Furthermore, cofilin-actin binding to mitochondrial outer membrane is an early step in apoptosis and is both necessary and sufficient to cause leakage of cytochrome c, the activator of the Apaf-1 complex that initiates mitochondrial-dependent apoptosis.[109] It thus seems likely that competition and cooperation between cofilin and different Tm isoforms in modulating actin filament stability and turnover also will impact cell survival and aging.

Nuclear Functions of Actin

Actin accumulation in the nucleus occurs in response to several different stressors including heat shock, exposure to high concentrations of DMSO and treatment with cytochalasin B, a fungal metabolite that blocks actin filament barbed-end dynamics. Only recently, specific roles for actin in nuclear events have been emerging. Actin in the nucleus is critical for telomere movement and clustering during prophase in meiosis, which could affect senescence of cells.[110,111] Actin interacts directly with all three RNA polymerases in eukaryotic cells and is required in early transcription.[112] Actin is part of SWI/SNF chromatin remodeling complexes and is necessary to recruit histone modifying enzymes for transcriptional activation.[113] Actin together with myosin 1β interacts with premessenger RNA binding proteins implicated in mRNA transport during transcription.[12] The conformation and polymerization state of actin in all these nuclear processes remains a mystery but is elemental to illuminate its roles.[114] Perhaps, the response of cells to sequester actin in the nucleus upon exposure to extrinsic stressors could arise from its vital role in maintaining transcription. Actin contains a nuclear export sequence but not a nuclear localization sequence (NLS). However ADF/cofilins in all higher eukaryotes have an NLS and can chaperone actin into the nucleus.[8,20] Since AC proteins are generally cytoplasmic, the NLS must be cryptic and only available to interact with other components of the nuclear import complexes when appropriately exposed. The mechanism by which this occurs is not yet clear, but extrinsic signals that alter the ratio and/or turnover of AC phosphorylation might be able to influence gene expression. Events that lead to the decoration of cytoplasmic actin filaments with AC could modulate expression of some genes in one direction whereas Tm-dependent displacement of AC could have opposing effects. Yet another connection between actin filament dynamics and gene expression has been reported. MAL proteins (myocardin family of transcription activators) are capable of transporting actin monomers into nuclei thereby relaying information regarding changes of the monomeric actin pool to gene expression.[115,116] Studies on serum response factor (SRF) demonstrated that specific MAL proteins are implicated in nuclear shuttling of actin thus directly relaying the degree of actin polymerization to transcription.

Conclusions and Perspectives

Two major cytoplasmic isoforms of actin, three isoforms of ADF/cofilin and >40 isoforms of tropomyosin allow for a large variety of different actin filament systems to co-exist within a cell. These allow the formation of regional actin superstructures that may be stable or undergo rapid interconversion. These superstructures may create unique cytoskeletal compartments, or provide overlapping superstructures with different dynamics. Competing activities of Tms and ACs allow for the dynamic interconversion of stable superstructures to those exhibiting rapid turnover. In each cell compartment, the molecular composition of actin filaments is influenced by the presence of a repertoire of Tm and AC isoforms resulting in an enormously complex regulatory system. These interactions generate synergy, cooperativity and reciprocity typical for complex systems of multiple protein interactions. For instance, a naïve actin filament presents a surface allowing interactions with all AC and perhaps Tm members. However, decoration of an actin filament with cofilin stabilizes a "twisted" form thus not only changing the surface of the actin filament for protein interactions but also establishing an additional interaction surface through the bound cofilin (cooperativity). This new interaction surface could either greatly increase or decrease binding affinity of one or several Tm isoforms as well as other actin binding proteins (synergy). Interaction with this new surface could further induce conformational changes in the bound Tm isoform and support or dismiss interaction with Tm targets (reciprocity). The conclusions drawn by many studies might suffer from their combinatorial use of proteins from different sources, some of which are expressed in a different host cell environment. In particular, Tm and AC isoforms exhibit non redundant distribution patterns and activities with respect to cell types and species. For instance, an analysis of a skeletal Tm isoform with actin dynamics in a nonmuscle cell could raise the principal question whether the observed effects reflect actual changes in actin dynamics of the test cell or the actual function of the Tm isoform of the host cell. However, the general picture of cooperation and antagonism between some Tms and ACs is likely to be upheld.

References

1. Chick JK, Lindberg U, Schutt CE. The structure of an open state of beta-actin at 2.65A resolution. J Mol Biol 1996; 263:607-623.
2. Otterbein LR, Graceffa P, Dominguez R. The crystal structure of uncomplexed actin in the ADP state. Science 2001; 293:708-711.
3. Holmes KC, Popp D, Gebhard W et al. Atomic model of the actin filament. Nature 1990; 347:44-49.
4. Lorenz M, Popp D, Holmes KC. Refinement of the F-actin model against X-ray fiber diffraction data by the use of a directed mutation algorithm. J Mol Biol 1993; 234:826-836.
5. Pollard TD, Blanchoin L, Mullins RD. Molecular mechanisms controlling actin filament dynamics in nonmuscle cells. Annu Rev Biophys Biomol Struct 2000; 29:545-576.
6. Carlier MF, Laurent V, Santolini L et al. Actin depolymerizing factor (ADF/cofilin) enhances the rate of filament turnover: implication in actin-based motility. J Cell Biol 1997; 136:1307-1322.

7. Carlier MF, Pantaloni D. Control of actin dynamics in cell motility. J Mol Biol 1997; 269:459-467.
8. Bamburg JR. Proteins of the ADF/Cofilin family: essential regulators of actin dynamcs. Annu Rev Cell Dev Biol 1999; 15:185-230.
9. Moseley JB, Goode BL. The yeast actin cytoskeleton: from cellular function to biochemical mechanism. Microbiol Mol Biol Rev 2006; 70:605-645.
10. Hehnly H, Stamnes M. Regulating cytoskeleton-based motility. FEBS Lett 2007; 581:2112-2118.
11. Pollard TD. Cellular motility powered by actin filament assembly and disassembly. Harvey Lect 2002-2003; 98:1-17.
12. Obrdlik A, Kukalev A, Percipalle P. The function of actin in gene transcription. Histol Histopathol 2007; 22:1051-1055.
13. Pak C, Flynn KC, Bamburg JR. Actin binding proteins take the reigns in growth cones. Nature Revs Neurosci 2008; 9(2):136-147.
14. Gunning PW, Schevzov G, Kee AJ et al. Tropomyosin isoforms: divining rods for actin cytoskeleton function. Trends Cell Biol 2005; 15(6):333-341.
15. Lappalainen P, Kessels MM, Cope MJTV. The ADF homology (ADF-H) domain: a highly exploited actin-binding module. Mol Biol Cell 1998; 9:1951-1959.
16. Puius YA, Mahoney NM, Almo SC. The modular structure of actin-regulatory proteins. Curr Opin Cell Biol 1998; 10:23-34.
17. Vartiainen MK, Mustonen T, Mattila PK et al. The three mouse actin-depolymerizing factor/cofilins evolved to fulfill cell-type specific requirements for actin dynamics. Mol Biol Cell 2002; 13:183-194.
18. Thirion C, Stucka R, Mendel B et al. Characterization of human muscle type cofilin (CFL2) in normal and regenerating muscle. Eur J Biochem 2001; 268:3473-3482.
19. Abe H, Nagaoka R, Obinata T. Cytoplasmic localization and nuclear transport of cofilin in cultured myotubes. Exp Cell Res 1993; 206:1-10.
20. Bamburg JR, McGough A, Ono S. Putting a new twist on actin: ADF/cofilins modulate actin dynamics. Trends Cell Biol 1999; 9:364-370.
21. Lappalainen R, Fedorov EV, Fedorov AA et al. Essential functions and actin-binding surfaces of yeast cofilin by systematic mutagenesis. EMBO J 1997; 16:5520-5530.
22. Galkin VE, Orlova A, Lukoyanova N et al. Actin depolymerizing factor stabilizes an existing state of F-actin and can change the tilt of F-actin subunits. J Cell Biol 2001; 153:75-86.
23. Hawkins M, Pope B, Maciver SK et al. The interaction of human actin depolymerizing factor with actin is pH regulated. Biochemistry 1993; 32:9985-9993.
24. Hayden SM, Miller PS, Brauweiler A et al. Analysis of the interactions of actin depolymerizing factor with G- and F-actin. Biochemistry 1993; 32:9994-10004.
25. McCough A, Pope B, Chui W et al. Cofilin changes the twist of F-actin: implications for actin filament dynamics and cellular function. J Cell Biol 1997; 138:771-781.
26. Andrianantoandro E, Pollard TD. Mechanism of actin filament turnover by severing and nucleation at different concentrations of ADF/cofilin. Mol Biol 2006; 24:13-23.
27. Pavlov D, Muhlrad A, Cooper J et al. Actin filament severing by cofilin. J Mol Biol 2007; 365:1350-1358.
28. Blanchoin L, Pollard TD, Mullin RD. Interactions of ADF/cofilin, Arp2/3 complex, capping proteins and profilin in remodeling of branched actin filament networks. Curr Biol 2000; 10:1273-1282.
29. Moriyama K, Yahara I. Two activities of cofilin, severing and accelerating depolymerization of actin filaments, are affected differentially by mutations around the actin-binding helix. EMBO J 1999; 18:6752-6761.
30. Chen H, Bernstein BW, Sneider JM et al. In vitro activity differences between proteins of the ADF/cofilin family define two distinct subgroups. Biochemistry 2004; 43:7127-7142.
31. Yeoh S, Pope B, Mannherz HG et al. Determining the differences in actin binding by human ADF and cofilin. J Mol Biol 2002; 315:911-925.
32. Nishida E. Opposite effects of cofilin and profilin from porcine brain on rate of exchange of actin-bound adenosine 5'-triphosphate. Biochemistry 1985; 24:1160-1164.
33. Moriyama K, Yahara I. Human CAP1 is a key factor in the recycling of cofilin and actin for rapid actin turnover. J Cell Sci 2002; 115:1591-1601.
34. Bertling E, Hotulainen P, Mattila PK et al. Cyclase associated protein 1 (CAP1) promotes cofilin-induced actin dynamics in mammalian nonmuscle cells. Mol Biol Cell 2004; 15:2324-2334.
35. Paavilainen VO, Bertling E, Falck S et al. Regulation of cytoskeletal dynamics by actin-monomer binding proteins. Trends Cell Biol 2004; 14:386-394.
36. Bertling E, Quintero-Monzon O, Mattila PK et al. Mechanism and biological role of profilin-Srv2/CAP interaction. J Cell Sci 2007; 120:1225-1234.
37. Agnew BJ, Minamide LS, Bamburg JR. Reactivation of phosphorylated actin depolymerizing factor and identification of the regulatory site. J Biol Chem 1995; 270:17582-17587.

38. Arber S, Barbayaniis FA, Hanser H et al. Regulation of actin dynamics through phosphorylation of cofilin by LIM-kinase. Nature 1998; 393:805-809.

39. Yang N, Higuchi O, Ohashi K et al. Cofilin phosphorylation by LIM-kinase 1 and its role in Rac-mediated actin reorganization. Nature 1998; 393:809-812.

40. LaLonde DP, Brown MC, Bouverat BP et al. Actopaxin interacts with TESK1 to regulate cell spreading on fibronectin. J Biol Chem 2005; 280:21680-21688.

41. Niwa R, Nagata-Ohashi K, Takeichi M et al. Control of actin reorganization by Slingshot, a family of phosphatases that dephosphorylate ADF/cofilin. Cell 2002; 108:233-246.

42. Huang TY, DerMardirossian C, Bokoch GM. Cofilin phosphatases and regulation of actin dynamics. Curr Opin Cell Biol 2006; 18:26-31.

43. Nishita M, Tomizawa C, Yamamoto M et al. Spatial and temporal regulation of cofilin activity by LIM kinase and Slingshot is critical for directional cell migration. J Cell Biol 2005; 171:349-359.

44. Yonezawa N, Nishida E, Iida K et al. Inhibition of the interactions of cofilin, destrin and deoxyribo-nuclease I with actin by phosphoinositides. J Biol Chem 1990; 265:8382-8386.

45. Gorbatyuk VY, Nosworthy NJ, Robson SA et al. Mapping the phosphoinositide-binding site on chick cofilin explains how PIP2 regulates the cofilin-actin interaction. Mol Cell 2006; 24:511-522.

46. Okada K, Blanchoin L, Abe H et al. Xenopus actin interacting protein (XAip1) enhances cofilin frag-mentation of filaments by capping filament ends. J Biol Chem 2002; 277:43011-43016.

47. Ono S. Regulation of actin filament dynamics by actin depolymerizing factor/cofilin and actin-interacting protein 1: new blades for twisted filaments. Biochemistry 2003; 42:13363-13370.

48. Okada K, Ravi H, Smith EM et al. Aip1 and cofilin promote rapid turnover of yeast actin patches and cables: a coordinated mechanism for severing and capping filaments. Mol Biol Cell 2006; 17:2855-2868.

49. Clark MG, Amberg DC. Biochemical and genetic analyses provide insight into the structural and mechanistic properties of actin filament disassembly by the Aip1 cofilin complex in Saccharomyces cerevisia. Genetics 2007; 176:1527-2539.

50. Hotulainen P, Paunola E, Vartiainen MK et al. Actin-depolymerizing factor and cofilin-1 play overlap-ping roles in promoting rapid F-actin depolymerization in mammalian nonmuscle cells. Mol Biol Cell 2005; 16:649-664.

51. Minamide LS, Painter WB, Schevzov G et al. Differential regulation of actin depolymerizing factor and cofilin in response to alterations in the actin monomer pool. J Biol Chem 1997; 272:8303-8309.

52. Bernstein BW, Painter WB, Chen H et al. Intracellular pH modulation of ADF/cofilin proteins. Cell Motil Cytoskeleton 2000; 47:319-336.

53. Estornes Y, Gay F, Gevrey JC et al. Differential involvement of destrin and cofilin-1 in the control of invasive properties of Isreco1 human colon cancer cells. Int J Cancer 2007;121:2162-2171.

54. Bernstein BW, Bamburg JR. Tropomyosin binding to F-actin protects the F-actin from disassembly by brain actin-depolymerizing factor (ADF). Cell Motil 1982; 2:1-8.

55. Bamburg JR, Bernstein BW. Actin and actin-binding proteins in neurons. In: Burgoyne RD, ed. The Neuronal Cytoskeleton. New York: Wiley-Liss, 1991:121-160.

56. Nishida E, Maekawa S, Sakai H. Cofilin, a protein in porcine brain that binds to actin filaments and inhibits their interactions with myosin and tropomyosin. Biochemistry 1984; 23:5307-5317.

57. McCough A. F-actin binding proteins. Curr Opin Struct Biol 1998; 8:166-167.

58. Lal AA, Korn ED. Effect of tropomyosin on the kinetics of polymerization of muscle actin. Biochemistry 1986; 25:1154-1158.

59. Blanchoin L, Pollard TD, Hitchock-DeGregori SE. Inhibition of the Arp2/3 complex-nucleated actin polymerization and branch formation by tropomyosin. Curr Biol 2001; 11:1300-1304.

60. Weinberger R, Schevzov G, Jeffrey P et al. The molecular composition of neuronal microfilaments is spatially and temporally regulated. J Neurosci 1996; 16:238-252.

61. Bryce NS, Schevzov G, Ferguson V et al. Specification of actin filament function and molecular com-position by tropomyosin isoforms. Mol Biol Cell 2003; 14:1002-1016.

62. Stehn JR, Schevzov G, O'Neill GM et al. Specialization of the tropomyosin composition of actin fila-ments provides new potential targets for chemotherapy. Curr Cancer Drug Targets 2006; 6:245-256.

63. Pittenger MF, Helfman DM. In vitro and in vivo characterization of four fibroblast tropomyosins pro-duced in bacteria: TM-2, TM-3, TM-5a and TM-5b are colocalized in interphase fibroblasts. J Cell Biol 1992; 118:841-858.

64. Yu R, Ono S. Dual roles of tropomyosin as an F-actin stabilizer and a regulator of muscle contraction in Caenorhabditis Elagans body wall muscle. Cell Motil Cytoskeleton 2006; 63:659-672.

65. Liu HP, Bretscher A. Disruption of the single tropomyosin gene in yeast results in the disappearance of actin cables from the cytoskeleton. Cell 1989; 57:233-242.

66. Moon AL, Janmey PA, Louie KA et al. Cofilin is an essential component of the yeast cortical cytoskel-eton. J Cell Biol 1993; 120:421-435.

67. Wen K-K, Kuang B, Rubenstein PA. Tropomyosin-dependent filament formation by a polymerization-defective mutant yeast actin (V266G, L267G). J Biol Chem 2000; 275:40594-40600.
68. Bharadwaj S, Hitchcock-DeGregori S, Thorburn A et al. N terminus is essential for tropomyosin functions: N-terminal modification disrupts stress fiber organization and abolishes anti-oncogenic effects of tropomyosin-1. J Biol Chem 2004; 279:14039-14048.
69. McKim KS, Matheson C, Marra MA et al. The Caenorhabditis elegans unc-60 gene encodes proteins homologous to a family of actin-binding proteins. Mol Gen Genet 1994; 242:346-357.
70. Ono S, Baillie DL, Benian GM. UNC-60B, an ADF/cofilin family protein, is required for proper assembly of actin into myofibrils in Caenorhabditis elegans body wall muscle. J Cell Biol 1999; 145:491-502.
71. Ono S, Ono K. Tropomyosin inhibits ADF/cofilin-dependent actin filament dynamics. J Cell Biol 2002; 156:1065-1076.
72. Ono S. Regulation of actin filament dynamics by actin depolymerizing factor/cofilin and actin-interacting protein 1: New blades for twisted filaments. Biochemistry 2003; 42:13363-13370.
73. Schevzov G, Gunning P, Jeffrey PL et al. Tropomyosin localization reveals distinct populations of microfilaments in neurites and growth cones. Mol Cell Neurosci 1997; 8:439-454.
74. Schevzov G, Bryce NS, Almonte-Baldonado R et al. Specific features of neuronal size and shape are regulated by tropomyosin isoforms. Mol Cell Biol 2005; 16:3425-3437.
75. Cooper J. Actin dynamics: tropomyosin provides stability. Curr Biol 2002; 12: R523-525.
76. Balasubramanian MK, Helfman DM, Hemmingsen SM. A new tropomyosin essential for cytokinesis in the fission yeast S. pombe. Nature 1992; 360:84-87.
77. Lin JJ, Warren KS, Wamboldt DD et al. Tropomyosin isoforms in nonmuscle cells. Int Rev Cytol 1997; 170:1-38.
78. Hughes JA, Cooke-Yarborough CM, Chadwick NC et al. High molecular weight tropomyosins localise to the contractile rings of dividing CNS cells but are absent from malignant paediatric and adult CNS tumours. GLIA 2003; 42:25-35.
79. Percival JM, Thomas G, Cock TA et al. Sorting of tropomyosin isoforms in synchronised NIH 3T3 fibroblasts: evidence for distinct microfilament populations. Cell Motil Cytoskeleton 2000; 47:189-208.
80. Schevzov G, Vrhovski B, Bryce NS et al. Tissue-specific tropomyosin isoform composition. J Histochem Cytochem 2005; 53:557-570.
81. Glotzer M. Animal cell cytokinesis. Annu Rev Cell Dev Biol 2001; 17:351-386.
82. Noguchi T, Mabuchi I. Reorganization of actin cytoskeleton at the growing end of the cleavage furrow of Xenopus egg during cytokinesis. J Cell Sci 2001; 114:401-412.
83. Pelham RJ, Chang F. Actin dynamics in the contractile ring during cytokinesis in fission yeast. Nature 2002; 419:82-86.
84. Marks J, Hyams JS. Localization of F-actin through the cell division cycle of Schizosaccharomyces pombe. Eur J Cell Biol 1985; 39:27-32.
85. Arai R, Nakano K, Mabuchi I. Subcellular localization and possible function of actin, tropomyosin and actin-related protein 3 (Arp3) in the fission yeast Schizosaccharomyces pombe. Eur J Cell Biol 1998; 76:288-295.
86. Arai R, Mabuchi I. F-actin ring formation and the role of F-actin cables in the fission yeast Schizosaccharomyces pombe. J Cell Sci 2002; 115:887-898.
87. Nagaoka R, Abe H, Kusano K. Concentration of cofilin, a small actin-binding protein, at the cleavage furrow during cytokinesis. Cell Motil Cytoskeleton 1995; 30:1-7.
88. Balasubramanian MK, Hirani BR, Burke JD et al. The Schizosaccharomyces pombe cdc3+ gene encodes a profilin essential for cytokinesis. J Cell Biol 1994; 125:1289-1301.
89. Gunsalus KC, Bonaccorsi S, Williams E et al. Mutations in twinstar, a Drosophila gene encoding a cofilin/ADF homologue, result in defects in centrosome migration and cytokinesis. J Cell Biol 1995; 131:1243-1259.
90. Abe H, Obinata T, Minamide LS et al. Xenopus laevis actin depolymerizing factor/cofilin: a phosphorylation-regulated protein essential for development. J Cell Biol 1996; 132:871-885.
91. Balasubramanian MK, Bi E, Glotzer M. Comparative analysis of cytokinesis in budding yeast, fission yeast and animal cells. Curr Biol 2004; 14:806-818.
92. Nakano K, Mabuchi I. Actin-depolymerizing protein Adf1 is required for formation and maintenance of the contractile ring during cytokinesis in fission yeast. Mol Biol Cell 2006; 17:1933-1945.
93. DesMarais V, Ichetovkin I, Condeelis J et al. Spatial regulation of actin dynamics: a tropomyosin-free, actin-rich compartment at the leading edge. J Cell Sci 2002; 115:4649-4660.
94. Gupton SL, Anderson KL, Kole TP et al. Cell migration without a lamellipodium: translation of actin dynamics into cell movement mediated by tropomyosin. J Cell Biol 2005; 168:619-631.
95. Dawe HR, Minamide LS, Bamburg JR et al. ADF/cofilin controls cell polarity during fibroblast migration. Curr Biol 2003; 13:252-257.

96. Bakin AV, Safina A, Rinehart C et al. A critical role of tropomyosins in TGF-beta regulation of the actin cytoskeleton and cell motility in epithelial cells. Mol Biol Cell 2004; 15:4682-4694.
97. Danuser G. Coupling the dynamics of two actin networks—new views on the mechanics of cell protrusion. Biochem Soc Trans 2005; 33:1250-1253.
98. Iwasa JH, Mullins RD. Spatial and temporal relationships between actin filament nucleation, capping and disassembly. Curr Biol 2007; 17:395-406.
99. Delorme V, Machacek M, DerMardirossian C et al. Cofilin activity downstream of Pak1 regulates cell protrusion effciency by organizing lamellipodium and lamella actin networks. Developmental Cell 2007;13:646-662.
100. Ikonen E, de Almeida JB, Fath KR et al. Myosin II is associated with Golgi membranes: identification of p200 as nonmuscle myosin II on Golgi-derived vesicles. J Cell Sci 1997; 110:2155-2164.
101. Heimann K, Percival JM, Weinberger R et al. Specific isoforms of actin-binding proteins on distinct populations of Golgi-derived vesicles. J Biol Chem 1999; 274:10743-10750.
102. Lorra C, Huttner WB. The mesh hypothesis of Golgi dynamics. Nat Cell Biol 1999; 1:E113-E115.
103. Pruyne DW, Schott DH, Bretscher A. Tropomyosin-containing actin cables direct the Myo2p-dependent polarized delivery of secretory vesicles in budding yeast. J Cell Biol 1998; 143:1931-1945.
104. Rosso S, Bollati F, Bisbal M et al. LIMK1 regulates Golgi dynamics, traffic of Golgi-derived vesicles and process extension in primary cultured neurons. Mol Biol Cell 2004; 15:3433-3449.
105. Gourlay CW, Carpp LN, Timpson P. A role for the actin cytoskeleton in cell death and aging in yeast. J Cell Biol 2004; 164:803-809.
106. Xu X, Forbes JG, Colombini M. Actin modulates the gating of Neurospora crassa VDAC. J Membr Biol 201; 180:73-81.
107. Maloney MT, Bamburg JR. Cofilin-mediated neurodegeneration in Alzheimer's disease and other amyloidopathies. Mol Neurobiol 2007; 35:21-44.
108. Roman I, Figys J, Steurs G et al. Direct measurement of VDAC-actin interaction by surface plasmon resonance. Biochim Biophys Acta 2006; 1758:479-486.
109. Chua BT, Volbracht C, Tan KO et al. Mitochondrial translocation of cofilin is an early step in apoptosis induction. Nat Cell Biol 2003; 5:1083-1089.
110. Scherthan H. Telomere attachment and clustering during meiosis. J Cell Biol 2005; 170:213-223.
111. Trelles-Stricken E, Adelfalk C, Loidl J et al. Meiotic teomere clustering requires actin for its formation and cohesin for its resolution. Nat Cell Biol 2004; 6:1165-1172.
112. Percipalle P, Visa N. Molecular functions of nuclear actin in transcription. J Cell Biol 2006; 172:967-971.
113. Miralles F, Visa N. Actin in transcription and transciption regulation. Curr Op Cell Biol 2006; 18:261-266.
114. Hofmann WA, de Lanerolle P. Nuclear actin: to polymerize or not to polymerize. J Cell Biol 2006; 172:541-542.
115. Wu JI, Crabtree GR. Nuclear actin as choreographer of cell morphology and transcription. Science 2007; 316:1710-1711.
116. Vartiainen MK, Guettler S, Larijani B et al. Nuclear actin regulates dynamic subcellular localization and activity of the SRF cofactor MAL. Science 2007; 316:1749-1752.

CHAPTER 19

Caldesmon and the Regulation of Cytoskeletal Functions

C.-L. Albert Wang*

Abstract

Caldesmon (CaD) is an extraordinary actin-binding protein, because in addition to actin, it also binds myosin, calmodulin and tropomyosin. As a component of the smooth muscle and nonmuscle contractile apparatus CaD inhibits the actomyosin ATPase activity and its inhibitory action is modulated by both Ca^{2+} and phosphorylation. The multiplicity of binding partners and diverse biochemical properties suggest CaD is a potent and versatile regulatory protein both in contractility and cell motility. However, after decades of investigation in numerous laboratories, hard evidence is still lacking to unequivocally identify its in vivo functions, although indirect evidence is mounting to support an important role in connection with the actin cytoskeleton. This chapter reviews the highlights of the past findings and summarizes the current views on this protein, with emphasis of its interaction with tropomyosin.

Introduction

Many important cellular processes involve changes of the actin cytoskeleton, which maintains and controls the cell shape in concert with activities of the contractile apparatus as a result of cell signaling. It is well established that polymerization and depolymerization of actin filaments plays a central role in controlling a wide spectrum of cellular phenomena including cell division and migration, in addition to exo- and endocytosis, apoptosis and inflammation, as well as vesicle trafficking and gene expression.[1,2] A large number of actin cytoskeleton proteins, including focal adhesion complex-associated adaptor proteins and actin-binding proteins (ABPs) are responsible for the organization and remodeling of the actin cytoskeleton. Malfunction of these processes leads to pathological consequences, but how actin-mediated motility is regulated is only beginning to be understood. With recent advances in the field, particularly in the elucidation of protein structures and their binding partners, the potential roles of the actin cytoskeleton in many diseases is becoming apparent. Two proteins, caldesmon (CaD) and tropomyosin (Tm), stand out as unique types of ABPs, because they are also integral components of the contractile apparatus. Both of them are the so-called "side-binders" of actin filaments, which stabilize the filamentous structure; their presence reinforces the stability of F-actin and therefore is intimately involved in the regulation of actin cytoskeleton assembly and organization. In this chapter we aim to describe the biochemical properties of CaD in the context of its relationship with Tm and discuss its biological functions. There is a vast amount of data in the literature on CaD. In an attempt to attain an overview and to derive new insights, some of the earlier observations, especially those controversial ones, will be discussed in comparison with more recent findings. However, it is not the intention of this

*C.-L. Albert Wang—Boston Biomedical Research Institute, 64 Grove Street, Watertown, MA 02472, USA. Email: wang@bbri.org

Tropomyosin, edited by Peter Gunning. ©2008 Landes Bioscience and Springer Science+Business Media.

article to make an exhaustive survey of the entire field. Interested readers are referred to many other excellent reviews that can be found elsewhere.[3-7]

Genes and Isoforms

Vertebrate CaD has a single gene that is alternatively spliced[8] to generate the smooth muscle h-CaD and the nonmuscle isoform (l-CaD),[9,10] the latter being present in almost all types of cells.[11] In the human CaD gene (7q33-q34) there is further isoform diversity in l-CaD. In addition to the first exon (exon1′) shared by h-CaD (793 residues) and l-CaD (termed WI38 l-CaD; 538 residues), another exon (exon 1) further upstream can be used as an alternative initiation site; the resulting isoform (HeLa l-CaD) contains a different N-terminal segment that is 6 residues longer than the WI38-counterpart.[12] Moreover, depending on whether exon 4 (coding for 26 amino acid residues) is incorporated or not, both HeLa- and WI38-l-CaD further exist in type-I and type-II, respectively, giving rise to a total of 4 isoforms of human l-CaD.[13] Exon 1, however, is never transcribed in h-CaD. During embryogenesis h-CaD appears at a later stage than do other smooth muscle markers such as smooth muscle actin,[14] but more parallel to smooth muscle α-Tm (Tm6).[15] It is generally assumed that h-CaD is a component of the contractile apparatus and l-CaD is a cytoskeleton protein.[4,16,17] The difference between the two isoforms is a highly charged repeating sequence, encoded by exon 3b and exon 4, that is only present in h-CaD (Fig. 1). This region forms a 35-nm long single helix (see below) known as the "spacer", which separates the more compact N-terminal myosin-binding domain from the C-terminal actin-binding domain of CaD.[18] It is curious why only h-CaD, but not l-CaD, needs such a spacer region. Presumably, the distance between the two end-domains in h-CaD is evolutionarily optimized to *fit* the specific spatial arrangement of myosin molecules in the smooth muscle thick filament. Such a requirement may not be present in nonmuscle cells. Recently, the expression of smooth muscle CaD was successfully abrogated in mice without blocking the expression of nonmuscle CaD.[19] Such a strategy was achieved by disrupting the CaD gene (on mouse chromosome 6) at exon 3 beyond the splicing site. The homozygous mice thus obtained indeed lack h-CaD, but still express l-CaD. The expression level varies with the tissue type: In tonic vascular smooth muscles the level of

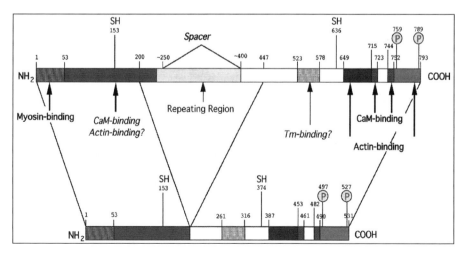

Figure 1. CaD has two isoforms resulting from alternative splicing. The domain structures of mammalian h-CaD (upper bar) and l-CaD (lower bar) indicate the common functional regions for myosin-binding (light green), CaM-binding (red) and actin-binding (blue and turquoise). All functional domains are shared between both isoforms, except that the central 'spacer' (yellow) is missing in l-CaD. Also shown are the two phosphorylation sites common for ERK and cdc2 kinase. A color version of this figure is available at www.Eurekah.com.

l-CaD is low in both the homozygote and the wild-type, whereas in the visceral smooth muscles of homozygous animals l-CaD is much more over-expressed. This appears to be true both at the protein level (by Western blot analysis; Fig. 2) and at the message level.[19] The fact that nonmuscle CaD is apparently able, at least in certain tissues, to "substitute" for h-CaD blurs the boundary between the contractile and cytoskeletal nature of the two isoforms; it also raises questions about the function of CaD in nonmuscle cells.

Smooth muscle cells gradually lose the contractile phenotype upon culturing and become dedifferentiated, fibroblast-like cells; at the same time, h-CaD is replaced by l-CaD.[20,21] Although a number of smooth muscle specific proteins undergo such a differentiation-dependent isoform switchover, including actin,[22] myosin heavy chain,[23] calponin,[24] vinculin[25] and Tm,[26] the expression of CaD and Tm are probably most closely related to each other. In fact, the same splicing machinery appears to work on both CaD and Tm, as the two α-Tm isoforms (α-Tm-SM or Tm6 and α-Tm-F1/2 or Tm2; for Tm nomenclature, see Gunning et al[27]) are expressed in a tightly coordinated fashion with the two isoforms of CaD both in vivo and in vitro.[26,28] Interestingly, when cells were forced to express Tm1 but not Tm2, there was also an up-regulation of CaD expression.[29] It has been shown that a serum response factor (SRF) is necessary but not sufficient to transactivate the CaD promoter.[30] Whether the same or additional factors are recruited for the Tm promoter is not known.

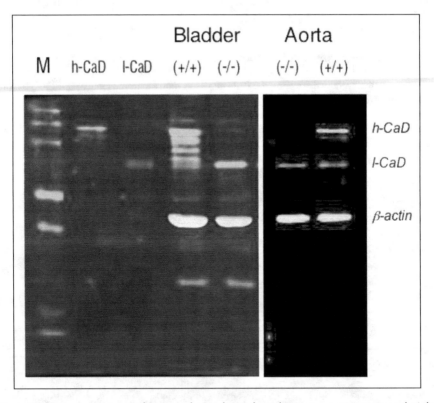

Figure 2. The compensatory isoform switchover depends on the tissue type. Western analysis by Odyssey imaging of tissue extracts from bladder and aorta of wild-type (+/+) and CaD-deficient (−/−) mice. Note that the up-regulation of nonmuscle CaD is more robust in bladder than in aorta. There appeared to be more severe proteolysis in bladder than in aorta. β-actin (green) was used as a reference. A color version of this figure is available at www.Eurekah.com.

Many actin-binding proteins, including CaD[31] and Tm,[32,33] are down-regulated in transformed cells and in certain, although not all, types of cancerous cells. In a sense, these ABPs may act as tumor suppressors. On the other hand, CaD has also been found to be a marker for other types of cancers.[34,35] HeLa-CaD, for example, was found in a number of tumor cells.[36-38] While the antibodies specific for the exon 1 of HeLa-CaD could serve as useful tools for diagnostic purpose, it is rather surprising that the replacement of the leading peptide in the N-terminus would make such a functional difference.

Cellular Content of h-CaD

There has been a controversy over whether the h-CaD content varies among different types of smooth muscles.[39-42] Using immuno-precipitated whole muscle extracts, quantified by Coomassie Blue staining in combination with Western blot analysis, Haeberle et al[39] found that phasic smooth muscles (rat uterus and guinea pig taenia coli, where CaD : actin = 1 : 22-28) have more CaD (8- and 5-fold using actin and myosin as references, respectively) than do tonic vascular smooth muscles (bovine aorta and porcine carotid artery). Lehman et al[42] on the other hand, reported that the two types of smooth muscles (sheep and rabbit aorta, versus rabbit stomach and uterus and chicken gizzard) have about the same level of CaD (~1 mol CaD per 34 mol actin or 5 mol Tm) in either isolated native thin filaments, or heat-treated or unfractionated tissue extracts. It was thought that immuno-quantification of CaD from different species could be difficult owing to differential reactivity toward the antibodies;[41] in the meantime, fractionation could also have left some proteins unaccounted for.[40] Still, the discrepancy is puzzling, because both groups seem to have had adequate controls and exercised stringent precautions. A simple, although unlikely, explanation is that different tissues were used. Other potential causes for the apparent disagreement include the estimated amount of reference proteins (such as actin) and differential degradation of CaD.

It was reported that the h-CaD content was more than twice higher in phasic opossum esophageal body than in the tonic sphincter.[43] Mice also have a lower h-CaD level in tonic vascular smooth muscles (aorta) than in visceral smooth muscles (bladder; Fig. 2). By Western blot analysis the ratios of h-CaD to β-actin staining in bladder and aorta were found to be 2.1 ± 0.4 and 0.33 ± 0.02, respectively. This would be more in agreement with Haeberle et al.[39] In addition, the nonmuscle isoform was also present in the smooth muscle tissues that were devoid of endothelial cells. In mouse aorta the amount of l-CaD was ~25% of that of h-CaD, but much less (<10% of h-CaD) in the urinary bladder. Previously, Gluhkova et al[44] had reported that 78.2% of the total immunoreactive CaD (both isoforms) in the media of human aorta was attributable to h-CaD, leaving 21.8% (or 27.8% of h-CaD) as l-CaD, in good agreement with these data. Interestingly, Lehman et al[42] also noted that they found a "degradation fragment" of 75 kDa in an unfractionated aorta sample, which may very well be l-CaD. Whether such a peptide had contributed to their overall estimation of CaD content is an intriguing question.

Since h-CaD is known to play an inhibitory role during muscle contraction, the higher expression level of h-CaD in visceral smooth muscles may be necessary to suppress contractility after reaching peak force, giving rise to the characteristics of transient contraction (hence phasic). When the expression of h-CaD was abolished in mice, l-CaD became up-regulated only in phasic muscles.[19] This may suggest that CaD (of either isoform) is "indispensable" in phasic smooth muscles and that l-CaD can at least partially substitute h-CaD for its function. On the other hand, tonic smooth muscles, which contain less h-CaD in the wild-type, did not show isoform switchover in the h-CaD-deficient animals, probably because the basal level of l-CaD was sufficient to carry out h-CaD's function. Although it is conceivable that the actin cytoskeleton exists in all cell types, the exact role of l-CaD in terminally differentiated smooth muscle cells remains an interesting subject of further studies.

Tissue Distribution and in Situ Localization

Immunostaining of isolated thin filaments from chicken gizzard indicated that h-CaD binds actin filaments with a periodicity of 38 nm,[45] similar to that of Tm. However, since the total CaD content is much less than that of actin (actin:Tm:CaD = 28:4:1), a "nonsaturating" model was proposed with staggered binding of CaD to the smooth muscle thin filaments. Interestingly, in such an arrangement the N-terminal end of all CaD molecules would naturally appear on the same side of an actin filament (Fig. 3).[46,47] This type of binding mode may facilitate interactions with the neighboring myosin filament (see below), which is presumably assembled in a side-polar fashion.[48] Furthermore, in order for h-CaD to function as a regulatory protein, the CaD-containing thin filaments must be "appropriately" located on the actin lattice to interact with the much fewer thick filaments.[45] Indeed, in situ immunostaining of gizzard sections demonstrated that h-CaD is associated with a subset of actin filaments and there are regions containing both actin and Tm but void of CaD.[49] A closer examination of these images revealed that CaD is distributed in clusters.[46] Such clustering was seen both in the sections and in isolated native thin filaments, thus ruling out antibody inaccessibility and rebinding of dissociated CaD. The discontinuous distribution was also apparent both along the thin filaments and along the thick filaments. The simplest explanation is that the two kinds of filaments are not parallel to each other, but rather intersect at a small angle (Fig. 4).[17] Since CaD is only needed in the regions that actin filaments overlap with myosin filaments, CaD would naturally appear in clusters along the actin filaments and, at the same time, along the myosin filaments as observed. This model accounts for the limited CaD needed to "saturate" actin and myosin present in much higher amounts and carry out its regulatory function. The obliquely arranged filaments also allow for a greater extent of shortening, which is characteristic for smooth muscles. The fact that smooth muscle myosin forms side-polar filaments[48,50] that are torsionally flexible[50] further supports this model, as the nonparallel filaments could maximize their interactions and facilitate contraction. So far this model remains speculative, but should be testable by mathematical modeling based on the geometrical parameters and more precise force measurements.

Nonmuscle CaD also binds to actin filaments along with Tm. It was reported that both proteins exhibit the same periodicity (~36 nm) on the microfilaments isolated from cultured rat embryonic fibroblasts.[51] Similar patterns of periodic distribution of CaD was also observed in human astroglia.[52] It was noted that such "cross striation" was not seen in gizzard filaments because of the sparse distribution. The similarity of the periodicities for CaD and Tm is striking. This suggests the two proteins not only interact with each other, but are also functionally related. l-CaD and Tm (in most cases, the high molecular weight Tm, HMW-Tm, which includes Tm1, 2, 3 and 6)[27] are normally present in the stress fibers of nonmuscle cells, but characteristically excluded from stable focal adhesions. On the other hand, both proteins as well as myosin II are found in nascent focal

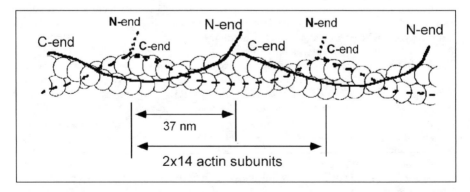

Figure 3. CaD binds actin longitudinally with the N-terminus appearing on one side of the actin filament. A model illustrates the position of h-CaD on the two-stranded actin filament. CaD molecules on one strand are shown in solid lines and those on the opposite strand in broken lines. Note that the ends of all CaD molecules appear on the same side of an actin filament. Such an arrangement is only possible with h-CaD. Taken from Mabuchi et al.[206]

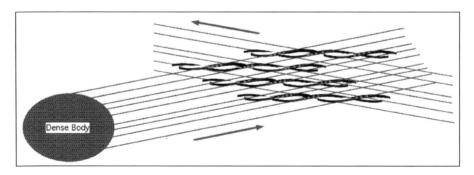

Figure 4. A model with obliquely arranged contractile units allows clustered distribution of h-CaD along both actin and myosin filaments. Actin filaments (thin lines attached to the dense body) and myosin filaments (thick lines with a helical twist to represent the side-polar filaments) intersect each other at an angle. Both the intersecting angles and the twist of myosin filaments are exaggerated in this drawing. The myosin heads on opposite sides of the myosin filament interact with two bundles of actin filaments in reverse orientation, allowing muscle shortening. As suggested by this model, because of the nonparallel alignment, a given myosin filament is bound to interact with multiple actin filaments in the same bundle. Assuming that h-CaD (red dots) is only present at the junctions of these filaments, it naturally has a clustered distribution along either the actin or the myosin filament. Taken from Wang.[6] A color version of this figure is available at www.Eurekah.com.

contacts and more dynamic structures such as podosomes[53] and neuronal growth cones.[54] It was thought that these contractile proteins are involved in the regulation of actomyosin activities (see below) and their presence therefore indicates the loci of cellular contraction. In fibroblasts l-CaD distinguishes itself from myosin II and HMW-Tms by the fact that it is primarily associated with short actin filaments in the core of the podosomes,[53] as well as ruffling membranes.[55] Curiously, low molecular weight Tms (LMW-Tms),[56] along with other cytoskeleton proteins including myosin I,[57] are also found at cell leading edges and growth cones. More recently, it was reported that in osteoclasts LMW-Tms are present in the podosomes with Tm4 in the actin core and Tm5a/5b in the ring that encircles the podosome core.[58] These findings suggest that by targeting a separate pool of actin filaments l-CaD and LMW-Tm are involved in another type of contractile activity.

When the N-terminal fragment of CaD was expressed in CHO cells, the expressed protein appeared in the nucleus.[59] Whether the positively charged amino acid stretches in this region serve as a nuclear localization signal is an intriguing question that remains to be answered. More recently, HeLa-CaD was also found to be present in the nucleus of tumor cells.[60] This finding raises interesting questions, e.g., whether l-CaD is involved in the contractile activities or some other functions in the nucleus.

Direct Interaction between CaD and Tm

Colocalization of CaD and Tm implies these two proteins interact with each other. The direct interaction between CaD and Tm was shown by binding studies[61] and by the salt-dependent enhancement in the viscosity of gizzard Tm in the presence of stoichiometric amounts of h-CaD.[62] Such binding was reversed by calmodulin (CaM) in the presence of Ca^{2+}.[63,64] This direct interaction may conceivably contribute to the observed increase in the inhibitory effect of CaD, although a more indirect route through actin cannot be ruled out.[65] Subsequently, it was determined that the Tm-binding sites were localized in the C-terminal region.[66-70] This region of the last ~300 amino acid residues not only contains the actin- and the CaM-binding sites, but also harbors TnT-analogous sequences that interact with Tm.[71] Apparently there are several peptide segments in this region that bind actin, Tm and CaM independently (see, for example, 72). The affinity between CaD and Tm at physiological ionic strength was estimated to be 2.5×10^{-5} M^{-1} and was enhanced by actin.[73]

Based on further binding studies a model was proposed in which CaD binds Tm in an antiparallel manner at sites near Cys-190 (residue 201-227).[74] This region probably is fairly sticky, because it also interacts with calponin.[75]

CaD and Tm enhance each other's affinity for actin. They also act synergistically on other actin binding proteins. For example, CaD and Tm together, but not separately, inhibit the actin-binding and actin-bundling activity of fascin, a protein involved in the formation of microspikes in cultured cells.[76] Clearly, the interaction between CaD and Tm plays a role in this effect, although the detailed mechanism requires further elucidation. In light of that l-CaD exhibits differential colocalizations with specific nonmuscle Tm isoforms (see above), it would also be interesting to compare the interactions between l-CaD and different Tm isoforms.

Molecular Shape and Domain Structure

Both h-CaD and Tm are elongated molecules. Hydrodynamic studies indicated that h-CaD is 74 nm in length,[77] about twice as long as Tm. While Tm forms an α-helical coiled-coil, h-CaD contains a long, single helix in the middle of the molecule.[78] It is interesting that this middle segment, which is encoded by exons 3b and 4 and is therefore missing in l-CaD, contains 11 repeats of a 15-amino acid residue motif of oppositely charged residues (Glu and Lys/Arg) and alanine. This unique sequence has long been thought to form a coiled-coil structure based on widely accepted algorithms (such as COILS[79] and Paircoil,[80]) but the lack of cooperativity in the thermal unfolding that is characteristic to Tm[81] clearly defies such a prediction. Instead, the periodically spaced charged residues form (i, i + 4) ion pairs and thus stabilize the single helical structure.[82] Under the electron microscope, h-CaD appears to be a rather rigid dumbbell, with the two end-domains separated by a fixed distance of 60 ± 3 nm.[83] The two domains at the N- and the C-termini are configurationally more compact, but lack well-defined secondary structures. They appear easily collapsible under rotary shadowing.[83] Indeed, structural studies showed the C-terminal region of CaD contains multiple β-turns, which allows for plenty of flexibility and facilitates docking on actin filaments.[84]

Functionally, the C-terminal region of CaD harbors actin-, CaM- and Tm-binding sites,[68,85-89] whereas the N-terminal domain contains the major myosin-binding sites[90-92] and also interacts with CaM and actin.[93,94] The actin- and myosin-binding capacity enables CaD to play a role in bringing the thin filaments close to the thick filaments (see below). Actin binding on both ends of CaD renders the molecule to lie down on the actin filament longitudinally. The fact that one of these two actin-binding sites is near the myosin-binding site is also consistent with the observation that myosin S-1 is able to change the orientation of bound CaD in the ternary complex without displacement.[95] However, the N-terminal actin-binding site apparently has a lower affinity for actin than the C-terminal ones and is heat labile.[96] After heat treatment, CaD no longer adheres to the actin filament, but only binds to the filament by its C-terminal end, leaving the N-terminal end sticking out.[97] This type of binding mode, termed as the mosaic multiple-binding model,[98,99] may also occur when CaD is added to actin in the absence of Tm under near saturating concentrations. That CaD contains multiple actin-binding sites (both in the full-length molecule and in the C-terminal fragment, see below) is consistent with its strong tendency to bundle actin filaments in vitro.[100,101] Tm seems to promote the dissociation of such bundles,[102] which could indicate that in the presence of Tm lengthwise binding is preferred.

CaD and Tm as Actin-Binding Proteins

The elongated shapes of CaD and Tm facilitate their binding to actin filaments as "side-binders". Upon binding, they stabilize the filamentous structure, increase the rigidity of the filament[103] and synergistically protect against gelsolin-mediated severing.[104,105] Tm is also known to enhance the affinity of CaD for actin by lowering the dissociation rate[106] and thereby to augment CaD's inhibitory action on the actomyosin ATPase activity.

Binding of CaD on actin filaments was visualized by 3D reconstruction studies. Helical reconstruction of negatively stained filaments decorated with a C-terminal CaD fragment (H32K) demonstrated density attributable to H32K on subdomain 1 of actin, consistent with earlier reconstructions of full length CaD[107] and with biochemical data.[84] In the reconstructed image H32K is localized on the inner aspect of subdomain 1, but instead of binding along the same genetic strand, it traverses the upper surface of the subdomain towards actin's C-terminus and forms a bridge to the neighboring actin monomer of the adjacent long-pitch helical strand, by connecting to its subdomain 3 (Fig. 5), thus "stapling" the two strands of actin filaments.[108] This "staple-like" binding mode suggests a mechanism by which CaD could stabilize actin filaments and resist F-actin severing or depolymerization in both smooth muscle and nonmuscle cells. In the image of ERK-phosphorylated H32K, which is less effective in inhibiting the ATPase (see below), the density over subdomain 1 is much less and the inter-strand connectivity is lost. The two-pronged attachment of CaD on actin was supported by intramolecular FRET coupled with mass spectrometric analysis.[109] It was shown that within the C-terminal region of CaD there exist multiple actin-binding segments that form two clusters, each constituting one actin-attaching site; when H32K is phosphorylated by ERK, only one of the two actin-binding clusters dissociates from F-actin.

The above model was further tested by crosslinking experiments using chicken mutants, H32Kqc (with Q766 replaced by Cys, thus containing 2 Cys) and H32Kqc/ca (a double mutant with the endogenous Cys595 also replaced by Ala; containing only one Cys at position 766). When both Cys residues were labeled with a photo-crosslinker, benzophenone maleimide, H32Kqc was

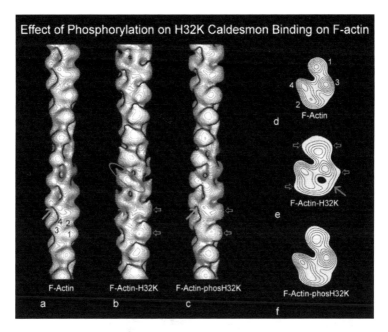

Figure 5. 3-D reconstruction shows an unusual binding mode of CaD on the actin filament. Surface views (a-c) of thin filament reconstructions showing the position of the C-terminal CaD fragment, H32K and phospho-H32K on F-actin and transverse sections (d-f) through maps of 3D reconstructions. The extra density (open bold arrows in b and c) contributed by H32K is associated with subdomains 1 and 2 of actin. In b the density that spans like a staple from the back of subdomain 1 to subdomain 3 of the neighboring actin monomer of the genetic helix (red ellipse). This inter-strand connectivity is present in b (red arrow), but is absent in a and c (green arrows). Open bold arrows in e indicate regions of significant H32K density and the red arrow points to the inter-strand density. Taken from Foster et al.[108] A color version of this figure is available at www.Eurekah.com.

capable of crosslinking actin subunits to form high molecular weight adducts, indicating that it spans at least 2 actin subunits when bound to F-actin. ERK-phosphorylated H32Kqc, however, no longer crosslinks actin to polymers.[108] Similar results were obtained by disulfide crosslinking between H32Kqc and actin (Fig. 6). The single-Cys mutant H32Kqc/ca only crosslinks to one actin monomer; such crosslinking is also diminished after phosphorylation by Erk. Furthermore, acrylamide quenching experiments showed that the solvent accessibility of probes attached to Cys766, but not to Cys595, was increased by ERK treatment.[108] These results are consistent with a phosphorylation-dependent conformational change that moves the C-terminal segment of CaD, but not the other binding site, away from F-actin, conferring the observed removal of its inhibitory effect.

The presence of multiple actin-binding sites in the C-terminal region is again consistent with the observation that even the CaD fragment bundles actin filaments.[110] The bundles formed by the fragment, however, are tight and straight, unlike the loose bundles derived from the full-length CaD (Fig. 7), indicating the relatively close proximity between the actin-binding sites in the fragment. Interestingly, it was noted that the bundling activity of the C-terminal half of CaD was diminished by the addition of the N-terminal fragment.[111] Although this may have been a charge effect exerted by the acidic N-fragment, as seen with polyanionic peptides,[112] it could also be due to the

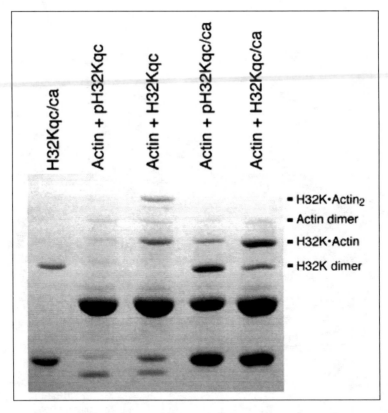

Figure 6. CaD is able to crosslink neighboring actin subunits. Disulfide crosslinking occurs between a C-terminal CaD fragment that contains two cysteine residues (at positions 595 and 766; H32Kqc), or its variant that contains only one cysteine residue (at position 766; H32Kqc/ca) and actin, as shown by the SDS-PAGE with Coomassie staining in the absence of reducing agent. Note that ERK-induced phosphorylation resulted in less H32Kqc/ca•actin crosslinking and almost no H32Kqc•actin₂ species.

N-terminal actin-binding site. That the C-terminal fragment of CaD binds two neighboring actin subunits also explains CaD's ability to act as a nucleator that promotes actin polymerization under the conditions actin normally exists as monomers.[113,114] On the other hand, we (Huang and Wang, unpublished observations) and others (Matsumura, personal communication) have found that CaD imposes some inhibition on actin polymerization when monitored by the pyrene fluorescence of labeled actin, although only a minimal effect was reported earlier.[115] This apparent paradox and how a "side-binder" inhibits the polymerization process remains to be reconciled.

Biochemical Properties and Regulatory Functions

Smooth muscle CaD inhibits the actomyosin ATPase activity[116] and Tm enhances such an inhibitory effect. A similar inhibitory effect of nonmuscle CaD has also been observed in resting

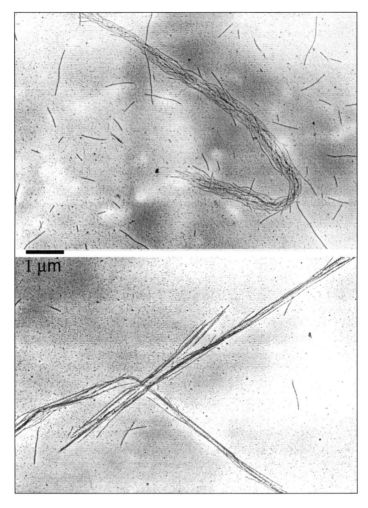

Figure 7. Actin filaments form bundles in the presence of CaD. CaD is known to bundle actin filaments owing to its multiple actin-binding sites. However, full-length h-CaD forms loose bundles (top panel), whereas the C-terminal fragment forms tight and straight bundles (bottom panel). Both samples were processed for rotary shadowing and viewed by electron microscopy. Scale bar: 1 μm. (Mabuchi and Wang, unpublished results).

platelets.[117] The molecular mechanism of the CaD-Tm inhibition has been a subject of great interest (see also Chapter 9). It has been shown that in the presence of Tm, the actomyosin ATPase activity was inhibited to a maximum (>80%) at a 1:10-13 molar ratio of CaD to actin monomer compared to only 50% inhibition for CaD alone.[101,118] This is not only because the enzymatic activity of actomyosin is enhanced by Tm owing to its activating effect at the myosin concentration used,[119-121] but more importantly, because there is a synergistic effect of Tm on CaD's action. CaD exerts its inhibitory effect by decreasing the V_{max}[122] and/or increasing the K_{ATPase}.[123] The latter is most likely due to a direct competition between CaD and weak myosin binding to actin (in the presence of ATP)[124] as their binding sites on the actin surface overlap.[107] It has been shown that competition between CaD and myosin alone can give rise to an apparent cooperative activation of the thin filament even in the absence of Tm,[125] although Tm enhances such a cooperativity.[126] This Competition Model, however, has been disputed, because there was a disagreement whether the concentration of CaD needed for the inhibition of myosin binding matches that for the inhibition of the ATPase activity.[127] Indeed it takes "unphysiologically" high ([CaD] : [actin] > 1 : 7) amounts of CaD to show a sigmoid-shaped binding isotherm, although there seems no such requirement to slow the myosin binding rate in the kinetic experiments.[126] On the other hand, it was argued that the reduced binding rate could be balanced out by a change in the dissociation rate, yielding a moderate (9%) overall maximum rate reduction that fails to account for the observed level of inhibition (75%) of the ATPase unless a higher concentration of CaD was used.[128] The discrepancy is difficult to reconcile, not only because of the subtle differences in the experimental conditions (such as ionic strength and temperature), but also due to the intrinsically complicated nature of the system that involves multiple, mutually interacting, protein species. However, it might be worthwhile to point out that the cellular contents of CaD and actin only give an averaged ratio between the two. Knowing that CaD has a clustered distribution in the smooth muscle,[46] one cannot rule out the possibility of a higher local concentration of CaD. Moreover, it is well known that there is a minimal level (10-15%) of myosin phosphorylation before tension is detected in smooth muscles.[129] Whether the blockage of myosin binding by CaD causes this threshold, which resembles the simulated coorperativity,[126] awaits further investigation.

An alternative interpretation of CaD's inhibition is primarily based on the observed change in the catalytic activity, which can be best explained by a switch of the thin filament state. Like troponin (Tn) in the striated muscle system, CaD at relatively low concentrations may alter the position of Tm on the actin filament depending on other regulatory factors such as Ca^{2+}/CaM or phosphorylation and thereby modulate the actomyosin interaction in a cooperative fashion.[130] So it can be Tm, instead of CaD, that blocks the binding of myosin. This Cooperative-Allosteric Model is supported by both structural[107] and biochemical data.[127,128] Two important pieces of evidence are that at low ratios (1:14) to actin, CaD was able to compete with not only weak, but also strong, myosin binding to actin[131] and that CaD was able to decrease the population of moving filaments without much changing the velocity in the in vitro motility assay.[132] These observations are indeed difficult to explain by the pure Competition Model. While in many cases CaD behaves similarly to Tn, there are differences. Kinetic experiments (using skeletal S1)[128] showed that CaD affects the cross-bridge cycling by mainly slowing down the rate of phosphate release, rather than that of the ADP release as in the case of Tn-Tm.[133] These results also suggested that CaD moves Tm between two states (open and closed), rather than three states (including a blocked state) as in the skeletal muscle system.[134] On the other hand, CaD itself may constitute a blocked state in smooth muscle as implied by the Competition Model and structural studies (see below).

Since CaD abolishes the effect of Tm to enhance the actomyosin ATPase activity (at high myosin concentrations) without dissociating bound Tm from F-actin,[117] it was thought that CaD could change the state of bound Tm along the actin filament, a conclusion reached indirectly by several other investigators.[61,118,135] This structural effect was later visualized in the 3D reconstruction from electron microscopic images of the smooth muscle thin filament. It was found that CaD "keeps" Tm at a position that is close to the inner domain of the actin subunit where it is away from the major myosin binding sites.[136] Upon addition of Ca^{2+}/CaM, CaD (the C-terminal part) is dissociated from the filaments and at the same time, Tm becomes dislodged and rolls to the outer domain of actin surface that usually is considered as the "closed" position.[137] While these studies confirm that CaD indeed alters the position of Tm on actin, such a movement is in sharp contrast to what has been observed for Tn-Tm in the striated muscle system,[138] suggesting that CaD regulates the actomyosin ATPase activity in a fashion different from that of Tn. The finding that Tm is situated in a position opposite to that predicted by the actomyosin ATPase activity in both activated and resting states is also surprising. This apparent paradox was reconciled as follows: In the resting state smooth muscle Tm lies in a position partially overlapping the strong myosin binding site, while CaD sterically blocks the weak myosin binding and results in inhibition.[107] When activated by Ca^{2+}/CaM, CaD is locally dissociated, allowing Tm to move to a closed position. In that position active myosin heads can move Tm to the open position, thereby activating neighboring actin subunits.[139] Smooth muscle Tm has a strong end-to-end interaction;[140] it would be easier for myosin to turn on more actin subunits than in the striated muscle, conferring a higher cooperativity. Thus it seems both the Competitive Model and Allosteric Model are partly correct. By either mechanism, CaD negatively regulates the actomyosin interaction and acts as a molecular brake.[141]

CaD also Binds to Myosin

Unlike Tm, CaD also interacts with myosin.[142,143] The primary myosin-binding sites are localized in the N-terminal region of CaD,[92] although a secondary site in the C-terminal region has also been reported.[144] The interaction site on myosin has been identified as being in the S-2 region.[142] Smooth muscle myosin is known to undergo a conformational change upon phosphorylation.[145,146] In the unphosphorylated state the myosin heads tend to fold back to the rod and assumes a compact configuration (the so-called 10S form). Upon phosphorylation the molecule prefers an extended configuration (the 6S form). The folded form of unphosphorylated myosin is enzymatically inactive and unable to form filaments. Electron microscopic imaging showed that the myosin heads in this inactive configuration "droop" down, whereas they are pointing more upward in the extended, active 6S configuration.[147] The heads-down configuration of the relaxed myosin was also demonstrated in a recent 3D image reconstruction of invertebrate thick filament,[148] where the unphosphorylated myosin heads appear to interact with the S2 region of the rod. Such potential interactions may be disrupted by the N-terminal region of CaD, shifting the equilibrium toward the "heads-up" configuration, thereby "activating" the myosin head without phosphorylation (Fig. 8). Indeed, it was observed that CaD promotes filament assembly of unphosphorylated myosin under the conditions that myosin otherwise stays soluble.[149] We have found that the actin-activated ATPase activity of unphosphorylated smooth muscle heavy meromyosin is increased by the N-terminal CaD fragment (by 46%), but not by the C-fragment (Huang and Wang, unpublished results). However, this effect may not manifest itself as true activation, because the C-terminal region of CaD would inhibit the ATPase activity under a condition when myosin is unphosphorylated.

Binding of myosin via the N-terminal end of CaD and binding of actin via the C-terminal end enables cross-linking of actin filaments to myosin filaments.[150] This may be structurally important for the maintenance of the intracellular filamentous organization, considering that smooth muscle cells do not contain sarcomeric compartments. At a low CaD concentration the tethering effect actually recruits myosin molecules and promotes in vitro motility.[151] The interaction between CaD and myosin is rather weak ($Ka{\sim}10^5\ M^{-1}$),[92] so that it does not impede the sliding movement of the filaments during contraction; on the other hand, the binding energy may be sufficient to dictate the localization of CaD and give rise to a discontinuous distribution.[17] It is also conceivable that the latch phenomenon known for tonic type of smooth muscles could result from the simultaneous binding of CaD to both actin and myosin.[152] That the unphosphorylated myosin exerts a mechanical load to shortening filaments suggests that tethering of thick and thin filaments by CaD might help in maintaining some basal force such as the vascular tone under resting conditions.[153] On the other hand, antisense knockdown of h-CaD in arterial smooth muscles showed that after the CaD content was decreased (by 78%) upon antisense oligodeoxynucleotide treatment, there was an apparent 62% decrease in contractility.[154] This was interpreted as an increased basal tone

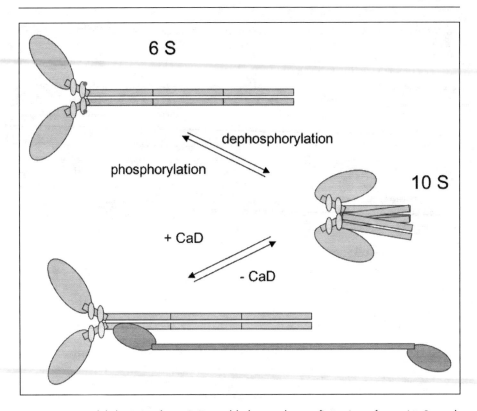

Figure 8. A model depicting how CaD could change the configuration of myosin. Smooth muscle myosin heavy chains (orange) undergo a conformational change upon phosphorylation (red dots) at the light chains (yellow) from an elongated (6S) to a compact (10S) configuration. In this model binding of the N-terminal domain of CaD (blue) to the S-2 region of myosin is thought to interfere with the head-rod interaction and shift the myosin conformation to the 6S form even in the absence of phosphorylation. A color version of this figure is available at www.Eurekah.com.

due to the loss of h-CaD. If true, this observation would imply that smooth muscle regulation includes a thin-filament-based disinhibition component by h-CaD. The in vivo function of CaD may thus be both inhibitory for the active tension and maintaining the passive tension. In non-muscle cells l-CaD most likely plays a similar role to regulate the cellular tension.[155] For example, CaD has been suggested to be involved in cell blebbing.[156] This interesting aspect also deserves more investigation.

Phosphorylation as a Regulatory Mechanism

Nearly all cytoskeleton proteins are substrates of one or more kinases. Phosphorylation by intracellular kinases downstream of Ras and Rac may in fact be one common feature shared by many ABPs. Through phosphorylation the actin-binding properties of these ABPs are altered, thus allowing actin cytoskeleton remodeling. For CaD, the inhibitory effect is diminished upon phosphorylation.[157] In intact smooth muscle the level of CaD phosphorylation indeed increases upon stimulation[158] and the responsible kinase has been identified to be MAPK.[159,160] Phosphorylation of CaD was also detected in cultured smooth muscle cells upon serum stimulation.[161] Such phosphorylation was markedly reduced by the MEK inhibitor PD98059, but not by the p38 MAPK inhibitor SB203580,[161] thus strongly pointing to ERK-induced phosphorylation during cell proliferation. With the use of mass spectrometry it was shown that phosphorylation at Ser759 and Ser789 of mammalian smooth muscle CaD (or Ser497 and Ser527 in nonmuscle CaD; Fig. 1) indeed dissociates one of the actin-binding sites of CaD and weakens its inhibitory effect on the actomyosin ATPase activity.[109] The regulatory role of CaD phosphorylation by MAPK in smooth muscle cells still remains controversial, because inhibition of MAPK failed to produce detectable differences in contractility of smooth muscle tissues;[162] however, there is little doubt that phosphorylation of CaD is involved in nonmuscle cell division and locomotion. As shown by Yamboliev and Gerthoffer,[163] inhibition of ERK phosphorylation slowed down the PDGF-induced migration of cultured smooth muscle cells by 50%.

For nonmuscle CaD a number of pioneering discoveries on phosphorylation were made by Matsumura's group. Of particular interest are the findings that CaD transiently dissociates from actin filaments during mitosis[164] and that p34[cdc2] is responsible for regulating this process.[165] In contrast to ERK, which phosphorylates CaD primarily at only 2 sites near one of the actin-binding sites, there are a total of 7 residues in the C-terminal region of CaD that can be phosphorylated by cdc2 kinase.[166,167] These residues encompass both actin-binding sites, such that when all are phosphorylated CaD dissociates from actin completely.[168] Immunofluorescence images indicate that, in contrast to other actin-binding proteins such as myosin, α-actinin and Tm, CaD is not concentrated at the cleavage furrow until the later stages of cytokinesis.[169] Based on this finding, it was postulated that CaD inhibits activation of the contractile ring at early stages of assembly, presumably by blocking either the actomyosin interaction, or the severing activities of gelsolin, both being required for cytokinesis. Upon phosphorylation by cdc2 kinase, CaD dissociates from actin filaments, thus removing the inhibitory effects and allowing activation of the contractile ring. Prevention of CaD phosphorylation at all potential cdc2 sites by mutagenesis indeed slows down progression through the cell cycle.[156,170] More direct evidence for CaD phosphorylation in individual cells at various cell cycle stages was obtained by immuno-staining studies. Anti-phosphopeptide antibodies revealed a dynamic change of CaD phosphorylation throughout the cell cycle progression, in a manner that is reciprocal to the change of actin stress fibers.[171] These results suggest that phosphorylation of CaD has a broad functional significance. It is more likely to be involved in the change of cell shape during cell division as well as in postmitotic spreading. Interestingly, the same residues of the major phosphorylation sites during mitosis[172] are also phosphorylated when cultured smooth muscle cells are stimulated to migrate.[173,174] Since both ERK and cdc2 kinase are simultaneously activated under a wide range of conditions,[175-177] CaD phosphorylation may thus provide a common mechanism to link cell proliferation and cell migration, both requiring cell shape changes.

When the cdc2-sites or the ERK-sites were blocked by mutagenesis, cell division and detachment were slowed down, but not stopped,[171,178] indicating that there must be alternative pathways that cells can adopt to circumvent the impediment. Indeed, CaD is also known to be phosphorylated by the p21-activated protein kinase (PAK).[179] The major PAK-phosphorylated sites (Ser672 and Ser702, in the chicken smooth muscle sequence)[180] are also in the C-terminal region, but different from the ERK sites. It was reported[181] that constitutively active PAK causes Ca^{2+}-independent contractility in smooth muscle fibers accompanied by an increase in the level of CaD phosphorylation at the same position as Ser672 in the chicken sequence. When these residues were mutated to Ala, CaD appeared to accumulate at cell leading edges, suggesting a potential role for phosphorylation in cell motility. Since PAK is a downstream effector in the Rac1/Cdc42 signaling pathways[182] under a variety of agonist stimulations, it is not at all surprising that PAK-induced phosphorylation affects migratory behaviors. Whether CaD is indeed subject to PAK regulation and the structural and functional consequences of this are of great interest. These issues have been addressed in parallel with the investigation of ERK-phosphorylation. An interesting cellular feature is the formation of podosomes, which exist in many cell types including smooth muscle cells.[183,184] In A7r5 cells podosomes are formed upon stimulation with phorbol dibutyrate (PDBu), which activates PKC. Interestingly, l-CaD is present in such podosomes[185] and is phosphorylated at ERK sites.[186] By over-expressing a phosphorylation-deficient CaD-GFP mutant it was found that, although both the size and the lifetime of the podosomes are modulated by ERK-mediated CaD phosphorylation, the modes of ERK and CaD in their modulation of the formation and dynamics of podosomes are different.[186] This suggests involvement of other players in addition to ERK. It turned out that the formation of podosomes was more tightly correlated with PAK mediated phosphorylation of CaD.[187] It was suggested that PAK phosphorylation renders CaD more effective in displacing Arp2/3[115] and thereby increases its ability to inhibit podosome formation. Such an effect should be readily testable by biochemical experiments. Another notable finding in these studies is that ERK-phosphorylated CaD (although not so clear about PAK-phosphorylated CaD) is localized at the ring of podosomes[186] where Tm5a/5b was found in the osteoclasts.[58] Whether such colocalization suggests interactions or common targets is worthy of further investigation.

Nonmuscle CaD and Its Roles during Cell Proliferation and Migration

Over-expression of CaD in nonmuscle cells has led to a number of conflicting phenotypes including stabilized or disrupted stress fibers, increases or decreases of focal adhesions and podosome structures, hampered or unaffected cell division process and enhanced or compromised cell motility.[155,156,171,185,188-192] These interesting yet confusing results may have stemmed from (i) the difference of cell types used, (ii) different stages of cells and (iii) different levels of over-expression. Nevertheless, several observations are particularly noteworthy. Antisense oligonucleotide targeted to CaD dramatically inhibited hormone-induced stress fiber formation.[193] Transfection of adenovirus l-CaD suppressed the growth and survival in vascular smooth muscle cells and inhibited neointimal formation after angioplasty.[194] Most recently it has been shown that ectopic expression of l-CaD suppresses the invasive activity of cancer cells.[195]

Based on the biochemical properties of CaD, it may be assumed that its primary function is to stabilize the actin filaments. Depending on the phosphorylation states and differential affinities toward HMW and LMW Tm isoforms, CaD may target different pools of actin filaments. Over-expression of CaD would be expected to reinforce the actin cytoskeleton. However, excess CaD may displace crosslinked actomyosin bundles and thereby disrupt stress fibers. Similarly, properly regulated CaD should enhance the actin meshwork and promote cell movement, but too much unphosphorylated CaD, as seen in the case of over-expression of the nonphosphorylatable mutant,[171] cell adhesion could be stifled and both cell migration and cell proliferation could be slowed down. This is consistent with the finding that during cell division l-CaD undergoes phosphorylation, which weakens actin-binding. Since Rho activation induces cell adhesion, it had been suggested that focal adhesion involves actomyosin-based contractility.[192] What was not addressed is how much CaD in the cell was phosphorylated. It was observed that phosphorylated, but not unphosphorylated, CaD colocalizes with vinculin.[171] It is thus possible that phospho-CaD recruits essential partners to the newly formed focal adhesions and this process may be blocked by unphosphorylated CaD when expressed in large quantities. By suppressing the expression of CaD in cells and monitoring the adhesion and migration properties, one may be able to assess its overall functions. Interestingly, hampered cytokinesis was also observed upon over-expression of a HMW-and-LMW chimeric nonmuscle Tm that exhibited a much higher affinity toward actin than the wild-type Tm,[196] indicating that disassembly of microfilament organization is an essential step during cell division. Evidently, both CaD and Tm are part of stabilizing factors for the actin cytoskeleton.

In addition to cell division and migration, a number of other functions for l-CaD have been previously suggested. It was reported[197] that a monoclonal antibody against the C-terminal region of CaD inhibited granular movement in fibroblast cells, similar to the effect of anti-Tm antibodies,[198] once again indicating that both CaD and Tm are involved in the organization of the cytoskeleton and trafficking. Furthermore, CaD is associated with Grb2, Shc and Sos; in this complex CaD was found to be tyrosine-phosphorylated.[199,200] More recently, it has also been suggested that the interaction between phospho-CaD and Tm is further influenced by Hsp27.[201] The significance of all these findings awaits further investigation.

Future Directions

Cytoskeleton remodeling involves numerous actin-binding proteins. The fact that all of them including CaD contain multiple target-specific domains suggests that cytoskeleton proteins work together as partners. CaD most likely works with other protein components in addition to Tm for synergistic maintenance and regulation of actin filament function. Many of these binding partners and structural/functional consequences of such interactions remain to be identified. Phosphorylation is also likely to have an effect on the interactions. One example is cortactin, which is an ABP mainly found in the cell cortex.[202] Cortactin is known to bind Arp2/3[203] and also interacts with CaD.[204] Not only was binding of CaD to cortactin demonstrated in vitro, but the two proteins were also shown to colocalize in cells at the cortex, where CaD was found to be phosphorylated.[171] The functional significance of this interaction needs further elucidation. Another prominent candidate is Arp2/3, which competes with CaD for actin binding.[115] Since cortactin promotes Arp2/3-mediated actin polymerization, it would be of interest to see how the interactions among CaD, cortactin and Arp2/3 play out in this process and what ERK- or PAK-phosphorylation would do to them. Myosin may also serve as a partner. Nonmuscle myosin II, like smooth muscle myosin, is activated through light chain phosphorylation.[205] It is possible that the N-terminal region of CaD binds the S2 region and stabilizes the elongated configuration of unphosphorylated myosin II in nonmuscle cells as well. Whether and how this interaction affects the behaviors of nonmuscle cells is not known and should also be tested.

All in all, the role of CaD in the regulation of actin cytoskeleton is still a fertile field. With recent advancement in cell biology, it is timely to perform more detailed biochemical and biophysical studies on cytoskeleton proteins. In light of the fact that both CaD and Tm are involved in cell growth and cell motility, new information should enhance our understanding of cell proliferation and metastasis and lead to development of novel therapeutic agents for the treatment of cancers.

Acknowledgements

The author wishes to thank Drs. Sherwin Lehrer, John Gergely and Jolanta Kordowska for critical reading of this manuscript and Drs. Fumio Matsumura, Katsuhide Mabuchi, Renjian Huang and Knut Langsetmo for valuable discussions and for sharing their unpublished results. This work is supported by the funding from NIH (P01-AR41637).

References

1. Pollard TD, Borisy GG. Cellular motility driven by assembly and disassembly of actin filaments. Cell 2003; 112:453-465.
2. Winder SJ. Structural insights into actin-binding, branching and bundling proteins. Current Opinion in Cell Biology 2003; 15:14-22.
3. Huber PA. Caldesmon. Int J Biochem Cell Biol 1997; 29:1047-1051.
4. Marston SB, Huber PAJ eds. Caldesmon. San Diego, CA: Academic Press, Inc; 1996. Bárány M ed. Biochemistry of Smooth Muscle Contraction. pp77-90.
5. Matsumura F, Yamashiro S. Caldesmon. Curr Opin Cell Biol 1993; 5:70-76.
6. Wang C-LA. Caldesmon and smooth-muscle regulation. Cell Biochem Biophys 2001; 35:275-288.
7. Hai CM, Gu Z. Caldesmon phosphorylation in actin cytoskeletal remodeling. Eur J Cell Biol 2006; 85:305-309.
8. Humphrey MB, Herrera-Sosa H, Gonzalez G et al. Cloning of cDNAs encoding human caldesmons. Gene 1992; 112:197-204.
9. Ueki N, Sobue K, Kanda K et al. Expression of high and low molecular weight caldesmons during phenotypic modulation of smooth muscle cells. Proc Natl Acad Sci USA 1987; 84:9049-9053.
10. Paul ER, Ngai PK, Walsh MP et al. Embryonic chicken gizzard: expression of the smooth muscle regulatory proteins caldesmon and myosin light chain kinase. Cell Tissue Res 1995; 279:331-337.
11. Bretscher A, Lynch W. Identification and localization of immunoreactive forms of caldesmon in smooth and nonmuscle cells: a comparison with the distributions of tropomyosin and alpha-actinin. J Cell Biol 1985; 100:1656-1663.
12. Novy RE, Lin JL, Lin JJ. Characterization of cDNA clones encoding a human fibroblast caldesmon isoform and analysis of caldesmon expression in normal and transformed cells. J Biol Chem 1991; 266:16917-16924.

13. Hayashi K, Yano H, Hashida T et al. Genomic structure of the human caldesmon gene. Proc Natl Acad Sci USA 1992; 89:12122-12126.
14. Duband JL, Gimona M, Scatena M et al. Calponin and SM 22 as differentiation markers of smooth muscle: spatiotemporal distribution during avian embryonic development. Differentiation 1993; 55:1-11.
15. Vrhovski B, McKay K, Schevzov G et al. Smooth Muscle-specific {alpha} Tropomyosin Is a Marker of Fully Differentiated Smooth Muscle in Lung. J Histochem Cytochem 2005; 53:875-883.
16. Matsumura F, Yamashiro S. Caldesmon. Curr Opin Cell Biol 1993; 5:70-76.
17. Wang C-LA. Caldesmon and smooth-muscle regulation. Cell Biochem Biophys 2001; 35:275-288.
18. Wang C-LA, Chalovich JM, Graceffa P et al. A long helix from the central region of smooth muscle caldesmon. J Biol Chem 1991; 266:13958-13963.
19. Guo H, Wang C-LA. Specific disruption of smooth muscle caldesmon expression in mice. Biochem Biophys Res Commun 2005; 330:1132-1137.
20. Owada MK, Hakura A, Iida K et al. Occurrence of caldesmon (a calmodulin-binding protein) in cultured cells: comparison of normal and transformed cells. Proc Natl Acad Sci USA 1984; 81:3133-3137.
21. Dingus J, Hwo S, Bryan J. Identification by monoclonal antibodies and characterization of human platelet caldesmon. J Cell Biol 1986; 102:1748-1757.
22. Owens GK, Loeb A, Gordon D et al. Expression of smooth muscle-specific alpha-isoactin in cultured vascular smooth muscle cells: relationship between growth and cytodifferentiation. J Cell Biol 1986; 102:343-352.
23. Rovner AS, Murphy RA, Owens GK. Expression of smooth muscle and nonmuscle myosin heavy chains in cultured vascular smooth muscle cells. J Biol Chem 1986; 261:14740-14745.
24. Shanahan CM, Weissberg PL, Metcalfe JC. Isolation of gene markers of differentiated and proliferating vascular smooth muscle cells. Circ Res 1993; 73:193-204.
25. Volberg T, Sabanay H, Geiger B. Spatial and temporal relationships between vinculin and talin in the developing chicken gizzard smooth muscle. Differentiation 1986; 32:34-43.
26. Kashiwada K, Nishida W, Hayashi K et al. Coordinate expression of alpha-tropomyosin and caldesmon isoforms in association with phenotypic modulation of smooth muscle cells. J Biol Chem 1997; 272:15396-15404.
27. Gunning PW, Schevzov G, Kee AJ et al. Tropomyosin isoforms: divining rods for actin cytoskeleton function. Trends Cell Biol 2005; 15:333-341.
28. Sobue K, Hayashi K, Nishida W. Expressional regulation of smooth muscle cell-specific genes in association with phenotypic modulation. Mol Cell Biochem 1999; 190:105-118.
29. Shah V, Bharadwaj S, Kaibuchi K et al. Cytoskeletal organization in tropomyosin-mediated reversion of ras-transformation: Evidence for Rho kinase pathway. Oncogene 2001; 20:2112-2121.
30. Momiyama T, Hayashi K, Obata H et al. Functional involvement of serum response factor in the transcriptional regulation of caldesmon gene. Biochem Biophys Res Commun 1998; 242:429-435.
31. Cerda-Nicolas M, Lopez-Gines C, Gil-Benso R et al. Solitary fibrous tumor of the orbit: morphological, cytogenetic and molecular features. Neuropathology 2006; 26:557-563.
32. Leonardi CL, Warren RH, Rubin RW. Lack of tropomyosin correlates with the absence of stress fibers in transformed rat kidney cells. Biochim Biophys Acta 1982; 720:154-162.
33. Ryan MP, Higgins PJ. Cytoarchitecture of Kirsten sarcoma virus-transformed rat kidney fibroblasts: butyrate-induced reorganization within the actin microfilament network. J Cell Physiol 1988; 137:25-34.
34. Watanabe K, Kusakabe T, Hoshi N et al. h-Caldesmon in leiomyosarcoma and tumors with smooth muscle cell-like differentiation: its specific expression in the smooth muscle cell tumor. Hum Pathol 1999; 30:392-396.
35. Comin CE, Dini S, Novelli L et al. h-Caldesmon, a Useful Positive Marker in the Diagnosis of Pleural Malignant Mesothelioma, Epithelioid Type. Am J Surg Pathol 2006; 30:463-469.
36. Zheng PP, van der Weiden M, Kros JM. Differential expression of Hela-type caldesmon in tumour neovascularization: a new marker of angiogenic endothelial cells. J Pathol 2005; 205:408-414.
37. Zheng PP, Hop WC, Sillevis Smitt PA et al. Low-molecular weight caldesmon as a potential serum marker for glioma. Clin Cancer Res 2005; 11:4388-4392.
38. Zheng PP, Luider TM, Pieters R et al. Identification of tumor-related proteins by proteomic analysis of cerebrospinal fluid from patients with primary brain tumors. J Neuropathol Exp Neurol 2003; 62:855-862.
39. Haeberle JR, Hathaway DR, Smith CL. Caldesmon content of mammalian smooth muscles [see comments]. J Muscle Res Cell Motil 1992; 13:81-89.
40. Haeberle JR, Hathaway DR. Correspondence. J Muscle Res Cell Motility 1992; 13:584-585.
41. Lehman W, Denault D, Correspondence. J Muscle Res Cell Motility 1992; 13:582-583.

42. Lehman W, Denault D, Marston S. The caldesmon content of vertebrate smooth muscle. Biochim Biophys Acta 1993; 1203:53-59.

43. Szymanski PT, Chacko TK, Rovner AS et al. Differences in contractile protein content and isoforms in phasic and tonic smooth muscles. Am J Physiol 1998; 275:C684-692.

44. Glukhova MA, Kabakov AE, Frid MG et al. Modulation of human aorta smooth muscle cell phenotype: a study of muscle-specific variants of vinculin, caldesmon and actin expression. Proc Natl Acad Sci USA 1988; 85:9542-9546.

45. Lehman W, Craig R, Lui J et al. Caldesmon and the structure of smooth muscle thin filaments: immunolocalization of caldesmon on thin filaments. J Muscle Res Cell Motil 1989; 10:101-112.

46. Mabuchi K, Li Y, Carlos A et al. Caldesmon exhibits a clustered distribution along individual chicken gizzard native thin filaments. J Muscle Res Cell Motil 2001; 22:77-90.

47. Katayama E, Ikebe M. Mode of caldesmon binding to smooth muscle thin filament: possible projection of the amino-terminal of caldesmon from native thin filament. Biophys J 1995; 68:2419-2428.

48. Craig R, Megerman J. Assembly of smooth muscle myosin into side-polar filaments. J Cell Biol 1977; 75:990-996.

49. Mabuchi K, Li Y, Tao T et al. Immunocytochemical localization of caldesmon and calponin in chicken gizzard smooth muscle. J Muscle Res Cell Motil 1996; 17:243-260.

50. Cooke PH, Fay FS, Craig R. Myosin filaments isolated from skinned amphibian smooth muscle cells are side-polar. J Muscle Res Cell Motil 1989; 10:206-220.

51. Yamashiro-Matsumura S, Matsumura F. Characterization of 83-kilodalton nonmuscle caldesmon from cultured rat cells: stimulation of actin binding of nonmuscle tropomyosin and periodic localization along microfilaments like tropomyosin. J Cell Biol 1988; 106:1973-1983.

52. Abd-el-Basset EM, Ahmed I, Fedoroff S. Actin and actin-binding proteins in differentiating astroglia in tissue culture. J Neurosci Res 1991; 30:1-17.

53. Tanaka J, Watanabe T, Nakamura N et al. Morphological and biochemical analyses of contractile proteins (actin, myosin, caldesmon and tropomyosin) in normal and transformed cells. J Cell Sci 1993; 104:595-606.

54. Kira M, Tanaka J, Sobue K. Caldesmon and low Mr isoform of tropomyosin are localized in neuronal growth cones. J Neurosci Res 1995; 40:294-305.

55. Bretscher A, Lynch W. Identification and localization of immunoreactive forms of caldesmon in smooth and nonmuscle cells: a comparison with the distributions of tropomyosin and alpha-actinin. J Cell Biol 1985; 100:1656-1663.

56. Lin JJ, Hegmann TE, Lin JL. Differential localization of tropomyosin isoforms in cultured nonmuscle cells. J Cell Biol 1988; 107:563-572.

57. Fukui Y, Lynch TJ, Brzeska H et al. Myosin I is located at the leading edges of locomoting Dictyostelium amoebae. Nature 1989; 341:328-331.

58. McMichael BK, Kotadiya P, Singh T et al. Tropomyosin isoforms localize to distinct microfilament populations in osteoclasts. Bone 2006; 39:694-705.

59. Warren KS, Lin JL, Wamboldt DD et al. Overexpression of human fibroblast caldesmon fragment containing actin-, Ca++/calmodulin- and tropomyosin-binding domains stabilizes endogenous tropomyosin and microfilaments. J Cell Biol 1994; 125:359-368.

60. Zheng PP, Weiden MV, Sillevis Smitt PA et al. Hela /-CaD Undergoes a DNA Replication-Associated Switch in Localization from the Cytoplasm to the Nuclei of Endothelial Cells/Endothelial Progenitor Cells in Human Tumor Vasculature. Cancer Biol Ther 2007; 6.

61. Smith CW, Pritchard K, Marston SB. The mechanism of Ca2+ regulation of vascular smooth muscle thin filaments by caldesmon and calmodulin. J Biol Chem 1987; 262:116-122.

62. Graceffa P. Evidence for interaction between smooth muscle tropomyosin and caldesmon. FEBS Lett 1987; 218:139-142.

63. Watson MH, Kuhn AE, Mak AS. Caldesmon, calmodulin and tropomyosin interactions. Biochim Biophys Acta 1990; 1054:103-113.

64. Czurlyo EA, Emelyanenko VI, Permyakov EA et al. Spectrofluorimetric studies on C-terminal 34 kDa fragment of caldesmon. Biophys Chem 1991; 40:181-188.

65. Nomura M, Yoshikawa K, Tanaka T et al. The role of tropomyosin in the interactions of F-actin with caldesmon and actin-binding protein (or filamin). Eur J Biochem 1987; 163:467-471.

66. Fujii T, Ozawa J, Ogoma Y et al. Interaction between chicken gizzard caldesmon and tropomyosin. J Biochem (Tokyo) 1988; 104:734-737.

67. Huber PA, Fraser ID, Marston SB. Location of smooth-muscle myosin and tropomyosin binding sites in the C-terminal 288 residues of human caldesmon. Biochem J 1995; 312:617-625.

68. Wang Z, Horiuchi KY, Chacko S. Characterization of the functional domains on the C-terminal region of caldesmon using full-length and mutant caldesmon molecules. J Biol Chem 1996; 271:2234-2242.

69. Lamb NJ, Fernandez A, Mezgueldi M et al. Disruption of the actin cytoskeleton in living nonmuscle cells by microinjection of antibodies to domain-3 of caldesmon. Eur J Cell Biol 1996; 69:36-44.
70. Hnath EJ, Wang CL, Huber PA et al. Affinity and structure of complexes of tropomyosin and caldesmon domains. Biophys J 1996; 71:1920-1933.
71. Hayashi K, Yamada S, Kanda K et al. 35 kDa fragment of h-caldesmon conserves two consensus sequences of the tropomyosin-binding domain in troponin T. Biochem Biophys Res Commun 1989; 161:38-45.
72. El-Mezgueldi M, Copeland O, Fraser ID et al. Characterization of the functional properties of smooth muscle caldesmon domain 4a: evidence for an independent inhibitory actin- tropomyosin binding domain. Biochem J 1998; 332:395-401.
73. Horiuchi KY, Chacko S. Interaction between caldesmon and tropomyosin in the presence and absence of smooth muscle actin. Biochemistry 1988; 27:8388-8393.
74. Watson MH, Kuhn AE, Novy RE et al. Caldesmon-binding sites on tropomyosin. J Biol Chem 1990; 265:18860-18866.
75. Childs TJ, Watson MH, Novy RE et al. Calponin and tropomyosin interactions. Biochim Biophys Acta 1992; 1121:41-46.
76. Ishikawa R, Yamashiro S, Kohama K et al. Regulation of actin binding and actin bundling activities of fascin by caldesmon coupled with tropomyosin. J Biol Chem 1998; 273:26991-26997.
77. Graceffa P, Wang C-LA, Stafford WF. Caldesmon. Molecular weight and subunit composition by analytical ultracentrifugation. J Biol Chem 1988; 263:14196-14202.
78. Wang C-LA, Chalovich JM, Graceffa P et al. A long helix from the central region of smooth muscle caldesmon. J Biol Chem 1991; 266:13958-13963.
79. Lupas A, Van Dyke M, Stock J. Predicting coiled coils from protein sequences. Science 1991; 252:1162-1164.
80. Berger B, Wilson DB, Wolf E et al. Predicting coiled coils by use of pairwise residue correlations. Proc Natl Acad Sci USA 1995; 92:8259-8263.
81. Graceffa P, Lehrer SS. Dynamic equilibrium between the two conformational states of spin-labeled tropomyosin. Biochemistry 1984; 23:2606-2612.
82. Wang E, Wang C-LA. (i, i + 4) Ion pairs stabilize helical peptides derived from smooth muscle caldesmon. Arch Biochem Biophys 1996; 329:156-162.
83. Mabuchi K, Wang C-LA. Electron microscopic studies of chicken gizzard caldesmon and its complex with calmodulin. J Muscle Res Cell Motil 1991; 12:145-151.
84. Gao Y, Patchell VB, Huber PA et al. The interface between caldesmon domain 4b and subdomain 1 of actin studied by nuclear magnetic resonance spectroscopy. Biochemistry 1999; 38:15459-15469.
85. Bartegi A, Fattoum A, Derancourt J et al. Characterization of the carboxyl-terminal 10-kDa cyanogen bromide fragment of caldesmon as an actin-calmodulin-binding region. J Biol Chem 1990; 265:15231-15238.
86. Fujii T, Imai M, Rosenfeld GC et al. Domain mapping of chicken gizzard caldesmon. J Biol Chem 1987; 262:2757-2763.
87. Riseman VM, Lynch WP, Nefsky B et al. The calmodulin and F-actin binding sites of smooth muscle caldesmon lie in the carboxyl-terminal domain whereas the molecular weight heterogeneity lies in the middle of the molecule. J Biol Chem 1989; 264:2869-2875.
88. Szpacenko A, Dabrowska R. Functional domain of caldesmon. FEBS Lett 1986; 202:182-186.
89. Wang C-LA, Wang L-WC, Xu SA et al. Localization of the calmodulin- and the actin-binding sites of caldesmon. J Biol Chem 1991; 266:9166-9172.
90. Velaz L, Ingraham RH, Chalovich JM. Dissociation of the effect of caldesmon on the ATPase activity and on the binding of smooth heavy meromyosin to actin by partial digestion of caldesmon. J Biol Chem 1990; 265:2929-2934.
91. Wang Z, Jiang H, Yang ZQ et al. Both N-terminal myosin-binding and C-terminal actin-binding sites on smooth muscle caldesmon are required for caldesmon-mediated inhibition of actin filament velocity. Proc Natl Acad Sci USA 1997; 94:11899-11904.
92. Li Y, Zhuang S, Guo H et al. The major myosin-binding site of caldesmon resides near its N-terminal extreme. J Biol Chem 2000; 275:10989-10994.
93. Wang C-LA. Photocrosslinking of calmodulin and/or actin to chicken gizzard caldesmon. Biochem Biophys Res Commun 1988; 156:1033-1038.
94. Wang C-LA, Wang L-WC, Lu RC. Caldesmon has two calmodulin-binding domains. Biochem Biophys Res Commun 1989; 162:746-752.
95. Szczesna D, Graceffa P, Wang C-LA et al. Myosin S1 changes the orientation of caldesmon on actin. Biochemistry 1994; 33:6716-6720.
96. Zhuang S, Mabuchi K, Wang C-LA. Heat treatment could affect the biochemical properties of caldesmon. J Biol Chem 1996; 271:30242-30248.

97. Mabuchi K, Lin JJ, Wang CL. Electron microscopic images suggest both ends of caldesmon interact with actin filaments. J Muscle Res Cell Motil 1993; 14:54-64.

98. Chen YD, Chalovich JM. A mosaic multiple-binding model for the binding of caldesmon and myosin subfragment-1 to actin. Biophys J 1992; 63:1063-1070.

99. Fredricksen S, Cai A, Gafurov B et al. Influence of ionic strength, actin state and caldesmon construct size on the number of actin monomers in a caldesmon binding site. Biochemistry 2003; 42:6136-6148.

100. Moody CJ, Marston SB, Smith CW. Bundling of actin filaments by aorta caldesmon is not related to its regulatory function. FEBS Lett 1985; 191:107-112.

101. Dabrowska R, Goch A, Galazkiewicz B et al. The influence of caldesmon on ATPase activity of the skeletal muscle actomyosin and bundling of actin filaments. Biochim Biophys Acta 1985; 842:70-75.

102. Cuneo P, Magri E, Verzola A et al. 'Macromolecular crowding' is a primary factor in the organization of the cytoskeleton. Biochem J 1992; 281:507-512.

103. Isambert H, Venier P, Maggs AC et al. Flexibility of actin filaments derived from thermal fluctuations. Effect of bound nucleotide, phalloidin and muscle regulatory proteins. J Biol Chem 1995; 270:11437-11444.

104. Ishikawa R, Yamashiro S, Matsumura F. Annealing of gelsolin-severed actin fragments by tropomyosin in the presence of Ca2+. Potentiation of the annealing process by caldesmon. J Biol Chem 1989; 264:16764-16770.

105. Ishikawa R, Yamashiro S, Matsumura F. Differential modulation of actin-severing activity of gelsolin by multiple isoforms of cultured rat cell tropomyosin. Potentiation of protective ability of tropomyosins by 83-kDa nonmuscle caldesmon. J Biol Chem 1989; 264:7490-7497.

106. Chalovich JM, Chen YD, Dudek R et al. Kinetics of binding of caldesmon to actin. J Biol Chem 1995; 270:9911-9916.

107. Lehman W, Vibert P, Craig R. Visualization of caldesmon on smooth muscle thin filaments. J Mol Biol 1997; 274:310-317.

108. Foster DB, Huang R, Hatch V et al. Modes of caldesmon binding to actin: sites of caldesmon contact and modulation of interactions by phosphorylation. J Biol Chem 2004; 279:53387-53394.

109. Huang R, Li L, Guo H et al. Caldesmon binding to actin is regulated by calmodulin and phosphorylation via different mechanisms. Biochemistry 2003; 42:2513-2523.

110. Mornet D, Harricane MC, Audemard E. A 35-kilodalton fragment from gizzard smooth muscle caldesmon that induces F-actin bundles. Biochem Biophys Res Commun 1988; 155:808-815.

111. Takiguchi K, Matsumura F. Role of the Basic C-Terminal Half of Caldesmon in Its Regulation of F-Actin: Comparison between Caldesmon and Calponin. J Biochem (Tokyo). 2005; 138:805-813.

112. Tang JX, Janmey PA. The polyelectrolyte nature of F-actin and the mechanism of actin bundle formation. J Biol Chem 1996; 271:8556-8563.

113. Galazkiewicz B, Mossakowska M, Osinska H et al. Polymerization of G-actin by caldesmon. FEBS Lett 1985; 184:144-149.

114. Makuch R, Kulikova N, Graziewicz MA et al. Polymerization of actin induced by actin-binding fragments of caldesmon. Biochim Biophys Acta 1994; 1206:49-54.

115. Yamakita Y, Oosawa F, Yamashiro S et al. Caldesmon inhibits Arp2/3-mediated actin nucleation. Journal of Biological Chemistry 2003; 278:17937-17944.

116. Ngai PK, Walsh MP. Inhibition of smooth muscle actin-activated myosin Mg2+-ATPase activity by caldesmon. J Biol Chem 1984; 259:13656-13659.

117. Onji T, Takagi M, Shibata N. Caldesmon specifically inhibits the effect of tropomyosin on actomyosin system in platelet. Biochem Biophys Res Commun 1987; 143:475-481.

118. Sobue K, Takahashi K, Wakabayashi I. Caldesmon150 regulates the tropomyosin-enhanced actin-myosin interaction in gizzard smooth muscle. Biochem Biophys Res Commun 1985; 132:645-651.

119. Chacko S, Conti MA, Adelstein RS. Effect of phosphorylation of smooth muscle myosin on actin activation and Ca2+ regulation. Proc Natl Acad Sci USA 1977; 74:129-133.

120. Chacko S, Eisenberg E. Cooperativity of actin-activated ATPase of gizzard heavy meromyosin in the presence of gizzard tropomyosin. J Biol Chem 1990; 265:2105-2110.

121. Dabrowska R, Hinssen H, Galazkiewicz B et al. Modulation of gelsolin-induced actin-filament severing by caldesmon and tropomyosin and the effect of these proteins on the actin activation of myosin Mg(2+)-ATPase activity. Biochem J 1996; 315:753-759.

122. Horiuchi KY, Samuel M, Chacko S. Mechanism for the inhibition of acto-heavy meromyosin ATPase by the actin/calmodulin binding domain of caldesmon. Biochemistry 1991; 30:712-717.

123. Hemric ME, Freedman MV, Chalovich JM. Inhibition of actin stimulation of skeletal muscle (A1)S-1 ATPase activity by caldesmon. Arch Biochem Biophys 1993; 306:39-43.

124. Chalovich JM, Cornelius P, Benson CE. Caldesmon inhibits skeletal actomyosin subfragment-1 ATPase activity and the binding of myosin subfragment-1 to actin. J Biol Chem 1987; 262:5711-5716.

125. Yan B, Sen A, Chalovich JM et al. Theoretical studies on competitive binding of caldesmon and myosin S1 to actin: Prediction of apparent cooperativity in equilibrium and slow-down in kinetics of S1 binding by caldesmon. Biochemistry 2003; 42:4208-4216.

126. Sen A, Chen YD, Yan B et al. Caldesmon reduces the apparent rate of binding of myosin S1 to actin-tropomyosin. Biochemistry 2001; 40:5757-5764.

127. Marston SB, Redwood CS. The essential role of tropomyosin in cooperative regulation of smooth muscle thin filament activity by caldesmon. J Biol Chem 1993; 268:12317-12320.

128. Alahyan M, Webb MR, Marston SB et al. The mechanism of smooth muscle caldesmon-tropomyosin inhibition of the elementary steps of the actomyosin ATPase. J Biol Chem 2006; 281:19433-19448.

129. Rembold CM, Wardle RL, Wingard CJ et al. Cooperative attachment of cross bridges predicts regulation of smooth muscle force by myosin phosphorylation. Am J Physiol Cell Physiol 2004; 287:C594-602.

130. Marston S, Burton D, Copeland O et al. Structural interactions between actin, tropomyosin, caldesmon and calcium binding protein and the regulation of smooth muscle thin filaments. Acta Physiol Scand 1998; 164:401-414.

131. Marston SB, Fraser ID, Huber PA. Smooth muscle caldesmon controls the strong binding interaction between actin-tropomyosin and myosin. J Biol Chem 1994; 269:32104-32109.

132. Fraser ID, Marston SB. In vitro motility analysis of smooth muscle caldesmon control of actin- tropomyosin filament movement. J Biol Chem 1995; 270:19688-19693.

133. Rosenfeld SS, Taylor EW. The dissociation of 1-N6-ethenoadenosine diphosphate from regulated actomyosin subfragment 1. J Biol Chem 1987; 262:9994-9999.

134. McKillop DF, Geeves MA. Regulation of the acto.myosin subfragment 1 interaction by troponin/tropomyosin. Evidence for control of a specific isomerization between two acto.myosin subfragment 1 states. Biochem J 1991; 279(Pt 3):711-718.

135. Horiuchi KY, Miyata H, Chacko S. Modulation of smooth muscle actomyosin ATPase by thin filament associated proteins. Biochem Biophys Res Commun 1986; 136:962-968.

136. Vibert P, Craig R, Lehman W. Three-dimensional reconstruction of caldesmon-containing smooth muscle thin filaments. J Cell Biol 1993; 123:313-321.

137. Hodgkinson JL, Marston SB, Craig R et al. Three-dimensional image reconstruction of reconstituted smooth muscle thin filaments: effects of caldesmon. Biophys J 1997; 72:2398-2404.

138. Lehman W, Vibert P, Uman P et al. Steric-Blocking By Tropomyosin Visualized In Relaxed Vertebrate Muscle Thin Filaments. Journal of Molecular Biology 1995; 251:191-196.

139. Lehrer SS, Geeves MA. The muscle thin filament as a classical cooperative/allosteric regulatory system. J Mol Biol 1998; 277:1081-1089.

140. Lehrer SS, Golitsina NL, Geeves MA. Actin-tropomyosin activation of myosin subfragment 1 ATPase and thin filament cooperativity. The role of tropomyosin flexibility and end-to-end interactions. Biochemistry 1997; 36:13449-13454.

141. Word RA, Stull JT, Casey ML et al. Contractile elements and myosin light chain phosphorylation in myometrial tissue from nonpregnant and pregnant women. J Clin Invest 1993; 92:29-37.

142. Ikebe M, Reardon S. Binding of caldesmon to smooth muscle myosin. J Biol Chem 1988; 263:3055-3058.

143. Hemric ME, Chalovich JM. Effect of caldesmon on the ATPase activity and the binding of smooth and skeletal myosin subfragments to actin. J Biol Chem 1988; 263:1878-1885.

144. Huber PA, Redwood CS, Avent ND et al. Identification of functioning regulatory sites and a new myosin binding site in the C-terminal 288 amino acids of caldesmon expressed from a human clone. J Muscle Res Cell Motil 1993; 14:385-391.

145. Onishi H, Wakabayashi T. Electron microscopic studies of myosin molecules from chicken gizzard muscle I: the formation of the intramolecular loop in the myosin tail. J Biochem (Tokyo) 1982; 92:871-879.

146. Suzuki H, Onishi H, Takahashi K et al. Structure and function of chicken gizzard myosin. J Biochem (Tokyo) 1978; 84:1529-1542.

147. Suzuki H, Stafford WF 3rd, Slayter HS et al. A conformational transition in gizzard heavy meromyosin involving the head-tail junction, resulting in changes in sedimentation coefficient, ATPase activity and orientation of heads. J Biol Chem 1985; 260:14810-14817.

148. Woodhead JL, Zhao FQ, Craig R et al. Atomic model of a myosin filament in the relaxed state. Nature 2005; 436:1195-1199.

149. Katayama E, Scott-Woo G, Ikebe M. Effect of caldesmon on the assembly of smooth muscle myosin. J Biol Chem 1995; 270:3919-3925.

150. Marston S, Pinter K, Bennett P. Caldesmon binds to smooth muscle myosin and myosin rod and crosslinks thick filaments to actin filaments. J Muscle Res Cell Motil 1992; 13:206-218.

151. Haeberle JR, Trybus KM, Hemric ME et al. The effects of smooth muscle caldesmon on actin filament motility. J Biol Chem 1992; 267:23001-23006.

152. Marston SB, Latchbridges J. Muscle Res Cell Motil 1989; 10:97-100.
153. Horiuchi KY, Chacko S. Effect of unphosphorylated smooth muscle myosin on caldesmon-mediated regulation of actin filament velocity. J Muscle Res Cell Motil 1995; 16:11-19.
154. Earley JJ, Su X, Moreland RS. Caldesmon inhibits active crossbridges in unstimulated vascular smooth muscle: an antisense oligodeoxynucleotide approach. Circ Res 1998; 83:661-667.
155. Numaguchi Y, Huang S, Polte TR et al. Caldesmon-dependent switching between capillary endothelial cell growth and apoptosis through modulation of cell shape and contractility. Angiogenesis 2003; 6:55-64.
156. Li Y, Wessels D, Wang T et al. Regulation of caldesmon activity by Cdc2 kinase plays an important role in maintaining membrane cortex integrity during cell division. Cell Mol Life Sci 2003; 60:198-211.
157. Ngai PK, Walsh MP. The effects of phosphorylation of smooth-muscle caldesmon. Biochem J 1987; 244:417-425.
158. Adam LP, Haeberle JR, Hathaway DR. Phosphorylation of caldesmon in arterial smooth muscle. J Biol Chem 1989; 264:7698-7703.
159. Adam LP, Gapinski CJ, Hathaway DR. Phosphorylation sequences in h-caldesmon from phorbol ester-stimulated canine aortas. FEBS Lett 1992; 302:223-226.
160. Childs TJ, Watson MH, Sanghera JS et al. Phosphorylation of smooth muscle caldesmon by mitogen-activated protein (MAP) kinase and expression of MAP kinase in differentiated smooth muscle cells. J Biol Chem 1992; 267:22853-22859.
161. D'Angelo G, Graceffa P, Wang C-LA et al. Mammal-specific, ERK-dependent, caldesmon phosphorylation in smooth muscle. Quantitation using novel anti-phosphopeptide antibodies. J Biol Chem 1999; 274:30115-30121.
162. Nixon GF, Iizuka K, Haystead CM et al. Phosphorylation of caldesmon by mitogen-activated protein kinase with no effect on Ca2+ sensitivity in rabbit smooth muscle. J Physiol (Lond) 1995; 487:283-289.
163. Yamboliev IA, Gerthoffer WT. Modulatory role of ERK MAPK-caldesmon pathway in PDGF-stimulated migration of cultured pulmonary artery SMCs. American Journal of Physiology—Cell Physiology 2001; 280:C1680-C1688.
164. Yamashiro S, Yamakita Y, Ishikawa R et al. Mitosis-specific phosphorylation causes 83K nonmuscle caldesmon to dissociate from microfilaments. Nature 1990; 344:675-678.
165. Yamashiro S, Yamakita Y, Hosoya H et al. Phosphorylation of nonmuscle caldesmon by p34cdc2 kinase during mitosis. Nature 1991; 349:169-172.
166. Mak AS, Carpenter M, Smillie LB et al. Phosphorylation of caldesmon by p34cdc2 kinase. Identification of phosphorylation sites. J Biol Chem 1991; 266:19971-19975.
167. Yamashiro S, Yamakita Y, Yoshida K et al. Characterization of the COOH terminus of nonmuscle caldesmon mutants lacking mitosis-specific phosphorylation sites. J Biol Chem 1995; 270:4023-4030.
168. Yamakita Y, Yamashiro S, Matsumura F. Characterization of mitotically phosphorylated caldesmon. J Biol Chem 1992; 267:12022-12029.
169. Hosoya N, Hosoya H, Yamashiro S et al. Localization of caldesmon and its dephosphorylation during cell division. J Cell Biol 1993; 121:1075-1082.
170. Yamashiro S, Chern H, Yamakita Y et al. Mutant Caldesmon lacking cdc2 phosphorylation sites delays M-phase entry and inhibits cytokinesis. Mol Biol Cell 2001; 12:239-250.
171. Kordowska J, Hetrick T, Adam LP et al. Phosphorylated l-caldesmon is involved in disassembly of actin stress fibers and postmitotic spreading. Exp Cell Res 2006; 312:95-110.
172. Yamashiro S, Yamakita Y, Yoshida K et al. Characterization of the COOH terminus of nonmuscle caldesmon mutants lacking mitosis-specific phosphorylation sites. J Biol Chem 1995; 270:4023-4030.
173. Yamboliev IA, Gerthoffer WT. Modulatory role of ERK MAPK-caldesmon pathway in PDGF-stimulated migration of cultured pulmonary artery SMCs. Am J Physiol Cell Physiol 2001; 280:C1680-1688.
174. Goncharova EA, Vorotnikov AV, Gracheva EO et al. Activation of p38 MAP-kinase and caldesmon phosphorylation are essential for urokinase-induced human smooth muscle cell migration. Biol Chem 2002; 383:115-126.
175. Manes T, Zheng DQ, Tognin S et al. Alpha(v)beta3 integrin expression up-regulates cdc2, which modulates cell migration. J Cell Biol 2003; 161:817-826.
176. Juliano R. Movin' on through with Cdc2. Nat Cell Biol 2003; 5:589-590.
177. Liu X, Yan S, Zhou T et al. The MAP kinase pathway is required for entry into mitosis and cell survival. Oncogene 2004; 23:763-776.
178. Yamashiro S, Chern H, Yamakita Y et al. Mutant caldesmon lacking cdc2 phosphorylation sites delays M-phase entry and inhibits cytokinesis. Molecular Biology of the Cell 2001; 12:239-250.
179. Van Eyk JE, Arrell DK, Foster DB et al. Different molecular mechanisms for Rho family GTPase-dependent, Ca2+-independent contraction of smooth muscle. J Biol Chem 1998; 273:23433-23439.

180. Guo H, Bryan J, Wang C-LA. A note on the caldesmon sequence. J Muscle Res Cell Motil 1999; 20:725-726.
181. McFawn PK, Shen L, Vincent SG et al. Calcium-independent contraction and sensitization of airway smooth muscle by p21-activated protein kinase. Am J Physiol Lung Cell Mol Physiol 2003; 284:L863-870.
182. Vidal C, Geny B, Melle J et al. Cdc42/Rac1-dependent activation of the p21-activated kinase (PAK) regulates human platelet lamellipodia spreading: implication of the cortical-actin binding protein cortactin. Blood 2002; 100:4462-4469.
183. Linder S, Kopp P. Podosomes at a glance. J Cell Sci 2005; 118:2079-2082.
184. Hai CM, Hahne P, Harrington EO et al. Conventional protein kinase C mediates phorbol-dibutyrate-induced cytoskeletal remodeling in a7r5 smooth muscle cells. Exp Cell Res 2002; 280:64-74.
185. Eves R, Webb BA, Zhou S et al. Caldesmon is an integral component of podosomes in smooth muscle cells. J Cell Sci 2006; 119:1691-1702.
186. Gu Z, Kordowska J, Williams GL et al. Erk1/2 MAPK and caldesmon differentially regulate podosome dynamics in A7r5 vascular smooth muscle cells. Exp Cell Res 2007; 313:849-866.
187. Morita T, Mayanagi T, Yoshio T et al. Changes in the balance between caldesmon regulated by p21-activated kinases and the Arp2/3 complex govern podosome formation. J Biol Chem 2007; 282:8454-8463.
188. Warren KS, Shutt DC, McDermott JP et al. Overexpression of microfilament-stabilizing human caldesmon fragment, CaD39, affects cell attachment, spreading and cytokinesis. Cell Motil Cytoskeleton 1996; 34:215-229.
189. Surgucheva I, Bryan J. Over-expression of smooth muscle caldesmon in mouse fibroblasts. Cell Motil Cytoskeleton 1995; 32:233-243.
190. Mirzapoiazova T, Kolosova IA, Romer L et al. The role of caldesmon in the regulation of endothelial cytoskeleton and migration. J Cell Physiol 2005; 203:520-528.
191. Helfman DM, Levy ET, Berthier C et al. Caldesmon inhibits nonmuscle cell contractility and interferes with the formation of focal adhesions. Mol Biol Cell 1999; 10:3097-3112.
192. Grosheva I, Vittitow JL, Goichberg P et al. Caldesmon effects on the actin cytoskeleton and cell adhesion in cultured HTM cells. Exp Eye Res 2006; 82:945-958.
193. Castellino F, Ono S, Matsumura F et al. Essential role of caldesmon in the actin filament reorganization induced by glucocorticoids. J Cell Biol 1995; 131:1223-1230.
194. Yokouchi K, Numaguchi Y, Kubota R et al. l-Caldesmon regulates proliferation and migration of vascular smooth muscle cells and inhibits neointimal formation after angioplasty. Arterioscler Thromb Vasc Biol 2006; 26:2231-2237.
195. Yoshio T, Morita T, Kimura Y et al. Caldesmon suppresses cancer cell invasion by regulating podosome/invadopodium formation. FEBS Lett 2007; 581:3777-3782.
196. Warren KS, Lin JL, McDermott JP et al. Forced expression of chimeric human fibroblast tropomyosin mutants affects cytokinesis. J Cell Biol 1995; 129:697-708.
197. Hegmann TE, Schulte DL, Lin JL et al. Inhibition of intracellular granule movement by microinjection of monoclonal antibodies against caldesmon. Cell Motil Cytoskeleton 1991; 20:109-120.
198. Hegmann TE, Lin JL, Lin JJ. Probing the role of nonmuscle tropomyosin isoforms in intracellular granule movement by microinjection of monoclonal antibodies. J Cell Biol 1989; 109:1141-1152.
199. Boerner JL, McManus MJ, Martin GS et al. Ras-independent oncogenic transformation by an EGF-receptor mutant. J Cell Sci 2000; 113:935-942.
200. Boerner JL, Danielsen AJ, Lovejoy CA et al. Grb2 regulation of the actin-based cytoskeleton is required for ligand-independent EGF receptor-mediated oncogenesis. Oncogene 2003; 22:6679-6689.
201. Somara S, Bitar KN. Phosphorylated HSP27 modulates the association of phosphorylated caldesmon with tropomyosin in colonic smooth muscle. Am J Physiol Gastrointest Liver Physiol 2006; 291(4):630-639.
202. Weed SA, Parsons JT. Cortactin: coupling, membrane dynamics to cortical actin assembly. Oncogene 2001; 20:6418-6434.
203. Daly RJ. Cortactin signalling and dynamic actin networks. Biochem J 2004; 382:13-25.
204. Huang R, Cao G-J, Guo H et al. Direct interaction between caldesmon and cortactin. Arch Biochem Biophys 2006; 456:175-182.
205. Totsukawa G, Yamakita Y, Yamashiro S et al. Activation of myosin phosphatase targeting subunit by mitosis-specific phosphorylation. J Cell Biol 1999; 144:735-744.
206. Mabuchi K, Li YH, Carlos A et al. Caldesmon exhibits a clustered distribution along individual chicken gizzard native thin filaments. J Muscle Res Cell Motil 2001; 22:77-90.

CHAPTER 20

Tropomyosins as Discriminators of Myosin Function

E. Michael Ostap*

Abstract

Vertebrate nonmuscle cells express multiple tropomyosin isoforms that are sorted to subcellular compartments that have distinct morphological and dynamic properties. The creation of these compartments has a role in controlling cell morphology, cell migration and polarization of cellular components. There is increasing evidence that nonmuscle myosins are regulated by tropomyosin in these compartments via the regulation of actin attachment, ATPase kinetics, or by stabilization of cytoskeletal tracks for myosin-based transport. In this chapter, I review the literature describing the regulation of various myosins by tropomyosins and consider the mechanisms for this regulation.

Introduction

Tropomyosins in muscle and nonmuscle cells are key regulators of myosin and actin interactions and dynamics.[1] The most studied tropomyosins are those that are expressed in striated muscle cells where they interact with actin and the troponin-complex to regulate active muscle contraction in a calcium-dependent manner [2 and Chapter 8]. However, tropomyosins are expressed in most tissues and cell types where they have defining effects on cell morphology, intracellular motility and cell migration.

Alternative splicing of the four tropomyosin genes in humans results in the expression of more than 40 isoforms.[1,3] Multiple isoforms are commonly expressed simultaneously in a single cell type and expression is developmentally regulated. Tropomyosin isoforms have discrete subcellular localizations, which results in the creation of distinct microfilament compartments.[4-6] For example, isoforms are differentially sorted in neurons resulting in distinct tropomyosin-actin filament populations in the axons and growth cones, each with different morphological and dynamic properties.[6,7] Cells also contain actin compartments that are notable for the absence of tropomyosin. These tropomyosin-free actins filaments are generally in regions of rapid actin assembly and disassembly.[8]

The presence of different microfilament compartments somehow plays a role in controlling cell morphology, motility and polarization of cellular components,[1] but how the compartments regulate these events in nonmuscle cells is not clear. What is known is that tropomyosin binding modulates actin dynamics by affecting the kinetics of actin polymerization and depolymerization and by regulating the association between actin and actin severing, capping, cross-linking and nucleating proteins.[9]

*E. Michael Ostap—Department of Physiology, University of Pennsylvania School of Medicine, B400 Richards Building, Philadelphia, PA 19104-6085, USA. Email: ostap@mail.med.upenn.edu

Tropomyosin, edited by Peter Gunning. ©2008 Landes Bioscience and Springer Science+Business Media.

Tropomyosin clearly regulates actomyosin interactions in striated muscle contraction, so it is an intriguing possibility that tropomyosin-defined microfilament compartments in nonmuscle cells also control nonmuscle myosins via the regulation of actin binding, ATPase kinetics, or by stabilization of cytoskeletal tracks for myosin-based transport.

Myosin Superfamily

The myosin superfamily consists of 40 genes in humans that sort into 12 phylogenetically distinct families,[10] with additional families present in lower organisms and plants.[11] Myosins are widely expressed and are found in nearly all tissue and cell types where they participate in diverse functions that include muscle contraction, organelle motility, cell adhesion and signal transduction. The subcellular distributions of different myosin isoforms are tightly controlled[12,13] by mechanisms that are not fully understood.

The tail domains are the most obvious structural feature that distinguishes the myosin gene families. These domains have evolved to mediate the specialized roles of the different myosins where they function in myosin-complex assembly or cargo attachment.[14] The motor domains of myosins bind to actin and ATP and generate force. The sequences of the motor domains are significantly more conserved across the myosin families than the tail domains, but differences do exist that result in kinetic and motile adaptations.[15]

All characterized myosins share the same ATPase mechanism that follows the same hydrolysis pathway with similar biochemical intermediates. However, different myosin isoforms (even within the same myosin family) have ATPase mechanisms with very different kinetic rate constants, which results in myosins with different motile properties tuned to specific cellular roles.[15] For example, the kinetic rate constants that define the ATPase mechanism of myosin-II isoforms in fast-twitch striated muscles are fast and allow rapid contractions, while cytoplasmic myosin-II molecules have slow rate constants that allow slow and sustained contractions.[16,17]

A consequence of myosins having diverse kinetic properties is that they have different predominant steady-state intermediates that have different kinetic lifetimes. For example, some myosins are "low-duty-ratio" motors that have predominant steady-state intermediates that are detached from actin, while others are "high-duty-ratio" motors that dwell in states that are strongly bound to actin for long periods of time.[15] These differences result in myosins with distinct steady-state mechanical properties which give them the ability to interact with and activate tropomyosin-actin filaments differently (see below).

Tropomyosin Regulation of Myosins

Members of the myosin superfamily are regulated by several different mechanisms that include one, or a combination of the following: modification of myosin structure and ATPase activity by phosphorylation or calcium binding; control of myosin localization or myosin assembly by protein-protein or protein-lipid interactions; blocking of the actomyosin attachment by actin-binding regulatory proteins; and spatial regulation of actin assembly. It is becoming apparent that both muscle and nonmuscle tropomyosins play roles in the latter two mechanisms.

The best characterized mode of myosin regulation is in striated muscles where myosin binding to actin is regulated by tropomyosin, the troponin complex and calcium (see Chapter 8). In the absence of calcium, actin-bound tropomyosin is in a position to block the myosin.ADP.P$_i$ state from entering its strong-binding state and undergoing a force-generating powerstroke. Calcium binding to the troponin complex stabilizes tropomyosin on the actin filament in a position that allows myosin to enter the strong-binding state. A three-state model for the regulation of myosin binding by tropomyosin has been proposed.[18,19] This model was developed for defining the regulation of striated muscle myosin, but it is likely to be applicable to all tropomyosin containing actin filaments, regardless of the tropomyosin isoform, the presence of troponin, or the myosin isoform.[20] Therefore, it is important to consider this model when investigating the roles of tropomyosin isoforms in nonmuscle myosin regulation.

In the three-state model, tropomyosin acts as a flexible cooperative unit in equilibrium among three states represented by three different positions on the actin filament (Fig. 1). The energy barrier between each of these positions is low. The three states are: the blocked state in which no myosin binding occurs, the closed state in which only weak binding occurs and the open state which allows strong binding. Myosin is catalytically activated by actin only when bound to the open state. The relative populations of the tropomyosin states in the absence of myosin are represented by the equilibrium constants K_B (between the blocked and closed states) and K_T (between the closed and open states). The binding of myosin to actin is represented by K_w (between detached and weakly bound states) and K_s (between the weakly-bound and strongly-bound states). Assuming the affinity of myosin for actin is high in the weakly-bound states and the blocked state is not significantly populated, the ratio of open to closed cooperative units depends on the fraction of actin sites occupied by strongly-bound myosin as defined by $K_T (1 + K_s)^m$ where m is the number of sites occupied by myosin within the cooperative unit (Fig. 1).[19,21] Since K_T is a property of the tropomyosin-actin filament and K_s is a property of the myosin and is dependent on the nucleotide state of the myosin, the activation of the tropomyosin-actin filament (i.e., population of the tropomyosin-actin open state) depends directly on the kinetic properties of both the tropomyosin and myosin isoforms that define these equilibrium constants. This dependence has important implications for understanding the regulation of all myosins, since a single myosin may be regulated differently due to tropomyosin isoform-specific differences in K_T and K_B. Additionally, because different myosin have very different kinetic properties, myosin isoforms will have varying abilities to activate the tropomyosin-actin filament due to differences in the myosins kinetic rate constants, which ultimately define K_w and K_s. For example, a high duty-ratio myosin (e.g., myosin-V) binds to actin tightly and dwells in the strong-binding states (large K_w and K_s),[22] so one would predict that it has a higher probability of binding to the open-state of a tropomyosin-actin filament than a

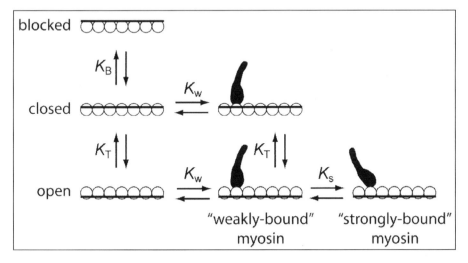

Figure 1. McKillop and Geeves model for activation of tropomyosin-actin filaments.[18] Tropomyosin acts as a flexible cooperative unit that is in equilibrium among three states (blocked, closed, open) with relative populations defined by the equilibrium constants K_B and K_T. K_B and K_T are defined by the intrinsic properties of the tropomyosin-actin filament and are dependent on the tropomyosin isoform. Myosin can not bind to the blocked state. Myosin binds weakly in the closed state and can only transition to the strongly-bound state when the tropomyosin-actin filament is in the open state. The equilibrium constants K_w (between the detached and weakly-bound myosin) and K_s (between the weakly- and strongly-bound myosin) are myosin isoform dependent.

low-duty-ratio myosin (e.g., myosin-I), which binds to actin weakly and dwells in the weak-binding states (small K_w and K_s).[23]

When considering the regulation of myosin by tropomyosin, it is also important to consider the possibilities that some myosin isoforms might interact directly with tropomyosin and different myosins might have slightly different actin binding sites. These differences may alter the myosin affinity and probability of binding to the open state. It is also possible that tropomyosin changes the structure of actin, so the "open state" is not equivalent to the tropomyosin-free state.[24] Finally, it is possible that any or all of these considerations may affect the ATPase kinetics of myosin once it is bound to actin (see below).

Tropomyosin Regulation of Specific Myosins

Myosin-I

Myosin-Is are the widely expressed, low-molecular-weight members of the myosin superfamily that play roles in regulating the structure and dynamics of cell membranes. Eight myosin-I isoforms are expressed in humans where they play crucial roles in a diverse array of essential cellular processes, including endocytosis, vesicle delivery, microvilli structure and dynamics, mechanosignal transduction and transcription.[25-28] All characterized vertebrate myosin-I isoforms bind weakly to actin filaments and are low-duty-ratio motors in the absence of external load, i.e., the predominant steady-state intermediates are weakly-bound to actin.[23,29,30]

Both the myosin-I motor and tail domains are necessary for the correct localization of isoforms to membranes, specialized membrane projections (e.g., microvilli, pseudopods and endocytic structures) and the actin-rich cell cortex.[31,32] The tail domains bind to cellular membranes and to other proteins that may direct myosin-I localization and the motor domains target the myosins to regions of high actin concentration. A key characteristic of myosin-Is is their exclusion from actin filament populations that contain tropomyosin, suggesting that tropomyosins may play a role in regulating myosin-I localization.[13,32,33]

It was suggested that nonmuscle tropomyosins regulate the activity and localization of myo1a (also known as brush border myosin-I) by Collins and Matsudaira[33] based on the exclusion of myosin-I from the terminal web of the apical brush border. Fanning et al[34] showed that vertebrate isoforms of tropomyosin recombinantly expressed in bacteria inhibit the actin-activated ATPase activity of myo1a by greater than 75% and completely inhibit actin gliding in an in vitro motility assay. Moreover, this inhibition was seen with tropomyosin isoforms that activate the ATPase activity of myosin-II isoforms (see below).

In vivo experiments have provided indirect evidence for the regulation of myosin-I based motility by nonmuscle tropomyosin. Microinjection of a tropomyosin isoform (Tm3) into normal rat kidney (NRK) epithelial cells was found to induce retrograde translocation of organelles into the perinuclear region.[35] Because myosin-I and dynein were found to redistribute with the translocated organelles, it was suggested that myosin-I normally inhibits dynein-mediated retrograde motion of these organelles and that the microinjected tropomyosin blocks the ability of myosin-I to interact with actin. Interestingly, microinjection of a low molecular weight tropomyosin isoform (Tm5) had no effect on organelle distribution, suggesting isoform-specific regulation of motor activity.[35]

Tang and Ostap[32] provided further in vivo evidence for tropomyosin regulation of myosin-I. GFP constructs of the widely expressed myosin-I isoform, myo1b, colocalize with dynamic actin filaments, most notably in membrane ruffles and not with actin bundles or stress fibers that contain tropomyosin (Fig. 2). However, a chimeric protein consisting of the tail domain of myo1b and the motor domain of nonmuscle myosin-IIb (which is catalytically activated by actin filaments that contain tropomyosin) concentrates on actin filaments in ruffles as well as on stress fibers and actin cables that contain tropomyosin. This suggests that the exclusion of myo1b from most actin structures is not due to the binding of the myosin-I tail domain to membranes or other receptors. Rather, the exclusion of myo1b from certain actin filament populations is due to regulation of the actomyosin interaction by tropomyosin. This finding is supported by in vitro sliding filament

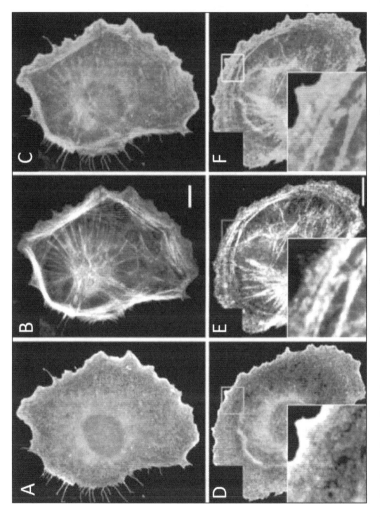

Figure 2. Subcellular localizations of myo1b, actin and tropomyosin. Fluorescence micrographs of a fixed NRK cell expressing (A) myo1b-eGFP labeled with (B) rhodamine phalloidin. C) A merged image showing relative distributions of (green) myo1b-eGFP and (red) F-actin. D) Myo1b-eGFP is not concentrated on (E) tropomyosin-containing actin filaments. Tropomyosin was visualized by indirect immunofluorescence using an anti-tropomyosin (36/39 kDa) monoclonal antibody. The different distributions are clearly seen in the (F) superimposed image and in the insets that show magnification of the cell margin. Myo1b is shown in green and tropomyosin is shown in red. The scale bars represent 10 μm. Figure is reprinted from Tang and Ostap.[32] A color version of this figure is available online at www.Eurekah.com.

assays that show myo1b is inhibited by the nonmuscle Tm2 tropomyosin isoform. This finding is significant because it suggests that myosin-I interacts preferentially with the dynamic and tropomyosin-free actin filament population. Therefore, tropomyosin and spatially regulated actin polymerization play key roles in regulating the activity and localization of myo1b.

The molecular mechanism of tropomyosin regulation of myosin-I has not been definitively determined. One possibility is that the actin-binding site of myosin-I is such that myosin can not bind to actin in the presence of tropomyosin, even when the tropomyosin is in the "open" state (Fig. 1). Kollmar et al[36] found that a surface loop on myosin-I (loop-4) is longer than in other myosin classes and they proposed that the loop would sterically clash with tropomyosin when myosin-I bound to actin. Lieto-Trivedi et al[37] replaced loop-4 in myo1b with the shorter loop of *Dictyostelium* myosin-II and found that this chimera was able to translocate actin filaments in an in vitro motility assay. However, this mutant did not localize to tropomyosin-containing filaments in vivo.

Another key factor in determining myosin-I localization may be the actomyosin-I ATPase and actin-binding kinetics. Myosin-I isoforms are low-duty-ratio motors[23,37] that do not assemble into filaments or other higher-order structures. Therefore, in terms of the model for activation of tropomyosin-actin filaments (Fig. 1), the equilibrium constants K_w and K_s are low (Fig. 1). Thus, the probability of myosin-I populating the strongly bound states in the presence of tropomyosin is low, which would result in no actin-activation of the ATPase activity. If the kinetics of the actomyosin-I interaction are a contributing factor to the regulation by tropomyosin, one would predict that increasing the effective duty ratio of myosin-I would allow the myosin to bind and activate the tropomyosin-actin filament. Tang and Ostap tested the possible contribution of the effective myosin-I duty ratio to actin binding by creating a myo1b protein construct that forms a tetramer, which is expected to have a higher effective duty ratio and larger values of K_s and K_w than the monomer. When the tetrameric construct is expressed in NRK cells, it localizes to stress fibers and actin cables that contain tropomyosin (Fig. 3). Therefore, even in the presence of a native loop-4, myosin-I is able to concentrate to tropomyosin-containing actin compartments.

To fully understand the role of tropomyosin regulation of myosin-I, further characterization of the kinetic relationship of myosin-I with various tropomyosin isoforms is required. For example, it is important to determine (a) if all myosin-I isoforms are regulated by tropomyosin, (b) how different tropomyosin isoforms regulate myosin motility and localization and (c) how actin filament activation is affected by myosin-I concentration. Finally, it is important to determine if tropomyosin and myosin-I can simultaneously bind to actin filaments, since it is possible that the exclusion of tropomyosin from some myosin-I-rich structures (e.g., microvilli) is due directly to competition between tropomyosin and myosin-I for actin binding.

Myosin-II

Myosin-II isoforms are the widely expressed two-headed myosins that assemble into bipolar filaments and are best known as the motors that drive the contraction of muscle cells. Myosin-II isoforms also have contractile roles in nearly all nonmuscle cells, where they function in cytokinesis, cell migration, endocytosis and maintenance of cell structure and tension. The troponin complex of proteins is not expressed in nonmuscle cells and myosin-II in these cells is generally regulated by phosphorylation of myosin light chain.[38] Myosin-II filaments in nonmuscle cells frequently colocalize with tropomyosin-bound actin filaments, so it is likely that tropomyosin has a direct role in modulating nonmuscle myosin-II activity or assembly.

The biochemical and mechanical effects of tropomyosins on myosin-II depend on both the myosin and tropomyosin isoform and the effects range from inhibition to activation of activity. For example, it was shown more than 25 years ago that the actin-activated ATPase activity of smooth muscle myosin-II increases in the presence of smooth muscle tropomyosin[39] and it was subsequently demonstrated that smooth muscle tropomyosin increases the rate of actin gliding in the in vitro motility assay.[40] Fanning et al[34] demonstrated that bacterially expressed *Xenopus* Tm4 (similar to human Tm5b) increases the rate of actin gliding in the presence of skeletal muscle myosin-II, while the chicken isoform Tm4 (similar to human Tm3) does not affect motility, but inhibits the ATPase

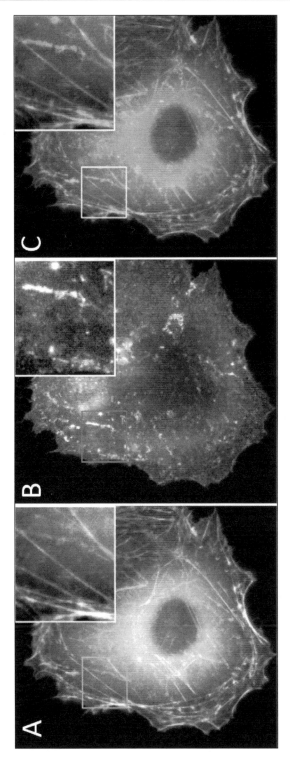

Figure 3. Subcellular localization of (A) GFP-actin and (B) tetrameric myo1b-DsRed in a live NRK cell. The tetrameric myo1b construct is not concentrated in membrane ruffles (compare with (Fig. 2), but is found on actin cables in the cell periphery and on stress-fiber-like structures. The distributions are clearly seen in the (C) superimposed image and in the magnified insets. GFP-actin is shown in green and myo1b-DsRed is shown in red. A color version of this figure is available online at www.Eurekah.com.

activity. Additionally, it has been shown that the mouse nonmuscle myosin-II isoforms show an increase in in vitro motility rates in the presence of smooth muscle tropomyosin.[16,40,41]

Tropomyosins, Tpm1p and Tpm2p, from budding yeast were found to moderately increase the actin gliding velocity in the presence of skeletal muscle myosin II and the velocity depends on the myosin concentration.[42] However, when the two yeast tropomyosins were tested with yeast myosin-II in the in vitro motility assay, it was found that the Tpm1p isoform does not affect the gliding velocity, while the Tpm2p isoform inhibits the velocity by 40% at the same myosin concentration.[43]

How tropomyosin isoforms inhibit or enhance the rates of myosin-II dependent actin gliding has not yet been determined directly. Since motility rates of myosin-II are limited by the rate of ADP release,[44] this step is likely accelerated in the presence of tropomyosin. It is also possible that tropomyosin limits the association of weak-binding crossbridges, which are known to put drag on the gliding filaments, resulting in a reduced velocity.[45]

The differential effects of the myosin and tropomyosin isoforms on motility are likely related to the kinetic properties of both isoforms as described above (Fig. 1). For example, cardiac tropomyosins spend more time in the "blocked state" than yeast tropomyosins,[20] which is consistent with the finding that higher concentrations of myosin are required to propel filaments with cardiac-tropomyosin at the same rates as filaments with yeast tropomyosin.[42]

The cellular consequences of the modulation of actomyosin-II activity by tropomyosin in vertebrate cells are largely unexplored, but it is clear that the differential expression of tropomyosin isoforms results in altered myosin-II localization. For example, Bryce et al[46] demonstrated that over expression of $Tm5_{NM1}$ resulted in the recruitment of myosin-II to stress fibers, while over expression of TmBr3 induced the formation of lamellipodia without increasing myosin-II filament levels. Additionally, over expression of $Tm5_{NM1}$ resulted in the recruitment of myosin-II to the cell margins and to the enlargement of growth cones.[7] Finally, it was found that microinjection of α-skeletal muscle tropomyosin into epithelial cells resulted in the loss of the cell's dynamic lamellipodium, an increase in the rate of cell migration and the alteration of the dynamics of focal adhesions.[47]

A revealing investigation of the roles of the two budding yeast tropomyosins, Tpm1p and Tpm2p, in actin cable dynamics supports a model in which the two isoforms modulate the in vivo myosin-II activity directly.[43] It was found that cells that express only Tpm2p have decreased rates of retrograde flow of actin filament cables, while cells that express only Tpm1p have normal retrograde-flow rates, which is consistent with the effect of the tropomyosin on the rates of actin gliding in the in vitro motility assay. Thus, yeast may control actin dynamics by regulating tropomyosin isoform binding to actin cables during polarized growth.

Myosin-V

Myosin-V is the unconventional myosin that processively transports vesicles and other cellular cargos on actin filaments.[48] Unlike myosins-I and -II, most characterized myosin-V isoforms are high duty ratio motors.[15,49] Detailed investigations of the effects of tropomyosin isoforms on myosin-V biochemistry and motility have not been published. However, it has been reported that tropomyosin does not affect the motility rates of myosin-V coated beads,[50] suggesting that tropomyosin does not play a role in modulating the mechanochemistry of myosin-V. The inability of tropomyosin to inhibit myosin-V is not unexpected, given the high probability of myosin-V activating tropomyosin-actin filaments due to the large K_s, but systematic biochemical experiments are required to determine if this is the case for all tropomyosin isoforms.

Despite the lack of an obvious effect on motility, tropomyosin does play a role in the regulation of myosin-V function. In budding yeast, tropomyosin stabilizes the actin cables that extend from the mother cell to the developing bud during growth. Myosin-V is crucial for the polarized delivery of cargo to the bud via transport along this cable.[51] When tropomyosin is lost, the actin cables disappear, resulting in the loss of the myosin-V cytoskeletal track and inhibition of cargo delivery. It will be of interest to determine if such a function is conserved in higher eukaryotes.

Future Directions

The role of tropomyosin in establishing microfilament compartments for the regulation of cytoskeletal dynamics, cell polarization and organelle dynamics is well established. However, there is much to be learned about how the scores of tropomyosin isoforms regulate, recruit and exclude the multiple members of the myosin superfamily. We have just scratched the surface in understanding how nonmuscle tropomyosins regulate the activities of this diverse motor family. Given the fact that we still do not know much about the cellular roles of many members of the myosin superfamily, there is much work to be done.

Acknowledgements

Supported by grants from the National Institutes of Health (GM57247 and AR051174). I would like to thank Dr. David Hokanson and Jennine Dawicki-McKenna for helpful comments on the manuscript.

References

1. Gunning PW, Schevzov G, Kee AJ, et al. Tropomyosin isoforms: divining rods for actin cytoskeleton function. Trends Cell Biol 2005; 15(6):333-41.
2. Greaser ML, Gergely J. Reconstitution of troponin activity from three protein components. J Biol Chem 1971; 246(13):4226-33.
3. Pittenger MF, Kazzaz JA, Helfman DM. Functional properties of nonmuscle tropomyosin isoforms. Curr Opin Cell Biol 1994; 6(1):96-104.
4. Gunning P, Hardeman E, Jeffrey P, et al. Creating intracellular structural domains: spatial segregation of actin and tropomyosin isoforms in neurons. Bioessays 1998; 20(11):892-900.
5. Lin JJ, Hegmann TE, Lin JL. Differential localization of tropomyosin isoforms in cultured nonmuscle cells. J Cell Biol 1988; 107(2):563-72.
6. Schevzov G, Gunning P, Jeffrey PL, et al. Tropomyosin localization reveals distinct populations of microfilaments in neurites and growth cones. Mol Cell Neurosci 1997; 8(6):439-54.
7. Schevzov G, Bryce NS, Almonte-Baldonado R, et al. Specific features of neuronal size and shape are regulated by tropomyosin isoforms. Mol Biol Cell 2005; 16(7):3425-37.
8. DesMarais V, Ichetovkin I, Condeelis J et al. Spatial regulation of actin dynamics: a tropomyosin-free, actin-rich compartment at the leading edge. J Cell Sci 2002; 115(Pt 23):4649-60.
9. Cooper JA. Actin dynamics: tropomyosin provides stability. Curr Biol 2002; 12(15):R523-5.
10. Berg JS, Powell BC, Cheney RE. A millennial myosin census. Mol Biol Cell 2001; 12(4):780-94.
11. Foth BJ, Goedecke MC, Soldati D. New insights into myosin evolution and classification. Proc Natl Acad Sci USA 2006; 103(10):3681-6.
12. Hasson T, Gillespie PG, Garcia JA et al. Unconventional myosins in inner-ear sensory epithelia. J Cell Biol 1997; 137(6):1287-307.
13. Heintzelman MB, Hasson T, Mooseker MS. Multiple unconventional myosin domains of the intestinal brush border cytoskeleton. J Cell Sci 1994; 107(Pt 12):3535-43.
14. Krendel M, Mooseker MS. Myosins: Tails (and Heads) of Functional Diversity. Physiology (Bethesda) 2005; 20(4):239-51.
15. De La Cruz EM, Ostap EM. Relating biochemistry and function in the myosin superfamily. Curr Opin Cell Biol 2004; 16(1):61-7.
16. Golomb E, Ma X, Jana SS, Preston YA et al. Identification and characterization of nonmuscle myosin II-C, a new member of the myosin II family. J Biol Chem 2004; 279(4):2800-8.
17. Kovacs M et al. Functional divergence of human cytoplasmic myosin II: kinetic characterization of the nonmuscle IIA isoform. J Biol Chem 2003; 278(40):38132-40.
18. McKillop DF, Geeves MA. Regulation of the interaction between actin and myosin subfragment 1: evidence for three states of the thin filament. Biophys J 1993; 65(2):693-701.
19. Maytum R, Lehrer SS, Geeves MA. Cooperativity and switching within the three-state model of muscle regulation. Biochemistry 1999; 38(3):1102-10.
20. Lehman W, Hatch V, Korman V et al. Tropomyosin and actin isoforms modulate the localization of tropomyosin strands on actin filaments. J Mol Biol 2000; 302(3):593-606.
21. Maytum R, Geeves MA, Konrad M. Actomyosin regulatory properties of yeast tropomyosin are dependent upon N-terminal modification. Biochemistry 2000; 39(39):11913-20.
22. De La Cruz EM, Wells AL, Rosenfeld SS et al. The kinetic mechanism of myosin V. Proc Natl Acad Sci USA 1999; 96(24):13726-31.
23. Lewis JH, Lin T, Hokanson DE et al. Temperature dependence of nucleotide association and kinetic characterization of myo1b. Biochemistry 2006; 45(38):11589-97.

24. Tobacman LS, Butters CA. A new model of cooperative myosin-thin filament binding. J Biol Chem 2000; 275(36):27587-93.

25. Sokac AM, Schietroma C, Gundersen CB et al. Myosin-1c couples assembling actin to membranes to drive compensatory endocytosis. Dev Cell 2006; 11(5):629-40.

26. Bose A, Robida S, Furcinitti PS et al. Unconventional myosin Myo1c promotes membrane fusion in a regulated exocytic pathway. Mol Cell Biol 2004; 24(12):5447-58.

27. Tyska MJ, Mackey AT, Huang JD et al. Myosin-1a is critical for normal brush border structure and composition. Mol Biol Cell 2005; 16(5):2443-57.

28. Holt JR, Gillespie SK, Provance DW et al. A chemical-genetic strategy implicates myosin-1c in adaptation by hair cells. Cell 2002; 108(3):371-81.

29. El Mezgueldi M, Tang N, Rosenfeld SS et al. The kinetic mechanism of Myo1e (human myosin-IC). J Biol Chem 2002; 277(24):21514-21.

30. Jontes JD, Milligan RA, Pollard TD et al. Kinetic characterization of brush border myosin-I ATPase. Proc Natl Acad Sci USA 1997; 94(26):14332-7.

31. Ruppert C, Godel J, Müller RT et al. Localization of the rat myosin I molecules myr 1 and myr 2 and in vivo targeting of their tail domains. J Cell Sci 1995; 108(Pt 12):3775-86.

32. Tang N, Ostap EM. Motor domain-dependent localization of myo1b (myr-1). Curr Biol 2001; 11(14):1131-5.

33. Collins K, Matsudaira P. Differential regulation of vertebrate myosins I and II. J Cell Sci Suppl 1991; 14:11-6.

34. Fanning AS, Wolenski JS, Mooseker MS et al. Differential regulation of skeletal muscle myosin-II and brush border myosin-I enzymology and mechanochemistry by bacterially produced tropomyosin isoforms. Cell Motil Cytoskeleton 1994; 29(1):29-45.

35. Pelham RJ Jr, Lin JJ, Wang YL. A high molecular mass nonmuscle tropomyosin isoform stimulates retrograde organelle transport. J Cell Sci 1996; 109(Pt 5):981-9.

36. Kollmar M, Dürrwang U, Kliche W et al. Crystal structure of the motor domain of a class-I myosin. EMBO J 2002; 21(11):2517-25.

37. Lieto-Trivedi A, Dash S, Coluccio LM. Myosin surface loop 4 modulates inhibition of actomyosin 1b ATPase activity by tropomyosin. Biochemistry 2007; 46(10):2779-86.

38. Bresnick AR. Molecular mechanisms of nonmuscle myosin-II regulation. Curr Opin Cell Biol 1999; 11(1):26-33.

39. Chacko S. Effects of phosphorylation, calcium ion and tropomyosin on actin-activated adenosine 5'-triphosphatase activity of mammalian smooth muscle myosin. Biochemistry 1981; 20(4):702-7.

40. Umemoto S, Bengur AR, Sellers JR. Effect of multiple phosphorylations of smooth muscle and cytoplasmic myosins on movement in an in vitro motility assay. J Biol Chem 1989; 264(3):1431-6.

41. Pato MD, Sellers JR, Preston YA et al. Baculovirus expression of chicken nonmuscle heavy meromyosin II-B. Characterization of alternatively spliced isoforms. J Biol Chem 1996; 271(5):2689-95.

42. Strand J, Nili M, Homsher E et al. Modulation of myosin function by isoform-specific properties of Saccharomyces cerevisiae and muscle tropomyosins. J Biol Chem 2001; 276(37):34832-9.

43. Huckaba TM, Lipkin T, Pon LA. Roles of type II myosin and a tropomyosin isoform in retrograde actin flow in budding yeast. J Cell Biol 2006; 175(6):957-69.

44. Siemankowski RF, Wiseman MO, White HD. ADP dissociation from actomyosin subfragment 1 is sufficiently slow to limit the unloaded shortening velocity in vertebrate muscle. Proc Natl Acad Sci USA 1985; 82(3):658-62.

45. Warshaw DM et al. Smooth muscle myosin cross-bridge interactions modulate actin filament sliding velocity in vitro. J Cell Biol 1990; 111(2):453-63.

46. Bryce NS, Schevzov G, Ferguson V et al. Specification of actin filament function and molecular composition by tropomyosin isoforms. Mol Biol Cell 2003; 14(3):1002-16.

47. Gupton SL, Anderson KL, Kole TP et al. Cell migration without a lamellipodium: translation of actin dynamics into cell movement mediated by tropomyosin. J Cell Biol 2005; 168(4):619-31.

48. Langford GM. Myosin-V, a versatile motor for short-range vesicle transport. Traffic 2002; 3(12):859-65.

49. Sellers JR, Veigel C. Walking with Myosin v. Curr Opin Cell Biol 2006; 18(1):68-73.

50. Wolenski JS, Cheney RE, Mooseker MS et al. In vitro motility of immunoadsorbed brain myosin-V using a Limulus acrosomal process and optical tweezer-based assay. J Cell Sci 1995; 108(Pt 4):1489-96.

51. Pruyne DW, Schott DH, Bretscher A. Tropomyosin-containing actin cables direct the Myo2p-dependent polarized delivery of secretory vesicles in budding yeast. J Cell Biol 1998; 143(7):1931-45.

Tropomodulin/Tropomyosin Interactions Regulate Actin Pointed End Dynamics

Alla S. Kostyukova*

Abstract

Dynamics of the slow-growing (pointed) end of the actin filament is regulated by tropomodulins, a family of capping proteins that require tropomyosin for optimal function. Tropomodulin is an elongated molecule with a molecular mass of about 40 kDa, containing the Tm-independent actin-binding site at the C-terminus. The highly disordered N-terminal half of tropomodulin contains two Tm-binding sites and a Tm-dependent actin-binding site. There are many Tm isoforms whose distribution varies in different tissues and cell compartments and changes during development of these tissues. Tropomyosin/tropomodulin interactions are isoform specific. Differences in Tm affinity for the two binding sites in Tmod may regulate its correct positioning at the pointed end as well as effectiveness of capping actin filament. The regulation of tropomodulin binding may have significant consequences for local cytoskeletal formation and filament dynamics in cells.

Introduction

Tropomodulin (Tmod) was found first in erythrocyte membranes as a tropomyosin (Tm) binding protein with a molecular mass of about 40 kDa.[1] Later, Tmod was shown to bind specifically to the pointed end of the actin filament, inhibiting polymerization and depolymerization of actin monomers.[2,3] The affinity of Tmod for the pointed end of actin is low in the absence of Tm ($Kd \sim 0.3\text{-}0.4\ \mu M$), whereas it increases substantially in the presence of Tm ($Kd \sim 50$ pM).[4] In in vitro experiments, actin capping is tight; however, in living myocytes capping is transient.[5] Actin capping is a dynamic process; in vivo, actin and Tmod molecules bound to the pointed end can exchange with free molecules. The mechanism by which Tmod capping may be downregulated in muscle is not known.

There are many Tm isoforms whose distribution varies in different tissues and cell compartments and changes during development of these tissues.[6] Tmod interactions with these Tm isoforms may regulate Tmod function as a capping protein for the pointed end.

At present, four Tmod isoforms are known.[7-9] Tmod1, previously E(erythrocyte)-Tmod, is found mainly in erythrocytes, heart and slow skeletal muscles, however, it may be detected in many other tissues. Tmod4, Sk(skeletal)-Tmod, prevails in fast skeletal muscles and replaces Tmod1 during development. Tmod2, N(neuron)-Tmod, was found in brains. Tmod3, U(ubiquitous)-Tmod, has been found in a variety of tissues. These isoforms are 60% identical and 70% similar in amino acid

*Alla S. Kostyukova—Department of Neuroscience and Cell Biology, Robert Wood Johnson Medical School, 675 Hoes Lane, Piscataway, NJ 08854, USA.
Email: kostyuas@umdnj.edu

Tropomyosin, edited by Peter Gunning. ©2008 Landes Bioscience and Springer Science+Business Media.

sequence. In addition, there are several homologues of Tmod, including the product of the *Sanpodo* gene in *Drosophila*, which is responsible for asymmetric cell division[10] and leiomodins, larger proteins with molecular masses of about 64 kDa.[9,11] There are three known leiomodin isoforms: Lmod1 is found mainly in smooth muscles, Lmod2 is found in heart and skeletal muscle and Lmod3 has unknown distribution. Although, Lmod function is not well studied, it is known that Lmods bind Tm.[11,12] There is evidence that Lmod2 may act as an actin filament nucleating factor.[13]

Little is known about Tmod2 and Tmod3. However, it is known that Tmod3 is able to sequester actin monomers, unlike Tmod1 and Tmod4.[14] Also, at low concentrations, Tmod3 increases actin polymerization by nucleating actin filaments; while at high concentration, it decreases actin filament polymerization, not only by capping the pointed end, but also by binding actin monomers.[15] Overexpression of Tmod3 leads to decreased endothelial cell motility.[16] Tmod2 causes decrease in steady state F-actin, therefore it is presumed that it also has a sequestering ability similar to Tmod3.[15] Altered Tmod2 expression was found in pathological conditions and human diseases, such as epilepsy or cerebral ischemia.[17-19]

In muscles, Tmod was immunolocalized not only at the pointed (free) ends of thin filaments,[20] but also in the Z-disc region.[21] This may reflect the presence of the Z-line associated filament network.[22] Tmod1 overexpression in mice myocardium causes myofibril degeneration, which leads to dilated cardiomyopathy.[23] In contrast, decreased Tmod concentration resulted in the formation of abnormally long actin filaments.[24] Overexpression of GFP-Tmod1 in cardiac myocytes resulted in shorter thin filaments[5] and in a Tmod1 knockout mouse, heart defects, including aborted development of the myocardium and inability to pump, led to embryonic lethality.[25] Finally, cardiomyocyte differentiation was studied in Tmod1 null embryonic stem cells and it was shown that Tmod1 function is critical for late stages of myofibrillogenesis.[26]

Tmod1 is the most studied of all Tmod isoforms. Its structure, function and interactions with other proteins have been studied in detail. The studies that follow were mostly done on Tmod1.

Tropomodulin Structure: Tmod1 Is an Intrinsically Disordered Protein

Numerous unsuccessful attempts to crystallize Tmod1[27] necessitated studying its structure using structural methods other than crystallography. Circular dichroism (CD), limited proteolysis, fluorescence, differential scanning calorimetry (DSC) and small-angle X-ray scattering were intensively used to understand the peculiarities of Tmod1 structure. Based on these data, N- and C-halves of the Tmod molecule were found to differ substantially in their structure.[27-29] The C-terminal half of the molecule is a stable compact cooperatively melting domain; whereas the N-terminal half is elongated and has a flexible structure. CD studies of Tmod N-terminal fragments, residues 1-92, 1-130 and 1-159, revealed no cooperatively melting structure and is mostly represented by random coil with small α-helical content.[27,30,31] Absence of definite tertiary structure in the N-terminal half of the Tmod molecule explains the failure in crystallization of full-length protein. Tmod is a striking example of an intrinsically disordered protein, an important feature of these proteins is that they become ordered during or prior to their biological function.[32]

The C-terminal domain was crystallized[33] and its atomic model was built and refined at a resolution of 1.45 Å.[34] The atomic structure of the C-terminal domain represents a right-handed super helix composed of alternate α-helices and β-strands, the helices' axes are slightly bent to the β-side (Fig. 1). This structure is typical for leucine rich repeat (LRR) proteins.[35] There are four amino acid repeats that contain a sequence that is characteristic for LRR proteins, axaLxxNxxaxxaxa, where L and N are conserved Leu and Asn, "a" is represented with Leu, Val, Ala, Ile, Phe or Met and "x" may be any residue (Fig. 2). Unlike other known LRR proteins, conserved asparagine residues are located at the beginning of αβ-loops but not in βα-loops. These residues form hydrogen bonds both with adjacent loops and with the main chain in the same repeat, forming the so called asparagine ladder.[36] The C-terminal α-helix (α6) is longer than other helices and its axis is bent further towards β-side than is common for other α-helices.

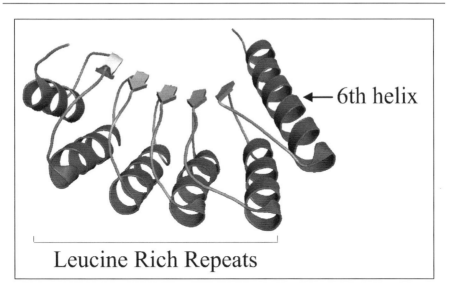

Figure 1. Ribbon presentation of crystal structure of Tmod1 C-terminal domain, a.a. 160-344, (PDB code 1IO0).

The solution structure of Tmod1 N-terminal residue fragment was solved using NMR[37] (Fig. 3). It confirmed the absence of definite tertiary structure predicted by other structural data. Residues 24-35 are helical but the rest of the peptide has no regular secondary structure. There are two regions with increased flexibility, residues 55-62 and 76-92.[37] These regions are important for proper positioning of Tmod at the pointed end.[38] The highly disordered Tmod N-terminal domain contains 3 of 4 known binding sites including two Tm-binding sites.[28,30,31,37-43]

Localization of Binding Sites in the Tmod Molecule

In spite of the fact that the Tmod N-terminal domain has no cooperatively melting structure, adding the Tmod1 N-terminal fragment (res 1-91) to high molecular weight (HMW) muscle Tm

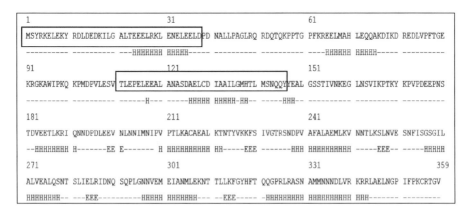

Figure 2. The amino acid sequence of Tmod1 aligned to the secondary structure obtained from NMR data (residues 1-92), secondary structure prediction (residues 93-159) and crystal atomic structure (residues 160-344). H-α-helix, E-β-strand. Residues in red were mutated in helical regions. Fragments containing Tm-binding sites are shown in boxes.

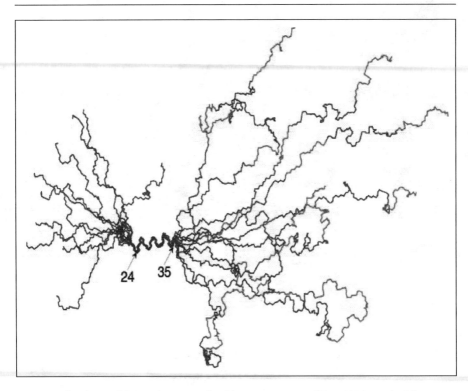

Figure 3. Alignment of the ten best NMR backbone structures of Tmod1 N-terminal fragment, a.a. 1-92, in solution.

drastically changed the melting curves as indicated by CD and DSC.[28] The heat denaturation of Tm is a multi-step process[44] and after forming the Tmod-Tm complex, major changes occurred in the high-temperature transition, which corresponds to Tm N-terminus. As a result of binding, the temperature of the transition and the excess heat of denaturation increased as well as α-helical content. Similar data were obtained when bigger N-terminal fragments (a.a. 1-130) of Tmod1 and Tmod4 were mixed with Tm peptides.[30] Complex formation between Tmod and Tm fragments resulted in increased α-helical content and stability. N-terminal acetylation that stabilizes the coiled coil of the N-terminus of HMW Tm was found to be essential for its interaction with Tmod.[30]

An earlier study suggested that the site of interaction of Tmod1 is dependent on the type of target Tm; the region of amino acids 6-94 of Tmod1 interacts with skeletal muscle Tm, whereas the region 90-184 interacts with low molecular weight (LMW) nonmuscle erythrocyte Tm (a heterodimer of α and γ LMW Tm).[40] This contradicts the fact that Tmod1 residues 95-359 exhibited a 160-fold increase in capping activity in the presence of skeletal muscle Tm and infers the presence of a second binding site for this Tm in the region.[41] Moreover, the Tmod1 N-terminal fragment, res. 1-92, was able to bind not only HMW skeletal α-Tm but also LMW nonmuscle α-Tm5a.[45] In recent studies Vera et al[42] mapped a binding site for Tm5 (a LMW erythrocyte Tm encoded by the γ-Tm gene) to residues 105-127 and Kong et al[43] found that residues L134 and L135 are crucial for Tm5 binding. However, in both studies, neither binding of γ-Tm to the first Tm-binding site, nor binding of HMW muscle Tm to the second Tm-binding site was found, confirming the suggestion of Babcock et al.[40] The questions how many Tm-binding sites does a Tmod molecule have and what is the specificity were still unanswered.

In addition to helix 24-35 which was determined by NMR, there are several predicted helical regions in the N-terminal half of Tmod1 (Fig. 2). While the α-helix formed with res. 24-35 has a

***

Table 1. Alignment of TmZip sequences

Peptide (Source)	Tropomyosin	GCN4
α-Tm1aZip (stTm)	MDAIKKKMQMLKLD	NYHLENEVARLKKLVGER
α-Tm1bZip (Tm5a)	AGSSSLEAVRRKIRSLQEQ	NYHLENEVARLKKLVGER
γ-Tm1bZip (Tm5NM1)	AGSTTIEAVKRKIQVLQQQ	NYHLENEVARLKKLVGER
δ-Tm1bZip (Tm4)	AGLNSLEAVKRKIQALQQQ	NYHLENEVARLKKLVGER
Heptad repeat	a d a d	a d a d a

Sequences of Tm chimeric proteins containing the N-termini of different Tm isoforms. Residues 20 to 37 of the peptides correspond to the last 18 C-terminal residues (264-281) of the yeast transcription factor GCN4. The residues that are coiled coil are labeled with the residue position of the heptad repeats.

***

high probability to form a coiled coil, the two other putative helices, res. 65-75 and res. 126-135, represent amphipatic helices. Correct folding of these helices is crucial for the formation of the binding sites. The L27E mutation destroys α-helix hydrophobic formation in the helical region, res. 24-35, located in the first Tm-binding site.[37] This mutation causes a loss of Tm-binding ability in this site. Mutation L71D inhibits formation of the hydrophobic surface in the amphipathic helix, res. 65-75, which is responsible for Tm-dependent capping activity.[38] The third mutation, I131D, postulated to destroy the hydrophobic surface in a putative helix, res. 126-135, caused a loss of Tm-binding in the second binding site.[31] Collectively, these three mutations cause a 30-fold decrease of capping ability.

Figure 4 shows the positions of Tm-binding and actin-capping sites that were determined using the pyrene-actin polymerization assay, native gel-electrophoresis and circular dichroism.[31,37,38,41,45] Two binding sites were localized for both LMW and HMW Tm isoforms on Tmod1 within res. 1-38 and 109-144 and a Tm-independent actin-capping site within res. 48-92. The Tm-independent actin-capping site is located at the C-terminus of the Tmod1 molecule. Tmod1 without 15 C-terminal residues has drastically lower ability to cap actin filaments in the absence of Tm.

Tm/Tmod Interactions Are Isoform Specific

Specificity of Tm binding to Tmod1 was first shown by Sussman et al with Tm isoforms from erythrocyte, brain, platelet and skeletal muscle tissue.[46] Tmod1 forms complexes with all of these isoforms, but binds preferentially to erythrocyte Tm. At that time, it was known that Tmod binds to the end of Tm,[47] therefore it was assumed that binding ability reflected the heterogeneity in the N- or C-terminal sequences characteristic of the different Tm isoforms. For the first time, it was suggested that isoform-specific interactions of Tmod with Tm may represent a novel mechanism for selective regulation of Tm/actin interactions.

Later it was shown that Tmod binds to the N-terminus of Tm.[48] Without the first 19 residues, LMW nonmuscle γ-Tm, Tm5, could not bind to Tmod.[49] The binding site was mapped to residues 7-14. The first 14 residues of HMW Tms are homologous to residues 6-19 of LMW Tm (Table 1) and contain a Tmod-binding site[30]. To measure the affinities of Tm isoforms to Tmod1, model peptides were used. These peptides contained the 19 N-terminal residues of LMW or the 14 N-terminal residues of HMW Tms. In addition to the Tm N-terminal region these peptides contain the 18 C-terminal residues of the GCN4 leucine zipper domain (Table 1), which help to stabilize the coiled-coil structure.[50] The validity of peptide models is well established. The structures of two of these peptides, α-Tm1aZip and α-Tm1bZip, are known[50,51] and they retain the major properties of full-length Tm's N-terminus: they bind Tmod,[30,37,41,45] bind C-terminal Tm fragments and form a ternary complex with troponin.[51]

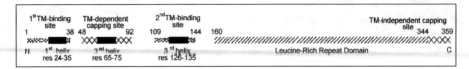

Figure 4. Schematic model of the Tm-binding and actin-capping sites.

Affinities to the individual Tm-binding sites were studied in detail using Tmod1 fragments, res. 1-38 and 109-144 and four Tm peptides representing different isoforms: HMW muscle α-stTm, α-TM1aZip and LMW-nonmuscle Tms: α-Tm5a, α-Tm1bZip, γ-Tm5NM1, γ-Tm1bZip and δ-Tm4, δ-Tm1bZip. Dissociation constants calculated from the CD unfolding curves are presented in Table 2.[12,31,52] N-terminal sequence of HMW muscle β-Tm encoded by exon 1a is identical to the α-Tm sequence and there is only one conservative replacement of Asp2 to Glu in HMW γ-Tm. No HMW Tm coded by δ-gene was found to be expressed. Therefore, dissociation constants determined for α-Tm1aZip/Tmod complexes should be the same or very similar in case of other HMW Tms. The N-terminal sequences of LMW Tms are similar and different from HMW Tm (Table 1). In spite of the similarity, the difference in binding abilities was striking (Table 2). While α-Tm1bZip and α-Tm1aZip both bind well to both sites in Tmod1 (though α-Tm1bZip binds with higher affinity) the peptides γ-Tm1bZip and δ-Tm1bZip bind only to the second binding site. On the contrary the N-terminal fragments of Lmod1, res. 3-40 and Lmod2, res. 5-42, which is highly homologous to Tmod1's first Tm-binding site, bind to γ-Tm1bZip and δ-Tm1bZip much tighter (Table 2). The binding can be easily detected either by native gel-electrophoresis or CD.[31]

Even though the γ-Tm1bZip peptide only binds the second Tmod1 binding site, full-length γ-Tm, γ-Tm5NM1, inhibits pointed end elongation in a pyrene-actin fluorescence assay with Tmod1 N-terminal fragment, res. 1-92, containing only first Tm-binding site and the Tm independent actin capping site, although with less effectiveness than with full-length Tmod.[52] To do this, there should be interaction of γ-Tm5NM1 with the first binding site. It was shown using cross-linking that there is an interaction of first Tm-binding site with γ-Tm1bZip. Increasing concentration of fragments in CD experiments also showed weak interaction with γ- and δ-Tm1bZip.

The residues responsible for isoform specificity of Tm's binding were determined.[52] Changing Ser4 of α-Tm1bZip to Thr as in γ-Tm1bZip decreased 4-fold the binding ability and changing Arg14 to Gln resulted in the loss of binding. These residues are not involved in coiled-coil formation, which is important for Tm-Tmod interaction.[37]

The analysis resolves a long-standing debate in the literature concerning the location of Tm binding sites on Tmod. All Tm isoforms bind to both Tm-binding sites on Tmod1; but LMW γ-Tm and δ-Tm bind to the first site with much lower affinity than α-Tms. Subtle sequence

---

Table 2. *Binding of tropomodulin and leiomodin fragments containing Tm-binding sites to Tm peptides. The Kd values (μM) were estimated from the thermodynamics of unfolding of the complexes compared with the Tmod/ Lmod fragments and TmZips alone. NC—K_d cannot be calculated in these conditions*

Tm Peptide	Tmod1, a.a.1-38	Tmod1, a.a. 109-144	Lmod2, a.a. 5-42	Lmod1, a.a. 3-40
α-Tm1aZip	1.1 ± 0.4	1.3 ± 0.3	0.8 ± 0.2	1.98
α-Tm1bZip	0.22 ± 0.10	0.003 ± 0.001	0.011 ± 0.008	0.016 ± 0.009
γ-Tm1bZip	NC	0.04 ± 0.03	0.6 ± 0.1	0.61 ± 0.07
δ-Tm1bZip	NC	0.09 ± 0.02	0.24 ± 0.07	0.43 ± 0.08

differences among Tm isoforms can have major effects on the affinity for the first Tmod1 binding site and thereby modulate the dynamics of the actin filament's pointed end.

A Model for Tmod/Tm/Actin Complex at the Pointed End

There are several possible models: One Tmod could bind two different Tm molecules at the same time; both sites could bind the same Tm molecule; the sites could be mutually exclusive so that Tm binding to one site makes binding to the other site impossible. In the first case, one Tmod molecule would bind two Tm molecules while in the other two cases a Tmod molecule would bind only one Tm molecule. The question now is: how many Tm molecules does one Tmod molecule bind?

Using titration of Tmod1 with α-Tm1bZip, it was shown that one Tmod1 molecule binds two Tm peptides in a cooperative manner.[31] The model was proposed for actin capping where one tropomodulin molecule binds two Tm molecules at the pointed end (Fig. 5A). This completely changed the previous concept of pointed end organization, whereby one molecule of tropomodulin binds to one molecule of Tm[53] and resolves a long-standing controversy in the field.

The NMR studies using α-Tm1bZip and Tmod1 fragments show that the Tm structures are different in the two complexes, therefore different in the two sites.[52] While the structures of Tmod1-Tm complexes remain to be solved, possible models of binding were offered. These models are based on circular dichroism spectra of the complexes, the effects of complex formation on the ^{1}H-^{15}N HSQC spectra of α-Tm1bZip and mutagenesis studies.[31,37,42,43,52]

For the first Tm-binding site residues 24-38 of Tmod1 are oriented parallel to residues 2-16 of α-Tm1bZip while residues 1-22 of Tmod1 interact in an antiparallel sense with residues 2-17 on the opposite side of the Tm coiled coil (Fig. 5B). Possible hydrophobic interactions are consistent

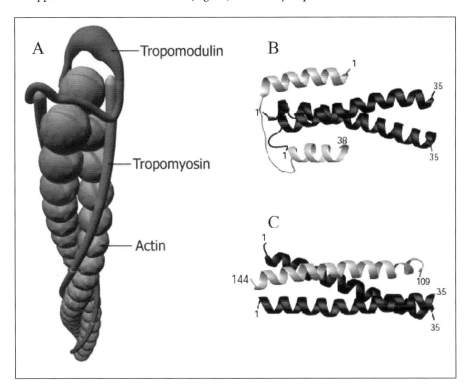

Figure 5. A cartoon representation of the pointed end. The N-terminal half of Tmod1 binds to both Tms and interacts with actin (A). Schematic of possible binding modes of α-Tm1bZip to two binding sites on Tmod1, residues 1-38 (B) and residues 109-144 (C).

with such a model. For the second Tm-binding site it was suggested that Tmod1 res. 109-144 and αTm1bZip form an antiparallel three-helix coiled coil that is interrupted at P114, near the C-terminal end of the GCN4 region (Fig. 5C). These figures illustrate hypothetical models; the arrangement of the helices and the significance of specific residues will be learned only by solving the structures of the complexes.

Conclusions

The position of a single tropomodulin molecule at the pointed end of the actin filament that forms fundamentally different complexes with the tropomyosin molecules on the two sides of the filament helix increases the asymmetry of the end. Differences in tropomyosin affinity for the two binding sites in tropomodulin may regulate its correct positioning at the pointed end. Isoform-specific differences in affinity for the two sites contribute to the efficiency in capping the pointed end of the actin filament. Since small sequence variations in the N-terminus of tropomyosin can have major affects on Tmod1 binding and the ability to cap the pointed end, the end becomes a significant regulatory site. Tropomyosins are recognized to be a major regulator of the actin filaments in cells, having the ability to protect filaments against severing and branching,[54-56] to recruit specific myosins,[57,58] alter cell shape and now to regulate the pointed end. Regulation of tropomodulin binding as well as the effectiveness of capping by specific tropomyosins may have significant consequences for local cytoskeletal formation and filament dynamics in cells.

Acknowledgements

I thank Dr. Sarah Hitchcock-DeGregori and Dr. Norma Greenfield for discussing this manuscript and Denise Dehnbostel for editing. Supported by the American Heart Association Grant 0535328N and UMDNJ Foundation Grant.

References

1. Fowler VM. Identification and purification of a novel Mr 43,000 tropomyosin- binding protein from human erythrocyte membranes. J Biol Chem 1987; 262(26):12792-12800.
2. Weber A, Pennise CR, Babcock GG et al. Tropomodulin caps the pointed ends of actin filaments. J Cell Biol 1994; 127(6 Pt 1):1627-1635.
3. Gregorio CC, Fowler VM. Mechanisms of thin filament assembly in embryonic chick cardiac myocytes: tropomodulin requires tropomyosin for assembly. J Cell Biol 1995; 129(3):683-695.
4. Weber A, Pennise CR, Fowler VM. Tropomodulin increases the critical concentration of barbed end-capped actin filaments by converting ADP.P(i)-actin to ADP-actin at all pointed filament ends [In Process Citation]. J Biol Chem 1999; 274(49):34637-34645.
5. Littlefield R, Almenar-Queralt A, Fowler VM. Actin dynamics at pointed ends regulates thin filament length in striated muscle. Nat Cell Biol 2001; 3(6):544-551.
6. Gunning PW, Schevzov G, Kee AJ et al. Tropomyosin isoforms: divining rods for actin cytoskeleton function. Trends Cell Biol 2005; 15(6):333-341.
7. Watakabe A, Kobayashi R, Helfman DM. N-tropomodulin: a novel isoform of tropomodulin identified as the major binding protein to brain tropomyosin. J Cell Sci 1996; 109(Pt 9):2299-2310.
8. Almenar-Queralt A, Lee A, Conley CA et al. Identification of a novel tropomodulin isoform, skeletal tropomodulin, that caps actin filament pointed ends in fast skeletal muscle. J Biol Chem 1999; 274(40):28466-28475.
9. Conley CA, Fritz-Six KL, Almenar-Queralt A et al. Leiomodins: larger members of the tropomodulin (tmod) gene family. Genomics 2001; 73(2):127-139.
10. Dye CA, Lee JK, Atkinson RC et al. The Drosophila sanpodo gene controls sibling cell fate and encodes a tropomodulin homolog, an actin/tropomyosin-associated protein. Development 1998; 125(10):1845-1856.
11. Conley CA. Leiomodin and tropomodulin in smooth muscle. Am J Physiol Cell Physiol 2001; 280(6): C1645-1656.
12. Kostyukova A. Leiomodin/tropomyosin interactions are isoform specific. Archives Biochem. Biophys 2007; 465(1):227-230.
13. Chereau D, Boczkowska M, Fujiwara I et al. Leiomodin: a novel actin filament nucleating factor. Paper presented at: 46th ASCB Annual Meeting 2006; San Diego, CA.
14. Fischer RS, Sept D, Weber KL et al. Tmod3 binds actin monomer in vitro and in vivo. Molecular Biology of the Cell 2004; 15:147a.

15. Fischer RS, Yarmola EG, Weber KL et al. Tropomodulin 3 binds to actin monomers. J Biol Chem 2006; 281(47):36454-36465. Epub 32006-36451.
16. Fischer RS, Fritz-Six KL, Fowler VM. Pointed-end capping by tropomodulin3 negatively regulates endothelial cell motility. J Cell Biol 2003; 161(2):371-380.
17. Yang JW, Czech T, Felizardo M et al. Aberrant expression of cytoskeleton proteins in hippocampus from patients with mesial temporal lobe epilepsy. Amino Acids 2006; 30(4):477-493.
18. Iwazaki T, McGregor IS, Matsumoto I. Protein expression profile in the striatum of acute metham-phetamine-treated rats. Brain Res 2006; 1097(1):19-25.
19. Chen A, Liao WP, Lu Q et al. Upregulation of dihydropyrimidinase-related protein 2, spectrin alpha II chain, heat shock cognate protein 70 pseudogene 1 and tropomodulin 2 after focal cerebral ischemia in rats-A proteomics approach. Neurochem Int 2007; 50(7-8):1078-1086.
20. Fowler VM, Sussmann MA, Miller PG et al. Tropomodulin is associated with the free (pointed) ends of the thin filaments in rat skeletal muscle. J Cell Biol 1993; 120(2):411-420.
21. Sussman MA, Ito M, Daniels MP et al. Chicken skeletal muscle tropomodulin: novel localization and characterization. Cell Tissue Res 1996; 285(2):287-296.
22. Kee AJ, Schevzov G, Nair-Shalliker V et al. Sorting of a nonmuscle tropomyosin to a novel cytoskeletal compartment in skeletal muscle results in muscular dystrophy. J Cell Biol 2004; 166(5):685-696.
23. Sussman MA, Welch S, Cambon N et al. Myofibril degeneration caused by tropomodulin overexpression leads to dilated cardiomyopathy in juvenile mice. J Clin Invest 1998; 101(1):51-61.
24. Sussman MA, Baque S, Uhm CS et al. Altered expression of tropomodulin in cardiomyocytes disrupts the sarcomeric structure of myofibrils. Circ Res 1998; 82(1):94-105.
25. Fritz-Six KL, Cox PR, Fischer RS et al. Aberrant myofibril assembly in tropomodulin1 null mice leads to aborted heart development and embryonic lethality. J Cell Biol 2003; 163(5):1033-1044. Epub 2003, 1031.
26. McElhinny AS, Schwach C, Valichnac M et al. Nebulin regulates the assembly and lengths of the thin filaments in striated muscle. J Cell Biol 2005; 170(6):947-957.
27. Kostyukova A, Maeda K, Yamauchi E et al. Domain structure of tropomodulin: distinct properties of the N-terminal and C-terminal halves. Eur J Biochem 2000; 267(21):6470-6475.
28. Kostyukova AS, Tiktopulo EI, Maeda Y. Folding properties of functional domains of tropomodulin. Biophys J 2001; 81(1):345-351.
29. Fujisawa T, Kostyukova A, Maeda Y. The shapes and sizes of two domains of tropomodulin, the P-end-capping protein of actin-tropomyosin. FEBS Lett 2001; 498(1):67-71.
30. Greenfield NJ, Fowler VM. Tropomyosin requires an intact N-terminal coiled coil to interact with tropomodulin. Biophys J 2002; 82(5):2580-2591.
31. Kostyukova AS, Choy A, Rapp BA. Tropomodulin binds two tropomyosins: a novel model for actin filament capping. Biochemistry 2006; 45(39):12068-12075.
32. Uversky VN. Natively unfolded proteins: a point where biology waits for physics. Protein Sci 2002; 11(4):739-756.
33. Krieger I, Kostyukova AS, Maeda Y. Crystallization and preliminary characterization of crystals of the C-terminal half fragment of tropomodulin. Acta Crystallogr 2001; D57(Pt 5):743-744.
34. Krieger I, Kostyukova A, Yamashita A et al structure of tropomodulin C-terminal half and structural basis of actin filament pointed-end capping. Biophysical J 2002; 83(5):2716-2725.
35. Kajava AV. Structural diversity of leucine-rich repeat proteins. J Mol Biol. 1998; 277(3):519-527.
36. Kobe B, Deisenhofer J. A structural basis of the interactions between leucine-rich repeats and protein ligands. Mol Cell Neurosci 1995; 6(2):97-105.
37. Greenfield NJ, Kostyukova AS, Hitchcock-Degregori SE. Structure and tropomyosin binding properties of the N-terminal capping domain of tropomodulin 1. Biophys J 2005; 88(1):372-383.
38. Kostyukova A, Rapp B, Choy A et al. Structural requirements of tropomodulin for tropomyosin binding and actin filament capping. Biochemistry 2005; 44(12):4905-4910.
39. Sung LA, Fowler VM, Lambert K et al. Molecular cloning and characterization of human fetal liver tropomodulin. A tropomyosin-binding protein. J Biol Chem 1992; 267(4):2616-2621.
40. Babcock GG, Fowler VM. Isoform-specific interaction of tropomodulin with skeletal muscle and eryth-rocyte tropomyosins. J Biol Chem 1994; 269(44):27510-27518.
41. Fowler VM, Greenfield NJ, Moyer J. Tropomodulin contains two actin filament pointed end-capping domains. J Biol Chem 2003; 278(41):40000-40009.
42. Vera C, Lao J, Hamelberg D et al. Mapping the tropomyosin isoform 5 binding site on human eryth-rocyte tropomodulin: Further insights into E-Tmod/TM5 interaction. Arch Biochem Biophys 2005; 444(2):130-138.
43. Kong KY, Kedes L. Leucine-135 of tropomodulin-1 regulates its association with tropomyosin, its cel-lular localization and the integrity o sarcomeres. J Biol Chem 2006; 281(14):9589-9599.
44. Potekhin SA, Privalov PL. Co-operative blocks in tropomyosin. J Mol Biol 1982; 159(3):519-535.

45. Kostyukova AS, Hitchcock-DeGregori SE. Effect of the structure of the N terminus of tropomyosin on tropomodulin function. J Biol Chem 2004; 279(7):5066-5071.
46. Sussman MA, Fowler VM. Tropomodulin binding to tropomyosins. Isoform-specific differences in affinity and stoichiometry. Eur J Biochem 1992; 205(1):355-362.
47. Fowler VM. Tropomodulin. a cytoskeletal protein that binds to the end of erythrocyte tropomyosin and inhibits tropomyosin binding to actin. J Cell Biol 1990; 111(2):471-481.
48. Sung LA, Lin JJ. Erythrocyte tropomodulin binds to the N-terminus of hTM5, a tropomyosin isoform encoded by the gamma-tropomyosin gene. Biochem Biophys Res Commun 1994; 201(2):627-634.
49. Vera C, Sood A, Gao KM et al. Tropomodulin-binding site mapped to residues 7-14 at the N-terminal heptad repeats of tropomyosin isoform 5. Arch Biochem Biophys 2000; 378(1):16-24.
50. Greenfield NJ, Montelione GT, Farid RS et al. The structure of the N-terminus of striated muscle alpha-tropomyosin in a chimeric peptide: nuclear magnetic resonance structure and circular dichroism studies. Biochemistry 1998; 37(21):7834-7843.
51. Greenfield NJ, Huang YJ, Palm T et al. Solution NMR structure and folding dynamics of the N terminus of a rat nonmuscle alpha-tropomyosin in an engineered chimeric protein. J Mol Biol 2001; 312(4):833-847.
52. Kostyukova A, Hitchcock-DeGregori SE, Greenfield NJ. Molecular basis of tropomyosin binding to tropomodulin, an actin capping protein. J Mol Biol 2007; 372(3):608-618.
53. dos Remedios CG, Chhabra D, Kekic M et al. Actin binding proteins: regulation of cytoskeletal microfilaments. Physiol Rev 2003; 83(2):433-473.
54. Bernstein BW, Bamburg JR. Tropomyosin binding to F-actin protects the F-actin from disassembly by brain actin-depolymerizing factor (ADF). Cell Motil 1982; 2(1):1-8.
55. DesMarais V, Ichetovkin I, Condeelis J et al. Spatial regulation of actin dynamics: a tropomyosin-free, actin-rich compartment at the leading edge. J Cell Sci 2002; 115(Pt 23):4649-4660.
56. Blanchoin L, Pollard TD, Hitchcock-DeGregori SE. Inhibition of the Arp2/3 complex-nucleated actin polymerization and branch formation by tropomyosin. Curr Biol 2001; 11(16):1300-1304.
57. Gupton SL, Anderson KL, Kole TP et al. Cell migration without a lamellipodium: translation of actin dynamics into cell movement mediated by tropomyosin. J Cell Biol 2005; 168(4):619-631.
58. Bryce NS, Schevzov G, Ferguson V et al. Specification of actin filament function and molecular composition by tropomyosin isoforms. Mol. Biol. Cell 2003; 14(3):1002-1016.

Emerging Issues for Tropomyosin Structure, Regulation, Function and Pathology

Peter Gunning*

Abstract

There is a growing awareness of the role of tropomyosin in the regulation of the actin filament. Work in the field is increasingly directed at understanding the mechanisms of function at both a molecular and atomic level and developing therapeutic strategies to treat tropomyosin-based pathology. This chapter highlights unresolved issues that cross the boundaries between individual chapters and are likely to be fertile areas of research in the future.

Introduction

Tropomyosin is remarkable for its deceptive simplicity. On the one hand, what could be simpler than a polymer of a coiled coil dimer running along the length of an actin filament? The perfect portrait of a filament stabiliser and steric inhibitor of the actin filament interaction with myosin. On the other hand, it is able to regulate many of the functional outputs of actin filaments in an isoform dependent manner. It is therefore surprising that diagrams of actin function, if they contain tropomyosin at all, consider it as one of many independent and different options rather than as a core component of the actin filament itself.[1,2] There are many reasons that may be raised to explain this situation but none are probably as relevant as the starting point; deceptive simplicity.

The aim of this chapter is not to cover that which the authors of this book have achieved with such elegance. Rather, I wish to raise five issues which cross the boundaries of the chapters and represent some of the challenges for the future.

What Is the Composition of the Actin Filament and How Is It Assembled?

This question epitomises the deceptive simplicity of both tropomyosin and actin. Put alternatively, are actin filaments heterogeneous polymers of actin and tropomyosin isoforms? Studies in skeletal muscle have indicated that skeletal actin is located in the thin filaments of the sarcomere, γ-actin is at the costamere and adjacent to the Z-line and β-actin is at the neuromuscular junction.[3-5] Thus, despite the similarity of the different actin isoforms, it is possible for different polymer populations to be composed largely of one isoform or the other. Similarly, over expression of γ-actin in C2C12 myoblasts can drive the HMW Tm2 but not the LMW Tm5NM1 out of stress fibres.[6] Finally, the observation of isoform sorting of tropomyosin means that homo-polymers of those

*Peter Gunning—Oncology Research Unit, Department of Pharmacology, School of Medical Sciences, University of New South Wales, Sydney, NSW 2052, Australia.
Email: p.gunning@unsw.edu.au.

Tropomyosin, edited by Peter Gunning. ©2008 Landes Bioscience and Springer Science+Business Media.

tropomyosin's must, to a certain extent, exist in different cell types (Chapter 15). The question can therefore be rephrased; to what extent are actin filaments composed of homo-polymers of a specific actin and tropomyosin isoform? This remains a very difficult question to answer but the fact that at least some primarily homogeneous polymers must be formed raises the questions of why and how?

Why form a homo-polymer of a specific tropomyosin along an actin filament? At its simplest a tropomyosin homo-polymer may be a mechanism of providing fidelity of function along the entire length of an actin filament. A single actin filament can traverse a substantial distance in a cell and differences in function along the length of a filament may result in cellular dysfunction. This is likely to be particularly true where contractile force is being generated or where a vesicle is being tracked along a filament by a myosin motor. The use of a single tropomyosin may promote homogeneous functional interactions along the length of the filament. In this light, the creation of chimeric tropomyosin by Jim Lin and coworkers is potentially most instructive (Chapter 16).[7] Whereas forced expression of Tm3 and Tm5NM1 were not found to be toxic, the expression of the Tm5/3 chimera was quite disruptive, particularly for cytokinesis.[7] It may be that the chimera disrupts homo-polymer formation and/or integrity of filament function.

How do you form a tropomyosin homo-polymer? Firstly, there are two types of homo-polymer, polymers of a homo-dimer and polymers of a hetero-dimer. In the case of skeletal- and smooth-muscle, it is the hetero-dimer which forms the homo-polymer whereas it is largely the homo-dimer in cardiac muscle and the cytoskeleton (Chapter 6). This is most easily explained by mass action where the vast excess of muscle tropomyosin over cytoskeletal tropomyosin and the intrinsic preference for muscle tropomyosin to form hetero-dimers inevitably drives homo-polymer formation with muscle actin filaments. But what happens in human cardiac muscle where there is likely coexistence of both α/β hetero-dimers and α/α homo-dimers? Are the polymers homogeneous or heterogeneous and what is the functional significance? The genetic manipulation of tropomyosin isoform composition in the mouse heart and the impact of mutations on tropomyosin dimerisation in nemaline myopathy indicate that this will be of functional significance (Chapters 11, 12). Secondly, how do the cytoskeletal tropomyosins associate with γ-actin containing filaments in skeletal muscle?[4,8] It seems likely that local activity of actin binding proteins must contribute to the assembly of specific filaments at these different locations (Chapters 5, 7, 14-21).

The challenge of formation of a homo-polymer is much more difficult to understand in the cytoskeleton. The recent data from Hitchcock-DeGregori and coworkers has provided an insight into the basis of the overlap between the N- and C-termini of adjoining tropomyosins which in turn is the basis for polymer formation (Chapter 5). Is there sufficient specificity in this overlap to favour the formation of homo-polymers or are other features of the molecule required or are local interactions with actin binding proteins contributing to the final assembly of the filament? Many of the cytoskeletal tropomyosins have very similar N- and C- termini (Chapter 2) and some of the LMW tropomyosins have the capacity to form hetero-dimers, at least in forced expression situations (Chapter 6). It therefore seems unlikely that just the overlap will be sufficient to entirely account for homo-polymer formation and this is in accord with the observed low affinity of the overlap (Chapter 7).

Finally, phosphorylation of tropomyosin has been implicated in polymer assembly and stability.[9-11] Recent studies suggest that phosphorylation of Tm1 is associated with its assembly into stress fibres and the phosphorylation is transient indicating a catalytic role for this modification.[9] This has the potential to link signalling cascades directly to isoform specific tropomyosin incorporation into actin filaments. Whether this will apply to other cytoskeletal isoforms remains to be determined.

As we move toward an understanding of the tropomyosin polymer at an atomic level the challenge will become integrating the series of low affinity interactions with the aggregate stability of these functionally specialised filaments. Long range cooperative interactions (Chapters 5, 7) involving actin, tropomyosin and actin binding protiens (Chapter 9, 17-21) are likely to provide an understanding that should approach our view of the archtypal model; the striated muscle thin filament (Chapter 8).

What Exactly Is Tropomyosin Doing to the Actin Filament?

On the one hand, the molecular characterisation of the mechanism of muscle contraction is one of the great achievments of biological research (Chapter 8.) On the other hand, it is also remarkable what we are yet to fully understand (Chapter 8). The nature of the interaction between tropomyosin and actin and the mechanism of coordinate structural regulation of the filament remain poorly understood (Chapters 7-9). The interaction between tropomyosin and actin more resembles one polymer 'floating' above the surface of the other than it does close protein-protein interactions. On the one hand, there are many actin-tropomyosin interactions at any one point in time along one filament and they involve a number of different residues in both molecules. At a molecular level it is easy to appreciate steric hindrance of the myosin interaction but it is quite another to understand what specific atomic interactions are responsible for this process (Chapters 8,9). By virtue of the dynamic nature of this interaction and the multiple residues involved, a solution at an atomic level seems distant at this time. It does, however, suggest the possibility that different isoforms with different atomic interactions may have quite different impact on actin filament function (Chapters 5-7).

The move from muscle function to the cytoskeleton is daunting because there are so many more isoforms and functional outputs to consider (Chapters 2, 4, 10, 15 and 16). The genetic analysis of yeast tropomyosin has provided unambiguous insight into fundamental aspects of its role in the cytoskeleton (Chapter 14). It is essential for actin filament stability, cytokinesis and vesicle transport. Similarly, genetic analysis of more complex organisms has demonstrated that tropomyosin is required for a wide range of cellular functions (Chapters 16-21).[12] These different functions are often associated with the use of different tropomyosin isoforms (Chapters 4, 15 and 16) (see next section). The challenge is therefore to understand how subtle changes in isoform structure can translate into quite different outcomes in filament function. The work of Bill Lehman and coworkers has suggested one way in which this may be achieved. They have shown that different isoforms of tropomyosin may occupy different positions in the groove of the actin filament.[13] However, it is not known at this time how these different positions could translate into specific and different functions.

In conclusion, despite substantial progress in understanding the molecular regulation of muscle contraction, we are at a very preliminary stage in understanding how cytoskeletal tropomyosin mediates its wide range of regulatory outcomes for actin filaments.

Why Are There so Many Isoforms of Tropomyosin?

The original expectation when the existence of tropomyosin isoforms was first discovered was that they would contribute functional diversity to the actin filament. Protein chemistry studies in the 1980s provided extensive support for the proposition that tropomyosin isoforms differ in their impact on actin filament stability and interactions with actin binding proteins (Chapters 17-21). Unfortunately it proved quite difficult to demonstrate functional differences between isoforms using molecular genetic manipulation of isoform expression whereas total ablation of tropomyosin provided compelling demonstrations of its essential role in organisms from yeast to mouse (Chapters 11, 14). Hence we were confronted with 'mechanisms of functional discrimination' in search of 'functional validation'; quite an unusual situation.

There is now compelling evidence that tropomyosin isoforms are functionally distinct and that in vivo studies have confirmed in vitro findings (Chapters 11, 16). This correlates very well with the observation that tropomyosin isoforms are spatially segregated to functionally distinct actin filament populations in many different cell types (Chapter 15). Attention is now focussed on understanding how specific filaments are tailor-made for specific localised function in terms of their biochemical properties. Hence it is likely that the generation of isoforms has provided diversification of actin filament function in time and space (12). The relationship between isoform number and organism complexity is certainly compatible with this proposition (Chapters 2, 4).

While the answer to the question posed above is therefore relatively straight forward, the mechanisms underlying the answer pose major challenges for the future. How are the isoforms sorted to different intracellular populations of actin filaments? Is sorting active or is it simply a manifestation of a preferred tropomyosin isoform being most compatible with the local concentrations and activities of actin binding proteins (Chapter 15)? But to really understand this, we need to answer the two questions posed above, how do the homo-polymers form and how do they bring different functional properties to the actin filament (Chapter 5)?

How Do Signalling Cascades Coordinate the Regulation of Tropomyosin Transcription and Splicing with Local Assembly of Different Filament Populations?

The transcription and splicing of the tropomyosin genes is tightly regulated and the impact of this regulation has far reaching consequences for actin filament function (Chapters 2-4 and see above). The signalling cascades responsible for this must provide tissue and cell type specific regulation. In some cases, tissue specific exons must be either masked or revealed (Chapter 3). Considerable insight into the principles of splicing regulation has come from tropomyosin genes but there is little knowledge of what specific signalling pathways are ultimately responsible for the tissue specific choreography of tropomyosin splicing (Chapter 3). However, there is also extensive regulation of transcription in both developmental and pathological conditions (Chapters 4, 10). Indeed, it seems likely that there may be some common pathway(s) which regulates HMW Tm expression during differentiation (Chapter 4). There is little knowledge of which signalling pathways are responsible for any of this regulation with the singular exception of Tm1 expression in cancer cells. In the case of Tm1 expression, there is some disagreement regarding the details of the specific pathway which may ultimately reflect differences in cell behaviour in culture (Chapter 10).[12]

David Helfman raises the interesting possibility that tropomyosins themselves may regulate oncogenic signalling cascades (Chapter 10). This is certainly not unreasonable in the context of cell transformation but does potentially highlight the practical difficulty of dissecting the role of a specific pathway independent of its impact on a molecule which may in turn regulate that pathway. Because tropomyosins are spatially segregated they could serve as templates for the binding of signalling complexes and changes in the existence of specific filaments could change the availability of these molecules to engage in signalling events.

The local assembly of specific actin filaments is likely to reflect the local activity of actin binding proteins which in turn is likely to reflect the local activity of signalling pathways (Chapter 15). For example, the local levels and activity of gelsolin (Chapter 17), ADF/Cofilin (Chapter 18), caldesmon (Chapter 19), myosin motors (Chapter 20) and tropomodulin (Chapter 21) are likely to determine the local preference for a specific tropomyosin.[12] It is not unreasonable to expect that this in turn will be coordinated with the expression of specific tropomyosins which would demand some coordination between local signalling and the regulation of transcription and splicing of tropomyosin. Integration of these pathways has major functional implications for cell specific structural domains and knowledge of these mechanisms has far reaching implications for cell and developmental biology.

What Are the Prospects for Treating Tropomyosin-Based Diseases?

The observation that HMW tropomyosins are commonly down regulated in avian and mammalian cancer cells has suggested a direct involvement in transformation (Chapter 10). This is reinforced by the demonstration that restoration of HMW tropomyosin expression, particularly of Tm1, can eliminate some transformed characteristics of cancer cells (14-16). This suggests the possibility that reversion of tropomyosin expression in a tumour may have therapeutic value. The difficulty with this approach is achieving efficient delivery and expression of Tm1 to all the tumour cells. This is not easily achieved and attention has turned to the mechanisms of Tm1 suppression. There is good evidence to support promoter methylation as one mechanism of Tm1 suppression (Chapter 10) and hence reversion of methylation is a possible anti-cancer strategy. One difficulty lies with using a global approach to reverting DNA methylation. In addition, there are concerns that reverting cancer cells, which carry many defects, is less desirable that achieving their permanent elimination.

Tropomyosin does, however, offer a potential strategy for cancer therapy. There is considerable interest in disabling the actin cytoskeleton of the cancer cell because of its involvement in cell growth and metastasis. The difficulty with anti-actin drugs is their cardiac and respiratory toxicity due to compromising contractile function. However, drugs which target the cytoskeletal tropomyosins would provide a means of disabling the cytoskeleton without compromising the function of the contractile apparatus. Furthermore, the cancer cell relies on only a small subset of cytoskeletal tropomyosins which provides a more specific target than the entire cytoskeleton.[17] Similarly, the treatment of ulcerative colitis may benefit from reduced expression of the auto-antigen Tm5NM1 (Chapter 13).

Therapeutic strategies for contractile apparatus dysfunction based on tropomyosin mutations are very challenging. Manipulating expression of isoforms to drive substitution of a mutated product with a normal isoform may be feasible but will present its own difficulties in terms of isoform function. For example, a mutation in β-Tm causing nemaline myopathy could be treated by either down regulating β-Tm expression and/or up-regulating α-Tm expression. This would lead to homo-polymers of α-Tm which are functionally distinct from the normal α-/β-hetero dimers found in skeletal muscle and may bring with it a different type of muscle dysfunction. Similarly, increasing β-Tm expression in the heart of patients with a cardiomyopathy-causing α-Tm mutation may give some alleviation of symptoms but the change from α-/α-homo-dimers to α-/β-hetero-dimers will also lead to a different type of cardiac dysfunction (Chapter 11). It is much more likely that the availability of animal models for these diseases of the contractile apparatus will be used to test different therapeutic strategies (Chapters 11, 12). Similar approaches have shown promise in defining treatment options for muscular dystrophy.

Acknowledgements

I want to thank both past and present members of the Oncology Research Unit for their contribution to our research. I am pleased to acknowledge support from the National Health and Medical Research Council of Australia (NHMRC) and the Oncology Children's Foundation. I am a Principal Research Fellow of the NHMRC.

I am extremely grateful to the authors of these chapters who have made this field so accessible to a broad readership. It is our collective hope that this monograph will promote research in this field and advance our understanding of the role of tropomyosin in actin filament function.

References

1. Alberts B, Bray D, Lewis J et al. Molecular Biology of the Cell, 3rd Ed. Garland Publishing Inc., New York: 1994; Fig 16-79.
2. Ayscough KR. In vivo functions of actin-binding proteins. Curr Opin Cell Biol 1998; 10:102-111.
3. Craig SW, Pardo JV. Gamma actin, spectrin and intermediate filament proteins colocalize with vinculin at costameres, myofibril-to-sarcolemma attachment sites. Cell Motil 1983; 3:449-462.
4. Kee AJ, Schevzov G, Nair-Shalliker V et al. Sorting of a nonmuscle tropomyosin to a novel cytoskeletal compartment in skeletal muscle results in muscular dystrophy. J Cell Biol 2004; 166:685-696.
5. Lubit BW. Association of beta-cytoplasmic actin with high concentrations of acetylcholine receptor (AChR) in normal and anti-AChR-treated primary rat muscle cultures. J Histochem Cytochem 1984; 32:973-981.
6. Schevzov G, Lloyd C, Hailstones D et al. Differential regulation of tropomyosin isoform organisation and gene expression in response to altered actin gene expression. J Cell Biol 1993; 121:811-821.
7. Wong K, Wessels D, Krob SL et al. Forced expression of a dominant-negative chimeric tropomyosin causes abnormal motile behaviour during cell division. Cell Motil Cytoskel 2000; 45:121-132.
8. Vlahovich N, Schevzov G, Nair-Shalliker V et al. Tropomyosin 4 defines novel filaments in skeletal muscle associated with muscle remodelling/regeneration in normal and disease muscle. Cell Motil Cytoskel 2008; 65:73-85.

9. Houle F, Rousseau S, Morrice N et al. Extracellular signal-regulated kinase mediates phosporylation of tropomyosin-1 to promote cytoskeleton remodelling in response to oxidative stress: impact on membrane blebbing. Mol Biol Cell 2003; 14:1418-1432.

10. Naga Prasad SV, Jayatilleke A, Madamanchi A et al. Protein kinase activity of phosphoinositide 3-kinase regulates beta-adrenergic receptor endocytosis. Nat Cell Biol 2005; 7:785-796.

11. Somara S, Pang H, Bitar KN. Agonist-induced association of tropomyosin with the protein kinase C-α in colonic smooth muscle. Am J Physiol Gastrointest Liver Physiol 2005; 288:G268-G276.

12. Gunning P, O'Neill G, Hardeman E. Tropomyosin-based regulation of the actin cytoskeleton in time and space. Physiol Rev 2008; 88:1-35.

13. Lehman W, Hatch V, Korman V et al. Tropomyosin and actin isoforms modulate the localization of tropomyosin strands on actin filaments. J Mol Biol 2000; 302:593-606.

14. Prasad GL, Fuldner RA, Cooper HL. Expression of transduced tropomyosin 1 cDNA suppresses neoplastic growth of cells transformed by the ras oncogene. Proc Natl Acad Sci USA 1993; 90:7039-7043.

15. Boyd J, Risinger JI, Wiseman RW et al. Regulation of microfilament organization and anchorage-independent growth by tropomyosin1. Proc Natl Acad Sci USA 1995; 92:11534-11538.

16. Gimona M, Kazzaz JA, Helfman DM. Forced expression of tropomyosin 2 or 3 in v-ki-ras-transformed fibroblasts results in distinct phenotypic effects. Proc Natl Acad Sci USA 1996; 93:9618-9623.

17. O'Neill GM, Stehn J, Gunning PW. Tropomyosins as interpreters of the signalling environment to regulate the local cytoskeleton. Seminars Cancer Biol 2008; 18:35-44.

INDEX